DEVELOPMENT OF THE UNIVERSITY HOSPITAL
OF THE
UNIVERSITY OF MICHIGAN
1891 – 1933

DRAWN BY THE
UNIVERSITY OF MICHIGAN
BUILDINGS & GROUNDS DEPARTMENT
CHRONOLOGICAL DATA SUPPLIED BY
PROFESSOR REUBEN PETERSON. JAN. 1933

LEGEND
EXISTING STRUCTURES
SITE OF FORMER STRUCTURES
SCALE-1"=50'

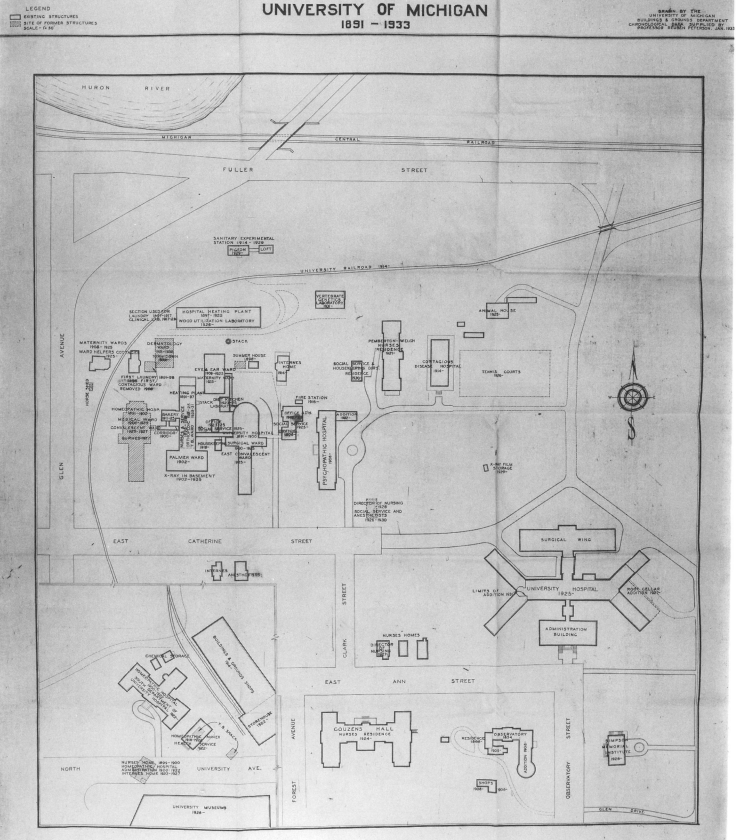

Not Just Any Medical School

DATE DUE

Not Just Any Medical School

The Science, Practice, and Teaching of Medicine at the University of Michigan 1850–1941

Horace W. Davenport

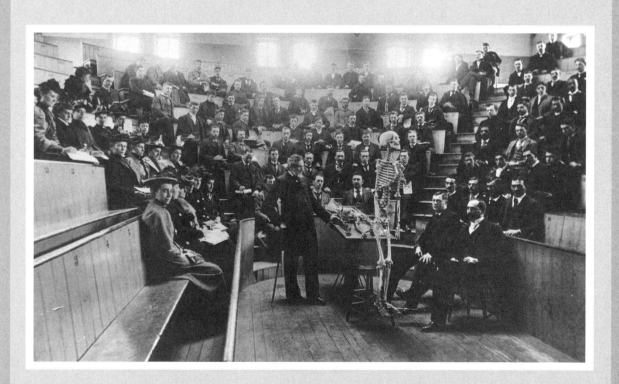

Ann Arbor
THE UNIVERSITY OF MICHIGAN PRESS

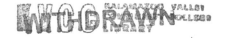

Copyright © by the University of Michigan 1999
All rights reserved
Published in the United States of America by
The University of Michigan Press
Manufactured in the United States of America
⊛ Printed on acid-free paper

2002   2001   2000   1999   4   3   2   1

A CIP catalog record for this book is available from the British Library.

Library of Congress Cataloging-in-Publication Data

Davenport, Horace Willard, 1912–
    Not just any medical school : the science, practice, and
teaching of medicine at the University of Michigan, 1850–1941 /
Horace W. Davenport
      p.   cm.
    Rev. ed. of: Fifty years of medicine at the University of
Michigan, 1891–1941. 1986, c1987.
    Includes bibliographical references (p.   ) and index.
    ISBN 0-472-11076-4 (acid-free paper)
    1. University of Michigan. Medical School—History. 2. Medical
colleges—Michigan—Ann Arbor—History. I. Davenport, Horace
Willard, 1912–   Fifty years of medicine at the University of
Michigan, 1891–1941. II. Title.
R747.U6834 D38   1999
610'.71'177435—dc21
                                                            99-6221
                                                              CIP

Endsheet maps drawn by the University of Michigan Building and Grounds
Department from chronological data by Professor Reuben Peterson, April
1933. (Courtesy of the Bentley Historical Library, University of Michigan,
Reuben Peterson Papers, Box 2.)

Foreword

Howard Markel

Not Just Any Medical School was begun by Professor Davenport as a "retirement project" in the early 1980s after he had stepped down from the chairmanship of the Department of Physiology and closed his gastrointestinal physiology laboratory. I use quotations around the term "retirement project" decidedly since Dr. Davenport has been more active in retirement than most practicing medical historians are during their working careers. Indeed, by most recent count, he has written six historical books and dozens of papers since 1983 when he officially became the William Beaumont Professor Emeritus of Physiology.

In point of fact, Dr. Davenport's historical works comprise only the most recent phase of his varied and brilliant career; at an imposing six feet six inches, he is both physically and intellectually one of the giants of the University of Michigan. He is a graduate of the California Institute of Technology and Oxford University, a former Rhodes scholar, and a member of the National Academy of Sciences (to name but a few of his academic achievements). After academic positions at Rochester, Yale, Pennsylvania, Harvard, and Utah, he settled into the chair of physiology at Michigan in 1956. Professor Davenport's international reputation flowed not only from his well-known elucidation of the role of carbonic anhydrase in the parietal cells of the stomach and the physiology of the gastric mucosal barrier, he was also the author of several major textbooks, including *The ABC of Acid-Base Chemistry,* a volume that generations of budding physicians read, memorized, and clutched to their chests during long and anguished nights before critical examinations.[1]

The original version of this book, *Fifty Years of Medicine at the University of Michigan,* covered the period between 1891 and 1941. In its revised version to commemorate the Medical School's sesquicentennial celebration, Dr. Davenport has incorporated new materials and photographs telling the story of the opening of the Medical School in 1850 and the decades that followed until the advent of World War II. The narrative stops at that point because, as he correctly asserts, the war and its aftermath signaled a watershed period in which the Michigan

Medical School, like most academic medical centers in the United States, changed and expanded markedly as a result of the postwar boom and the rise of government-funded research and medical care. Such a story requires a different historiographic approach that centers on the social, economic, political, and cultural aspects of what Paul Starr once referred to as "the social transformation of American medicine."[2] Happily, not a few medical historians at work today are studying the University of Michigan Medical School's more recent history as a means of understanding the social context of medical education, research, treatment, and the "medical marketplace." Undoubtedly, such historical works will broaden our view of the role Michigan continues to play in the world of medicine and biomedical research.[3] An epilogue by Janet Tarolli appears at the end of this volume and should serve as a brief summary of the remarkable medical expansion that took place during the fifty-nine years after Dr. Davenport's narrative ends.

The book you are about to read not only reflects Dr. Davenport's historical scholarship but also how seriously he always took his role as teacher and mentor—a role that many Michigan Medical School faculty, both past and present, have played in the lives of their students. If I may take a purposefully unorthodox approach to a book's introduction, I will illustrate this point with a personal example.

My first acquaintance with Dr. Davenport was, fittingly, as a member of the audience of one of his lectures. It was the induction of students into the Michigan chapter of Phi Beta Kappa in May 1981, and he was invited to speak. Calling his address "A Non-Oration," in literary deference to Emerson's more famous Phi Beta Kappa "Oration," Dr. Davenport began in his booming, deep voice: "If you people think you are special just because someone awarded you a tiny, metal-alloy Phi Beta Kappa key— think again." Speaking loudly over the gasps of visiting parents and not a few undergraduates, Dr. Davenport explained what he thought constituted an educated person: unquenchable curiosity and the energy and discipline to find out about those things you do not know much about.

The following year, at the time of the book's original composition, I was a first-year medical student at Michigan and working in the renal physiology laboratory of Professor Arthur Vander. As a former English major driven almost to madness by the medical school treadmill of rote memorization and multiple choice examinations, I found the first semester especially angst ridden. Perhaps to help channel some of my nervous energy, Professor Vander suggested that I introduce myself to Dr. Davenport in order to make his acquaintance and, if possible, inquire if I could help him in his historical research. It was a request that ultimately resulted in the most seminal relationship of my academic career. I should add that I am hardly alone in making such a claim— there are, literally, legions of physiologists, surgeons, physicians, and historians who benefited from Horace's erudition and scholarship over the past seven decades.

Dr. Davenport then occupied a small, two-room office in Medical Science Building II that was loaded with books, file cabinets, and the standard metallic Steelcase of Grand Rapids, Michigan, desk. As I mentioned, Dr. Davenport is a rather tall man and, as a result, given to stretching his long body, legs, and arms while working at his desk. He was engaging in precisely such a stretching maneuver as I summoned up the courage to knock softly on his open door on a November afternoon some sixteen years ago. Dr. Davenport, who worked facing the window and, hence, with his back to potential visitors, did not look up but responded in his twangy baritone that pronounced affirmative responses as a long and dragged out, "Ye—eessss?"

I had interrupted Professor Davenport precisely as he was reviewing the clinical notes of Dr. George Dock, who was chairman and professor of medicine at Michigan from 1891 to 1908. Dock, who was one of William Osler's prized students at the University of Pennsylvania, left behind sixteen volumes (more than sixty-eight hundred pages) of clinical notes. They were transcriptions of his biweekly medical diagnostic clinics in which everything Dock, the students, and occasionally the patients said each Tuesday and Friday afternoon was recorded by a faithful stenographer. Dr. Davenport handed me the transcript for a poorly attended clinic of 12 May 1905 that began with Dock's opening line to his students that day: "We can pick out those who are neither lovers of music or baseball."

"What do you think this means?" he queried, pointing to the passage about the music lovers. Fate was smiling on me that day. As an undergraduate, I had long served as a voluntary usher for the University Musical Society and correctly guessed that Dock must have been alluding to the May Festival—an annual series of grand orchestral concerts held in Ann

Arbor from 1891 until selling its final ticket in 1994. Davenport smiled and exclaimed a gleeful "That's absolutely right" before going on to explain that it was, in fact, the *second* concert of the May Festival and the concert was being given that very afternoon.

"What about the baseball lovers?" he continued. "What do you make of that?" Now, in medical school, there is an old adage that it is far more important to look like you know what you are doing than to actually know what you are doing; never has that axiom rung more loudly for me. So in my most confident tone and posture, I boldly but wildly speculated: "Michigan must have been playing baseball that afternoon." More than mildly impressed—not an easy thing to do to Dr. Davenport—he again enthusiastically rejoined: "Absolutely right. That's really fine. In fact, Michigan played Wisconsin that afternoon and won four to three." My pulse immediately slowed down as I came to the conclusion that, at the very least, Dr. Davenport would not have the opportunity to ask me the score of that long-forgotten athletic event. Almost two decades later, as I reflect on our friendship and, for me, profound intellectual relationship, I actually shudder to think what might have happened if I had gotten the questions wrong.

Dr. Davenport then asked me what I planned on becoming when I "grew up." I quickly replied, "a pediatrician"—and just as swiftly Dr. Davenport assigned me to research the life and work of David Murray Cowie, Michigan's first professor of pediatrics. At the time, I knew next to nothing on how to conduct historical research but recall fondly Dr. Davenport taking me to the Taubman Medical Library and, by campus bus, to the Bentley Historical Library, where he patiently introduced me to the task at hand. Each week, we would spend several hours discussing what I had found and, far more impressive, the twentyfold volume of materials he was researching. Dr. Davenport would also assign books he thought I should read, ranging from U.S. history to literature. I soon learned that keeping up with Dr. Davenport was not an easy task. Horace always chose to teach research by example; it would be an understatement to note that his prodigious energy and attention to detail were inspiring. Well into the early 1990s, it was not uncommon to see Dr. Davenport in the stairwell of the Taubman Medical Library, climbing up the stairs three or four at a time with his white lab coat flapping in his wake, in search of a forgotten paper by Victor Vaughan, Frederick Novy, Warren Plimpton Lombard, John Alexander, Reuben Peterson, or some other Michigan luminary.

What remains most valuable of the book Dr. Davenport has written is that it is a scholarly tour de force: a narrative chronicle of what was taught, researched, and practiced at an excellent U.S. medical school between 1850 and 1941. And as we face increasing challenges of the medical marketplace in the next millennium, Dr. Davenport reminds us all that it was not through mere bricks and mortar that the Michigan Medical School achieved its heritage of excellence but, instead, through its most important resource—talented and dedicated individuals. But perhaps the greatest strength of this book is that it is written in the witty voice of one of the Medical School's most distinguished scholars and teachers.

Preface

The University of Michigan Medical School was founded 150 years ago. The date of founding was 1848 if you count the year the university's regents began to appoint its faculty, or it was 1850 if you count the date the faculty began to teach. In order to contribute to the celebration of the sesquicentennial of the school in 1998 and 2000 the University of Michigan Press has agreed to reprint a corrected edition of my *Fifty Years of Medicine at the University of Michigan, 1891–1941*[1] with a new first chapter relating the history of the school from 1850 to 1891. In addition the book has been given a new title.

Gert Brieger, the distinguished historian of medicine, said: "Michigan was just not any school. It was one of only a handful of truly important centers of medical education in the years around 1900."[2] It was just not any school at the time it was founded, for the men constituting the original medical faculty had one characteristic that distinguished them from teachers in all other U.S. medical schools: they were university professors paid professorial salaries. That meant that a medical student did not need to buy a ticket from a professor in order to be allowed to hear his lectures. Once a student had paid his university fees, admission to lectures and clinical demonstrations was free. It also meant that the professors had obligations as university employees: the triad of teaching, research, and service. Four of the first five professors had private practices as well, and so have many of their successors. Over the years there has sometimes been tension between the distractions and rewards of private practice and professorial obligations, but throughout the period covered by this book it is remarkable that even those professors who most jealously guarded their right of private practice were among the most diligent and effective teachers, investigators, and bedside physicians.

The story related in the first version of this book began in 1891 when Victor Vaughan was appointed dean of the Medical School, and it emphasized his role in making the University of Michigan a truly important center of medical education between that date and 1918. In this expanded version I describe how Vaughan had already become an effective leader of reform before 1891. Nevertheless, anyone who has participated in the governance of a progressive school knows Victor Vaughan could not have done it alone. Vaughan's achievements were founded upon antecedent conditions and events, and they could not have been accomplished without substantial help from many others. In the first place, there was the context of the state of Michigan. The Northwest Ordinance laid the foundation for a thoroughgoing system of public education in Michigan capped by a state-supported university. The early inhabitants of Michigan, chiefly literate migrants from New England and New York and immigrants from Germany anxious to obtain the privileges of education denied them in their homeland, understood the need for higher education, and the legislators they elected were with occasional reluctance willing to pay for it. Michigan citizens also understood the need for advanced professional education, and the University of Michigan early in its existence established schools of law, engineering, and pharmacy as well as of medicine. Although some physicians thought the state had no business spending money to support medical education, the legislature continued to appropriate money for buildings for preclinical and clinical instruction and money for faculty salaries and equipment. The first University Hospital, established in 1869, was a mere dormitory for patients to be demonstrated before the class in the lecture room of the Medical Building, but in 1875 the legislature appropriated eight thousand dollars to which the citizens of Ann Arbor added five thousand dollars to construct a pavilion hospital with wards and an operating room where students like Will Mayo could learn the elements of their profession. Again in 1888 the state of Michigan and city of Ann Arbor voted money to build the Catherine Street hospitals that served the Medical School until 1925 when its thousand-bed replacement was provided by much larger appropriations. Between 1875 and 1890 the University of Michigan rose to eminence among U.S. universities, private as well as public, and President Angell and the regents supported the physical and intellectual development of the Medical School as well as that of other units of the university. Finally, members of the Michigan medical faculty at the time Victor Vaughan was a child in Missouri were well aware of the deplorable state of U.S. medical education. As officers of the American Medical Association they proposed substantial reforms, and in their own school they extended the curriculum to nine months and replaced the established system of repeated lectures, occasional clinical demonstrations, and apprenticeship to a practicing physician with a three-year graded curriculum for students entering in 1877. That was three years after Vaughan came to the University of Michigan as a graduate student. When Vaughan was only an assistant professor the faculty recognized the need to add a full-time, thoroughly trained professional physiologist to its ranks, and it did so by hiring Henry Sewall. At the same time the school obtained microscopes and a qualified instructor for a course in clinical microscopy. Consequently, the state of Michigan, the university, and the Medical School were ready to participate in more thorough reforms introduced when Vaughan became acting dean in 1887 and dean in 1891.

Vaughan, who remained dean for the next three decades, began by establishing a four-year curriculum similar to those concurrently adopted by Harvard, Columbia, and Pennsylvania, and he assembled an unrivaled preclinical faculty that included John Jacob Abel, Arthur Robertson Cushny, J. Playfair McMurrich, George Linius Streeter, G. Carl Huber, and Frederick G. Novy in pharmacology, anatomy, and bacteriology. Vaughan believed a man he recruited should be trained in research and should be likely to continue to do it, and his recruits' research at the University of Michigan was internationally recognized for its importance. Vaughan, in a fashion uncharacteristic of deans, himself worked in the laboratory almost to the end of his career.

The University Hospital was completely in the hands of the faculty, and the university, unlike Harvard, did not have to depend on the good graces of busy physicians and surgeons in private or municipal hospitals for the clinical training of its students. After 1892 third- and fourth-year students worked on the wards under preeminent physicians such as George Dock and A. Walter Hewlett. Dock's and Hewlett's junior colleagues became professors in other medical schools, and Hewlett's protégé, Frank Wilson, became a famous electrocardiographer. In Vaughan's time pediatrics, otolaryngology, roentgenology, urology, and neurology became newly established specialties in the University Hospital, and each was directed by a man whose qualifications ranged from adequate to outstanding. At the same time a Michigan surgeon and a dentist collaborated in the country's largest clinic for the repair of cleft palate and harelip. In 1901 Vaughan and his colleague William J. Herdman convinced the legislature to found the Psychopathic Hospital for research on the cause and cure of mental diseases, anticipating by fifty years the establishment of a Mental Health Research Institute on the medical campus.

Vaughan admitted students, men and women alike from all over the country, on the basis of their academic qualifications. As a consequence of Jewish academic achievements the proportion of Jewish students in the classes between 1890 and 1930 exceeded that in the national population. Vaughan recruited African Americans, as his correspondence with the president of Lincoln University in Pennsylvania shows. Consequently, the University of Michigan Medical School was unique among white U.S. medical schools in having a succession of African American students, who struggled against the disadvantages of poverty to achieve doctor of medicine degrees.

Differentiation of the specialties within and among departments occurred in the 1920s as it did in other leading medical schools. For example, when Hugh Cabot became professor of surgery in 1920 he made individual men responsible for general surgery, orthopaedic surgery, neurosurgery, urological surgery, and thoracic surgery. All the clinical departments established formal training programs in which interns rose through the ranks to become chief residents. Many who completed a residency went on to further training in specialties with the result that the hospital's professional staff became several times larger than it had been a few years earlier. Preclinical departments were no longer one-man affairs, and they established graduate programs leading to the doctor of philosophy degree.

Long before Cabot came to Michigan in 1920 he had been deeply concerned with the problem of how the ordinary wage-earning citizen could get competent medical care without bankrupting him- or herself. He thought that the relatively progressive state of Michigan, less hidebound than his native Massachusetts, and a university medical establishment responsible to a lay board of university regents could be the places where he could develop a system of full-time, hospital-based group practice where patients would pay according to their means and where all would receive the same high-quality care. Cabot succeeded Vaughan as dean in 1921, but with all the power of his deanship, his department chairmanship, and his aggressive personality he failed. When he was abruptly dismissed in January 1930 the Michigan faculty with the regents' approval established a pattern in which the heads of each clinical department and section were allowed the privilege of almost unlimited, highly remunerative private practice and complete control of their departments or sections. That pattern survived until well after the period covered by this book, but it did not prevent privately practicing surgeons such as Reed Nesbit and Frederick Coller from achieving research results that profoundly influenced practice of medicine here and

abroad. Michigan clinicians became presidents of their elite societies, editors of the best journals, and members of the boards that established specialty qualifications, and they trained students in their image.

In the text of this book I have not explicitly placed the University of Michigan Medical School within the context of U.S. medicine and medical education of the period by describing how other medical schools met the challenge of reform. That context is now well known to serious students of the subject. Kenneth Ludmerer's often quoted book, *Learning to Heal: The Development of American Medical Education*,[3] provides the early context up to about 1910, and it places Michigan in the "second tier," immediately below Johns Hopkins. The histories of other occupants of that tier, Harvard, Columbia, and Pennsylvania, have been recorded in numerous readily available books and journal articles, and there are many places in my narrative in which comparison of Michigan with those schools will be obvious to the well-informed reader. For example, one who learns that Michigan *graduated fourteen women* in 1893 will remember that Johns Hopkins *admitted three women* to its first class in the same year. It is possible to name the top twenty schools of the eighty or so in the country between 1920 and 1941 when my narrative ends. Michigan has always been among the top twenty, but the rank order of schools within that list has changed frequently as circumstances within each school have changed. Circumstances have changed for better or worse at Michigan as well, and it would be ridiculous to try to specify Michigan's position precisely at every instant.

In telling this story I have tried to do more than give a list of names and dates together with an uncritical account of some of the faculty's accomplishments. I have endeavored insofar as the archival record and books and journals in a good university library permit to describe much that was said and done in the classroom, the laboratory, and the hospital, but I have not written an exhaustively comprehensive account of everything that was done by everyone at Michigan. I have concentrated upon what I thought was important, interesting, and, on occasion, amusing. In particular I have tried to avoid the institutional prejudice common to histories of U.S. medical schools, and I have seldom expressed opinions about what I thought was good, bad, or mediocre. An informed reader can make his or her own judgment.

The place of the University of Michigan in the early history of U.S. medical education was not generally known until Kenneth Ludmerer's book was published in 1985. I had begun my accounts of Michigan medical science a few years earlier with my "Physiology, 1850–1923: The View from Michigan" published by the American Physiological Society in 1982.[4] My *Fifty Years of Medicine at the University of Michigan, 1891–1941,* published in 1986, was followed in 1987 by my *Doctor Dock: Teaching and Learning Medicine at the Turn of the Century,* an account of George Dock's clinical teaching at the University of Michigan from 1899 through 1908.[5] I have also published *University of Michigan Surgeons, 1850–1970: Who They Were and What They Did*[6] and *Victor Vaughan: Statesman and Scientist.*[7] The former book describes the work of University of Michigan surgeons between 1850 and 1970. The latter book on Victor Vaughan contains a far more comprehensive account of his career than does this present book. Recently Joel D. Howell has edited *Medical Lives and Scientific Medicine at Michigan, 1891–1969,*[8] the story of the careers of seven eminent University of Michigan internists, including several described less completely in this book. As a result, the history of Michigan medical education at Michigan from its earliest days to near the present time is available.

My largest debt of gratitude is to the University of Michigan for giving me the freedom and opportunity to write this book and for allowing me to use its libraries and an office long past my retirement from its faculty so that I could enrich my knowledge of the history of its medical school.

I am deeply indebted to all those who over the last 150 years have brought the University Libraries, and in particular the Taubman Medical Library and the Bentley Historical Library, to their present state of usefulness. As one of his last acts as dean, John Gronvall transferred the accumulated files of his office to the Bentley Historical Library. Without access to them my work would have been much poorer. It would have been richer had not Victor Vaughan's documents before 1915 disappeared. The librarians of the several libraries have been unfailingly courteous and helpful.

Interim Dean A. Lorris Betz made publication possible by generous support of the Historical Center for the Health Sciences, where editing of my manuscript and its final preparation for press occurred, and then by pledging purchase of printed copies for use in the sesquicentennial celebrations. I hope that the quality of my book justifies his confidence in its worth. Rebecca McDermott of the University of Michigan Press has efficiently guided the negotiations preceding publication.

My book has benefited from the review comments and suggestions for illustrations from a number of former colleagues. I gratefully acknowledge the contributions of Doctors Gerald D. Abrams, Robert H. Bartlett, A. Kent Christensen, Edward F. Domino, Charles N. Ellis, Lazar J. Greenfield, John W. Henderson, Joel D. Howell, Donald F. Huelke, Timothy R. B. Johnson, Richard D. Judge, C. F. Koopmann Jr., Charles J. Krause, Bert N. Ladu Jr., Paul R. Lichter, William Martel, George Morley, Henry H. Swain, Jeremiah G. Turcotte, Arthur J. Vander, and Frank Whitehouse.

Janet Tarolli, assisted by Carol Shannon, has edited this book with superb skill. She has corrected and transformed my amateur manuscript to a professional text ready for the press, and my gratitude to her is beyond expression. I must also thank Barbara E. Cohen for the index and an editor for the University of Michigan Press who made many corrections and provided important suggestions for improvement of my text.

Howard Markel, the director of the Historical Center for the Health Sciences, initiated the project of enlarging and republishing a corrected version of my history of fifty years of medicine at the University of Michigan, and he has skillfully managed the undertaking from beginning to end. He and I began to collaborate on the history of medicine at the University of Michigan when he was a first-year medical student, and since then we have kept ourselves intimately informed of each other's diverse labors on medical history. As I thank Howard Markel for his labors during this current collaboration I add affection to gratitude.

Contents

1
The First Forty Years, 1850–90

When it opened its doors in October 1850 the University of Michigan Department of Medicine and Surgery differed from the many other medical schools in the country in having its building on the campus of the university whose name it bore and from all others in having professors who were paid salaries as professors in the university. The latter meant that medical students did not have to buy tickets from the professors to be admitted to the lectures and demonstrations that constituted the curriculum.[1]

In 1850 the university had seventy-three students, chiefly headed for careers in law or the church, and they were taught Greek, Latin, perhaps some Hebrew, and moral philosophy by a handful of professors who had graduated from church-related eastern colleges or universities that were themselves struggling to become something more than elementary academies.[2] The medical faculty taught courses in geology, chemistry, zoology, and botany.

The three-story Medical Building was on a dirt road at the eastern edge of the university campus, a forty-acre pasture on the outskirts of Ann Arbor (fig. 1–1). The building contained lecture rooms required by the curriculum, offices for the five professors, a small chemical laboratory, and a room under a dome on the roof dedicated to anatomical dissections when a cadaver was available.

To be admitted a student had to present evidence of a good moral character and sufficient knowledge of Greek and Latin to understand the technical language of medicine. The average student had not graduated from a college or a university, and he had probably learned his letters and a smattering of the classical languages in a village school. The most important requirement was that a student have an apprenticeship to a respectable physician for three years before or during the periods between the Ann Arbor terms. The qualification "respectable" meant that the physician must not be a member of one of the numerous heretical medical sects: homeopathic, eclectic, or Brunonian. The student's duties as an apprentice might include hitching the physician's horse to his buggy, compounding prescriptions, and helping hold a patient undergoing an operation without anesthesia. The Medical School had no means of judging the mentor's ability as a physician or the quality of the student's experience.

The medical faculty (fig. 1–2) consisted of

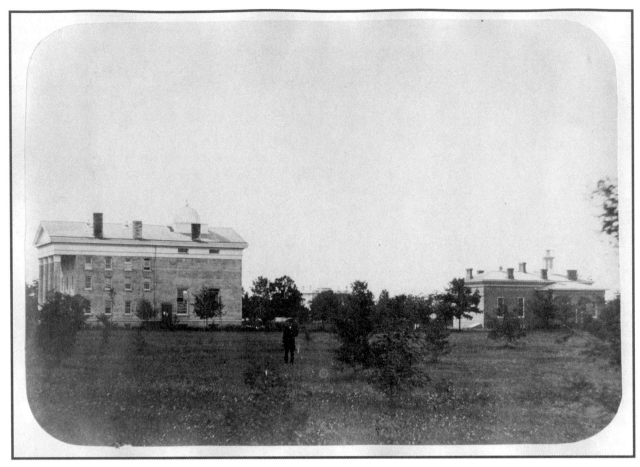

Fig. 1–1. Original Medical Building *(left)* and Chemical Laboratory *(right)*. (Courtesy of the Department of Anatomy, University of Michigan.)

Abram Sager, dean and professor of obstetrics and diseases of women and children,
Silas Douglas, professor of chemistry,
Samuel Denton, professor of medicine and pathology,
Moses Gunn, professor of surgery and anatomy,
Jonathan Adams Allen Jr., professor of physiology, materia medica, and therapeutics.

Abram Sager was the best educated man on the faculty.[3] He had graduated from Rensselaer Polytechnic Institute in 1831, and he had obtained his medical education at the Castleton Medical College in Vermont.[4] That school had two lecture courses, spring and fall, to accommodate two fee-paying classes, and the lectures had to be attended twice to qualify for graduation. There were occasional clinical demonstrations, and some anatomical dissection might be done in cool weather when a barrel labeled "Pork" had recently been delivered to a local grocer who was a trustee of the academy. Examinations were

oral and short, and a student never failed if he paid his diploma fee. Sager knew some embryology and enough botany to be responsible for that subject in the Michigan State Geological Survey. He kept up with European scientific literature, and he wrote articles summarizing French, German, English, and Irish papers on obstetrics.

Silas Douglas had obtained his medical qualification by apprenticeship, and he had been granted a doctor of medicine degree by a county medical society. He did not practice medicine as Sager, Denton, Gunn, and Allen did, but he was a consulting geologist in Michigan's Upper Peninsula mining district. Denton had also graduated from Castleton, and he had long practiced medicine in Ann Arbor. He had been a state senator from 1845 to 1848. Moses Gunn had graduated from the Geneva Medical College in upstate New York,[5] an institution much like Castleton, in 1846, and Allen had graduated from Castleton, also in 1846. Cory-

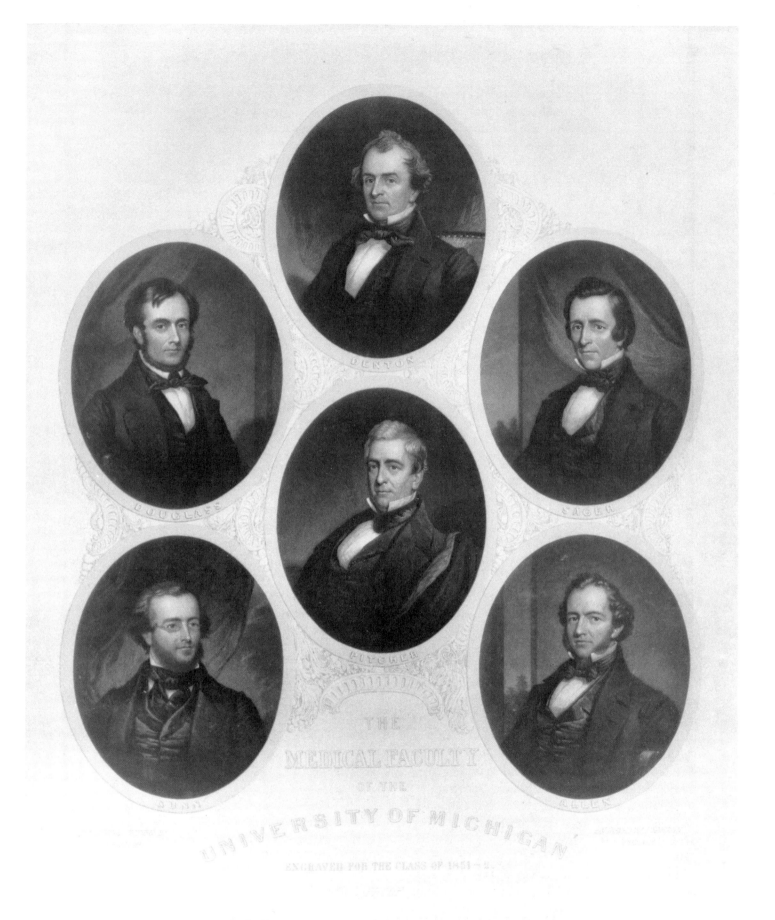

Fig. 1–2. Medical faculty in 1851–52 consisted of *(from left)* Moses Gunn, Silas Douglas, Samuel Denton, Abram Sager, Jonathan Adams Allen Jr., and *(center)* Regent Zina Pitcher. (Courtesy of the Bentley Historical Library, University of Michigan, UAm Collection, Box 18, "Sartain.")

don Ford, another Geneva graduate, succeeded Gunn as professor of anatomy in 1854, and Alonzo B. Palmer, who taught medical students continuously from 1854, became responsible for internal medicine on Denton's death in 1860 (fig. 1–3).

The medical faculty settled the curriculum at a meeting on 23 September 1850. There were to be four lectures a day, Mondays through Fridays. Clinical demonstrations would be given on Saturday mornings. The course would last from the first Wednesday in October to the third Wednesday in April. During that period the faculty gave between six hundred and seven hundred lectures. Students were required to attend two full courses of lectures and to present a thesis to qualify for graduation.

In 1850 the quality of the University of Michigan Medical School was far below the standard set by French and German schools, which had high entrance requirements, four- or six-year curriculums, professors distinguished for their research accomplishments, and access to large hospitals,[6] but between 1850 and 1890 it underwent a slow transformation that made it ripe for rapid and radical reform. That transformation is the subtext of this chapter. After 1890 the school began to meet French and German standards.[7]

The Chemical Laboratory: Silas Douglas and His Faculty

Silas Douglas had a small laboratory in the Medical Building, and he gave chemical demonstrations before the class. He soon persuaded the regents to appropriate money to build the Chemical Laboratory in 1855–56, the first building in any U.S. university to be solely devoted to chemistry. Douglas was in charge of the university's building program, and he placed the Chemical Laboratory immediately behind the Medical Building. The two were connected by a wooden walkway spanning the mud.

Silas Douglas and his staff taught chemistry to the rest of the university, and the Chemical Laboratory was repeatedly enlarged to accommodate growing programs. At first Preston B. Rose taught toxicology and the elements of analysis of urine to medical students, but the latter subject was soon included in a course in physiological chemistry taught by Victor Vaughan. Albert Benjamin Prescott taught the practical aspects of materia medica and the elements of pharmacy to medical students, who often had to be

their own pharmacists when in practice in the countryside. His program grew into a full-fledged college of pharmacy housed in the Chemical Laboratory. Engineering students studied inorganic analysis and metallurgical chemistry, and Literary College students learned organic as well as inorganic chemistry when the scientific course leading to the bachelor of philosophy degree was eventually added to the older classical course. There were 26 tables in the original building, and the number was raised to 190 by 1894. Because Silas Douglas and his staff were members of the medical faculty, the Chemical Laboratory was administratively part of the Medical School, and it remained so until 1910.

Victor Vaughan said that although Douglas was not a great teacher in the lecture room or laboratory he deserved credit for building the Chemical Laboratory and seeing that it functioned. The only traces of Douglas's lectures are in medical student notebooks. In 1860 one student recorded Douglas's advice on how to keep plants from freezing, and in 1866 another student heard Douglas distinguish between the properties of red and white phosphorus.[8] Students learned more at the laboratory benches, where they used successive editions of Douglas's *Guide to a Systematic Course of Qualitative Chemical Analysis* and his later *Qualitative Chemical Analysis,* written in collaboration with Prescott.[9] The latter book's 261 pages contain a thorough synopsis of the properties of metals, nonmetallic elements, and acids together with clear directions for their identification. Courses were elective, and these are the numbers of students who took them in 1871–72.

abridged analysis, 142
qualitative analysis, 60
quantitative analysis, 31
toxicology, 18
urinalysis, 143
pharmaceutical manipulations, 22
determinative mineralogy, 5
assaying, 2
organic analysis, 7

The average cost was $1.10 per week.

Poisons were everywhere. Lead was in cider and in the municipal water supply if there were one. Alum adulterated flour. Arsenic was in green wallpaper and available over the counter for a husband or wife anxious to end marital discord. In 1868–69, fifty-one medical students, well over half the class, took the

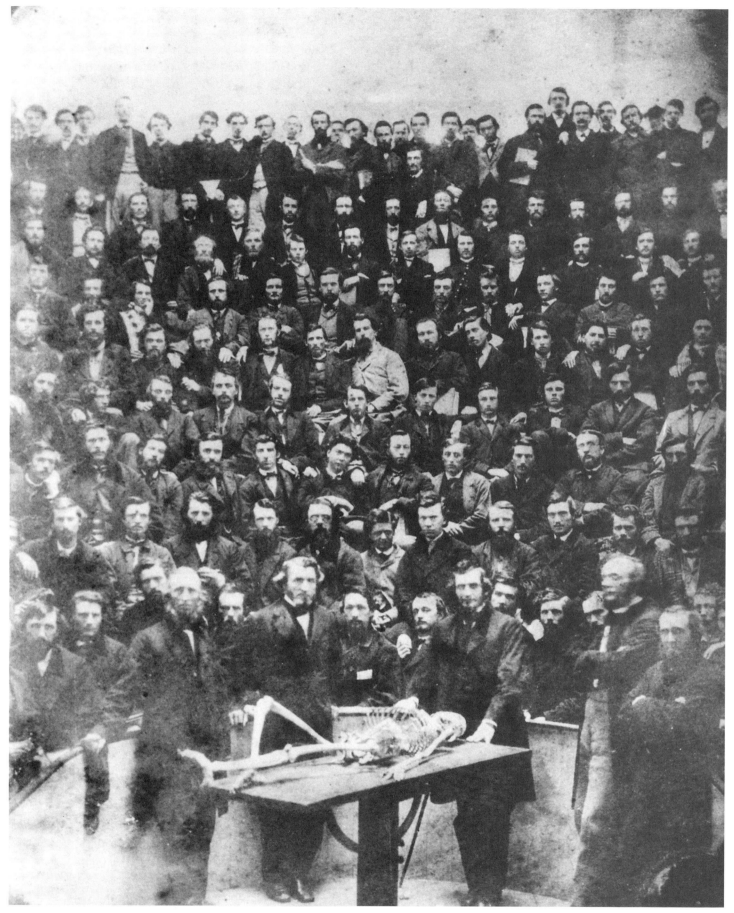

Fig. 1–3. Medical faculty and students, March 1865. Standing in front of the class *(from left)* are Abram Sager, Alonzo Palmer, Corydon Ford, Moses Gunn, and Silas Douglas. (Courtesy of the Bentley Historical Library, University of Michigan, Medical School Records, Box 136, "Classes by Subject, Surgery and Anatomy Amphitheater Views.")

course in toxicology. Preston B. Rose taught it, using his *Hand-Book of Toxicology*.[10] He told students how to collect evidence in a case of suspected poisoning, first by careful observation of the patient and his or her surroundings and then by determining whether anyone had shown a disposition to prepare the food or medicine and to wait upon the deceased to the exclusion of others during the fatal illness. He gave explicit directions on how to conduct the postmortem examination and how to find metals, alkaloids, or acids during subsequent chemical analysis of the tissues. He concluded by describing stains made by blood or semen. Health officials throughout Michigan regularly sent parts obtained at autopsy of suspicious cases to the Chemical Laboratory for analysis.

Rose also taught the course in urinalysis, and many medical students took it, 55 in 1868, 41 in 1869, and 143 in 1871. The textbook the faculty recommended was George Harley's *The Urine and Its Derangements*, an up-to-date book of 334 pages describing the physiological and pathological constituents of the urine.[11] In the laboratory students used a manual published by Silas Douglas that contained ten tables of directions for analysis of metals and acids and two for identifying inorganic and organic poisons. In table 13, "Systematic Course of Chemical Examination of the Urine," students were directed to evaporate a sample of urine to dryness over a water bath, boil the residue with alcohol, and identify constituents, including hippuric acid, mucus, calcium oxalate, bile pigments, oil, and purpurine.[12]

Rose was given the title assistant professor of physiological chemistry in 1875, and this is said to be the first use of that title in the country. There is no trace of what he taught, but he did not teach it for long. Rose collected the fees paid by the students and turned them over to Douglas to be transferred to the university treasurer. In October 1875 Douglas reported he had found a shortage of $831.10 in the laboratory accounts. Rose was blamed and at once dismissed. The ensuing controversy among Rose, Douglas, and the university lasted for years, reaching the Michigan Supreme Court in 1881 and costing everyone involved time, money, and reputation. The immediate effect was that Victor Vaughan, a laboratory teaching assistant, was told to teach Rose's course in physiological chemistry.

Vaughan had taught himself the elements of inorganic chemistry at a backwoods Missouri college, and he had come to the Chemical Laboratory in 1874 for graduate training in chemistry.[13] At the time of Rose's dismissal he was working on his doctor of philosophy thesis on the quantitative separation of arsenic from each of the metals precipitated by hydrogen sulfide in acid solution. The degree was granted in 1876, one of the first two doctoral degrees given by the University of Michigan. Douglas told Vaughan to take over the teaching of physiological chemistry, and Vaughan retained responsibility for that subject until he retired in 1921. Vaughan expanded both laboratory work and lectures. In 1878 he began an extended, optional laboratory course on physiological and pathological chemistry that included analysis of blood, urine, gastric juice, bile, brain, bone, and muscle. He printed his lecture notes in 1878, 1879, and 1880.[14] Some students complained that they were required to buy the books. Each edition contained many descriptions, apparently derived from a German text, of the composition but not the function of compounds isolated from animal tissues. The 1879 version of 315 pages began with a long section on the collection and analysis of saliva, gastric juice, pancreatic juice, intestinal juice, and feces. The properties and functions of hemoglobin were well covered in 44 pages. After a brief description of muscle, cartilage, and fat Vaughan devoted 160 pages to urine, its composition and diurnal variation observed in himself. He described the physiology and pathology of each constituent and ended with advice on detection of drugs in the urine.

Newell Martin in reviewing the book complained that Vaughan had paid little attention to the important work on metabolism done by Max Pettenkofer and Karl Voit in Germany.[15] Had Martin read the 1880 edition he might have been shocked by Vaughan's treatment of glucose metabolism. Vaughan rejected the claim of Claude Bernard that glucose is formed in the liver, and he accepted Frederick Pavy's belief that the liver is a glucose-assimilating organ.[16] Pavy, an English clinician, had found no difference in the glucose concentration of arterial and venous blood of dogs, and he concluded that glucose is not used by the tissues. Glucose absorbed into portal blood is prevented from entering the general circulation by being converted to glycogen in the liver.[17] Vaughan, following Pavy, wrote: "In health the liver prevents the larger portion of the sugar reaching the blood and thus prevents diabetes. If the sugar reaches the blood, as sugar, it cannot be oxidized and consequently is excreted in the urine."[18]

Vaughan thought the most plausible explanation of the fate of liver glycogen is that it is converted into fat. Vaughan changed his opinion later, and in the meantime medical students, who time out of mind have been confidently taught erroneous theories, were probably not harmed by this one.

Vaughan gave up his assistantship in the Chemical Laboratory in 1876 to enter medical school. After he received his doctor of medicine degree in 1878 he gradually became busy with the private practice of medicine, toxicology, bacteriology, immunology, medical administration, and many state and national medical affairs.[19] He was away from Ann Arbor weeks, months, and years at a time, and although he remained responsible for physiological chemistry, the subject was poorly taught until the year after his retirement, when a department of physiological chemistry was established at Michigan.

Public Health: Victor Vaughan

Victor Vaughan began a career in public health in the Chemical Laboratory. He was soon appointed by the governor to the Michigan State Board of Health, and he remained a member, sometimes as chairman, for almost thirty years. That involved many trips to meetings in Lansing and numerous ones investigating health problems throughout Michigan. He was often an expert witness on long civil and criminal trials involving matters of health. Immediately after the Spanish-American War he was one of the two civilian members of Walter Reed's Typhoid Commission, and he wrote most of its two-volume report and saw it through the press.[20] In World War I he was a member of the Executive Committee of the Army Medical Board with responsibility for health in all camps. He wrote four editions of a book on poisonous ptomaines and leukomaines and at the end of his career, a two-volume textbook of public health and epidemiology.[21]

An epidemic of cheese poisoning beginning in 1883 affected hundreds of persons in widely scattered parts of Michigan, and it was followed by an epidemic of poisoning by ice cream in 1886.[22] Samples of the poisonous products were sent to the Chemical Laboratory, and Vaughan had the responsibility of identifying the poison and determining its source. Vaughan isolated needle-shaped crystals he called tyrotoxicon. A drop of an aqueous solution placed on Vaughan's tongue caused a burning sensation, constriction of the throat, nausea, a gripping pain in the bowels, and diarrhea. He said: "This was tried several times, not only upon myself, but upon some of my students, who kindly offered themselves for experimentation."[23]

Vaughan went to a cheese factory in Lenawee County, Michigan, that had been identified as one of the sources of the poisonous cheese. Cheese makers blamed the cows' fodder, but Vaughan dismissed that for the reasons that no two agreed on the plant and that poisonous cheese had been produced in all seasons of the year. The dye used to color the cheese was free of adulterants, and the rennet produced by scraping salted and dried gastric mucosa had been used to produce nonpoisonous as well as poisonous cheese. Vaughan's own theory was that "tyrotoxicon may originate in milk on long standing in closed vessels. As the putrefactive changes in the milk are due to the growth of minute organisms, the introduction of these organisms into the milk may hasten its putrefaction, and consequently, the formation of the ptomaine. . . . When cows are kept in filthy stalls, the milk is likely to undergo speedy putrefaction."[24] Until the origin of tyrotoxicon was more clearly identified, he suggested that people test their cheese with litmus paper. Any cheese that was strongly acidic should be regarded "with suspicion."[25]

Improper care of milk was implicated in an investigation of milk-borne illness at three hotels in Long Branch, New Jersey, in 1886. Tyrotoxicon crystals were identified in the milk, which came from cows milked "at the unusual and abnormal hours of midnight and noon, and the noon's milking—that which alone was followed by illness—was placed, while hot, in the cans, and then, without any attempt at cooling, carted eight miles during the warmest part of the day in a very hot month."[26]

Victor Vaughan joined the American Public Health Association soon after he was appointed to the Board of Health. He was made a member of a committee whose chairman was George Miller Sternberg, the codiscoverer of the pneumococcus and the future surgeon general of the army. Thus began a friendship with one of the few men in the United States who knew about bacteriology in the 1880s. Many years later Sternberg's widow annually gave a medal honoring her husband to the member of Michigan's graduating class who had most distinguished himself in the study of public health.

In 1885 Vaughan won the Lomb Prize offered by the association for an essay called "Healthy Homes and Foods for the Working Classes."[27] He gave sound if rather presumptuous advice on how to build a house and how to install its plumbing and make other sanitary arrangements, all based on his own experience in villages and small towns such as Ann Arbor. Vaughan inspected the local markets, and he and his students analyzed many samples of food bought in the grocery stores. As a result his advice on how to select foods is a horrifying catalog of pervasive fraud and adulteration. Fishmongers hide evidence of decomposition by removing the fish's eyes and coloring the gills with blood. Dairy operators skim cream from milk and add an adulterant to restore bulk. They also add sodium bicarbonate to neutralize lactic acid as fast as it is formed. Measly pork is ground up for sausage to conceal its content of cysticerci (tapeworm larvae), and the sausage is often adulterated with cornmeal and doctored with fuchsin to give it a red color. All samples of ground coffee Vaughan bought in grocery stores were adulterated with chicory, pease, wheat, acorns, or corn. The only way to get unadulterated coffee is to buy the beans and grind them oneself.

In 1886–87 the legislature proposed to appropriate money to construct a building for the University of Michigan Physics Department, and a group of Michigan businessmen persuaded the legislature to add forty thousand dollars to add and equip a laboratory of hygiene. The result was the Physics-Hygiene Building, ready to be occupied when Vaughan and his student Frederick G. Novy returned in the autumn of 1888 from learning biological technique in Germany. The Hygienic Laboratory of the University of Michigan was in fact the state health laboratory until 1907. During the first seven years there were two to three thousand cases of typhoid fever in Michigan each year with a death rate of about 30 percent. Vaughan undertook to identify the bacteria in drinking water from affected areas.

Vaughan sent clean carboys to physicians in affected towns, and the physicians returned them to Ann Arbor filled with water suspected of causing the disease. Vaughan cultivated bacteria in the samples and identified them by reference to James Eisenberg's *Bakteriologische Diagnostik*.[28] He had brought an authentic sample of the typhoid bacillus back from Germany, but he never found the bacillus in 148 samples of drinking water from typhoid fever areas. Instead, he found several other pathogenic bacteria, and he concluded that the typhoid bacillus is not a specific microorganism but a modified form of a number of related pathogens. When Vaughan reported his findings at a meeting of the Association of American Physicians, William Henry Welch, who was present, would have none of it. Welch said: "Unless one adopts the view of Dr. Vaughan, which is at present hardly likely to obtain general acceptance, that typhoid fever is not due to any one specific germ but to a variety of more or less related germs, it is difficult to see what the bearing of these experiments is upon the etiology of typhoid fever. I am not prepared to go to the length of thinking that all these germs can be changed over into germs that may produce the same results as the typhoid bacillus, and still less that they may, under certain conditions, acquire all the morphological and cultural properties of the [typhoid] bacillus."[29]

Vaughan countered by saying that "I do believe . . . that typhoid fever may originate without a preexisting case of typhoid fever. . . . Most of you see this disease in the city. I see it principally in the country. I have seen cases of typhoid fever scattered among the farming population, among men, women, and children who have not been off their farms for weeks; and it would take a good deal to convince me that there was a common source of infection in these cases."[30]

Vaughan quietly dropped this idea when he was a member of the Typhoid Commission.

Gross Anatomy: Corydon L. Ford

Moses Gunn was professor of anatomy as well as of surgery when the Medical School opened in 1850. He had been teaching anatomy in his private office in Ann Arbor for the previous two years while he angled for an appointment on the medical faculty. Surgery was his primary interest, and he could turn his anatomical duties over to Corydon L. Ford in 1854. Gunn and Ford had been close friends at the medical institution of Geneva College, and when they heard the University of Michigan was planning a medical school they determined to become its professors of surgery and anatomy. Gunn came to Ann Arbor immediately after graduating from Geneva, but Ford stayed behind until 1854. Ford had an appointment on the Geneva faculty, and he had to wait for an opening at Michigan. Ford's career as professor of anatomy at Michigan covered almost all the first forty years of the school and extended briefly into the next fifty. He had a fatal stroke on 12 April 1894 while walking home from what he had intended to be his last lecture.

Ford was born on a farm in upstate New York in 1813, and an attack of poliomyelitis in his childhood gave him a limp that made him unfit for farm labor. At seventeen he became a schoolmaster, and in 1834 he began a four-year apprenticeship under a physician in Niagara County while continuing to teach school. When Ford moved to Canandaigua, New York, he was befriended by a physician who was a trustee of the Geneva medical school and who urged him to attend it. Ford graduated from Geneva in 1842. He had taught himself gross anatomy with the help of a cadaver and a textbook, and he was appointed to the Geneva faculty as a demonstrator in anatomy immediately upon graduation. He continued to teach anatomy at Geneva until he was summoned to Michigan, and he was kind to Elizabeth Blackwell when she was the lone woman medical student there.

In the custom of the day Ford also taught at Castleton, Bowdoin, Long Island Hospital College of Medicine, and the Berkshire Medical College. Despite repeated complaints to the Michigan regents that he was underpaid, Ford saved enough from his numerous jobs to leave three thousand dollars to a Christian society and twenty thousand dollars to the university library.[31]

Ford taught dissection in a room under a dome in the attic of the Medical Building, and his office was on the third floor. He lived in his office until 1865, when he married at the age of fifty-two. Dissection was moved to the top floor of the four-story addition constructed in 1864–65, and it was moved again in 1889 to a building constructed solely for dissection (fig. 1–4). Male medical students then dissected in a large room constituting the second floor of the building, and women students, who since their admission in 1870 had dissected in what had been

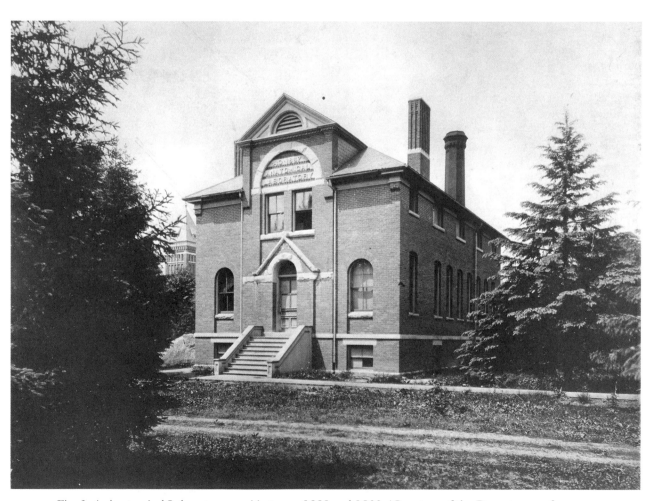

Fig. 1–4. Anatomical Laboratory, used between 1889 and 1903. (Courtesy of the Department of Anatomy, University of Michigan.)

Ford's office in the old Medical Building, worked on the ground floor. In the early years the bones of dissected cadavers were thrown into a ditch in back of the Medical Building, and their discovery during an excavation in the early 1990s aroused consternation in the tender minded. Ford always had a demonstrator to help him, one to six assistants who were usually recent medical graduates on their way to other careers, and the bell ringer, janitor, and unofficial demonstrator of anatomy Gregor "Doc" Nagele.

There was no effective anatomy act in Michigan until 1875, and the demonstrator's chief task was to obtain cadavers. In 1866, 15 to 25 cadavers were enough, but as classes enlarged after the Civil War, 125 to 140 were required each year. The demonstrator seldom robbed graves himself, but he bought cadavers from those who did. Edmund Andrews, an early demonstrator, described his methods.

After some study of the subject I settled on a few simple moral principles.

1. Nobody will spend money over the loss of a pauper cadaver. Therefore obtain *material* only from potter's fields and almshouse cemeteries.
2. The receiving point at Ann Arbor must be kept perfectly calm and friendly. Therefore I allowed no cadaver to be exhumed in Ann Arbor in any circumstances.

I then obtained an agent, in Buffalo, giving him $25 for every specimen sent by express. . . .

I also employed the sexton of the potter's field in Detroit, paying him a less price.

Next I got Dr. ——, of the almshouse at Wayne, to notify me of all specimens buried there, and sent after them by teams hired from the sheriff of Washtenaw county, who kept the livery stable. Lastly I established a flourishing agency in Chicago. It was pretty hard work at first, and I had to get up thirteen cadavers with my own hands the first winter. I was chased sometimes by constables but never caught, and I supplied the University.[32]

Such practices continued even after amendments to Michigan's Anatomy Act in 1875, which were intended to provide for an adequate supply of bodies by legal means. When in January 1878 three professional body snatchers were arrested in Toledo, Ohio, the authorities discovered they had a contract with an Ann Arbor firm to ship 130 bodies to Michigan.

Cadavers were expensive. In 1866 Ford estimated that the total cost was twenty-seven to forty-three dollars: initial cost, twenty to thirty dollars; trans-

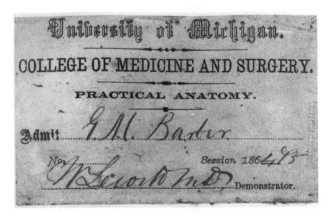

Fig. 1–5. Ticket of admission to dissecting room in 1864 signed by Dr. Lewitt, demonstrator of anatomy. (Courtesy of the Department of Anatomy, University of Michigan.)

portation, five to ten dollars; and injection material, two to three dollars. They were expensive for a student as well, for he paid five dollars for the use of the dissecting room (fig. 1–5) and forty dollars for use of the cadaver. This was at a time when a university professor could maintain himself and a large family on less than thirty dollars a week.

Ford lectured three or four times a week, and by all accounts he was an eloquent and convincing lecturer. He spent many hours preparing dissections that he used to illustrate his lectures, but one wonders how much a student could see from a seat thirty or forty feet away. Throughout his Michigan career Ford had at one time or another the title of professor of physiology, and he had the title at the end of his life although he had long since given up teaching the subject. Warren Lombard, who really was professor of physiology, said:

I had the pleasure of being present at the last lecture given by Doctor Ford to the students in the upper lecture room of the Old Medical Building. All of the faculty would have been there had he allowed it to be known in advance. He was then eighty-one years old, but he gave a great lecture. It was a masterpiece. Ford was without doubt the finest of the Old School lecturers on anatomy in this country and probably in the world. In those days the cadaver was brought into the lecture room, and the lecture was largely a demonstration of a dissection. Ford did this to perfection. He was a large man, of fine presence, dignified in his carriage, graceful in his movements, using a fine choice of language, and thoroughly at home in his subject. I shall never forget the ease and grace with which he handled forceps and scalpel, and the clearness with which he demonstrated to the students the structure and significance of the part he was considering. The following is an illustration of the way he brought physiology into his anatomical lectures.

Using an ox heart, he dissected the root of the aorta with the aortic ring free from the heart, thus exposing the curtains of the aortic valve from the heart side. Then he tied a cork, through which a tube passed, to the peripheral end of the piece of artery, and blew air into the artery, distending it and causing the aortic valve to close. One could readily see the valve curtains and their method of action. He then slid a finger between the curtains, and rapidly withdrew it, when one heard the sound caused by the snapping together of the valve curtains. It was a clever use of dead material to demonstrate the function which it possessed during life.[33]

Internal Medicine: Alonzo B. Palmer

Alonzo B. Palmer joined the faculty in 1854, and he remained a member until he died in 1887. For most of the time he was professor of internal medicine and pathology. He was also in private practice, where he was eminently successful. Palmer's large Victorian gingerbread house, called a "stately mansion" by Victor Vaughan, still stands opposite the Episcopal church on Division Street. Palmer paid for the erection of the tower on the church, and his widow gave the university twenty thousand dollars to construct the Palmer pavilion between the two major buildings of the University Hospital on Catherine Street. The Palmer pavilion was intended for pediatric patients, but it was inevitably used for other things as well, including the hospital's first X-ray laboratory and a nurses' dormitory.

Palmer was the most enthusiastic lecturer on the faculty, and he is said to have given more than a hundred lectures during an academic year. Someone said he would get up in the middle of the night to lecture if he were asked. Palmer's career began when auscultation, palpation, and percussion were coming into use among the better U.S. physicians, and sometime after 1860 he added clinical thermometry to his practice. He died before the sphygmomanometer was introduced, and he confessed to an inability to master the sphygmograph, a device for recording the pulse at the wrist. He depended upon the character of the pulse felt at the wrist to judge the state of the heart and circulation. The strength and frequency of the impulsion of the blood by the heart, he said, is shown by a pulse that is strong, weak, jarring, rapid, quick, slow, unequal, intermitting, or fluttering. The volume of blood flowing through the artery is shown by a pulse that is full, large, or small, and the force of the heart, the volume of blood, and the state of the circulation in general are revealed by a pulse that is thready, gassy, firm, or tense.

Palmer went to Europe in 1880 to visit physicians and hospitals in Great Britain, France, and Germany in order to prepare his two-volume textbook, *A Treatise on the Science and Practice of Medicine, or the Pathology and Therapeutics of Internal Diseases,* published in 1883.[34] It was up-to-date, for it quotes the opinions of such luminaries as Julius Cohnheim, whom Palmer obviously met. It was, however, soon swept into the dustbin by William Osler's book. The following summaries of Palmer's discussion of three representative diseases, scurvy, diphtheria, and typhoid fever, will show what Palmer taught Michigan medical students.[35]

Palmer defined *scurvy* as a condition of general malnutrition produced by a deficiency of fresh vegetables and organic acids in the diet. It is not caused by other dietary peculiarities, particularly not by salted meat, and it never occurs if the supply of fresh vegetables is sufficient. Fresh vegetables and fruit are required for prophylaxis and treatment, but in their absence lemon juice or a preparation that retains the natural properties of lemons is effective. Palmer gave a succinct but adequate description of symptoms and complications and said the disease is progressive, leading slowly to death. Its diagnosis on shipboard or among badly fed troops is easy, but isolated cases may not be recognized. If suspected, a minute inquiry into the patient's diet must be made. There has been much speculation about the special preventive and curative elements in fresh vegetables, but because no satisfactory conclusions have been reached, Palmer thought it unnecessary to detain the student with an account of the theories. Palmer himself had no experience as a practicing pathologist, and his account of the morbid anatomy of patients dying of scurvy is perfunctory. Palmer concluded with explicit directions for the care of a scorbutic patient, and he briefly mentioned the importance of the scorbutic state in other diseases (1:471–75).

Palmer said *diphtheria* is an acute, infectious, and contagious disease, generally occurring epidemically. It affects the whole organism but with particular local symptoms: the formation of a membrane resembling parchment in the fauces, nares, larynx, and trachea. That the disease depends upon a specific poison has been proved, and its contagious character is demonstrated by its production by inoculation with matter of the membrane. It is generally communicated through the atmosphere; therefore the poison must be capable of volatilization. Many low vegetable organisms, bacteria and micrococci, have been found in the membrane, and many competent observers believe them to be the essential contagious material. Others of equal authority have sought them unsuccessfully. Palmer knew the poison is in the membrane, but he did not know whether it is produced by the bacteria. The contagion is not only carried directly from the sick to the well in air, but it may be communicated by fomites, any morbific matter of disease, where it may be dormant for considerable periods. The disease prevails in all seasons and in persons of all ages. It is more common among young children, especially those between the ages of three and six years, and is more fatal in them than in older persons. Palmer gave a long description of the symptoms of nine varieties of diphtheria, ranging from mild to malignant, and he concluded by saying the prognosis must be guarded. If the patient recovers, temporary paralysis of the soft palate and other muscles of the throat occurs in a small proportion of cases. Because diphtheria is likely to be confused with other diseases of the throat, Palmer published a two-column table comparing diphtheria point by point with scarlatina, croup, tonsillitis, and erysipelas of the throat (1:315–16).

Preventive treatment requires isolation, disinfection, and cleanliness. Curative treatment is general or local, antidotal or symptomatic. There is no specific antidote certain to neutralize the poison and arrest the disease. On the supposition that bacteria are concerned in causing the disease, and because they abound in the membrane and its exudates, it is probable that the poisonous material produced locally enters the blood and when absorbed causes general septic effects. Palmer thought it logical to destroy the parasites or the septic material in the throat, whatever it may be, by local, antidotal treatment. He published eight prescriptions for mixtures that could be used as a gargle or could be brushed lightly on the lesion. The active ingredients included chlorine, carbolic acid, potassium permanganate, sodium or magnesium hyposulfite, salicylic acid, iodine, or a mixture of potassium permanganate and potassium chlorate. Flowers of sulfur might be blown into the throat through a squill (1:321–22).

The exudate appearing in the larynx and trachea suffocates, particularly in children, and when suffocation threatens an attempt might be made to remove the membrane. With an angular blunt brush and with the aid of a laryngoscope, the membrane might be caught near the glottis, and with a rapid rotary motion of the brush portions of the membrane might be removed. Another mechanical method is to induce vomiting by which a loosened membrane might be expelled. A spray of 5 to 10 percent lactic acid might loosen the membrane, or a spray of six ounces of limewater with fifteen minims of carbolic acid might be tried. In the last resort tracheotomy may be done. Conditions for success of tracheotomy are most unfavorable, for as suffocation approaches the system has already suffered severe shock. The operation itself is an additional shock, and experience shows that in a large proportion of cases death follows although relief of obstruction to breathing has been obtained.

After a long and gloomy discussion of means by which the general state of the patient may be supported, Palmer ended by saying: "We should not abandon the hope that the nature of this, as well as of specific diseases depending on organic poisons, parasitic or otherwise, may hereafter be better understood, and more effectual antidotes discovered" (1:330).

Palmer defined *typhoid fever* as "a specific fever produced by a peculiar poison usually found in connection with putrefying organic substances, particularly fecal matters in privies and sewers; the poison being conveyed to the system sometimes by means of water and other ingesta, and sometimes through the air. This poison has a period of incubation, in which there is probably multiplication of its amount, and possible changes in its quality; and it produces phenomena of various kinds, but essentially those of a fever, which usually comes on gradually with languor, *malaise,* feebleness, moderate chills, headache, and general pains, especially in the abdomen, back, and limbs, with a tendency to diarrhœa, and soon to tympanitis, tenderness and gurgling on pressure in the right iliac region. As the disease advances, in the early part of the second week, a characteristic slight rose-colored eruption generally appears, showing itself first and chiefly on the abdomen, coming in successive crops, each small spot being visible about three days; there is often slight epistaxis; more or less ringing in the ears, and deafness; the face is often purplish and irregularly flushed; the tongue coated and sometimes dry, and, not unfrequently, toward the latter stages, red and glazed; there is more or less restlessness, but sometimes somnolence; frequently mild delirium, especially in a half-sleeping condition; there is commonly a slight stuffy cough, which will be developed by a full inspiration, with dryness of the throat and thirst not satisfactorily allayed by drinking. These symptoms commonly come on and disappear gradually, continuing about three weeks, the case terminating in recovery in five or six weeks" (1:226). The mortality is between 16 and 25 percent (1:249).

Palmer said the temperature is important for diagnosis, prognosis, and treatment. In a typical case it is as follows (1:229).

Day	Morning	Evening
1	98.6°	100.8°
2	99.4°	101.4°
3	100.4°	102.6°
4	101.6°	104.0°
5	103.5°	104.4°
6	103.6°	104.6°
7	103.6°	104.6°

In most cases the temperature is maintained and possibly becomes higher. The rash continues; the tympanitis becomes greater; the diarrhea persists; the tongue becomes dryer and harder; it is protruded with difficulty, is often fissured, sometimes glossy and red, at other times nearly covered with a thick, black coat; delirium, stupor, or wakefulness is present; and blood may be passed by stool in small or large amounts. The patient may remain in this condition for a week or more; then the symptoms gradually abate; and convalescence is finally established. In other cases matters go unfavorably. Tremors, involuntary discharges, coma, failure of the heart's action occur, and death ensues.

Specific lesions seen at autopsy are congestion, swelling, ulceration, and sloughing of Peyer's patches, generally near the ileocecal valve. Swelling attains its full development by the ninth or tenth day, and, instead of resolution from the ninth to the twelfth day when swelling is at its maximum, ulceration occurs. The bottoms of some ulcers are covered with a brown, gray, or yellow granular mass; others are more clean and red; while in other cases the ulceration extends to the peritoneal coat, which may rupture. Then intestinal contents pass more or less freely into the peritoneal cavity causing great shock, violent peritonitis, and death.

Treatment of typhoid fever is expectant or positive (1:270). Palmer said expectant treatment had long prevailed in Germany but had recently been replaced by positive treatment. He cited the advice of Wünderlich and many others to use mercury in the early stages. Dr. Harley in London said mercury increases and modifies the secretions of the liver, improving its general function. Quinine in large doses may have an abortive effect, but it generally does not succeed in arresting the disease. Palmer diligently described at length the remedies other physicians found useful, and he gave some prescriptions. Those included carbolic acid, acetate of lead, aconite, potassium bromide, potassium chlorate, silver nitrate, and turpentine. Palmer, who was strongly opposed to the use of alcohol, thought that the good in some cases might outweigh its evil. It may diminish abnormal waste of tissue, soothe the nervous system like opium or chloral, and by inducing sleep prevent exhaustion.

Long-continued fever is of itself exceedingly disastrous, and this is most to be dreaded in typhoid fever. The two principal methods of reducing fever are abstraction of heat by cold baths and prevention of heat production by medicinal agents supposed to work on the heat-producing centers. Cold baths are particularly favored in Germany. When the temperature rises to 104 degrees Fahrenheit the patient is put into a full-length bath at 94 degrees Fahrenheit, and while the patient is gently rubbed the bath temperature is reduced to 68 degrees (1:288). The patient is kept in the bath for twenty or thirty minutes and then removed to a comfortably warm bed. The bath is repeated when the temperature rises again. Antipyretic medication consists in giving free doses of "quinine, salicylate of soda, salicylic acid, digitalis, veratrum viride, aconite, or gelseminum" (1:289). Palmer thought the last three objectionable, but he cited with approval reports of the use of salicylate of soda in German, Swiss, and Austrian hospitals.

Although the cause of typhoid fever has given rise to much investigation, professional opinion is at variance. Palmer confined himself to stating the conclusions to which long-continued study and observation had brought him. He was convinced that a single, living, germinal poison capable of preserving its vitality over long periods is the cause of typhoid fever, but the origin of the material is involved in the obscurity that pertains to the origin of all the lowest forms of life. The poison is harbored and multiplied in the bodies of persons with the fever, but it has little power of producing the disease in the form in which it is excreted. However, it is capable of multiplying in fecal matter and other forms of filth and becomes active again when taken into the body by way of ingesta or of the air. Palmer was impressed by the recent discovery in Germany that a disease of cattle is caused by "a rod-like bacteridia" and by Pasteur's demonstration that chicken cholera is caused by a similar specific organism. Something like this may occur in typhoid fever (1:265).

Physiology: Jonathan Adams Allen Jr. and Henry Sewall

Jonathan Adams Allen Jr. was professor of physiology, materia medica, and therapeutics between 1850 and 1854.[36] He had graduated from Castleton Medical College in Vermont in 1846, and he had taught briefly in a short-lived proprietary medical school in La Poste, Indiana, before coming to Michigan.

Allen was an elegant and scholarly exponent of the poetry of materia medica, and he taught students about motor and secretory reflexes. Allen was summarizing one of the major physiological discoveries of the first half of the century, that movement and secretion are independent of consciousness and volition, and he probably learned what he taught from an English translation of Johannes Müller's textbook. Otherwise, there is no trace of Allen's teaching.

Allen was abruptly dismissed by the Board of Regents on 4 May 1854.[37] There is no documentary evidence whatever revealing the reason. For example, Alexander Winchell was secretary of the board, and as a signer of the statement denouncing Allen, he must have known the details. On the day the board dismissed Allen, Winchell wrote in his diary only that he would leave the next day for New York to spend five hundred dollars appropriated by the regents to buy civil engineering equipment, that his daughter was 2 feet 8 5/16 inches tall, and that his rheumatism had moderated a bit.[38] He wrote nothing about what must have been an exciting meeting of the Board of Regents.

A plausible explanation of Allen's dismissal can be deduced from a letter quoted in an editorial published in the contemporary *Peninsular Journal of Medicine* that said Allen had "made himself obnoxious to . . . a body of as high-minded and honorable gentlemen as can be found in any other university."[39] Allen was certainly not obnoxious before 1854, and he was not obnoxious afterward. He went into private practice in Kalamazoo, Michigan, and he was soon elected president of the Michigan State Medical Society. He moved to Chicago, where he was professor of medicine and then president of Rush Medical College. The reason he was obnoxious in 1854 and not before or afterward lies in the date. The year 1854 was the one in which Senator Stephen Douglas introduced the Kansas-Nebraska Act, which if passed would repeal the Missouri Compromise and allow Kansas to be admitted as a slave state. Northerners were outraged, and the Republican Party was founded in protest, in part at a meeting in Jackson, Michigan, thirty miles from Ann Arbor, at which members of the Michigan faculty spoke. Allen, like the Democratic president Franklin Pierce, who had been elected chiefly by votes of the slave states, was from Vermont and a Democrat. In the spring of 1854 Allen was Democratic candidate for mayor of Ann Arbor, and the local Whig newspaper said that Allen was among the men "who employ their insidious wiles for the purpose of prostrating that in which we have a vital local interest; who will stoop to any means for the accomplishment of sinister purposes."[40] In short, Allen was dismissed because his politics were wrong.

After Allen left the professorship of physiology was passed around within the faculty, but sometimes outsiders were hired for a term to teach the subject. A few student notebooks preserved in the Bentley Historical Library record what the professors taught. On 14 December 1869, Vincent S. Lovell wrote under the heading "The Lungs" that carbonic acid is made in the lungs and that the symptoms of carbonic acid poisoning are headache, slowed pulse, and slowed respiration. John W. Bartlett's notebook shows that Burt Green Wilder, who was professor of neurology and vertebrate zoology at Cornell University, devoted a third of his lectures beginning 4 December 1874 to comparative anatomy and physiology and another third to neurology and criticism of phrenology.

This was obviously an unsatisfactory situation, and the medical faculty were becoming ready to make a radical change. In the first place the Medical School was now a part of a progressive university. Henry Philip Tappan, inaugurated president in 1852, promoted scholarship and research in order to transform the university into one on the German model. He raised money for the university library, and he instituted courses in physics and engineering and established the Law School. The Chemical Laboratory was built during his administration. Tappan solicited money for the university observatory, and he staffed it with capable astronomers. His successor, Erastus O. Haven, who was only briefly president, enlarged the Chemical Laboratory and the Medical Building. Haven hesitated to admit women to the university, but immediately after he left in 1870 women were admitted to the University of Michigan and the Medical School on the same terms as men. Haven's successor, James B. Angell, made the university what could unblushingly be called in 1890 the best of the state universities.

In 1872 Henry Sylvester Cheever, a rising young Michigan medical graduate, was asked to teach physiology as well as materia medica. Most of his colleagues taught at other medical schools when Michigan was not in session, and Cheever taught physiology several times at the Long Island Hospital College of Medicine. He had been preceded in that job by John Call Dalton Jr., whose primary position was professor of physiology at the New York College of Physicians and Surgeons. Dalton had studied under Claude Bernard, and he was the first full-time physiologist in the United States.[41] He taught physiology with many demonstrations to accompany his lectures. Traces of Dalton's teaching methods survived in Brooklyn, and it is possible that Cheever took the ferry to New York to learn directly from Dalton. Cheever transferred Dalton's methods to Ann Arbor, where he enlisted the help of medical students. Cheever had tuberculosis, and when he was dying in 1876 he wrote a long letter[42] to President Angell telling him that Michigan must have a professionally qualified physiologist and give him adequate facilities and assistance. Michigan must do the same for materia medica.

Harvard had done what Michigan was thinking of doing, for in 1871 President Charles Eliot had appointed Henry Pickering Bowditch assistant professor of physiology with the charge to teach physiology and begin research along German lines. Bowditch had studied under Carl Ludwig in Leipzig, where he had discovered the all-or-nothing behavior of heart muscle and treppe. In 1877 Dean Palmer, while on his way to teach at Bowdoin, stopped in Boston to see what Bowditch was doing. Palmer did not think much of what he saw, but he wrote President Angell a long letter saying: "I think we had better begin Cautiously even if the appropriation proposed by the . . . Committee passes the Legislature—and chiefly at first in the Study of Histology and the use of the Microscope in examining Physiological and Pathological products &c. *Numbers* will take and be profited by a course of that kind, but numbers will not work at experimental physiology and for the advancement of knowledge.—A taste and zeal in that direction must be developed—We must have Men or at least a *Man* with intelligence sufficient and a desire to work in that field or expensive apparatus will get out of order as I found it at Boston—We must have a Man to desire instruments and Means, and then they should be furnished."[43]

Palmer's prescription was followed. The university bought fifteen microscopes, and Charles Stowell taught a short course in histology with the help of his wife. The course was so successful that it had to be repeated five times in a term.

In December 1880 the full professors constituting the governing body asked Charles Stowell and Victor Vaughan, both junior faculty members with no vote, to report on the state of physiology teaching at Michigan. As a consequence of the report and of Palmer's visit to Boston Vaughan was commissioned to find a physiologist. Bowditch recommended Charles Sedgwick Minot, and Newell Martin at Johns Hopkins recommended Henry Sewall. Minot had been trained in Germany, and he considered himself to be a biophysicist. Sewall was the first person in the United States to earn a doctor of philosophy in physiology, and he had worked under Carl Ludwig in Leipzig, Willy Kühne in Heidelberg, and J. N. Langley in Cambridge. Each was well qualified, but Vaughan persuaded the faculty to elect Sewall by a vote of four to three. Sewall arrived in Ann Arbor for the 1881–82 term.

Henry Sewall had a lot of teaching to do when he arrived in Ann Arbor. There were 127 medical students in the 1882–83 class, including Franklin P. Mall, who became a famous anatomist and embryologist after study under Wilhelm His in Germany. Another was Will Mayo, who revered Donald Maclean as his mentor in surgery. Medical students attended the full two-term course of Sewall's lectures, but students of dentistry, pharmacy, and homeopathic medicine attended for only one term. The regents gave Sewall money for equipment, and he was able to illustrate his lectures to the medical students with many demonstrations, seventeen of them on the circulation alone. Sewall was never able to mount a laboratory course in which all students did the work themselves, but he did give an optional course. He also had students as research assistants.

Henry Sewall had done a large range of physiological experiments during his European trip in

1879–80, and he continued the practice at Johns Hopkins before he was recruited for Michigan. In Ann Arbor he had to work in a room under a lecture hall that Frederick Novy said was not fit for a dog, but he was able to determine the natural stimulus for the depressor reflex, detect the uneven flow of air in the lungs during normal breathing, and study color vision.

Beginning on 6 November 1886 Sewall injected several pigeons with different doses of rattlesnake venom diluted in glycerin. Those injected with small doses survived; those injected with large doses did not. Late in November he found that two pigeons who had survived injection of small doses remained alive after being injected with doses of venom previously determined to be fatal. Sewall's paper describing these results was published in the British *Journal of Physiology* in 1887.[44] His work is recalled by a bronze plaque affixed to the wall of a corridor in the East Medical Building in 1933. The plaque was moved to the wall of a seventh-level corridor in Medical Science Building II when East Medical Building was turned over to nonmedical departments.

COMMEMORATING
THE PIONEER WORK OF
HENRY SEWALL
PROFESSOR OF PHYSIOLOGY
AT THE UNIVERSITY OF MICHIGAN
FROM 1882 TO 1889
HIS WORK IN IMMUNIZING ANIMALS AGAINST SNAKE VENOM DEMONSTRATED THE PRINCIPLE OF ANTITOXIN PRODUCTION

Emil Behring and Shibasaburo Kitasato published a short paper in the *Deutsche medizinische Wochenschrift* in 1890 describing their evidence that the serum of guinea pigs immunized against tetanus toxin contains a characteristic that protects other animals against tetanus toxin.[45] Behring and Kitasato also found that the serum of animals immunized against diphtheria toxin contains a corresponding substance. They had demonstrated the principle of antitoxin production; Henry Sewall had not. Behring was awarded the Nobel Prize and was ennobled by the German emperor. During a useful career in the Japanese Health Service Kitasato was made Baron

Kitasato with a seat in the Japanese House of Lords. When Albert Calmette, who had worked with snake venom as well as with bacille Calmette-Guérin (BCG), visited Ann Arbor in 1908 or 1909, he wanted to see where Sewall had done his snake venom work, but otherwise no one except the Michigan faculty that commissioned the plaque paid any attention to Sewall's work. Late in life Sewall believed he had been deliberately cheated of credit by Behring.

Sewall had to take several leaves of absence on account of his tuberculosis, and he resigned in 1889. He went to Denver, where he obtained a doctor of medicine degree and practiced medicine. He died at the age of eighty-one after a distinguished second career in medicine and public health. He and Vaughan met frequently at the Association of American Physicians, and the two were members of the committee that founded the Board of Medical Examiners in 1915.

The Three-Year Curriculum, 1877–90

Most of Michigan's medical faculty were members of the American Medical Association, and they attended its meetings. The association from its founding in 1847 had campaigned for reform in medical education. Alonzo B. Palmer, Michigan's dean and professor of internal medicine, was for a time chairman of the association's Committee on Medical Education, and his report repeated what every chairman had been saying: the medical course should be extended to three or four years, and it should include not less than two years of clinical instruction in a well-regulated hospital. Michigan's faculty reacted slowly, but a three-year curriculum was substituted for the two-year course in October 1877 (table 1–1). Students already matriculated could choose between the two- and three-year curriculums, but after 1879–80 the two-year course would not be offered.[46]

The regents appointed a committee of local physicians in practice to evaluate the success of the new curriculum. The committee prepared an examination in anatomy, physiology, obstetrics, and diseases of women and children. They were particularly interested in the responses of women graduates, who, they thought, had a more thorough education than the men. Many of the women were college graduates. The committee wished they could fail the students who had gone through the two-year curriculum.

TABLE 1.1. The Three-Year Curriculum, 1887

Subjects in the First Year	Lectures
Descriptive anatomy	90
Comparative embryology	20
Histology and microscopy	40
*Physiology	80
*General chemistry	48
*Organic chemistry	25
Botany	20
Bacteriology	10
Sanitary science	20
Physiological chemistry	60
*Materia medica and therapeutics	60

Laboratory Work in the First Year
Qualitative analytical chemistry, afternoons, 12 weeks
Urinalysis, afternoons, 12 weeks
Practical histology, afternoons, 15 afternoons
Practical anatomy, afternoons until dissection complete

Subjects in the Second Year	
Descriptive anatomy, continued	90
*Physiology	80
*Materia medica and therapeutics	60
*General pathology	20
Pathological anatomy	30
*Physical diagnosis	16
*Medical jurisprudence	15
*Practice of medicine	90
*Systematic surgery	80
*Obstetrics	60
Physiology and pathology of menstruation	20
*Diseases of women and children	45

Optional Courses in the Second Year
Laboratory work in physiology
Electrotherapeutics, 12 lessons
Advanced histology, 30 afternoons
Pathological chemistry, continuing through a college
  year
Extended course in analysis and toxicology, continuing
  through a college year

Subjects in the Third Year	
*Practice of medicine	90
*Systematic surgery	80
Surgical anatomy, weekly	
*Obstetrics	60
*Diseases of women and children	45
Clinical medicine	148
Clinical surgery	72
Clinical gynecology and diseases of children	72
Diseases of the skin (20), ophthalmology and otology (24), laryngology (24), eye and ear clinic (72), minor surgery (36)	176

Optional Courses in the Third Year	
Extended course in clinical surgery	128
Clinical ophthalmology	128

Source: University of Michigan Department of Medicine and Surgery, *Annual Announcement 1887–88,* 13–17 *ff.*

Note: Students were required to attend lectures on subjects marked with an asterisk at least twice. The three-year curriculum was in force until 1890 beginning with students entering in 1877 and evolving over the years.

The Medical School *Annual Announcement* for the year 1889–90 contained a stern warning in sixteen-point italics.

All students entering after July 1st, 1890, will be required to spend four years in professional study, including the time spent in attendance upon lectures, before presenting themselves as candidates for the degree of Doctor of Medicine.[47]

The medical curriculum had finally become mature, and Michigan in the next few years became a member of the top tier of U.S. medical schools.[48]

Surgery: Moses Gunn and Donald Maclean

Moses Gunn was a close friend of Corydon Ford when he was a student at the Geneva medical school in 1844–46. They roomed together, and Gunn assisted Ford in preparing dissections to be demonstrated. Gunn and Ford planned their futures together at Michigan as well.[49]

Gunn had been born in a village between Rochester, New York, and Canandaigua, and he had early determined to become a surgeon. He served his apprenticeship with the same Canandaigua physician who had befriended Corydon Ford and who encouraged him to attend the Geneva medical school. Geneva was able to get unclaimed bodies from the Auburn State Prison, and at the end of the 1845–46 term the school received the body of an African American man. The school being closed had no immediate use for the body. Gunn bundled it into a trunk and took it with him by stagecoach to Detroit and by the recently completed railroad to Ann Arbor, where he gave a series of lectures on anatomy with demonstrations illustrated by dissections of his cadaver. Ann Arbor and its surroundings, like much of the Midwest, had been settled by German immigrants, and Gunn learned German so that he could deal with the immigrants in Washtenaw and Livingston Counties. Gunn found that the Germans paid better and more quickly than the others.

When the regents began to plan the Medical School in 1848 Gunn saw to it that they did not lack his advice. When the Medical Building was completed in 1850 Gunn at the age of twenty-eight was the school's professor of anatomy and surgery, but he turned anatomy over to Ford in 1854. Gunn moved to Detroit in 1853, where he began a successful practice, and he commuted by railroad to Ann Arbor to give his lectures and demonstrations. The trip took three hours each way.

At first Gunn taught surgery only by lectures. A student notebook from the 1852–53 session records that Gunn gave a systematic exposition of surgical problems and how to deal with them. In twenty-six lectures Gunn progressed from treatment of hernias through injuries of the head, amputations, dislocation of joints, fractures, gangrene, caries, venereal diseases, and cancer.[50] Students were supposed to provide themselves with textbooks, but the student's notes reveal that Gunn, in the immemorial custom of teachers of medicine, told the students everything he thought they ought to know, whether or not it had been written down. Eventually the Medical School attracted patients for diagnosis and treatment by its faculty, and in 1869 a house on North University Street was converted into a dormitory where patients could stay before being shown to the students in the Medical Building or could recover from an operation done before the students. The building was called University Hospital, but it had no operating or dressing rooms and no place where a student could study a patient closely.

A student notebook also records that one day in 1865 Gunn showed the students a patient with a gunshot wound of the thigh in whom previous attempts to remove the ball-shaped bullet with a probe were unsuccessful. Nothing was done with the patient because "it is not safe to cut and explore for a ball unless its locality has been pretty well ascertained." On the same day Gunn performed surgery on a twenty-year-old patient with severe convergent strabismus but was not confident sight could be restored in the crooked eye. Other physicians had declared that the swelling beside the trachea of a third patient was a fatty tumor, but Gunn deduced it was an enlarged thyroid gland, a goiter, not a tumor. Ford, who was present, agreed, but Gunn did not venture to excise the growth, although two prescriptions for goiter were suggested. On another day late in 1865 or early in 1866, Gunn demonstrated a boy of five with an enlarged lymphatic gland on the back of his neck extending under the edge of the trapezius muscle: "Chloroform was administered and the tumor was removed."[51] Chloroform was also used the same day when Gunn chiseled necrotic bone from a patient's elbow joint. Anesthesia was probably used in earlier operations before the class, for Gunn had used it for operations on his private patients since 1850.

Teaching surgery by lecture and demonstration continued throughout most of the rest of the first forty years, and it did not stop altogether until 1925, when the new hospital was occupied. It stopped then only because there were no seats for the class in the operating theaters. Teaching how to become a surgeon could not occur until a student stood beside his mentor as he worked. In the school's early days there was no operating room and few patients. The population of Washtenaw County in 1850 was 27,560 and that of Ann Arbor only a few thousand. Gunn and other members of the medical faculty campaigned vigorously to move the Medical School to Detroit, where the population grew from about 50,000 in 1850 to 65,000–70,000 in 1856 to 80,000 in 1858 and where there were hospitals. As editor of several short-lived medical journals Gunn wrote intemperate editorials saying that a full year of hospital instruction, unavailable in Ann Arbor, should be made one of the conditions of graduation. He said that medical colleges elsewhere than in large cities are an anachronism, and he concluded one editorial in which he described English bedside teaching by writing: "The question, then, next suggested, is: Can the Medical Department attain this high ground in its present locality? There can be but one answer: *Never.*"[52]

The regents refused to move the school to Detroit, and Gunn, disappointed in his failure to organize an adequate surgical clinic in Ann Arbor, moved to Chicago in 1867 to become professor of surgery at Rush Medical School. Rush was opposite Cook County Hospital, and Gunn did have an adequate clinic there.

In the five years 1867–72 four men held the position of professor of surgery. All taught elsewhere as well, and all were in private practice.[53] Only the last, Theodore McGraw, had anything to distinguish himself from the general run of contemporary surgeons. He was the first man on the Michigan faculty to have European experience and the first surgeon to do research. His clinical experience and his experiments on animals convinced him that it is safer to let gunshot perforations of the intestine heal themselves than to cause surgical shock by handling the intestine in order to find and sew up the perforations. He returned to his Detroit practice, and later Frederick Coller learned to admire him as "a master surgeon."

Donald Maclean taught surgery at Michigan for seventeen years, 1872–89. He had been born in Canada of Scottish parents who sent him to Edinburgh for his medical education after he had graduated from Queen's College in Kingston, Ontario. Maclean returned to be professor of surgery at Queen's, but he moved to the University of Michigan in 1872 and set up practice in Detroit. In his clinical years in Edinburgh Maclean had assisted James Syme, and he had become proficient in amputations and excisions for which Syme was famous. Syme told Maclean to pay attention to Joseph Lister and his antiseptic doctrine: "There is something in it." In October 1877 Maclean used Lister's carbolic acid spray in two operations before the class, but he soon abandoned the spray, citing deaths from car-

bolic acid poisoning. Instead, he urgently advocated "perfect cleanliness," and Will Mayo, who was Maclean's student, said that Maclean's insistence on cleanliness anticipated Lister's aseptic surgery. Nevertheless, in a series of twelve ovariectomies performed by Maclean three patients died of peritonitis.

The Pavilion Hospital (fig. 1–6) of sixty beds was completed in 1876, and an operating room was added three years later. At last the University of Michigan had a place where its students could gain some clinical experience and Will Mayo could stand beside Maclean at the operating table. Mayo would also have experience giving anesthesia. There were no anesthesiologists, and chloroform was given by anyone handy. He might also have the responsibility for postoperative care, for after completing his work Maclean left for Detroit, where he lived and practiced. The surgical service was busy. In 1883 Maclean published a list of 324 patients seen in the academic year 1881–82, and he published a similar report of 324 patients seen the next year.[54] A sample of the 1881–82 list is shown in table 1–2.

The future of clinical teaching was hotly debated

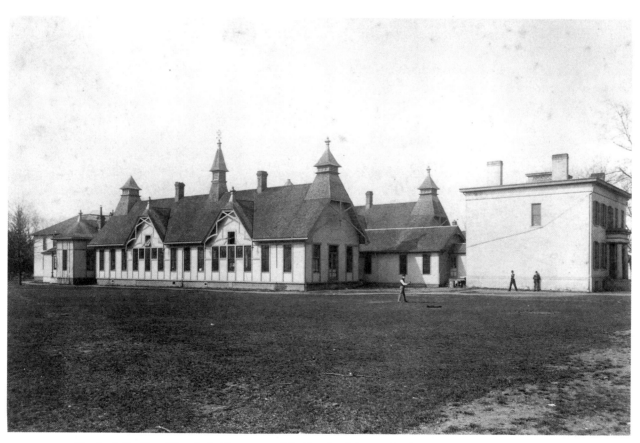

Fig. 1–6. Pavilion Hospital. (Courtesy of the Bentley Historical Library, University of Michigan.)

TABLE 1.2. Some Cases Seen by Donald Maclean in the University Hospital, 1881–82

Age	Diagnosis	Treatment	Result
14	necrosis of tibia	removal of bone and drainage	improved
21	harelip	operation	cure
20	malformed tooth	extracted	cure
26	malignant tumor of perineum	unfit for operation	
38	scirrhus of breast	excision of breast	death
19	sciatica	stretching of nerve	cure
21	stone in the bladder	left lateral lithotomy	cure
25	gonorrhea	zinc sulfate injection	cure

Source: D. Maclean, "A Tabular Statement of the Surgical Work Done in the Department of Medicine and Surgery of the University of Michigan during the School Year of 1881 and 1882," *Physician Surg.* 5 (1883): 387, 388, 391, 392, 393, 394, 396.

in 1885. The argument for moving to Detroit, where there were hospitals and numerous patients, was that Ann Arbor was too small ever to provide an adequate number of patients for teaching. Those who wanted clinical teaching to remain in Ann Arbor cited the advantage of continued association with the university, and they said the quality of teaching depended upon how the patients were used, not upon their number. Patients were now coming from all over Michigan and surrounding states, and their number would increase as the university's reputation spread. Even Maclean, an ardent supporter of the move, admitted patients were coming from almost every state in the Union.

President Angell and the regents ruled in 1888 that clinical teaching would remain in Ann Arbor.[55] The president said the move would be followed by agitation to move the preclinical years and then the School of Dentistry. Detroit physicians, no matter what they said, would not serve the university without adequate salaries. Furthermore, there was no hospital in Detroit that was properly equipped and had money enough to pay its running expenses.

Victor Vaughan and William Herdman appeared before a legislative committee to ask for an appropriation to build a university hospital in Ann Arbor.

Donald Maclean appeared before the same committee and intemperately denounced the university's request. Vaughan wrote: "Next morning the walls of Herdman's house and my own were covered with posters denouncing us as mountebanks, and one of these was found on the desk of each member of the legislature. Resort to this undignified and unwise procedure had just the opposite effect to that intended by [Maclean] who had resorted to it. The bill making the appropriation was immediately introduced, passed by a large majority and signed by the Governor."[56]

The bill appropriated fifty thousand dollars on the condition that the citizens of Ann Arbor contribute twenty-five thousand dollars. The local vote on the Ann Arbor bond issue was 936 ayes and 30 nays. The regents forced Maclean to resign. He continued to practice in Detroit, where he repeatedly expressed his bitter hostility to the Medical School and to Victor Vaughan. President Angell insisted that the hospital be built as far from the central campus as possible, and it was completed on Catherine Street and occupied in 1892. The first forty years of the Medical School were over. Michigan had a four-year curriculum and its own hospital where students could be trained at the bedside.

2
The First Years of Victor Vaughan's Deanship

Alonzo B. Palmer, dean and professor of medicine, died in December 1887, and the faculty elected Corydon Ford, at seventy-four its oldest member, dean. Ford allowed Victor Vaughan to exercise fully the dean's powers. In June 1891 the Board of Regents accepted Ford's resignation as dean, deprived the medical faculty of the right to elect its own dean, and appointed Vaughan.

Edward Dunster, professor of obstetrics and diseases of women, died in May 1888. Henry Sewall, professor of physiology, had to resign early in 1889 on account of his tuberculosis. Donald Maclean, professor of surgery, and George E. Frothingham, professor of ophthalmology and aural surgery, were dismissed at the same time. Vaughan had four major professorships to fill. He had to consider appointments in microscopic anatomy, bacteriology, pharmacology, dermatology, and neurology, and he had to deal with the problem of an incompetent professor of pathology. He was largely responsible for the faculty of the Medical School for the next decade or more (table 2–1).

Vaughan's success in finding George Dock to succeed Palmer will be described now, and other appointments will be described in succeeding chapters.

The Search for a Professor of Medicine

Victor Vaughan was legitimately proud of his success in recruiting faculty, and he listed them in his memoirs.[1] He did not list his failures. Frederick Novy did that, writing the names in pencil in his copy of Vaughan's autobiography, *A Doctor's Memories.* Next to George Dock's name Novy wrote: "Lyster 88, Georg—87—Christopher = failure 1 yr dropped 90–91."

Henry Francis Lyster was not really a failure; he was a Michigan graduate so well regarded in Ann Arbor that he was frequently called upon to fill a gap in the faculty. He had gone into practice in Detroit immediately after graduating in 1860, and he returned to Detroit after being wounded in the Wilderness in the Civil War. He was asked to teach surgery in 1868–69,

TABLE 2.1. Michigan Medical Faculty in the Early Years of Victor Vaughan's Deanship

Preclinical Faculty

Corydon Ford, professor of gross anatomy, died 1894
  Replaced by *J. Playfair McMurrich,* 1894–1907

Charles Stowell, microscopic anatomy, resigned 1889
  Replaced by *G. Carl Huber,* microscopic anatomy and neuroanatomy, 1892–1934

Victor Vaughan, professor of hygiene and physiological chemistry, retired 1921

Frederick G. Novy, professor of bacteriology, 1891–1935

Henry Sewall, professor of physiology, resigned 1889
  Replaced by *William H. Howell,* 1889–92
  Replaced by *Warren P. Lombard,* 1892–1923

John Jacob Abel, professor of pharmacology, 1891–93
  Replaced by *Arthur R. Cushny,* 1893–1905

Heneage Gibbes, professor of pathology, forced to retire, 1895
  Replaced by *George Dock* assisted by *Aldred Scott Warthin,* 1895–1903
  Replaced by *Aldred Scott Warthin,* 1903–30

Clinical Faculty

Alonzo B. Palmer, professor of internal medicine and dean, died 1887
  Replaced by *Henry Lyster,* 1888–90
  Replaced by *Walter S. Christopher,* 1890–91
  Replaced by *George Dock,* 1891–1908

Edward Dunster, professor of obstetrics and diseases of women and children, died 1888
  Replaced by *James Martin* and *James Lynds,* 1888–1901
  Replaced by *Reuben Peterson,* 1901–31

Donald Maclean, professor of surgery, dismissed 1889
  Replaced by *Charles B. Nancrede,* 1889–1917

George E. Frothingham, professor of ophthalmology and aural surgery, dismissed 1889
  Replaced by *Flemming Carrow,* 1889–1904
  Replaced by *Walter R. Parker,* professor of ophthalmology, 1904–32, and by *Roy Bishop Canfield,* professor of otolaryngology, 1904–32

William F. Breakey, professor of dermatology and syphilology, 1890–1912
  Replaced by *Udo Wile,* 1912–47

William J. Herdman, professor of neurology, electrotherapeutics, and diseases of the mind, 1888–1906

Note: Vaughan's appointments are in italics.

and he taught it again in 1877–78. He substituted for Palmer when Palmer went to Europe in 1880, and he was back teaching internal medicine in 1888–90 after Palmer's death. He then withdrew, pleading the exigencies of his Detroit practice. He died four years later of pernicious anemia on the train near Niles, Michigan, while going west to seek his health.

Vaughan had the help of Regent Hermann Kiefer. Kiefer had been born in Germany, and in the German fashion he had obtained his medical education in Freiburg, Heidelberg, and Vienna. Because he took part in the revolutions of 1848 and 1849 he had to flee to the United States. He set up practice in Detroit, and he soon became a leader in Michigan medicine and a leader in the Republican Party as well. As a regent he devoted his full time to the university's medical affairs, and he traveled with Vaughan to Philadelphia, Boston, and New York in search of men to fill the vacancies.

Vaughan listed his requirements in his memoirs.[2] The man selected must be broadly cultivated, and he must be a gentleman. Cultivation was desirable in the small academic community of Ann Arbor, and a gentlemanly physician was more likely to be popular than an abrasive one. In addition the man chosen must be a productive scholar and likely to remain one. This was a new requirement in the Medical School. To be sure, President Tappan long before had started Michigan on its way to becoming a real university by promoting research. He said that a university professor should "assist the student . . . by lectures which treat of every subject with the freshness of thought not yet taking its final repose in authorship" and should be qualified for "learned investigation and philosophical experiment."[3] But until Vaughan's time the medical faculty had done little research.

In July 1890 the regents appointed William Cecil Dabney of the University of Virginia the professor of the theory and practice of medicine and clinical medicine, but the next September they took note that Dabney had written President Angell declining the appointment. Neither Vaughan nor anyone else mentioned this transitory appointment, and its only record is a couple of sentences in the *Regents' Proceedings*.[4]

Vaughan and Kiefer must have had the thirty-one-year-old Walter S. Christopher on the string, for he was appointed professor of medicine as soon as Dabney's withdrawal became known. At the time Christopher was called to Michigan, he practiced in

Cincinnati, where he had been educated, and he was pediatrician to the General Hospital. He had published three papers, two of them on summer diarrhea.[5] Christopher thought the anatomical lesion insufficient to explain the complex of symptoms, and he blamed absorption of ptomaines. It is not the frequent stools that cause the child to have sunken eyes and fontanelle and a rapid pulse; those are caused by poisons of intestinal fermentation. The damage can be repaired by hot baths, opium, or belladonna, but the germs producing fermentation should be starved by proper diet and eliminated. Christopher distinguished between an acid stool and a putrid one, the results of different kind of fermentation. If the stool is acid, fermentation of carbohydrates is at fault, and only albumin, an egg white with a bit of salt, should be fed. If the stool is putrid, proteins should be restricted and only carbohydrates fed. If possible, get fluid into the child by mouth, because when it comes out the other end it will wash away the poison.

Then and for long afterward an initial appointment at the University of Michigan was for only one year at the rank of instructor. If the incumbent were satisfactory, the appointment was made permanent. Christopher was not reappointed, and he left for Chicago in 1891.

George Dock

The standards of Vaughan and Kiefer rose, and George Dock, the man they brought to Michigan in 1891, was an altogether different kind. Dock had graduated from the University of Pennsylvania Medical School in 1884. At that time Penn, like Michigan, was slowly transforming itself. In Dock's student days the dominating character at Penn was William Pepper, a clinician of the old school. He "with great dignity but conveying the impression of having no time to spare, . . . would enter the classroom while taking off gloves and coat, and immediately begin a brilliant discourse on some topic, not always related to his prescribed subject."[6] Then Pepper leaped into his carriage to visit his fashionable patients.

The year Dock graduated a death on the faculty left the professorship of clinical medicine vacant, and Penn acquired William Osler to fill it. Osler always maintained a private practice, but he did not disappear from the school as Pepper did. Instead, Osler took students onto the wards of the University Hospital and of Old Blockley and into the autopsy room. Dock

stayed in Philadelphia for a year's internship, and somehow he became Osler's friend and disciple. Dock learned conversational German from the nuns who were nurses in the Catholic hospital where he interned, and in 1885 he went to Germany and Vienna, where he studied under internists and pathologists: Krehl, Romberg, Virchow, Ehrlich, Paltauf, and Weigert. Osler called Dock back to Philadelphia to take charge of the new clinical laboratory in the University Hospital. Dock became a competent clinical pathologist and a thoroughly competent clinician. When Dock was established at the University of Michigan he took "braindusting" trips to Europe with Osler, and together they made a pious trip to Boerhaave's house. Like Osler, Dock bought rare books and wrote on the history of medicine. Dock became one of Osler's young men whose direct influence on U.S. medicine did not die out until the 1970s.[7]

In a contest for a professorship at Michigan there is usually an insider versus an outsider. When Vaughan presented Dock's name to the faculty on 11 June 1891, the insider was Osbourne F. Chadbourne, a University of Michigan graduate of 1883 who had been Palmer's assistant in practice. The faculty voted four to three in favor of Dock.

Admission Requirements

Vaughan stiffened admission requirements. Graduation from high school was still enough, but now diplomas were accepted only from the schools that had been certified by the University of Michigan Literary Department. Alternatively, a certificate from the Board of Regents of the State University of New York qualified a student for admission. Two years' work in a college was recommended but not required. Nineteen of the 128 students entering in 1903 had graduated from college, and that was a characteristic proportion for many years.

At that time only a small fraction of students attended high school, but the standards of a good Midwestern high school were high. The teachers might be graduates of Harvard or Oberlin. A high school graduate had studied mathematics through trigonometry and had probably taken courses in physiology, geography, and physics. He or she could write simple Greek and Latin prose and had read some Caesar, Cicero, Virgil, Xenophon, and Homer. The high school graduate knew U.S. history and could write an essay on *Macbeth*.[8]

For admission after 1892 algebra and geometry were absolute requirements, but a student could make up trigonometry after admission. The student had to be able to read French and German and must have read Caesar's *Gallic Wars*. A student with deficiencies in biology or chemistry could make them up in a summer course before Medical School classes started. For a student wishing to be licensed to practice in Michigan the school's requirements were reinforced by those set by the State Board of Registration.

The Curriculum

A student entering in 1890 took the new four-year curriculum. Because most students entered directly from high school, eighteen of thirty-five lectures in the first year were devoted to general and analytical chemistry and to physics (fig. 2–1). Likewise, twenty-six to thirty-two hours a semester were spent in the

Chemical Laboratory. The only medical subjects dealt with in lecture were osteology, descriptive anatomy, and materia medica. There were lectures on pharmacy, because doctors dispensed drugs.

College subjects, general and analytical chemistry, continued into the second year along with laboratory work in qualitative analysis. Strictly medical subjects, gross anatomy, histology, physiological chemistry, and physiology, began in the second year. Lectures on physiology continued in the third year when lectures on medicine, pediatrics, and obstetrics were introduced. Third-year afternoons were spent on laboratory work in gross anatomy (figs. 2–2 and 2–3), physiological chemistry, hygiene, physiology, and pathology. Lectures on medical subjects continued in the fourth year, and in the first semester of that year students began practical work in physical diagnosis and obstetrics. Not until the second semester of the fourth year did students attend outpatient clinics and work on the wards.

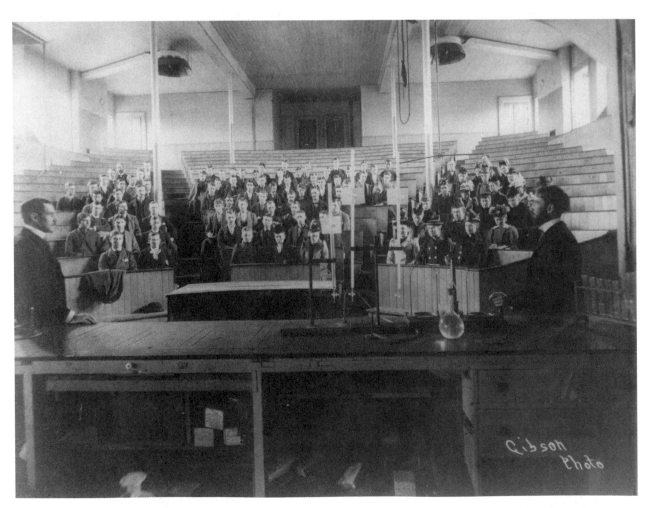

Fig. 2–1. Chemistry lecture. (Courtesy of the Department of Pharmacology, University of Michigan.)

Not Just Any Medical School

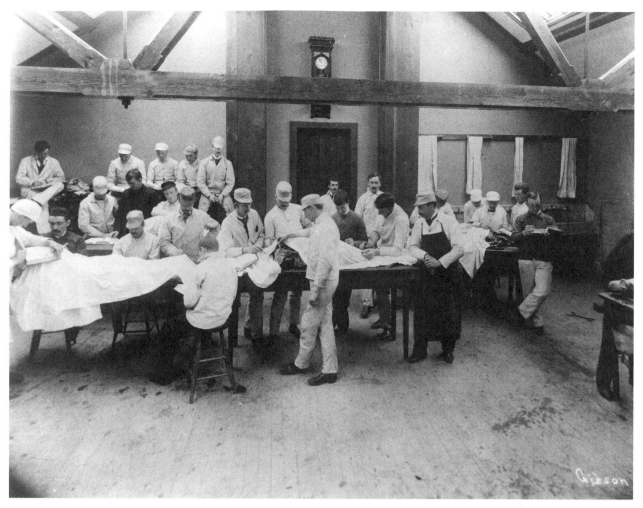

Fig. 2–2. Dissection room for male students, second floor of the Anatomical Laboratory, used between 1889 and 1903. (Courtesy of the Department of Anatomy, University of Michigan.)

In 1907 the Medical School announced that no student would be admitted to the Medical Department, beginning with the fall of 1909, unless he can "bring from the Dean of the Literary Department credits for at least 60 hours, the equivalent of two years' work in that department."[9] Students still had to meet the specific requirements in science, mathematics, and languages previously in force. College work was now removed from the medical curriculum.

When the requirement of two years of college work became effective in 1909 the entering students faced an almost solid block of gross anatomy lectures and dissection, lightened only by some lectures in physiology and bacteriology and by a little laboratory work in bacteriology in the second semester. Their second year was occupied by lectures and laboratory work in bacteriology, physiological chemistry, pharmacology, and pathology. In the third year there

were still some pharmacology and pathology, but most of the year and all of the fourth year were given over to medicine and surgery and the specialties.

The New Medical Building

The cornerstone of the new Medical Building (fig. 2–4) was laid with appropriate ceremony on 15 October 1901, but the building was not ready to be occupied until 1903. As so often happens, construction of a university building was delayed by an economic depression. When completed, the building offered more than adequate space for some of the preclinical departments. Only the Departments of Physiology and Pharmacology had to be content with remodeled rooms in the old Medical Building.

The new Medical Building had a high basement,

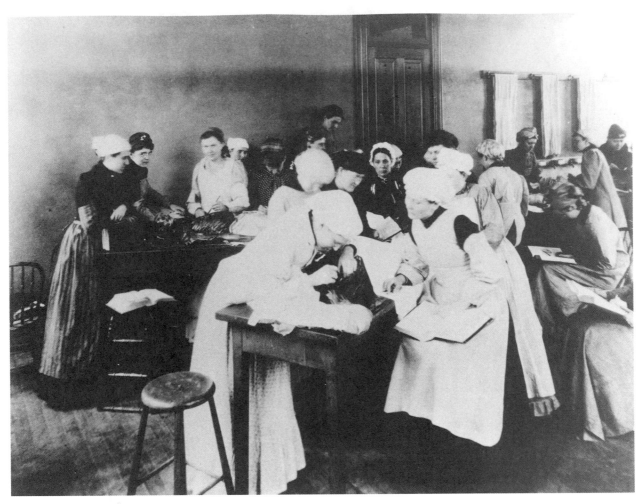

Fig. 2–3. Dissection room for female students, called hen medics, first floor of the Anatomical Laboratory. The women had separate dissection rooms until 1908. (Courtesy of the Department of Anatomy, University of Michigan.)

only partially underground, and there were three floors over the basement. It was built around an open court, and a narrow carriageway into the court allowed cadavers to be brought to the receiving and preparation rooms. The carriageway and its door also facilitated collection of dogs for research and teaching. When dogs were needed, the school's diener (laboratory man-of-all-work) would parade through the neighborhood leading a bitch in heat. Loudly admonishing the males to "go away, go away" he would lead the bitch through the carriageway into the court. When he slammed the door he had completed his primitive version of animal procurement.[10]

The building contained two large lecture rooms, several large classrooms for recitation, and laboratories for "elementary," that is, practical, teaching. Ser-

vice rooms included a photographic darkroom, an operating room for surgical anatomy, and animal quarters for all departments. Each senior member of the faculty, Vaughan, Novy, McMurrich, Warthin, and Huber, had his own office and research laboratory, and there were offices and laboratories for junior staff and advanced students. The dean's office adjoined a faculty room a short distance down the hall from Vaughan's private office, but Vaughan had in addition his own laboratory in which he worked until he retired in 1921 (fig. 2–5).

The old Medical Building was declared unsafe for classes in 1906, perhaps because students made it shake by marching in unison. It was damaged by fire in 1911, abandoned altogether, and torn down. Some alumni wanted to preserve the building as his-

Not Just Any Medical School

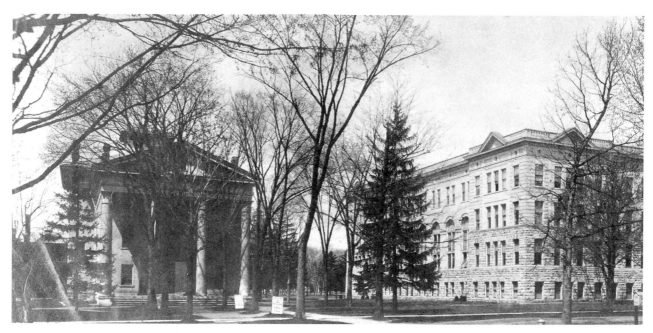

Fig. 2–4. Old Medical Building *(left)* and new Medical Building *(right)*. (Courtesy of the Department of Anatomy, University of Michigan.)

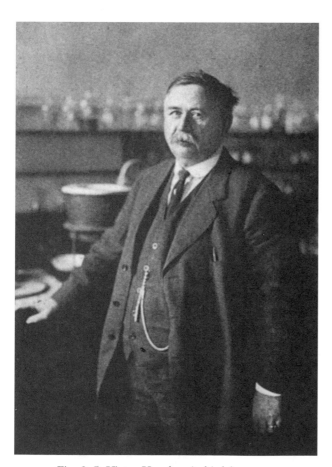

Fig. 2–5. Victor Vaughan in his laboratory

torically important, but a thorough engineering survey showed that was impractical.[11] The Departments of Physiology and Pharmacology were allocated more suitable space in the Chemistry-Pharmacy Building, the old Chemical Laboratory enlarged as chemistry as a university discipline expanded and as the College of Pharmacy was established under Albert B. Prescott.

The clinical departments moved into the University Hospital on Catherine Street in 1892, and Aldred S. Warthin used part of the old Pavilion Hospital as a pathology museum. No matter what the physical shortcomings of the Catherine Street Hospital, it had one great virtue: it was entirely under control of the university. The university authorities did not have to debate with boards of trustees of charity hospitals or with mayors and other politicians about appointments of professional and ancillary staff or about expenditures related to teaching. Abraham Flexner inspected the hospital in 1909 (fig. 2–6), and he wrote in his report: "The school is fortunate in the possession of its own hospital, every case in which can be used for purposes of instruction. . . . The thoroughness and continuity with which the cases can be used to train the student in the technique of modern methods go far to offset defects due to limitations in their number and variety."[12]

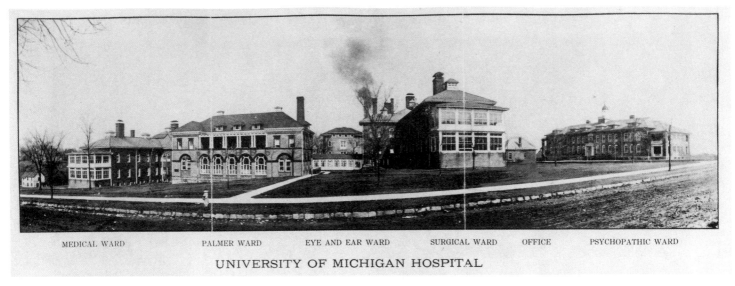

MEDICAL WARD   PALMER WARD   EYE AND EAR WARD   SURGICAL WARD   OFFICE   PSYCHOPATHIC WARD

UNIVERSITY OF MICHIGAN HOSPITAL

Fig. 2–6. Catherine Street Hospital, ca. 1910. (Courtesy of the Bentley Historical Library, University of Michigan, Medical School Records, Box 136, "Medical School Photographs, Laboratories.")

Victor Vaughan's Achievement

By the turn of the century the preclinical faculty, McMurrich, Huber, Novy, Cushny, Lombard, and Warthin, was as good as any in the country, and the clinical faculty, Dock, Nancrede, Peterson, and others, although it did little or no research, was distinguished for its practice. The school buildings ranged from adequate to excellent, and the students were well prepared and well taught. Victor Vaughan was largely responsible for this state of affairs, but he did not do it alone. He had a faculty willing to cooperate, a sympathetic university president and board of regents, a local population willing to vote bond issues for the good of the school and indirectly for its own good, and a state legislature and governor willing to support the school, sometimes reluctantly, with appropriations. It was a fortunate combination.

3
Students

The University of Michigan had a large number of medical students between 1850 and 1890. One hundred two students completed the three-year curriculum in 1891, but when the four-year curriculum was introduced in 1890 enrollment fell off sharply. Only fifty-two students graduated in 1896. Eventually faculty anxiety was allayed as enrollment increased.

Quotas

On 22 June 1927, Dean Hugh Cabot wrote to President C. C. Little asking the president's advice. There was no limit on the number of students admitted to the first-year class; selection was solely on the basis of the applicant's academic record. Dean Cabot said that although requirements had been raised, more than two hundred students had recently entered the freshman class. The preclinical faculty complained, and there was much discussion of imposing a limit. There was another problem: each class had a large number of students whose parents came from central or southern Europe. Their proportion in the medical class far exceeded their proportion in the population in general. The trouble was that their academic qualifications were so far higher than the average, and if students were admitted on the basis of those qualifications, there would be too many undesirables in the school. What did the president think about imposing racial and religious quotas? There is no record of the president's reply.

Cabot was worrying about Jews. The magnitude of the "invasion" Cabot was arming himself to repel is known. Rabbi Morris Lazaron of Baltimore circularized medical schools for information about numbers of Jewish students and attitudes toward them. Arthur Curtis, then secretary of the faculty, went to a great deal of trouble assembling data, and on 20 February 1934 he sent them to Rabbi Lazaron (table 3–1). Curtis also told Rabbi Lazaron where Michigan Jewish graduates interned (table 3–2).

Curtis said that Michigan tried to choose the best Jewish students from metropolitan centers but it distinctly limited the number from any one center. In response to the rabbi's plea for a frank description of Michigan's attitude toward Jews, Curtis distinguished between those whose ancestors had been residents of the United States for several generations and those

TABLE 3.1. Michigan Jewish Graduates, 1922–33

Year	Size of Graduating Class	Number of Jews in Class	Percentage
1922	70	2	3
1923	115	7	6
1924	139	12	9
1925	155	16	10
1926	116	9	8
1927	115	6	5
1928	107	6	6
1929	160	25	16
1930	162	13	8
1931	163	18	11
1932	130	28	22
1933	136	26	19

TABLE 3.2. Internship Locations of Jewish Graduates of the Medical School, 1930–33

Year	In Jewish Hospitals	In Christian Hospitals
1930	5	8
1931	3	15
1932	5	23
1933	3	23

whose parents were recent immigrants. The former were preferable to the latter, who were perceived to be radical and abrasive. Curtis thought that many of the Jewish students were brilliant, and he said there was no doubt that many of the best minds in medicine were Jewish. He hoped there would be a time when Jewish students of that caliber would be encouraged rather than discouraged in applying to medicine.

Beginning in 1927 all applicants with satisfactory credentials were told they must be interviewed. Those from the Midwest came to Ann Arbor. Others saw Michigan faculty or graduates in New York, Denver, and Los Angeles. At the interview applicants were asked to take a standardized vocabulary, reading, and interest test, and they were required to write a short essay on a nonmedical subject. In the first year 589 applied, but only 300 presented themselves for interview and examination. The reduction was particularly noticeable in New York, a major source of Jewish applicants.

There was the opposite problem with Catholics. In the 1920s the president of the University of Detroit, a Catholic school, was angry because none of his students was admitted. Dean Cabot wrote him that Michigan would take students from his university only after the most rigid examination of their credentials, and in 1940 Dean Furstenberg said that it was a matter of public record that students from the University of Detroit did not do well in medical school. He was referring to the American Medical Association composite report on student accomplishment. Of 203 students admitted to U.S. medical schools from the University of Detroit in 1930–35, only 104 had clear records. Forty-four had encumbered records, 40 had failed, and 12 had withdrawn. In fact, the dean said, Michigan would not accept credits from that school. Regent Murfin took up the problem with the dean, saying he had no intention of exerting pressure, but hardly a day passed when he did not get an appeal from a parent.

The academic standard of denominational schools and not religion was the problem. In 1938 Dean Furstenberg, in extensive correspondence with the president of Calvin College (a Christian liberal arts school), said that of the nine students admitted from Calvin in 1937, six were on probation and the remaining three were in the middle of the class. James Bosma from Calvin, however, was outstandingly good.

Admissions had always been handled by the dean's office, but Cabot appointed a faculty advisory committee. Between 1930 and 1935 the Executive Committee acted as an admissions committee, and when Furstenberg became dean in 1935, he, his confidential secretary, Vera Cummings, and Marvin Pollard, the secretary of the faculty, made the decisions. If quotas were imposed, they were the ones who did it.[1]

Out-of-State and Foreign Students

There had never been any geographical restriction; new students came from every state in the Union and from many foreign countries. In 1887 President Angell told the regents: "Nor in considering this subject [out-of-state tuition] can we ever permit ourselves to forget that our original and chief permanent endowment was the gift of the United States, and that therefore there rests on us the obligation to treat generously students from all parts of the Union."[2]

Over the years there would be at least one student from every state, but most came from the populous Northeast or Midwest. After 1898 there were always two or three from Puerto Rico and the Philippines. Because there was no limit on class size, Michigan students constituted only half the entering class until 1930. Then class size was unofficially limited to 120 students. Because all qualified Michigan students were admitted, out-of-state students were squeezed out. At the end of the decade entering class size was 140 as the United States prepared to enter the war, and then only 25 percent of the class was from out of state.

There were always two or three in each class from foreign countries: Nicaragua, China, Germany, Hungary, the Netherlands, Australia, South Africa, Manchuria, or Switzerland. Vaughan once told the faculty that many students from India who already had an Indian doctor of medicine degree wanted to come to Michigan to get a U.S. one. He had written the Indians that they could earn a Michigan medical degree in one year by satisfactory work in the senior class, and the faculty, with what reluctance the record does not show, approved his action. In 1915 Jokichi Takamine, who had worked with Parke, Davis and Company in isolating Adrenalin,[3] wrote Vaughan, saying that on account of the war, Japanese students would probably not be going to Germany any more. He hoped Michigan would take them. Vaughan replied they had always been welcome. The dean was ex officio a member of the Barbour Scholarship Committee, and a few Asian women supported by Barbour Scholarships earned doctor of medicine degrees in Ann Arbor.

Women

When the regents voted in January 1870 to admit women to the university on the same terms as men, the medical faculty marshaled arguments against their admission to medical school.[4] Women are qualified mentally and emotionally to tend the sick, but they are semi-invalids a large fraction of the month. There is the danger they would practice abortion to avoid having pregnancy, and childbearing would interfere with their medical careers. When the medical faculty found admission of women inevitable, they agreed to teach women in classes separate from men for an additional five hundred dollars of salary. Segregation by sex eventually disappeared, as photographs taken in the early 1890s show women mixed with men in medical and surgical clinics. George Dock's clinical notes show that he treated women like men in internal medicine.[5]

Many women intending to be medical missionaries received training at Michigan in the early days. At another social level the wealthy Alice Hamilton came to Ann Arbor after studying at Miss Farmer's School in Connecticut and left in 1893 after graduating for a famous career in industrial medicine (fig. 3–1). After she retired she wrote to ask if she could return to Michigan to teach a brief course for junior or senior medical students. Dean Furstenberg declined her offer; there was no room in the curriculum or money in the budget.

When Victor Vaughan became dean women constituted 25 percent of the medical classes, but the percentage fell to as low as 2 percent in 1910. Thereafter until 1941 women made up 5 percent to 10 percent of the classes. In 1926 Arthur Curtis found that, between 1916 and 1924, 924 men and 61 women had graduated.[6] Whereas 40 percent of the men prepared at other institutions, 76 percent of the women had studied at the University of Michigan Literary Department. Women were better prepared, for 85 percent of them had a bachelor's degree as compared with only 44 percent of the men. Women did about 10 percent better than men in the first two years and as well as men in the last two. The same proportion of women graduated as entered the school.

African Americans

The Medical School kept no record of race, and the only way to identify African American medical students is by examination of class pictures. Twenty-four of the fifty classes graduating before 1942 had one or two African American members. The high point was reached in 1931 when four African Americans graduated. Arthur Curtis had written that the class contained an unusually fine group of African Americans, one of whom was the first to be elected to Alpha Omega Alpha.[7]

There is no way of knowing how many African Americans were admitted and failed to graduate. Promotion Committee records occasionally note that a student of color was in trouble and working hard to support himself or herself. Dean Vaughan wrote to the president of Lincoln University, saying that African American medical students were handicapped by poverty; one was working four hours a day waiting on tables.

There were the inevitable charges of prejudice. In

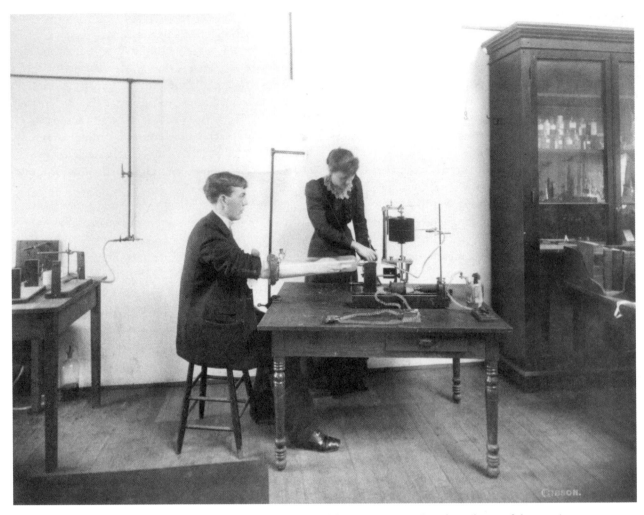

Fig. 3–1. Alice Hamilton *(standing)* in physiological laboratory, measuring the volume of the arm in relation to circulation and respiration. (Courtesy of the Bentley Historical Library, University of Michigan, Medical School Records, Box 136, "Gibson #3.")

1928 President Little wrote to a professor at Howard University, whose son had not been given an internship in the University Hospital after graduating from Michigan, that appointment "will not be denied on any grounds of race or creed," and he demanded proof of prejudice, something impossible to provide. There were occasional hints of prejudice in the opposite direction. A decade earlier two students had been caught cheating in a laboratory examination in pathology. The Honor Council recommended the African American student merely be required to repeat the course, because he "is well liked by his classmates being a good student, self-supporting and in our estimation will make a good practitioner among his race." The other, a white, was dismissed.

Immediately after Dean Cabot was himself dis-

missed in 1930, the Executive Committee rescinded his order that men of color not be allowed to examine women patients in the University Hospital, but when arrangements were made in 1931 for University of Michigan students to obtain additional obstetrical experience by spending a week at Detroit's Woman's Hospital, African American students and women students were excluded.

Costs

When the Medical School first opened students paid only a $10 registration or matriculation fee. By the time Vaughan became dean the matriculation fee was the same for Michigan residents but $25 for students

Not Just Any Medical School

from out of state. Michigan students were assessed an annual fee of $25, and tuition rose slowly over the next fifty years until it was $250 in 1940, when Harvard tuition was $400 and Johns Hopkins tuition $600. In the first fifteen years of Vaughan's deanship, students were required to pay laboratory and demonstration fees totaling $136 over the four years. Anatomy was the most expensive, costing $21 in 1914, but $10 was asked for the demonstration course in nervous diseases. Those fees were eventually incorporated into the tuition, but students were always required to make deposits in laboratory courses.

The real value of those dollar amounts can be judged by comparison with other costs. In 1893 a student paid $3 to $5 a week for room and board. If the student clubbed with others the cost of board was less than $2.50 a week. In 1931 room and board was $12 to $15, and it remained the same for the rest of the decade. In 1940 the secretary of the school estimated that total yearly expenses for a Michigan student were $400 beyond tuition. In 1892 an assistant professor of anatomy could marry and begin to raise a family on $1,600. In 1940 an assistant professor might be paid $3,500.

There were no solid data on student employment until replies to a questionnaire sent out in 1937 were tabulated. Of the 396 students replying, 136 were working an average of eighteen hours a week for room and board or as laboratory assistants. Fifty of those working were receiving $15 a month from the National Youth Administration. The percentage of students working rose from 10.7 percent of the freshman class to 33.3 percent of the senior class.

Loan funds gradually accumulated, and in 1924 Dean Cabot wrote that no request for a loan had been refused. By 1940 the money available was substantial. There were thirty thousand dollars from a woman physician who had graduated from the University of Michigan, ten thousand dollars from another graduate, and many smaller sums. A notable source was the medical students themselves. The Galens Medical Society had been founded in 1914, chiefly to be a liaison between students and faculty. In 1927 the Galens began to collect money for charitable purposes by means of its Christmas Tag Day. In the 1930s Galens established a loan fund of eight hundred dollars a year, specifying no loan should be greater than one hundred dollars. There was never any scholarship for entering students; the few there were went to upperclassmen. Here, too, Galens filled

a gap by providing scholarships not to exceed four hundred dollars a year.

The Combined Course

The University of Michigan never required a bachelor's degree before admission to the Medical School. Students entering in 1909 must have completed sixty semester hours, or two years, of college work. That included courses in English, history, mathematics, chemistry, physics, biology, Latin, and French or German.[8] Nevertheless, an increasing number of entering students were college graduates, for the additional work gave them an advantage in competition for admission. Of the 170 members of the first-year class in 1920, 36 had a degree, whereas 66 of the 121 first-year students in 1940 had one.

From the time the four-year curriculum was introduced in 1890 students could earn a college degree and shorten their medical course by enrolling in the combined literary and medical course. For example, in 1909–10 all courses in the first two years of the medical curriculum were open to students in the Literary Department, and students could register in the Department of Medicine and Surgery (Medical School) at the end of their third year when they had accumulated credits for ninety semester hours. They were eligible for a bachelor of arts degree at the end of the fourth year, provided the following course work was completed.[9]

Rhetoric—6 hours
French and German—16 hours of either and 8 of the other
English—6 hours
Psychology—6 hours
Physics—10 hours, including 2 hours of laboratory
Chemistry—12 hours for those with chemistry in high school, otherwise 16 hours
Biology—8 hours
Zoology—6 hours
Total—78 or 82 hours

The Medical School suggested that students fill the cracks in the combined course with eight hours of elementary Greek or Latin, eight hours of history, political economy, or philosophy, and four hours of qualitative analysis or five hours of organic chemistry. Sixty semester hours of college work were rigidly specified in the combined bachelor of science and doctor of medicine curriculum, which took six years.

Students could satisfy the college requirements of the combined course in colleges approved by the Literary Department. Many in the area were approved: Albion, Hope, and Earlham (Richmond, Indiana) but not Kalamazoo College.

In speeches, letters, and publications Deans Cabot and Furstenberg repeatedly deplored the emphasis on science to the exclusion of most liberal arts subjects. In 1926 Cabot agreed with a faculty committee that students needed more humanities: anthropology, ethnology, a more rounded knowledge of abnormal psychology, a broader understanding of sociology, and a better grasp of history. There should not be too much science, but more physical chemistry and biophysics were desirable. To allow time, the modern language requirement might be omitted, for translations were available.[10]

Preceptorships and Tutorials

The preceptorship originally required was abolished in 1877, but toward the end of the 1920s Dean Cabot wrote to a large number of Michigan physicians, inquiring if each would be willing to take a student in the summer between the junior and senior years for a preceptorship. The physician would provide minimal room and board and expose the student to the problems of practice. Many physicians were willing, and in 1929 twelve students had such preceptorships. Most of the physicians reported that the students were highly satisfactory, but some said they were not. Cabot said all students "wagged their tails" when they returned.

At the same time Cabot asked the clinical faculty if they were willing to take students for tutorials. Six students would be assigned to each, two from the top of the class, two from the middle, and two from the bottom. Most clinicians were pleased to cooperate, but the project soon died.

Grading and Promotion

When Victor Vaughan became dean grades given students were merely "passed," "conditioned," or "not passed." Students had to pass all courses in order to graduate, and they were given the opportunity to remove conditions or failures by taking a new examination or by repeating the course. In 1903 "incomplete" and "absent" were added with regulations for

their removal. Then in 1915 the faculty switched to letter grades: A, B, C, D, and E. At Michigan a D was not a very low pass as it was elsewhere, but it signified a condition that had to be removed. Pluses and minuses were given each grade with the result the faculty graded students on a thirteen-point scale. Numerical values were given to each grade, and because the calculator in the dean's office had four decimal places, students' grade point averages were calculated to four decimal places. Class standing was then determined with precision.

A student absent from an examination could make it up under suitable conditions, but the story was different when the faculty failed to show up to give an examination. In the late 1920s there was a rash of such instances; students came to a properly scheduled and advertised examination to find no examination to be taken. Dean Cabot reprimanded Doctors Cowie and Peterson for such neglect, and he ruled that students, having appeared and remained throughout the examination period, must be considered to have passed the phantom examination.

At first all students with academic deficiencies were discussed by the entire faculty, but subcommittees for preclinical and clinical years were established in the 1910s. Those became a full-fledged promotion committee in the 1920s. A typical meeting of that committee was held on 12 February 1926. Fifty-one students were considered. Ten freshmen were dropped from registration or advised to withdraw, and seven were placed on probation. Four sophomores but no juniors or seniors were dropped, and three seniors had their probation removed.

The Promotion Committee often allowed a student to clear his or her record on the condition that the student apply to another medical school. The dean sometimes went out of his way to secure a place for a failing student elsewhere. The University of Michigan Medical School refused to admit another school's failures, but it was sometimes the victim of fraudulent credentials. The faculty invariably accepted the committee's recommendations, but sometimes at a later date the faculty changed its mind in the direction of leniency. The committee always, or almost always, resisted pressure from an important person.

After a vast amount of discussion in 1928 the faculty instituted a comprehensive examination in all subjects in the curriculum to be given to senior medical students. Dr. Sturgis was put in charge. At first each student had to write an examination paper of a very general character for three successive mornings. Examination books were read by a committee of six members of the clinical faculty, each reading about twenty books. The faculty found students bewildered when asked to survey a broad field. The second part of the examination was oral, a student being examined at the bedside of a patient.

Dr. Sturgis told the dean the comprehensive examination was a burden and had to be modified. After successive changes it was dropped in 1940.

In the early days attrition was always high, and before 1914 more than 47 percent of the entering class failed to graduate. The greatest mortality was at the end of the first year, and a substantial loss occurred at the end of the second. In 1914 it dawned on the faculty that a student who failed probably entered with a poor academic record. The faculty voted to deny admission "to those who had not given evidence of good scholarship in college." In the next fifteen years 60 to 80 percent of the entering class graduated, and the percentage rose above 70 when the size of the entering class was limited in 1930.

The Honor System and Discipline

In 1927 a psychiatrist teaching in another school said that faculty and students were engaged in a perpetual war with each other. Therefore, students thought cheating a perfectly legitimate tactic, and they felt no guilt or shame when caught.[11] In the early days at Michigan an occasional student was expelled for cheating, but there is no evidence of the prevalence of the practice. In 1916 the Medical School *Announcement* contained this paragraph.

Honor System. For a number of years all the examinations in this School have been under student control. Under this "Honor System" the faculty turns over to the students the complete supervision of all examinations. Each class elects an Honor Committee which has charge of this matter and which is responsible to the faculty. In case there is any infraction of rules, this committee tries the offender, and if necessary makes recommendations to the faculty for official action.[12]

As a further refinement, numbers instead of names were used on examination papers after 1922. On several occasions when a faculty member appeared to proctor an examination he was reprimanded by the dean.

The trouble with the honor system was that each class was free to make its own rules or to abandon the system altogether. In one year sophomores and juniors had the system, and the freshmen and seniors did not. The faculty discussed this problem at length, and in 1925 it imposed a uniform honor system on all classes. Thereafter the system worked reasonably well, and once a new dean coming from the outside had to be told that recommendations for discipline came from the students.

There were the standard problems: students who drank, gambled, or fought. Sometimes a male student had a girl, not a relative, in his room. Once a girl from the Literary Department appeared to become pregnant, and her father demanded vengeance. When the girl herself was disciplined for cheating on a language examination and when the appearance of pregnancy mysteriously disappeared, Dean Cabot took no action against the medical student and said the girl's father was a crook. A particularly troublesome problem in the 1920s and 1930s was violation of the university's ban on driving an automobile. Sometimes a male student caught driving his girl home from a dance had to write an essay or do extra work in, appropriately, obstetrics and gynecology. Dean Furstenberg sometimes disciplined the offender with a reprimand and a smile.

Student Housing

President Tappan, as one of his first acts in 1854, took the university out of the dormitory business, and medical students lived off campus. The Medical School *Annual Announcement* always told prospective students how much they might have to pay for room and board. In 1882 Nu Sigma Nu was organized with Will Mayo as a charter member, and Phi Rho Sigma and Phi Chi followed as places for medical students to live. How they lived is described in *Arrowsmith*.

Digamma Pi was housed in a residence built in the expansive days of 1885. The living-room suggested a recent cyclone. Knife-gashed tables, broken Morris chairs, and torn rugs were flung about the room, and covered with backless books, hockey shoes, caps, and cigarette stubs. Above, there were four men to a bedroom, and the beds were iron double-deckers, like a steerage.

For ash-trays, the Digams used sawed skulls, and on the bedroom walls were anatomical charts, to be studied while dressing. In Martin's room was a complete skeleton.[13]

When a fraternity gave a party during Prohibition, faculty guests did not notice that there was alcohol in the drinks they were served.

In 1937, 176 students were living in fraternity houses, 80 in rooming houses, 64 in apartments, 41 at home, and 28 in private homes. The next year the university, with the help of the Public Works Administration and a two hundred thousand dollar loan from the Ann Arbor Trust Company, built Victor Vaughan House on the site of the old Medical Ward that had been destroyed by fire in 1927. In the summer of 1938 Vera Cummings wrote frantic daily letters to Dean Furstenberg, who was on vacation in Frankfort, Michigan, telling him that only one or two more students had signed up for Victor Vaughan House. The dean wanted to require freshmen students to live in it, and he polled the Executive Committee on that point. Cyrus Sturgis voted in favor and H. B. Lewis against the requirement. The house was filled, but when the war came a little later it was requisitioned by the navy and never again served its original purpose.

Tuberculosis

In the twentieth century medical students and faculty were no longer dying left and right of tuberculosis as they had in the nineteenth century, but the disease continued to be a serious problem. Medical students were exposed to tuberculous patients, and they were exhausted by hard work. Between 1917 and 1939 there were thirty-seven cases of tuberculosis, some fatal, among 9,988 medical students. The case rate among students in the College of Literature, Science, and the Arts and the Law School was lower, but it was 75 percent higher among students in the Graduate School.

The Summer Session

There was always substantial enrollment in the Medical School's summer session. In 1910, 104 students, including 14 doctors of medicine and 1 doctor of osteopathy, registered. In 1920 the total was 174, with 7 doctors of medicine, and in 1930 and 1940 there were 248 and 221 students, respectively.

The preclinical departments' summer courses were, in theory at least, equivalent to those taught in the academic year, and they carried equal credit.

They served three purposes. Students in the combined course might take medical subjects in anticipation of admission to medical schools or to lighten their load as medical students. For example, Carl Vernon Weller took a summer course in 1910. Later, biological chemistry was one course students liked to get out of the way before the regular term began. Some junior faculty members from Michigan or other schools, having only the doctor of philosophy degree and believing that the doctor of medicine degree was essential for academic advancement, took medical courses in the summer. When Elizabeth Crosby (fig. 3–2) achieved international renown, doctors of philosophy and doctors of medicine from all over came to Ann Arbor to take her summer course in neuroanatomy. Michigan students who failed a course were allowed to attempt to make up the deficiency by repeating the course in the summer. Likewise, failing students from other schools came to Michigan for the same purpose (table 3–3). In fact, a

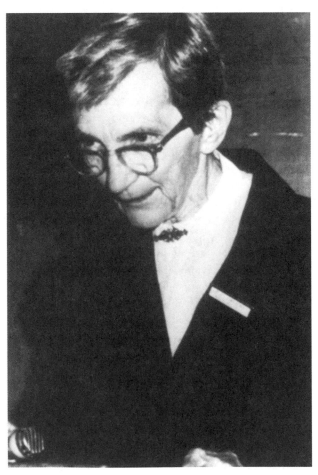

Fig. 3–2. Elizabeth Caroline Crosby. (Courtesy of the Department of Surgery, University of Michigan.)

TABLE 3.3.   Enrollment in the Summer Session for 1939

Reason for Enrollment/ Student Status	Students from Michigan	Students from Other Schools	Student Total
To clear academic record	55	81	136
On reduced schedule	5	?	5
In good standing	11	67	78

student might repeat the same course several summers in a row at different medical schools. Enrollment in the summer session for 1939 was typical. Twenty-four students took gross anatomy, twenty took bacteriology, sixty-six took biological chemistry, and thirty-one took pathology.

Makeup courses relieved the Promotion Committee of the responsibility of dropping a failing student. As a result many marginal students squeaked through to a doctor of medicine degree, or, as Dean Furstenberg said, "were saved for medicine."

History of Medicine and the Victor Vaughan Society

In the 1900s Aldred Scott Warthin began the practice of asking junior students who had done best in his sophomore course to be members of a journal club. Two students reported at each of seven monthly meetings on the evolution of medicine as a science. In January 1913, for example, Mr. Getty reported on the primitive period of Roman medicine, and Mr. Munson talked on Galen and the post-Galenic period. In May Mr. Weller, the second speaker, presented "Modern Medicine (Broussais, Laënnec, Magendie, etc., in France, English Medicine, Italian, German, Physiology, Pathology, Etiology)." Warthin's journal club expired in the 1920s.

Faculty encouragement revived in the late 1920s when Cyrus Sturgis and James Bruce helped senior students found the Victor Vaughan Society. From 1929 to the disastrous period of student revolt in the early 1970s some dozen or more seniors met once a month to hear one of their number read a paper on medical history. The meeting was at a faculty member's home, and a particularly knowledgeable faculty member was invited to discuss the paper. Typewritten copies were bound and deposited in the medical

library, and in 1932 twelve essays were published to show what the students were doing.[14]

The papers were often on some medical figure: Samuel D. Gross Sr. or William Pepper. Others were on the history of trephining, osteopathy, or bloodletting. For the most part the essays were based on secondary sources, but occasionally they were surprisingly substantial documents. Those essays themselves were primary sources, for they were about persons the students and faculty knew: Murray Cowie or Albert Barrett.

As soon as Frederick Coller became professor of surgery he inserted a weekly lecture on the history of medicine into his second-year course on surgery. Soon the lectures on surgery were dropped, but the lectures on the history of medicine lasted as long as Coller did. Coller's fifteen lectures were designed to effect a closer relation between the abstract sciences and the clinical years and to impress students with the ever progressive character of medicine.[15] Students could prepare for change by understanding medicine's background: where, for example, digitalis and quinine came from and how the cure for scurvy was discovered. The social relations of medicine are important; students would see every day in their patients the survival of folklore, and they would feel the influence of religion in the constant desire for a miracle. So Coller justified his course. Then, in eleven superficial lectures Coller raced through the Greco-Roman period, the Dark Ages, the Renaissance, the sixteenth, seventeenth, and eighteenth centuries to the modern period. Before ending with a lecture on religion and medicine Coller devoted one each to anesthesia, antisepsis, and hemostasis, and each year the students were required to "discuss fully" one of the three on the final examination. Another examination question required students to identify the contributions of the following.

Edward Jenner	Thomas Addison	Crawford Long
John Hunter	Leonardo da Vinci	Ignaz Semmelweis
William Harvey	Michael Servetus	Rudolf Virchow
William Halsted	William Beaumont	Vesalius

Although the lectures were chiefly lists of names and dates drawn from secondary sources, a student committee of which William Robinson, later chair of the Department of Internal Medicine, was a member had high praise for the course when it reported on the curriculum in 1934.

Students and Faculty

At Michigan the main body of students may have been at war with the faculty, but in many instances a student found a substitute parent among the faculty.

As soon as the faculty began to give demonstrations in the 1870s students were hired as assistants, and as laboratory courses grew in importance as many as six medical students would help teach a particular course each year. Such students may have been cheap labor, but they had a special opportunity for learning while they taught. When faculty members began to conduct research, students spent time in research, more collaborators than assistants and getting their names on papers. Some, like Carl Wiggers with Lombard and Charles Edmunds with Cushny, were deflected into scientific careers by the experience.

In the 1880s Maclean left his patients in the care of students when he went back to Detroit after operating, but soon Nancrede and Dock had graduate assistants who moved up in rank and importance. Most went into practice, but a number, Roger S. Morris, James Arneill, Frank Wilson, and A. C. Furstenberg among them, stayed in academic life and became professors in their specialty. The result was that for a while Michigan ranked just behind Harvard, Johns Hopkins, Columbia, and Pennsylvania in the number of its graduates in academic positions.

4
Bacteriology, Hygiene, and Physiological Chemistry to 1921

Victor Vaughan was officially a physiological chemist after 1890, and his protégé Frederick Novy was the bacteriologist. Nevertheless, Vaughan's research until he retired in 1921 dealt largely with the chemistry of bacteria.[1] He became very busy in national affairs, and he seriously neglected teaching physiological chemistry in Ann Arbor. Thus, Novy taught physiological chemistry (fig. 4–1) as well as bacteriology.

Ptomaines

Vaughan said the tyrotoxicon he had isolated from spoiled cheese is "only one of a large class of bodies that are produced by putrefaction."[2] Those are the ptomaines and leukomaines, intermediate products formed when bacteria degrade proteins to carbon dioxide, ammonia, and water.

Vaughan divided diseases into the infectious and the autogenous. Autogenous diseases "owe their existence to disturbances between tissue metabolism and excretion,"[3] and he ignored them for a while. Infectious diseases occur when "a specific, pathogenic microörganism, having gained admittance to the body, and having found the conditions favorable, grows and multiplies, and in so doing elaborates a chemical poison [derived from protein] which induces its characteristic effects."[4] Cholera infantum is an example of a disease produced by such a poison. Vaughan and Novy published a book called *Ptomaines and Leucomaines* in 1888, and the book established ptomaine poisoning as a clinical entity.[5]

By the time Vaughan and Novy wrote the fourth edition of their book in 1902 they had modified their opinion.[6] Microorganisms do produce ptomaines and leukomaines as transition products of putrefaction of proteins, and Vaughan and Novy described the products in great detail. However, there are other forms of toxins. One, such as diphtheria toxin, is synthesized and excreted by a pathogenic organism. The other is the protein poison, a constituent of cells.

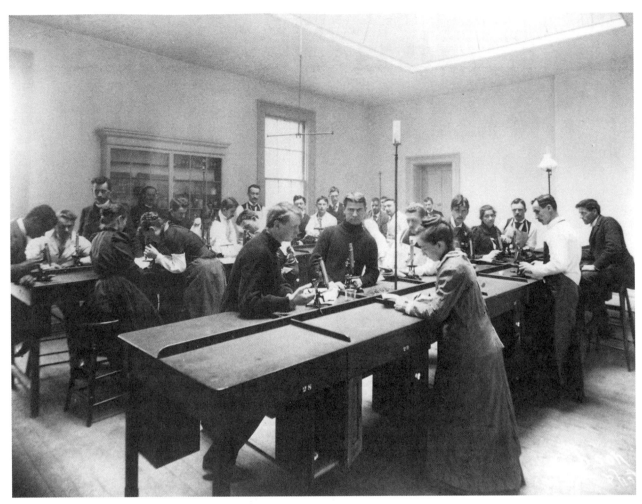

Fig. 4–1. Microscopic work in physiological chemistry. (Courtesy of the Bentley Historical Library, University of Michigan, Medical School Records, Box 136, "Gibson #3.")

The Protein Poison

Vaughan wrote:

Bacteria are particulate proteins containing, at least two carbohydrate groups, a nuclein group and one or more protein groups; consequently when bacteria cells are disrupted they supply carbohydrates, nuclein bodies and amino acids.[7]

As soon as a molecule becomes the seat of assimilation and excretion it is no longer dead; it lives. . . .
. . . The atomic groups taken into living molecules enter into new combinations. . . .
It is probable that in the absorption of energy by the living molecule oxygen is relieved from its combination with carbon or hydrogen and is attached to nitrogen, while in the liberation of energy the reverse takes place. Nitrogen and phosphorus, sometimes with iron and manganese,

seem to be, as it were, the master elements within the living molecule. It is by virtue of their chemism that groups are torn from extra-cellular matter, taken into the living molecule and assimilated by an atomic rearrangement.[8]

The keystone or archon of the protein molecule is the protein poison. It is common to all protein molecules. Physiologically it is the same in all molecules; i.e., when set free it is a poison and it is a poison on account of its intense chemism which enables it to tear off groups from other proteins.[9]

At the end of his book on cellular toxins Vaughan returned to the problem of autogenous diseases. He said that the body during its normal processes of metabolism produces poisons. A man may eat a perfectly innocuous diet, yet there are poisons in his urine. Perhaps autogenous diseases result from excessive production or inadequate elimination of the poisons. In gout, for example, uric acid accumulates. Mucus is a poison, and the "probabilities are that myxedema is a form of mucinæmia, and that the introduction of excess mucus into other tissues is prevented by the normal action of the thyroid gland."[10] Even glucose is a poison. In diabetes mellitus "cells which are accustomed to absorb and utilize the sugars find themselves unable to accomplish this duty, and the unused sugar acts as a poison to other tissues."[11]

Vaughan was invited to tell this story in many named lectures: Herter, Shattuck, and Harvey among them.

Vaughan as an Immunologist

The protein poison was the keystone of Vaughan's theory of immunity and disease. When a foreign protein enters the body, it stimulates cells to produce an enzyme that destroys the protein and liberates its poison. These enzymes remain intracellular until a second invasion occurs. The secondary groups attached to a foreign protein stimulate production of the proteolytic enzymes and are responsible for the specificity of the response. The foreign protein may be a simple one, such as egg white, or it may be a bacterium. Consequently, there is no fundamental difference between development of sensitivity to a protein and development of immunity to a bacterium; each results from induction of cellular ferments in the host. Then during a second invasion by the foreign protein or bacterium the enzymes induced by its first invasion are liberated and attack the protein or bacterium. If the second invasion is small, the invader is destroyed with no harm to the host. That is the process of immunity. Vaughan scorned Ehrlich's word *antibody*. "It would be equally rational," he said, "to speak of pepsin as an antibody of beefsteak, because the former digests the latter. . . . To say that anaphylaxis is the result of protein-antiprotein reaction is to talk jargon."[12]

When bacteria, living proteins, find their way to the tissues of the body, they feed upon the body's proteins, converting them to their own use. During the period of incubation when the invader is multiplying and stimulating the host's cells to produce intracellular proteolytic enzymes the invader does no harm to the host. There are no signs or symptoms of disease, and the host is not feverish. The crisis occurs

when the newly developed enzymes are liberated and attack the bacteria protein, liberating the protein poison. The faster the bacteria are destroyed, the more damage is done to the host. Then fever occurs. One source of fever is heat released during cleavage of foreign proteins, but Vaughan thought the most important cause of increased heat production is the reaction between protein digestion products and tissues. He did not consider heat conservation as one cause of fever.

Vaughan thought that "[t]he number of pathogenic bacteria which produce toxins, at least in appreciable quantity, is small, and the action of toxins and antitoxins in infections . . . is of minor importance."[13] Nevertheless, he fitted toxins into his scheme of protein poisons. The diphtheria bacillus grows in the upper air passages, and it might kill by mechanical obstruction. But "[i]t produces its soluble, diffusible toxin, which has the properties of a ferment and splits up the proteins of the body, setting free the protein poison. In the case of recovery or in the production of antitoxins in animals, the body cells elaborate an antiferment or antitoxin which neutralizes the toxin and prevents its cleavage action. . . . It is not, in our opinion, the toxin itself which kills, but a cleavage product which results from the action of the toxin on the proteins of the body."[14] Vaughan had no experimental evidence for this statement.

Vaughan's Nuclein Therapy

In 1893, after a long review of the literature, Vaughan became convinced that the germicidal power of serum is a property of its cell-free, soluble components and that it must belong to the proteins.[15] Because peptic digestion destroys albumin but not the germicidal action, "the only proteid [protein] likely to be present in the blood-serum and which is not destroyed by peptic digestion is nuclein."[16] Vaughan asked whether serum does contain nuclein and whether nuclein free from serum is germicidal. Vaughan and his pupil, Charles McClintock, accordingly prepared nuclein from the blood of dogs and rabbits. They collected blood aseptically and decanted the serum after the cells had settled. When they mixed the serum with ten volumes of an equal mixture of ether and absolute alcohol they obtained a voluminous precipitate. They digested the precipitate with pepsin in 0.2 percent hydrochloric acid until the fluid failed to give the biuret reaction for peptones. The small, gray undigested residue was collected on a sterile filter and washed with acid and then with alcohol. After it had dried, the residue was dissolved in sterile 0.6 percent sodium chloride. The fluid was then filtered through a Chamberland filter and stored in sterile flasks. Vaughan said: "We have now answered the first question. Blood-serum contains a nuclein."[17]

Vaughan and McClintock tested their nuclein for germicidal action by inoculating five-milliliter portions of the nuclein solution with various bacilli and plating the mixture at intervals. The counts with two strains are shown in table 4–1. Vaughan, McClintock, and Novy prepared large amounts of nuclein by exhaustive digestion of spleen, testes, thyroid, and eggs. Yeast-nuclein was their favorite preparation. Yeast cells, washed with water, were extracted with dilute alkali. The precipitate obtained when the solution was acidified was once more dissolved in 0.25 percent alkali. Vaughan admitted this was impure nuclein, "not free of albuminous bodies," but he used large amounts of it.[18]

Vaughan tested his nuclein by injecting rabbits or guinea pigs with nuclein and then challenging them with bacteria. He asked whether the favorable effects of nuclein depend upon its germicidal action or upon stimulating "the activity of those organs whose function it is to protect the body against [infectious] diseases."[19] He decided it is the latter. Vaughan thought nuclein stimulates production of polynuclear white corpuscles. He did no white cell counts himself. Carl Huber did a few for him and found that white cell counts did rise after nuclein treatment. George Dock, who was a real expert, found no leukocytosis in patients treated with nuclein.[20]

Vaughan found that nuclein injections retarded but did not prevent tuberculosis in guinea pigs, but four of six rabbits were made immune to tuberculosis by previous injections of nuclein. He gave rabbits an intravenous injection of nuclein and then inoculated them with a suspension of anthrax bacilli. Eight of ten rabbits survived, but only three of fifteen controls survived. When Vaughan presented these data to the Association of American Physicians someone said the survival of the controls showed the anthrax suspension to be too dilute. Vaughan lamely replied: "Of course this work will have to be gone over. It is simply suggestive."[21]

Vaughan had a private practice, and he immediately tried nuclein on his patients.[22] A ten-year-old girl with membranous tonsillitis gargled a 2 percent solution and was cured in a day. A three-year-old boy with "streptococcus diphtheria" would not gargle, but he was cured in three days by a spray of nuclein solution from an atomizer. An indolent ulcer on the leg was cured by eight injections of nuclein. Vaughan began to treat patients with tuberculosis on 1 May 1893, and in the next year he reported the results obtained with twenty-four patients.[23] Vaughan persuaded himself that nuclein had improved the condition for a while of those who subsequently died of the disease and that there had been a temporary cure in one patient in the early stages of pulmonary tuberculosis. He was more confident that in the cases of urinary tuberculosis he had treated "the results have been remarkably satisfactory."[24] One patient with tuberculosis of the left kidney was given injections of nuclein deeply into the muscles on each side of the spine over the kidneys. The left kidney decreased in size, but tubercle bacilli did not disappear from the patient's urine by the time Vaughan published. Archibald Muirhead, John Jacob Abel's assistant in pharmacology, discovered tubercle bacilli in his urine in 1892, and he consulted Vaughan on 21 June 1893. Vaughan began nuclein treatment the same day. Muirhead left to practice in Nebraska, but he continued to treat himself as well as his patients with nuclein. By the next year he had used four gallons of nuclein solution on himself, mostly by direct irrigation of his bladder. He may have been cured, for he lived until 24 April 1921.

Vaughan's most positive conclusion, with his emphasis, was that "[e]ven when the tuberculosis is of long standing, and when the extent of tissue involved is great, *so long as secondary infection with pyogenic germs has not occurred*, the proper use of the

TABLE 4.1. Germicidal Action of Nuclein

Asiatic Cholera Bacillus		*Staphylococcus aureus*	
Time	Colonies	Time	Colonies
Immediately	2,100	Immediately	Countless
5 min.	43	1 hr.	22,000
15 min.	54	5 hrs.	2,525
30 min.	71	19 hrs.	155
1 hr.	90	24 hrs.	0
1½ hr.	115		
22 hrs.	1,200		

Source: V. C. Vaughan and C. T. McClintock, "The Nature of the Germicidal Constituent of Blood-Serum," *Med. News* 63 (1893): 706.

remedy may *retard* (I do not say arrest) the progress of the disease.[25] Parke, Davis and Company sold Vaughan's nuclein solution for a while (fig. 4–2).

Vaughan's Public Work

Vaughan was a member of the Michigan State Board of Health for nearly thirty years and its president much of the time. Toward the end of his life he wrote a two-volume textbook, *Epidemiology and Public Health,*[26] and in its preface he described the unsanitary conditions prevailing in his boyhood and youth that made typhoid fever epidemic in the United States. Vaughan himself did much to clean up the water supply in the Midwest. He told how at the time of the Chicago World's Fair in 1893 "the fact that the water supply of this city was badly and specifically polluted was so well known, both in this country and in Europe, that this ill repute threatened the success of the exposition. The management appointed a commission [of which Vaughan was a member] to make a survey and report. At that time thirty public, and innumerable private, sewers poured their contents into the city's water supply. The commission found the city supply so badly contaminated that it recommended the laying of a pipe line from a spring near Waukesha, Wis., to the Fair Grounds, and this was done."[27]

As a teacher of toxicology with a firsthand knowledge of inorganic and organic poisons, Vaughan frequently testified in criminal cases. By 1910 his fee was five hundred dollars plus two hundred dollars a day or fraction thereof, and he once threatened to sue when payment was delayed. He earned one thousand dollars in a civil case testifying to the wholesomeness of corn syrup.

Teaching and Practicing Hygiene

As early as 1881 Vaughan began to lecture on sanitary science, and as professor of hygiene he continued to teach the subject until he retired. When the Hygienic Laboratory opened in 1888 Vaughan and his staff taught advanced and special courses in bacteriology, water analysis, and food analysis. Until the State Board of Health Laboratory was started in Lansing in 1907, the Hygienic Laboratory did the diagnostic work for Michigan physicians. He and Novy lectured around the state to promote public health inspection of water and public awareness of disease control. Vaughan learned the technique of the Wassermann reaction from Wassermann himself in Berlin, and he brought the test to Michigan.

Vaughan and Novy established a Pasteur Institute as part of the Hygienic Laboratory in 1903 for diagnosis and treatment of rabies. By 1941, 2,815 per-

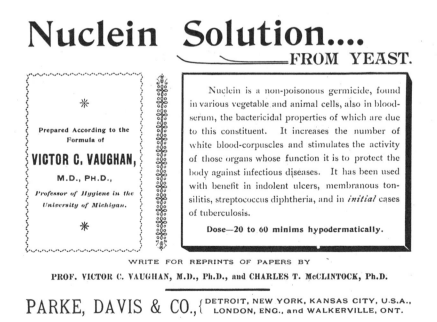

Fig. 4–2. Victor Vaughan's nuclein solution sold by Parke, Davis and Company. (From *Index Medicus* 7, no. 3 [1895].)

sons had been treated with no instances of paralysis or death.

Until he retired Vaughan gave annual lectures on sex hygiene for university students. Attendance was required for men, but hundreds of women voluntarily went to lectures given especially for them. Vaughan thought that attitudes toward sex had been fixed by moral teaching, medical instruction, and social propaganda, all based on only a slight foundation of fact. Vaughan gave students authentic information on venereal diseases and about sexual behavior in general in a nonminatory fashion with the result that students felt free to approach him about their problems. For example, one former student wrote Vaughan a frantic letter, saying that he had left Vaughan's lecture some years before determined never again to masturbate. He could not stop, and he appealed for help. Vaughan replied simply that it is a nasty habit; after a while marry some nice girl and forget about it.

The Spanish-American War

Vaughan said that typhoid fever was always present. The Spanish-American War of 1898 gave Vaughan the opportunity to deal with typhoid fever on a national scale. Immediately after the declaration of war Vaughan was appointed surgeon to a Michigan volunteer regiment, and he soon achieved the rank of major and division surgeon. He went with his regiment to Cuba, where he was under fire at the battle of Santiago and where he contracted yellow fever. Major William Gorgas, who several years later stamped out yellow fever in the Canal Zone, took care of him during the acute phase of his illness. When Vaughan was convalescent, so weak he could not walk unaided from one side of the deck to the other, he was put in charge of a troopship carrying other convalescent fever victims to Florida and northern hospitals.

The war was a medical disaster. Fighting in the Caribbean was over before most of the volunteer regiments could see action, and in the meantime they were shuttled from one southern U.S. camp to another where fever epidemics decimated the troops. The disease was typhoid fever, but it was generally diagnosed as typhoid, malaria, or typhomalaria.[28]

The adjutant general in the War Department appointed Vaughan as a member of a three-man commission to report on the origin and spread of typhoid fever in the national camps. The other civilian member was Edward O. Shakespeare, a Philadelphia ophthalmologist-bacteriologist-pathologist who had made a name for himself as an epidemiologist investigating Asiatic cholera in Italy, Spain, and India during the 1883 epidemic.[29] He had also identified the source of an epidemic of typhoid fever in Pennsylvania. Major Walter Reed was head of the commission, and as a regular army officer he could "damn a colonel" of volunteers and see to it that the commission's recommendations were heeded.[30]

The commission traveled from one camp to another by train in the luxury of a private car, complete with servants and a chef, provided by the manager of the Southern Railroad. They quickly found that the malarial-type fever was, in fact, typhoid fever. Every regiment in the six regular army corps contracted it within eight weeks of arrival at camp, and all the volunteer regiments within ten weeks. Minimal numbers of cases were reported in regiments whose line officers, instead of considering the medical officers' recommendations for sanitation as a "fad of the doctors," had enforced sanitary measures. The correct diagnosis, typhoid fever, had been made in about half the cases. George Dock was called from Ann Arbor as acting assistant surgeon to confirm the diagnosis. He took over a bacteriological laboratory at the Sternberg Hospital in Chickamauga Park, Georgia, on 9 September 1898, and he examined the sick and did autopsies there and in Knoxville, Tennessee, and Camp Meade, Pennsylvania. Dock found that the nomenclature of fevers in the camps was on the whole irrational and arbitrary. He discovered only one case of malaria, and he concluded that there was no such thing as typhomalaria.[31]

The commission came down hard on the fact that the spread of fever in the camps was facilitated by wretched sanitary practices for which "superior line officers can not be held blameless."[32] They calculated that if a regiment of thirteen hundred men were assembled, the chances were that one or more men already had typhoid fever when they arrived in camp. Reed, Vaughan, and Shakespeare also identified carriers of typhoid fever who themselves showed no signs of the disease. Contagion from feces spread at once, and with an incubation period of ten and a half days, typhoid fever eventually developed in one-fifth of the soldiers. The death rate among cases of typhoid fever was 7.61 percent, and typhoid fever was responsible for 86.24 percent of all military deaths.[33]

By the time the official report was published in the

names of Reed, Vaughan, and Shakespeare, Walter Reed was dead of peritonitis following an appendectomy, and Shakespeare was also dead. Vaughan had stayed in Washington, D.C., letting Michigan's Medical School take care of itself, while he completed the two massive volumes filled with utterly detailed tables and maps.

Teaching Bacteriology

In 1891 Novy took over the formal teaching of bacteriology, and he continued to lecture to medical students until he retired in 1935. He was an excellent showman, and his dramatic but sometimes wandering lectures were filled with comments on history, art, and mythology.[34] A laboratory course was given after completion of the Physics-Hygiene Building in 1888. The course, occupying twenty-four hours a week for three months, was at first elective for medical students, and it was open to students in the Literary Department. When the four-year curriculum was started in 1890 the laboratory course became required for medical students.

The nature of the course can be deduced from the 202-page *Directions for Laboratory Work in Bacteriology* that Novy published in 1894.[35] Students were drilled in preparation and examination of cultures of bacteria, molds, and yeast. The characteristics of nineteen were listed, a page for each, and on the opposite blank page students sketched the form of the colonies. Students were taught to examine water and air and how to detect tubercle bacilli in sputum. In his introduction Novy defended his use of pathogens, saying that any accident was the result of inexcusable carelessness, and he demonstrated postmortem examination of a guinea pig infected with anthrax. Novy gave directions for cultivation of anaerobes and for hardening, cutting, and staining tissues. Novy's laboratory class procedures were said by one who knew him to be disorganized, his assistants never knowing what he would require next.

By 1899 Novy's *Directions* had grown to a book of 563 pages that was actually an elementary textbook of bacteriology. The size of the book reflected the dominating position bacteriology had assumed in the second half of the first year. Students were kept in class every afternoon, far beyond the time allotted, by the simple device of a quiz given at the end of the period. Perhaps this accounts for the fact some students told George Dock that the first thing they would do when they had graduated was to kill Dr. Novy.

Novy as a Microbiologist

Novy receives polite but cursory mention, if any, in histories of microbiology or medicine. He is sometimes remembered as the inventor of the "Novy jar," a glass vessel in which anaerobic bacteria can be cultivated (fig. 4–3).[36] Otherwise, Novy is remembered for having isolated some trypanosomes and a spirochete.

Novy developed anaerobic methods in 1893 when something unexpected turned up. He and Vaughan were preparing nuclein by digesting casein. The reason was that Vaughan thought that because casein contains phosphorus it must be a nucleoprotein. The precipitate, filtered and dissolved in 0.5 percent sodium carbonate solution, was injected into three guinea pigs who all died within twenty-four hours of bloody edema. Novy isolated a motile, spiral, anaerobic trypanosome.[37]

Novy frequently found *Trypanosoma lewisi* in the blood of wild or laboratory rats, and he succeeded in cultivating it on blood-agar slants.[38] His success in this and subsequent isolations of trypanosomes was the result of perseverance. He made as many as one hundred cultures, and he found that in one or two of them the organism survived and could be carried

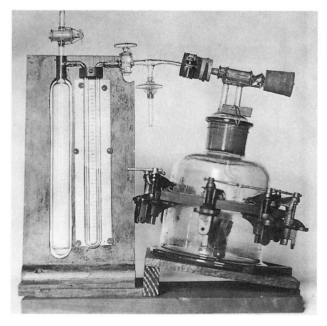

Fig. 4–3. Novy jar

into subsequent cultures. Novy thought this process selected one strain that could survive under artificial conditions out of many that could not. Having isolated *T. lewisi,* Novy carried it through more than one hundred generations.

David Bruce had identified *T. brucei* as the cause of tsetse fly disease, or nagana, in Zululand in 1895, but Novy was the first to cultivate it. The organism had been carried from one laboratory animal to another, and Novy was given infected blood by a friend at McGill University. One culture out of many made on blood-agar slants survived, and Novy found that once a culture had been obtained succeeding ones were easier to make. A culture grown at thirty-four degrees centigrade was less virulent than the original one, and Novy wondered whether it might impart immunity.[39] Thereafter Novy isolated trypanosomes of surra, a disease of cattle,[40] and he was able to illustrate his Harvey Lecture of 1905 with a large number of slides showing photomicrographs of trypanosomes he had found in birds.[41]

Novy used an ingenious method to cultivate the spirillum of relapsing fever when others had failed. The organism could be carried in successive passages through rats, but Novy's many hundreds of attempts to cultivate it on slants were unsuccessful. Novy made a collodium sac holding 2.5 to 3.0 milliliters of uncoagulated blood. This, when inoculated with blood from an infected rat, was at once placed in the peritoneal cavity of an uninfected one. When Novy removed the sac three days later he found it contained a flourishing colony, and he carried the organism through twenty passages in sixty-eight days.[42]

Novy tried to raise immunity against his cultures of trypanosomes. He succeeded in 1912 with the relatively harmless *T. lewisi.* The organism, after years of cultivation on blood-agar slants, had become noninfectious. Twenty-one of thirty-three rats tested with the virulent strain after being treated with the aviru-

lent one survived. Six had a very mild infection and six a rich one. Immunity lasted up to 159 days.[43]

Novy and the Plague

By 1901 Novy had a sufficient national reputation to be appointed by the secretary of the treasury as the bacteriologist on a commission to investigate the outbreak of bubonic plague in San Francisco. The local coroner had detected plague in a Chinese man who had died unattended in March 1900, and his report precipitated a characteristic controversy. Local authorities denied the existence of plague in San Francisco for the reason that it would be bad for business. State and national authorities took the other side with the result that Simon Flexner as a pathologist and Lewellys Barker as a clinician were dispatched along with Novy to investigate in January 1901. They inspected thirteen dead, confirmed the coroner's diagnosis, and isolated the organism.[44] Novy brought a culture back to Ann Arbor. On 3 April a medical student contracted the pneumonic form of plague while attempting to prepare a vaccine. The student rolled his own cigarettes, and he apparently contaminated one while handling a culture.[45] He was treated by Novy with antiplague serum and on 26 April 1901 he was described to the class in George Dock's medical clinic. He survived with a damaged heart.

Those plague germs carried from San Francisco to Ann Arbor were later carried to the Caribbean island of St. Hubert, where they killed Leora Arrowsmith. She too was infected by a contaminated cigarette. Sinclair Lewis got his medical information from Paul de Kruif, and when Lewis needed to know about a devastating epidemic, de Kruif told him about bubonic plague as he told him about the wonders of the McGurk Institute.

5
Bacteriology after Vaughan's Retirement, 1921–41

Paul de Kruif returned to the University of Michigan from the army as an assistant professor in 1919.[1] The next year on Donald Van Slyke's recommendation he became an associate at the Rockefeller Institute in Simon Flexner's division of bacteriology. In the next two years de Kruif worked on the problem that was to dominate Michigan's bacteriology for at least a decade and was to obsess Philip Hadley, de Kruif's successor in Novy's department. De Kruif gave the problem its name when he headed his first Rockefeller paper: "Dissociation of Microbic Species."[2]

Dissociation of Microbic Species

De Kruif isolated the bacillus of rabbit septicemia, and he found that his cultures contained two types of bacteria. One grew diffusely and was very virulent. De Kruif called this the D type. The other, the G type, readily flocculated in a liquid medium and was only slightly virulent. De Kruif demonstrated that he had not started with a mixed culture by growing both strains from a single D bacterium. He concluded that a D bacterium had changed to G and had become the parent of the second strain. De Kruif consulted Jacques Loeb, who agreed that the change from D to G was a mutation in the sense De Vries had used the word.

The phenomenon of dissociation, as de Kruif called it, had been known to bacteriologists ever since they were able to grow pure cultures. Members of a pure culture would undergo a spontaneous change; progeny of capsulated bacteria in a smooth colony would become non-capsulated in a rough colony. Consequently, the term *S to R* (smooth to rough) was used to denote the appearance in a pure culture of types differing in several characteristics from the parent type. Hadley listed twenty-four such differences that might include a change in virulence, pigment production, or ability to agglutinate. A variant might be sufficiently stable to maintain its characteristics over many generations; it might give rise to still other types; or it might revert to the parent type. There were several explanations for dissociation.[3] De Kruif thought that the change resulted from mutation and selection. Others thought that bacteria have some inherent flexibility to adapt to a multitude of environmental conditions. Hadley adopted the idea of cyclogenicity as described by Günther Enderlein of Berlin.[4]

According to Enderlein and Hadley, when bacteria grow on a medium to which they are well adapted they multiply by binary fission, and they possess a high degree of uniformity in all their characteristics. If the environment becomes unfavorable, binary fission is suppressed, and sexual reproduction by conjugation occurs. This produces new generations having highly variable characteristics, and some may be filterable. The change from the original type is not a mutation, because one of the new generation, even a filterable one, can revert to the original type.

Philip Hadley and His Experiments

Philip Bardwell Hadley, born in 1881, had earned his doctor of philosophy degree at Brown University in 1908, and thereafter he worked on animal husbandry at the Rhode Island Agricultural Experiment Station. At the same time he was professor of bacteriology at the Rhode Island State College. Hadley's publications reflect the concerns of agriculture: fowl cholera, egg production, hemorrhagic septicemia in lambs, trichinosis in turkeys and diseases of fox pups.[5] Novy brought him to Michigan in 1920 as an assistant professor to replace de Kruif, and Hadley quickly became an intellectual force in the department. He had many student assistants who did the vast amount of laboratory work required by his research, and at least five students, including Walter Nungester, earned a doctor's degree under him.

Dissociation could be forced by unfavorable conditions. Hadley grew Shiga dysentery bacilli in a broth medium containing 0.5 percent lithium chloride, and after twenty-four hours he transferred an inoculum from the broth to another tube also containing broth with 0.5 percent lithium chloride. At each transfer Hadley plated some of the culture on beef broth and agar plates and observed the nature of the colonies developing during incubation. Dissociation into an R form occurred at the fourth serial transfer, and when this R form was carried through more than fifty serial transfers into lithium-containing broth still another variant appeared at the tenth transfer and then repeatedly through more transfers.

Colonies of this new type were minute, the largest being 0.2 millimeter in diameter and the smallest being 0.004 millimeter. Hadley was able to touch one of the minute colonies with a fine, sterile, glass thread, and when the tip of the thread was dipped into 2 milliliters of broth a new culture was established. When the culture was plated, only a uniform, glassy sheen appeared on the agar, and an individual could be seen only at the limit of oil immersion microscopy. Fermentation characteristics of the new strain were different from those of the parent R strain, and the new strain was not toxic to a rabbit. Because Hadley thought that this minute organism was the sexual form of the Shiga bacillus, he called it G for "gonidium."

When Hadley passed a G culture through a Berkefeld filter, he obtained optically clear fluid containing a multitude of cultivable bodies that gave G colonies on plating. On continued cultivation seven strains of G reverted to R or S. For example, when a pure stock of G sealed in an ampoule for months was plated, reversion occurred. Hadley selected the largest of these colonies, and after four months of serial transfer he had S-type colonies whose members were agglutinated by S-type antiserum, were toxic for rabbits, and were susceptible to Shiga bacteriophage. G was, therefore, a filterable form of Shiga bacillus. Hadley found filterable forms of eleven other bacteria.

Filterable bacteria were nothing new at the time. Hadley cited demonstrations in Brazil, France, and Sweden of filterable forms of the tubercle bacillus and of *Bacillus typhosus*.[6] Long before in Ann Arbor, Novy had found that cultures of *Trypanosoma lewisi* contained small organisms and that a perfectly clear filtrate, when injected into a white rat, caused a typical infection.[7]

In an enormously long description of the Shiga bacillus work, "The Filterable Forms of Bacteria," Hadley made it clear that he had done all the thinking and that his assistants had done the laboratory work.[8] He also made it clear that he knew the validity of his conclusions depended upon his assistants' impeccable technique, and he cited numerous control experiments.

Hadley and Bacteriophage

Hadley grew two types of colonies of *B. pyocyaneus* from a lesion on the forehead of a patient. The first, obtained in ninety-nine of one hundred times, was a rich blue-green colony with irregular outlines and punched-out areas of lysis. The other, grown either as a streak or a discrete colony, did not produce pigment and had no areas of lysis. This second was the R type produced by dissociation, but Hadley was more interested in the areas of lysis in the S-type colonies. He showed that bacteria of the S type produced a "lytic principle" that passed through a Berkefeld filter and that was destroyed by heating to seventy degrees centigrade for thirty minutes. It was not in solution but was a discrete entity. When a suitably diluted aliquot of the filtrate was spread over an agar plate seeded with the susceptible parent strain, characteristic plaques of lysis appeared, and the number of lytic particles in the filtrate could be enumerated by counting the plaques. Hadley's lytic principle behaved like the bacteriophage described first by Twort and then by d'Herelle.[9]

Hadley grew *B. coli* on broth to which pancreatin (E. R. Squibb and Sons), sterilized by filtration, had been added. The filtrate obtained from the fifth passage contained the lytic principle that could be identified and assayed by plaques formed on plates evenly seeded with the bacterium. He showed that it was not the enzymes in pancreatin that induced the lytic principle by autoclaving the pancreatin solution and clearing it by Berkefeld filtration. A small amount of autoclaved pancreatin added to broth tubes forced appearance of the lytic principle in the eighth serial passage of Shiga bacillus.

Hadley believed that the bacteriophage does not destroy the bacterium; rather it causes a sort of fragmentation of the sensitive cells into minute particles that can pass through a filter and then regenerate into microscopically visible forms.

In 1933 President Ruthven ordered Hadley dismissed on unspecified charges of impropriety. Although Hadley protested that he had merely been indiscreet with the young women in his laboratory, he was not allowed to confront his accusers. He went quietly to become bacteriologist for the Western Pennsylvania Hospital in Pittsburgh.

Novy's Department after Vaughan's Departure

Vaughan retired from all his university positions in 1921, and hygiene and public health became an independent department under John Sundwall. At the same time H. B. Lewis was brought to Ann Arbor to head an independent department of physiological chemistry. Consequently, Novy's staff shrank

to Novy himself, Herbert W. Emerson as director of the Pasteur Institute, and Hadley as an assistant professor. Malcolm Soule became an instructor in 1924, and in 1930 Reuben Kahn became director of the hospital's serological laboratory and was nominally attached to the department as an assistant professor. Throughout this period and until 1941 there were from three to fourteen assistants in bacteriology, chiefly medical students, recent medical graduates, and graduate assistants working for advanced degrees. Eighteen of those students earned the doctor of philosophy degree between 1921 and 1941.

The assistants were needed to teach the laboratory course for medical students that occupied all afternoons five days a week and Saturday mornings in the second semester of the first year. When one medical student reported to begin his assistantship and asked what he should do, Novy merely peered at him over his half-moon glasses and said: "Robinson, your duty is to anticipate the students' needs." In the mid-1920s the secretary of the Association of American Medical Colleges on an accreditation visit was horrified to discover that bacteriology occupied 384 hours in the curriculum, whereas at other Class A medical schools, Harvard, Pennsylvania, and Columbia, it used 150 to 160 hours. Dean Cabot plaintively replied that he could not do much to control Novy. As soon as Novy retired in 1935 the academic vultures demanded that time for bacteriology be cut in half, but it was only reduced to 337 hours by 1939.

Microbic Respiration

Work on bacterial respiration ended Novy's research career (fig. 5–1). By the time he finished laboratory work he was well over sixty, and when Dean Cabot was dismissed in 1930 Novy first became a member of the Executive Committee running the school and then dean until he retired in 1935 at the age of seventy. Hadley was eventually replaced by Walter Nungester, brought back to Michigan from Northwestern University, and Malcolm Soule was made head of the department.

In the 1920s biologists were busy measuring respiration of cells and tissue slices over minutes or hours by means of Barcroft's differential blood-gas apparatus[10] or a simpler version devised by Warburg.[11] Novy and his students undertook to measure the much slower respiration of bacterial cultures over a period as long as fifty-six days. Novy said: "In the

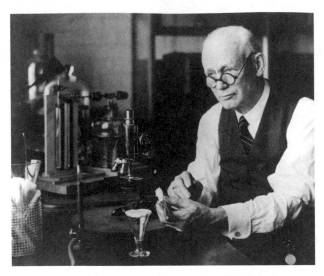

Fig. 5–1. Frederick Novy. (Courtesy of Dr. Frank Whitehouse.)

current methods of studying [micro]organisms, stress is placed on the medium, its composition and reaction, and on the chemical changes which it undergoes. The oxygen requirements, as expressed in Pasteur's terms, aerobe and anaerobe, are supplied somewhat mechanically, and little or no attention is given to the gaseous products of cell activity unless the organism happens to evolve considerable quantities of gas. The result is the misleading classification of organisms into aerogenic or gas-producing, and nonaerogenic or no gas producers. The truth is that all living organisms are actively engaged in gas production."[12]

In addition to determining gas exchange, Novy wanted to compare the composition of the gas phase under which microorganisms grow or do not grow with the partial pressures, or tensions, of carbon dioxide and oxygen existing in the body of their animal host.

Novy and his students constructed a differential manometer that was a crude version of Barcroft's. One arm of a mercury-containing U tube was attached to a closed vessel whose accurately determined volume was about 100 milliliters. The other arm was connected with the closed vessel in which the organisms grew, either a tube containing the culture growing on a slant of medium or a Novy jar containing several culture tubes. There were T tubes and stopcocks on the culture side so that gas over the culture could be sampled for analysis or renewed. When the level of the mercury in the manometer was read the volume of gas given off or taken up by the

culture could be calculated. Novy used a version of the Henderson-Haldane apparatus to measure oxygen, carbon dioxide, nitrogen, and hydrogen in the gas over the culture, and because he was able to extract carbon dioxide from the culture medium, he was able to determine the total carbon dioxide production. Consequently, he could calculate the respiratory quotient (RQ) for carbon dioxide production divided by oxygen consumption or the analogous quotient, HQ, when the culture produced hydrogen gas.

Malcolm Soule as Novy's research assistant and graduate student demonstrated the importance of paying attention to the gas phase when he measured the growth and respiration of the tubercle bacillus.[13] The bacillus was known to be an obligate aerobe, but nothing was known about the oxygen and carbon dioxide tensions required for optimal growth. It was customary to seal a culture tube on the assumption that the tube contained all the oxygen the culture would need. Soule found that good growth in a single tube of glycerol agar required 100 to 150 cubic centimeters of oxygen, far more than the sealed tube contained. The culture grew until the last atom of oxygen was consumed, and consequently growth in a sealed tube was poor. Best growth occurred when the tube was periodically refilled or when the culture tube was blown with a large bulb so that there was an adequate volume of gas in the tube before it was sealed. Optimal oxygen concentration was 40 to 50 percent, which, in a moist atmosphere at a barometric pressure of 740 millimeters of mercury, was a tension of 277 to 347 millimeters of mercury. When Soule ran up the scale of carbon dioxide tension, he found that 10 to 20 percent carbon dioxide did not inhibit growth and that fair growth occurred at 90 percent carbon dioxide. Thereafter Michigan bacteriologists routinely used an atmosphere of 40 percent oxygen and 10 percent carbon dioxide when growing tubercle bacilli.

Novy and Soule concluded that "[t]he slow multiplication of the tubercle bacillus in the body is explainable from the standpoint of growth in diminished O_2 tension. An indefinite supply of O_2 under a tension corresponding to a few mm. of Hg will probably enable the organism to grow, though very slowly. The 'rest cure' and rich diet in checking the progress of the disease probably act by reducing to a minimum the available O_2 supply in the tissues."[14]

The results of years of work reported in more than two hundred pages of print sank almost without a trace. If the work was mentioned at all, it was in relation to culture conditions. Anaerobes had been known to grow best in mixed cultures with aerobes. In commenting on this in her *Bacterial Metabolism* Marjory Stephenson said: "Novy, however, finally disposed of this theory [that enzymes secreted by aerobes enable anaerobes to grow] by showing that aerobes can bring about growth of anaerobes even when grown apart from them in a separate limb of a closed H tube; in such circumstances the aerobe develops first, completely removing the oxygen from the air space and hence from the culture media; the development of the anaerobe in the other limb of the H tube then follows."[15]

This Novy referred to by Stephenson in the preceding quote, however, is not Professor Frederick G. Novy but Frederick G. Novy Jr. passing through his father's laboratory on his way to becoming a dermatologist.[16]

Walter J. Nungester's Work to 1941

As a graduate assistant in the student laboratory in the 1920s Walter Nungester prepared for routine inoculation of guinea pigs by plating anthrax bacilli. Novy had brought the culture back from Koch's institute in 1888, and it had remained pure. Nungester fortuitously observed that the culture dissociated into a second strain, and this started him on work resulting in his doctor of philosophy thesis and first paper.[17] Nungester obtained six new culture types of *B. anthracis*, some practically avirulent, and in the manner of Hadley, he caused them to revert to the original type. Being in Novy's department, he also measured the respiration of each strain.

While working at Northwestern University after obtaining his University of Michigan degrees, Nungester found that by adding sterilized mucus to bacterial cultures he enabled the bacteria to survive longer and to be more infectious.[18] This observation allowed Nungester to produce pneumonia in the rat, a disease more like human pneumonia than pneumonia in the rabbit or guinea pig.[19] As few as one hundred pneumococci, injected intrabronchially along with 0.1 cubic centimeter of sterilized mucus, caused a typical fatal infection. When he returned to Michigan in 1936 Nungester used this model to study the mode of action of antiserum. Antiserum given immediately after intrabronchial inoculation gave 100 percent survival, but given twenty-four hours later it was only 50 percent effective.[20] Nungester showed by means of thorium dioxide (Thorotrast) infusion and X-ray photography that circulation persisted in the infected lung, but only a very small amount of antibody crossed the capillary wall into the parenchyma.[21] Pneumococci present in the tissues were not affected by the antiserum. The antiserum did, however, reduce the number of bacilli in the blood, and Nungester concluded that it is effective because it stops blood-borne dissemination of pneumococci. He supported his conclusion about blood-borne spread by showing that intravenous injection of pneumococci, otherwise ineffectual, caused pneumonia after intrabronchial injection of sterile mucus.[22]

There may be many pneumococci in the upper respiratory tract of a person not immune but free from pneumonia. Nungester thought the fact demands explanation. Perhaps aspiration of mucus determines infection. He found that exposure to cold and alcoholic intoxication, the predisposing factors in Skid Row victims of lobar pneumonia, prevent closure of the glottis and favor aspiration of mucus along with pneumococci.[23]

Malcolm Soule's Work to 1941

While Earl Baldwin McKinley was a medical student in 1912 he had been assistant in bacteriology. He did advanced work with Bordet, and he rose rapidly to become professor of bacteriology at Columbia University.[24] When Columbia assumed responsibility for establishing the School of Tropical Medicine in San Juan at the request of the Commonwealth of Puerto Rico, McKinley became the school's director. Somehow Soule began to work with McKinley in the early 1930s, first in San Juan and then in the Philippines.

The Puerto Rico leper colony had sixty patients, and authorities guessed there were forty more lepers on the island not under treatment. Soule and McKinley reviewed at length the problems of cultivation and identification of the bacillus causing leprosy.[25] Then they attempted to transfer the disease from humans to monkeys, to cultivate what was presumed to be Hansen's bacillus and to reproduce the disease with organisms grown in culture. After many failures they managed to produce leprouslike lesions in monkeys by intradermal injections of emulsions from human lesions. Soule cultivated the bacillus in Novy jars under 40 percent oxygen and 10 percent carbon dioxide and obtained reasonable growth for a few generations. The bacteria cultivated under atmospheric air did not grow. On intradermal injection, a culture produced a granulomatous lesion, but there was no evidence that the bacterium multiplied in the host. After the ninth serial transfer the culture failed even to produce those lesions.[26]

The work of Soule and McKinley had been criticized, chiefly on the ground that debris, not growing colonies of bacteria, had been inoculated. Soule went to the Culion leper colony in the Philippines, a colony containing more than sixty-seven hundred patients, where he was supported by the Leonard Wood Memorial for the Eradication of Leprosy. There he repeated the work with adequate controls. Once more he grew the organism in Novy jars, but he could not demonstrate infectivity of cultures.[27]

Wassermann and Kahn tests were often positive in leprous patients, and recognition of syphilis on a background of leprosy was virtually impossible. Philippine laboratory workers were convinced that leprosy per se does not interfere with the specificity of tests for syphilis, but clinicians and Soule were skeptical. Soule selected 615 cases with negative histories of syphilis or yaws, and he found that most sensitive tests for syphilis were positive in 64 to 75 percent. The Kahn test, for example, was "strongly positive" in 121 of 424 instances and "positive" in others.[28] McKinley died in 1938 when the Pacific Clipper in which he was flying from Guam to Manila disappeared leaving only an oil slick, and Soule returned to Ann Arbor to work on poliomyelitis. Soule and a student isolated three strains of poliomyelitis virus from feces of eighteen patients in the 1939 Detroit and Buffalo epidemics.[29]

Soule succeeded Novy as head of the department in 1935, and he continued his enterprising career until he resigned on 13 July 1951.[30]

Reuben Kahn and the Hospital Clinical Laboratories

Novy, Hadley, and Soule were members of a basic science department whose aim was to produce scientific knowledge. In contrast Reuben Kahn as director of the University Hospital Clinical Laboratories had the practical job of providing service, but by 1941 Kahn's accomplishments overshadowed those of Novy, Hadley, and Soule.

Kahn was brought to Ann Arbor in 1928 to reor-

ganize the hospital's diagnostic services.[31] The laboratories in the new hospital were inconveniently placed, the bacteriological laboratory being on the ground floor of the surgical wing and the subbasement for the rest of the hospital. When the laboratory's windows were open in hot weather, Kahn complained, contaminants drifted in from the surrounding fields. The serological laboratory was on the floor above, and the biochemical laboratory was somewhere else.

Kahn directed a staff of three bacteriologists and two biochemists assisted by technicians. He himself was responsible for serology, and he had two assistant serologists and a technician to help him. The work was mostly routine diagnostic service, but as Kahn said: "When laboratory findings, however, do not correspond to clinical findings, we immediately have before us a research problem." By 1930 Kahn himself had three research assistants paid from outside grants.

Kahn had a faculty appointment as assistant professor of bacteriology, and he taught a voluntary course in clinical laboratory methods to junior and senior medical students who had time and inclination to take it. He also taught serology technicians.

The Kahn Test

Reuben Kahn had been brought to the United States at the age of eleven by his immigrant parents. He earned a doctor of science degree in 1916 from the Department of Bacteriology and Hygiene of New York University with a thesis on complement fixation.[32] He showed that vegetable proteins, edestin (the main protein of hemp seed) for example, as well as animal proteins, when injected into rabbits call forth production of complement-fixing antibodies. Gelatin, protein racemized by digestion in normal sodium hydroxide solution, and Vaughan's protein poison do not. Kahn's thesis director, William H. Park, was also director of the Bureau of Laboratories of the Health Department of the City of New York, and he gave Kahn a job as a research chemist. In 1920 Kahn moved as a serologist to the laboratories of the Michigan Department of Health in Lansing.

A major task of the Health Department's laboratories was to perform Wassermann tests on thousands of serum samples submitted by doctors throughout the state. By 1920 the several variations of the

Wassermann reaction had reached a high degree of sensitivity and specificity, but the procedure was complex and time consuming.[33] Many persons had attempted with equivocal results to substitute a simpler, faster test, and in 1921 Kahn succeeded in doing so.

Kahn prepared his antigen by grinding at least three fat-free beef hearts in a meat chopper. He air dried the paste and then reduced it to a powder. Kahn thought that drying the paste was the crucial step in which his method differed from unsuccessful efforts of those who had used a wet paste. Kahn extracted his powder four times with ether and twice with ethyl alcohol. He added six milligrams of cholesterol to each cubic centimeter of extracted material, and when he suspended it in saline he had his opalescent antigen solution, which he then standardized. Serum to be tested was "inactivated" by brief heating to fifty-six degrees centigrade, and a small sample, suitably diluted, was added to a diluted sample of the standardized antigen. When the tubes containing the mixture were shaken mechanically the mixture positive for syphilis flocculated, whereas negative samples remained opalescent.[34]

Harry Eagle said: "For years after its description, the Kahn reaction was by far the best flocculation reaction, which not only combined some of the best features of . . . other technics which preceded it, but also made definite advances which underlie every test subsequently developed."[35] The advantages of the Kahn test were its simplicity and rapidity. If a blood sample were delivered to the University Hospital serological laboratory by 10 A.M., the result could be returned by noon.

Validation of the Kahn Test

On 1 July 1922, the Kahn test was added to the Wassermann test in the Michigan State Laboratories, and for years the results of both tests were reported to the referring physicians. Soon tens of thousands of comparisons of the two tests were made all over the world, and by 1928 there were publications on the subject from Great Britain, Germany, Italy, Russia, Japan, India, Columbia, and Brazil. Antigen, Kahn tubes, racks, and shakers were commercially available. In 1928 the League of Nations Health Committee assembled serologists in Copenhagen to compare the Wassermann test with the Kahn test and its variations. A similar assay was performed in Montevideo in 1930 and later in the United States. The numerous published summaries of validating tests showed the Kahn test to be sensitive and specific and to give no more doubtful, false-negative, or false-positive results than the Wassermann test. The Kahn test replaced the Wassermann test for most routine work by 1941.

Reuben Kahn took leaves of absence from Michigan to attend syphilology conferences in Europe, South America, and the United States. He traveled to lecture and to receive gold and bronze medals and honorary doctoral degrees in law, science, medicine, and philosophy. He had to rebut Dean Furstenberg's criticism that he was too frequently away from Ann Arbor.

6
Physiological Chemistry, 1921–41

Until he retired in 1921 Victor Vaughan was scheduled to give lectures in physiological chemistry, and Frederick Novy, with the help of an assistant, was responsible for laboratory work. In the last six or so years of his tenure Vaughan was increasingly busy with administrative affairs and was frequently out of town. His lectures were taken over by Novy and the assistants. When he did lecture, Vaughan gradually corrected the faults criticized by Newell Martin, for the topics covered became more physiological. When he set an examination Vaughan expected a student to give in detail the chemistry of blood but also to "give in detail the metabolism of carbohydrate in the body in health and disease."[1] Unfortunately no graded examinations survive to demonstrate the detail that satisfied Vaughan.

Laboratory work in physiological chemistry (fig. 6–1) was derived directly from the course in urinalysis that had been given in the Chemical Laboratory since the 1860s. Novy wrote a laboratory manual, which was used until he ceased to be responsible for the subject in 1922.[2] Students were drilled in the chemical properties of and tests for carbohydrates, fat, and protein, and they analyzed saliva, gastric juice, pancreatic secretion, bile, blood, and milk. After learning how to use a balance and to make standard solutions, students analyzed twenty-four-hour samples of urine for specific gravity, total solids, acidity or alkalinity, chloride, sulfate, phosphate, glucose, and urea. At the end of the course they had to demonstrate their competence by determining the composition of twenty-five unknown samples containing one or more abnormal constituents.

Vaughan's research in physiological chemistry stopped in 1917 when he went to Washington, D.C., as a member of the Executive Committee of the Army's General Medical Board, and Novy was busy with bacteriology. Few students received advanced degrees in physiological chemistry in Vaughan's later days. One was the notorious William Frederick Koch, who earned the degree of doctor of philosophy from the University of Michigan and the degree of doctor of medicine from the Detroit College of Medicine. Koch, who practiced in Detroit, devised a "cure" for cancer, and his advertisements for it in the 1920s implied that it was sponsored by the University of Michigan. Indignant alumni wrote to the dean of the Medical School to ask why the school was promoting the sale of such a product, and for years the school tried to dissociate itself from Koch's quackery.[3]

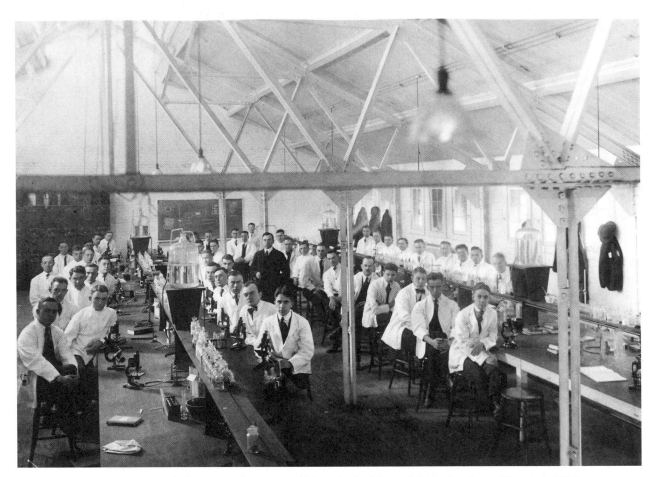

Fig. 6–1. Physiological chemistry laboratory, old laundry building of Catherine Street Hospital, 1918. (Courtesy of the Bentley Historical Library, University of Michigan, Medical School Records, Box 136, "Classes by Year, 1919.")

The university must have sensed that physiological chemistry was not what it should be at Michigan, for in 1916 the Graduate School recommended the establishment of a university department of biochemistry. Vaughan was away at the time, but as soon as he returned he protested furiously that he and Novy taught physiological chemistry, the same thing as "biochemistry." The matter was dropped then, but immediately after Hugh Cabot succeeded Vaughan as dean in the summer of 1921 Cabot began to look for a physiological chemist. In the meantime Earl Baldwin McKinley was promoted to instructor and given responsibility for teaching the subject. In November 1921 the regents created a chair of biochemistry in the Medical School, but in response to protests from Novy they changed its name to physiological chemistry. In order to indicate the subject's wider scope the name was again changed to biological chemistry

in 1935. The chair was filled in 1922 by Howard Bishop Lewis (fig. 6–2), who held it until he died in 1954, two years after an incapacitating stroke.[4]

Recruitment of H. B. Lewis

Early in the autumn of 1921 Dean Cabot asked advice of Graham Lusk, Donald D. Van Slyke,[5] and Otto Folin, and he accumulated a long list of candidates, including William C. Rose, E. A. Doisy, and H. B. Lewis. On 17 May 1922 the faculty voted to ask the regents to appoint Lewis, and the regents duly complied. At the same meeting Novy moved

[t]hat the Board of Regents be requested to ask Dr. Lewis to come here as Professor of Physiological Chemistry but that all matters pertaining to the Administration of the

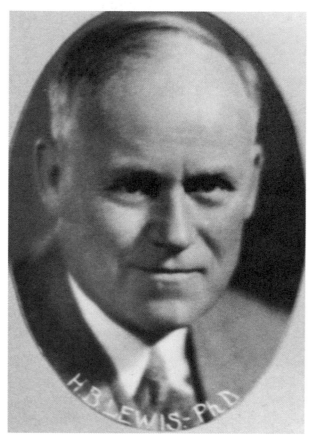

Fig. 6–2. Howard Bishop Lewis. (Courtesy of the Bentley Historical Library, University of Michigan, Medical School Records, Box 136, "Biochemistry Department.")

H. B. Lewis's Preparation

Lewis had taught himself Greek so that when he entered Yale College in 1904 he was awarded highest honors in the subject, but he turned to physical science. After teaching for two years he entered Yale's graduate school as a candidate for the doctor of philosophy degree in physiological chemistry. He was a student of Russell H. Chittenden, Thomas Osborne, and, in particular, Lafayette B. Mendel. The three had put Yale's physiological chemistry in parallel with the position occupied by Cannon's Harvard Department of Physiology. Yale was then, and would long remain, the first place one turned when seeking to fill a job in physiological chemistry.

After receiving his doctorate Lewis spent two years as an instructor at Pennsylvania, and in 1915 he was drafted by W. A. Noyes of the Department of Chemistry at the University of Illinois to establish a program of teaching and research in physiological chemistry.

At Yale Lewis learned the two major techniques then available for the study of intermediary metabolism. The first was to put something into an animal, by injecting or feeding it, and to see what came out in the urine. The method was useful if the something injected or fed had, like benzoic acid, a structure that was conserved in metabolism or if it contained a traceable element such as sulfur. The other technique was to feed an animal a defined diet, with or without supplements, and to see what happened to its growth.

Hydantoin is a five-membered ring, NH-CO-NH-CO-CH$_2$, that can be made to look something like pyrimidine, creatinine, allantoin or imidazole. Someone had thought it stimulates or inhibits nerves. Mendel and Lewis injected hydantoin into rabbits, cats, and dogs, and Lewis found it was excreted unchanged in the urine, giving no evidence of either toxic effects or a place in metabolism.[7] Lewis displayed competence in organic chemistry by preparing esters of hydantoic acid, and he began his long study of sulfur metabolism by making and using thiohydantoin and other sulfur derivatives. These latter turned out to be toxic, but their sulfur atom was not oxidized. At Pennsylvania Lewis learned another technique, for there he perfused dog and rat livers to discover that parabanic acid, another hydantoin derivative, is largely converted to urea.[8] He also learned to measure glucose excretion in phlorhizinized dogs.

Department of Physiological Chemistry be under the supervision of the Director of the Hygienic Laboratory [Novy himself].[6]

The motion was seconded by Lombard, but it failed to pass.

Novy had taken over Vaughan's space without consulting anyone, and when Lewis was negotiating with Michigan in the summer of 1922 he attempted to come to an agreement with Novy about squeezing his new department into the Medical Building. As early as 18 September 1922, Lewis discovered he could not share the stockroom with Novy, and he asked the dean for a partition and a separate storekeeper. Lewis's problems were partially relieved when Novy and the Department of Bacteriology moved into the new East Medical Building in 1925, but his department housed in the West (old) Medical Building was always cramped for space.

Benzoic acid was freely used as a preservative, and as a result of the clamor about food additives during Theodore Roosevelt's administration the Yale physiological chemists had confirmed that it is quantitatively conjugated with glycine and harmlessly excreted in the urine as hippuric acid. Lewis used this fact and the Yale technique of feeding deficient diets to show that the body can provide an essentially inexhaustible amount of glycine. Casein contains no glycine, and when Lewis fed a rabbit a milk diet and benzoic acid the animal excreted hippuric acid with no extra nitrogen in the urine. Lewis deduced that the nitrogen of glycine was the product of the deviation of normal metabolism and not of a process mobilized to deal with benzoic acid. He placed himself on a diet of milk, cane sugar, and butter for three days and then took six to ten grams of sodium benzoate. He excreted 85 to 90 percent as hippuric acid in fifty-six hours, and he, like the rabbit, had a correspondingly smaller amount of urea and ammonia in his urine.[9]

When Lewis was chosen at Michigan he had displayed exemplary industriousness as a biochemist, using techniques available in his day. So far he had done nothing of lasting importance, but neither had the rival candidates. Rose had been at Yale and at Pennsylvania in the years immediately before Lewis,[10] and in 1921 he was a professor of biochemistry in Texas, studying creatine metabolism as many of his contemporaries did. He replaced Lewis at Illinois, and his important work, developing a major school of biochemistry, identifying threonine, and quantifying amino acids essential for humans,[11] was yet to come. Doisy, who had been a student of Lewis at Illinois, had just gone to Washington University in St. Louis to begin his collaboration with Edgar Allen that resulted in the isolation of estrogens,[12] and he received the Nobel Prize for work done many years later. In 1921 there was no reason for Michigan to prefer Rose or Doisy to Lewis, but taking Lewis instead of one of the others was bad luck.

H. B. Lewis at Michigan

Lewis always had a small staff, and accreditation visitors in 1935 thought the department had too few personnel. There were always Adam Christman, whom Lewis had brought from Illinois, and H. C. Eckstein, both slowly climbing the professorial ladder. They taught medical and graduate students, and Lila Miller, always an instructor, took care of students of nursing, dentistry, and physical education. Sometimes there was another instructor or assistant professor. Forty-six students earned the doctor's degree before 1942, and most of them served as assistants in the laboratory courses. All these were squeezed into 16,500 square feet in the West Medical Building, and the accreditation visitors said the department was a "mess."

Because anatomy and bacteriology dominated the first year when Lewis arrived, physiological chemistry was taught in the second year where the dominating department was pathology. At first Lewis gave only 48 hours of lecture to sophomore students, and the number grew only to 60 in the early 1930s. In those days the 142 hours of laboratory were taught on the block system, one half the class being in the laboratory for eight weeks and the other half in a second eight weeks, both blocks alternating with the physiology laboratory. Lewis said: "One of the most important functions of our laboratory training in chemistry in the medical school is, in my opinion, not to make trained chemists or technicians of our medical students, but to seek to instill in them some critical judgment so that they are capable of discrimination between good and poor laboratory work. The fundamentals of good analytical technic, neatness, accuracy and good judgment, can be acquired by every medical student. Then and only then can he appreciate and demand intelligently a high type of technical assistance in his chemical diagnostic work. . . . I would not plead for more chemistry. In the crowded medical curriculum, that can not reasonably be expected at the present time. I do, however, plead for a more thoughtful chemistry."[13]

The senior students who surveyed the curriculum in 1934 reported that Lewis's course was a model of organization properly serving the needs of the medical students. They were particularly pleased that his laboratory course, in contrast with physiology's, was free from irksome detail in writing up experiments.

After Novy retired in 1935 bacteriology began to be gently cut down to size, and Lewis could give sixty-two, growing to eighty-five, lectures in the first semester of the first year. By 1938 his laboratory course was moved to the first year as well.

Lewis was liked and trusted by his colleagues, and he was given many committee assignments: the

Administrative Board under Dean Cabot; the Executive Committee under Dean Furstenberg; the Library, Scholarship, and Student Affairs Committees; and the Promotion Committee. In 1933 he was made director of the College of Pharmacy, a post he retained until 1947.

At Michigan the department, or more particularly the department chair, has always been the sole arbiter of course content, and Lewis, as chairman of the Curriculum Committee for many years, confined himself to shuffling hours between departments. Where could the Department of Internal Medicine find the time for the whole-class lectures it thought it needed? How could the Department of Psychiatry have a few more hours in the senior year, and how could rotation through the specialties be arranged if some of their time was to be made elective?

Although Lewis was also busy on the national scene with now forgotten tasks, membership on editorial boards and committees on nutrition and the like, he performed one service that should be remembered. Single-handedly he provided a placement service for the Federation of American Societies for Experimental Biology. By means of an enormous correspondence and by manning an office at the annual meetings Lewis helped many youngsters, chiefly recent doctors of philosophy, to meet prospective employers.

H. B. Lewis and Sulfur Metabolism

Lewis did a considerable amount of miscellaneous work on glycogen deposition, uric acid excretion, and amino acid metabolism. For example, he and his students found that a young white rat fed gliadin, a protein low in lysine, is unable to convert α-hydroxy-ε-amino-caproic acid to lysine.[14] In a similar fashion he found that phenylpyruvic acid cannot replace tyrosine. Phenylpyruvic acid appears in the urine when phenylalanine is fed, demonstrating, he thought, that α-oxidation occurs after deamination to give a product not further metabolized.[15] However, Lewis was known for his work on sulfur metabolism, for he published thirty papers on the subject before 1942. When the laboratory work was done by a student working for a doctor of philosophy degree, Lewis put the student's name first on the paper, but Lewis's position was recognized by his invitation to write three papers for *Annual Review of Biochemistry,*

one for *Physiological Reviews,* and a Harvey Lecture.[16] All the work was done cheaply, for Lewis, who had no outside grants, supported the work on the department's meager budget.

The sulfur and nitrogen atoms of proteins can be identified in the urine, and Lewis like many others thought that a study of the ratio of sulfur to nitrogen in the urine would reveal something of the metabolism of the protein molecule. Lewis fed and fasted a white female bulldog over seventy-eight days, and he found that sulfur was excreted before nitrogen.[17] Another dog maintained on a low protein diet went into negative nitrogen balance, but addition of 0.5 to 1.0 gram of cystine per day returned the animal to positive balance. Lewis concluded, in agreement with Osborne and Mendel,[18] that there is a specific demand for cystine as an essential amino acid. When he compared the feeding of serum albumin, high in cystine, with casein, low in cystine, he found that dogs remained in nitrogen balance on albumin but not on casein unless the casein was supplemented by cystine. Therefore, cystine is necessary for maintenance as well as growth.

By the time Lewis delivered his Harvey Lecture on 20 February 1941, the principles of sulfur metabolism had been defined. Lewis had accepted the mistaken conclusion that cystine is an essential amino acid, but by 1941 he had learned that methionine or homocystine supplemented by choline is the essential source of sulfur. Cystine is dispensable, but if the minimum requirement for methionine is met, cystine can supply additional sulfur. The essentiality of methionine had been demonstrated by Rose, using diets of purified amino acids,[19] and the role of cystine plus methionine and the synthesis of cystine from methionine had been established by Lewis's former pupil, Abraham White, after White had gone to Yale.[20] For all his thirty papers Lewis had made no contribution to this story. He had shown that taurine cannot replace cystine in the diet, that cystine oxidation is prevented if its amino groups are benzoylated, that the cystine content of the diet has no influence upon the concentration of cystine in tissue proteins, and that although growth of hair is related to cystine intake the cystine demand for growth of hair is secondary to the demand of more essential tissues. In those days sulfur and molasses was one of Grandmother's favorite spring tonics, but Lewis found that flowers of sulfur are toxic to the growing rat because they give rise to hydrogen sulfide.

H. B. Lewis and Cystinuria

Cystinuria is one of Archibald Garrod's inborn errors of metabolism.[21] Cystine is poorly soluble in acid urine, and the amino acid gets its name from the fact that it was first identified as a constituent of a bladder stone. Lewis studied a cystinuric patient on Reed Nesbit's urological service at the University Hospital. By testing 10,534 samples of urine of students at the University of Michigan, at Ypsilanti State Normal School, and at Albion College he found four others who excreted about a gram of dissolved cystine and cystine crystals a day. There were fourteen students whose urine gave a strong positive test for cystine but contained no crystals, and twenty-two more whose urine was weakly positive for cystine.[22]

Lewis studied the Michigan patient for years. Garrod had cited copious evidence purporting to show that dietary cystine is not the source of urinary cystine, and Lewis thought he had confirmed this.[23] In 1934 Lewis measured the daily excretion of cystine while his subject ate a "moderate" protein diet. Then he switched to a "high" protein diet and back again. For each period he averaged the cystine output on the control days. In the first period the cystine output averaged 0.66 gram a day; in the second it was 0.84 gram; and in the third it was 0.73 gram. Lewis did not report the daily excretions he had averaged, and he made no statistical analysis of his data. When he had substituted the high protein diet for the moderate protein diet nitrogen excretion rose from 7.7 grams a day to 15.0 grams, sulfate excretion rose from 0.39 to 0.70 gram, and cystine excretion rose from 0.18 to 0.22 gram. Lewis was so impressed by these data that he concluded cystine feeding does not increase cystine output in a cystinuric patient. He came to the same conclusion in 1935 when he supplemented a constant diet of 56 grams of protein with 2 grams of cystine. During control days cystine output was 0.76 to 0.80 gram. On the first day of supplementation it was 0.72 gram and on the second day 0.73 gram.[24] Lewis wrote that his results indicated "that the cystine excretion is largely endogenous in origin and is independent to a considerable extent of the cystine present in the protein element of the diet. . . . We would not be inclined to attribute this [increase in organic sulfur, presumably cystine sulfur, excretion] directly to the content of cystine in the diet, but rather to the effect of protein in stimulating some unknown endogenous metabolic process, whose abnormality in the cystinuric results in the excretion of a considerable portion of the cystine, which plays a rôle in body processes, unoxidized."[25]

Garrod had come to a similar conclusion: "The fact that in ordinary cases of cystinuria swallowed cystin is burned to sulphate, as by normal persons, certainly lends support to the view that the cystin which the patients excrete unchanged has its origin in the breaking down of the tissue proteins and not of those of the food."[26]

Garrod cited the fact that someone had shown that when cystine is injected into a systemic vein of an experimental animal cystine appears in the urine, but when cystine is injected into the portal vein it does not. Garrod did not exploit this fact, and Lewis paid no attention to it. The year 1908 was probably too early for Garrod to worry about glomerular filtration and tubular reabsorption of cystine, but 1935 was certainly not too early for Lewis to question the means by which cystine is excreted in the cystinuric person and conserved by a normal person. The isotopic work of Schoenheimer and Rittenberg destroyed the concept of exogenous and endogenous metabolism, but Lewis did not need an isotope to solve the problem of cystinuria.

Lewis's department at Michigan was a branch of the Yale tree of biochemistry, and the tree became barren. Between 1911 and 1941 European biochemistry far outshone U.S. biochemistry, and one who studied the subject at the end of the period remembers almost at random Engelhardt, Fischer, Hopkins and his Cambridge school, Embden and Meyerhof, Keilin, Lipmann, Linderstrøm-Lang, Peters, Szent-Györgyi, Sørensen, Theorell, Willstätter, and Warburg. There was nothing in the United States to match their work, but outside Michigan U.S. biochemists, not counting the refugees of the 1930s, were perfecting methods universally used in the clinic as well as in the preclinical laboratory, defining acid-base equilibria and mineral metabolism, identifying and isolating vitamins and hormones, determining the composition and structure of proteins, studying the specificity of proteases, crystallizing enzymes, and beginning to use deuterium and nitrogen 15. None of this occurred at Michigan, and Lewis ended thirty years of work with the same methods and outlook as he began.

7
Physiology

Henry Sewall recommended William H. Howell, his junior Johns Hopkins colleague, as his successor when he had to resign as professor of physiology on account of his tuberculosis in 1889. President Angell offered Howell the job at a salary two hundred dollars below Sewall's. Howell protested, and Angell, after a regent said the higher salary was little enough, raised the offer to twenty-two hundred dollars.[1] Although Howell was obliged to give Johns Hopkins six months' notice, Newell Martin arranged for Howell's early release, and Howell came to Ann Arbor in the autumn of 1889 to be professor of physiology and histology. Howell found time to do the clinical work for his doctor of medicine degree as a member of the class of 1890.

W. H. Howell's Preparation

Howell, a Baltimore boy, had graduated from the newly founded Johns Hopkins University in 1881, and he immediately became a graduate student, studying biology under Newell Martin and W. K. Brooks and chemistry under Ira Remsen.

Henry Sewall had helped Newell Martin make the first successful mammalian heart-lung preparation. Sewall and Martin did little with it, but early in his graduate work Howell and another student, F. A. Donaldson Jr., used the heart-lung preparation to determine effects of variations in arterial and venous pressure on stroke volume and cardiac work. The rate of the isolated heart was constant, and Howell and Donaldson found that over a wide range of arterial pressure stroke volume remains constant. Consequently, cardiac work rises in direct proportion to arterial pressure. When arterial pressure was held constant and venous pressure increased, both stroke volume and work rose in parallel until maxima were reached. Howell and Donaldson satisfied themselves that left atrial pressure, the factor determining left ventricular filling, varied over a physiological range as they changed venous pressure, and they concluded "that the most direct factor influencing the quantity of blood sent out from the ventricle, and hence the work done by the ventricle, is the intra-ventricular pressure by which the ventricle is distended during diastole . . . and that for the heart muscle the energy liberated as external work bears a direct proportion to the tension exerted by the load."[2] That was thirty years before the same facts were rediscovered at University College London by Ernest Starling.

In the fashion of the day Howell worked on diverse physiological problems, and his doctor of philosophy thesis was on coagulation of the blood of that Chesapeake delicacy, the terrapin. As he rose from graduate student to associate professor, Howell taught animal physiology, vertebrate histology, and mammalian anatomy. His responsibilities increased as Martin's health failed, and toward the end of his Baltimore period he could do little research. He told President Angell that he would not neglect his teaching duties at Michigan but it would be a bitter disappointment to him if his class work left no time for research.

W. H. Howell at Michigan

Starting from almost nothing, Sewall had gradually accumulated equipment for teaching and research. When Howell arrived in Ann Arbor he found five Du Bois-Reymond induction coils, two rotating cylinders with clockwork for smoked-paper recording, one Ludwig kymographion for registering blood pressure, a Browning spectrograph, a Thompson's galvanometer, a Roy-Gaskell heart tonometer, Zeiss microscopes, and machine and woodworking tools. With these Howell could mount a full demonstration course in physiology for medical students and resume research. Like Sewall, Howell also gave a course in physiology for students in the Literary Department who intended to become teachers of biology or psychology, and for them a required laboratory course was provided. There is some evidence that laboratory work was also required for medical students in Howell's third and last year at Michigan, but immediately upon his departure the requirement, if it existed, was abolished by faculty members greedy for time in the curriculum.

At Michigan Howell continued the work on hematopoiesis he had begun at Johns Hopkins. He made cats of all ages anemic by severe bleeding, and he found that in the early embryo red blood cells are formed in many tissues and in the second half of embryonic life in the liver, spleen, and bone marrow. After birth they are formed only in the bone marrow, but in profound anemia the spleen may resume production. The nucleus of the red blood cell is lost by extrusion, but in severely anemic animals a large frag-ment of nuclear material, now known as the Howell-Jolly body, persists until the cell disappears.[3] Howell did less well with white blood cells, for he seems to have misinterpreted their progenitors.[4]

Like Sewall, Howell had student assistants in his teaching and research. One Literary Department student and one medical student earned masters' degrees helping him demonstrate that it is the inorganic salts of plasma, not the proteins, that maintain the beat of the heart. The medical student did a particularly good job demonstrating that proteins are not consumed by the beating heart over a period of fourteen hours.[5] Again working with students, Howell attempted to determine the nature of conduction by a cooled segment of nerve in a nerve-muscle preparation. He concluded that "[a] nerve impulse in passing into a stretch of fibre of different temperature may suffer an increase or a diminution in force, according as the temperature of this portion of the nerve is above or below that in which the impulse originated."[6] Howell was handicapped by having to judge the "force" of a nerve impulse by the magnitude of the contraction of the muscle innervated. Howell did much better in a study of nerve regeneration, which will be described in chapter 10.

In 1892 first-year medical students at Harvard were required to do one hundred laboratory exercises in physiology, and Henry P. Bowditch, professor of physiology at Harvard, needed help. He hired Howell away from Michigan, but he could keep him only a year. Newell Martin resigned just as the Johns Hopkins School of Medicine opened, and Howell returned to Johns Hopkins as its first professor of physiology. Much later at a festive occasion in Ann Arbor Howell said: "It is true that when I was called to another position I accepted, and severed my connections here in an easy and friendly way. I have since come to recognize that, so far as I was concerned, this separation was effected without proper consideration, for I have not found elsewhere better opportunities for work nor any pleasanter or more stimulating environment for living."[7]

Howell's Replacement

When Howell was making up his mind to leave for Harvard, Warren Plimpton Lombard was looking for a job. For the last three years Lombard had been an assistant professor of physiology at G. Stanley Hall's Clark University in Worcester, Massachusetts. In

1889 Hall had gathered a faculty of extraordinary distinction at what he intended to be a "purer Hopkins," a research university. Jonas Gilman Clark, on whom Hall depended for money, was secretive and capricious, and dissension rapidly divided Hall, the faculty, and the trustees.[8] On 21 January 1892, most of the faculty resigned as of the first of next September. The academic world knew about Hall's problems, and William Rainey Harper hired a house in Worcester so that he could sign Albert Michelson, Charles O. Whitman, John U. Nef, and Franklin P. Mall for his new University of Chicago. Angell merely wrote a letter: Howell was thinking of leaving; was Lombard interested in coming to Ann Arbor? Lombard was, and in June Vaughan told him that the salary was twenty-two hundred dollars, that it was cheaper to live in Ann Arbor than in Massachusetts, and that Michigan had good laboratory facilities. President Angell told Lombard that the regents had accepted the faculty's recommendation that he be appointed professor of physiology and histology, and on 9 July Lombard wrote from Woods Hole accepting the appointment.

Lombard's Preparation

Warren Plimpton Lombard was a well-connected Bostonian who had played football as an undergraduate at Harvard College. As a medical student at Harvard Lombard received honorable mention in surgical anatomy, and he did a trivial piece of research in Bowditch's laboratory. After he graduated in 1881 Lombard served for a while in Boston hospitals and then went to Europe determined to study obstetrics in Vienna. In the summer of 1883 he attempted to perfect his German, first in Weimar and then in Leipzig. In Leipzig Lombard somehow wandered into Carl Ludwig's Institute of Physiology, and he immediately determined to devote his life to physiology.

In 1883 Ludwig was sixty-six years old and at the height of his powers. Years before Ludwig and his fellow students, Emil Du Bois-Reymond and Hermann Helmholtz, had determined to build physiology upon a foundation of physics and chemistry, and they had made Germany the world center of the science. Ludwig had more than 250 advanced students from all over the world, and they dominated physiology for the next fifty years.[9] Lombard along with all the others venerated his lovable master.

Ludwig set Lombard the task of determining how the spinal cord converts an afferent impulse into an appropriate movement. The machinists on the ground floor of Ludwig's institute made Lombard a "muscle harp" with which he could record the coordinated contractions of nineteen muscles of the right leg of a decerebrated frog on smoked paper carried on a kymograph drum (fig. 7–1). Lombard was afraid to stimulate the frog with electric current for fear of damaging the afferent nerves, so he applied a thermal stimulus to the left side of the frog. When the temperature of a copper bulb was raised from room temperature to forty-seven to fifty degrees centigrade the muscles of the right leg contracted. Lombard carefully tabulated the order in which they contracted, and he measured the latent periods. When he had accumulated a vast amount of data he wrote up his results in English and turned the manu-

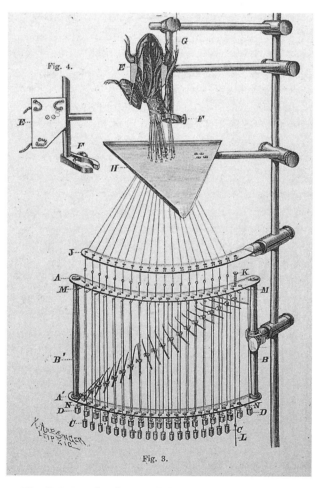

Fig. 7–1. Lombard's muscle harp. (From Lombard, "Die räumliche und zeitliche Aufeinanderfolge reflectorisch contrahirter Muskeln," *Arch. Physiol.* [1885]: fig. 3.)

script over to Ludwig. Ludwig rewrote it in German whose clarity was inferior to Lombard's English, and he saw that it was published, as was his custom, with only his student's name on it.[10]

For all his greatness Ludwig was lost in the spinal cord, and Lombard was lost with him. The work contributed nothing to understanding spinal reflexes. Only a few years later C. S. Sherrington, with no more apparatus than was available to Ludwig and Lombard but with incomparably greater insight, tackled the same problem with well-known results. Lombard demonstrated the same inferiority when he returned to the United States. There were no jobs open, so John Curtis, professor of physiology at the College of Physicians and Surgeons in New York, gave Lombard a place to work. Lombard arranged to measure his own knee jerk after his patella was struck uniformly by a swinging hammer released from a catch by his wife. In a period of six weeks in the late winter and early spring of 1887 Caroline Lombard tapped her husband's tendon 6,639 times while Warren Lombard recorded his state of mind, the cigars he smoked, and the meals he ate. Lombard found the magnitude of his knee jerk was closely dependent upon the weather, that it was reinforced by irritation of the skin or by reciting to himself "How They Brought the Good News from Ghent to Aix," or by a dream about football. On the other hand his knee jerk was profoundly depressed on the morning of 11 April 1887; early that morning Lombard had a seminal emission. Lombard said his wife helped him with his experiments, but he did not say whether she had helped him with his emission.[11]

At that time some thought that although the knee jerk is affected by events in the spinal cord, the response is too rapid to be a reflex. Efferent impulses merely alter the "tone" of the muscle, thus influencing its intrinsic response to stretch. Lombard came down on both sides of the question, publishing one paper declaring the knee jerk as a reflex and another declaring it is not.[12] Nearly twenty years later Lombard gave the same problem to Carl Wiggers though it had been solved by Sherrington.

Lombard's paper on his own knee jerk was the first to be published in G. Stanley Hall's new *American Journal of Psychology*, and Lombard had occasion to know Hall as a fellow founder of the American Physiological Society. When Hall offered Lombard a job at Clark University Lombard immediately went to work for a while with Angelo Mosso in Turin. Then he settled down at Clark to study fatigue in his own voluntary muscles and variation in blood flow in Franklin P. Mall's arm.

Lombard's Teaching at Michigan

Lombard had a lot of teaching to do. His lecture course for medical students extended over two semesters. Dental and homeopathic students took it for one semester. Lombard like Howell gave a course in physiology for Literary Department students, and they were given laboratory work as well as lectures. That much of Lombard's teaching was highly practical and aimed to satisfy the needs of medical students can be seen from typical examination questions.

> Describe the digestion of a ham sandwich.
> Where are the different sounds of the heart best heard? Explain their relation to the different phases of the cardiac cycle.
> Explain the effects of movements of the diaphragm upon the lung.[13]

Unfortunately Lombard's universal reputation was as an intolerably dull teacher. All that students remembered with pleasure was his lecture on defecation. He demonstrated the proper angle to assume at stool, and he unfolded and pretended to read a newspaper to show the technique of leisurely evacuation. He told the students that "if you have to catch a train or empty your bowels, miss the train."

Both matter and manner were the source of Lombard's reputation for dullness. He wrote a very detailed chapter on the biophysics of nerve and muscle for the first edition of Howell's *American Text-Book of Physiology*[14] in which he described such things as "anode opening contraction" and "kathode opening contraction," topics almost meaningless even then, and he drilled and examined his students on them. As for manner, Sinclair Lewis described him as the stuffy Boston Brahmin, John Aldington Robertshaw.

[His lectures] were held in an amphitheater whose seats curved so far around that the lecturer could not see both ends at once, and while Dr. Robertshaw, continuing to drone about blood circulation, was peering to the right to find who was making that outrageous sound like a motor horn, far over on the left Clif Clawson would rise and imitate him, with sawing arm and stroking of imaginary whiskers. Once Clif produced the masterpiece of throwing a brick into the sink beside the platform, just when Dr.

Robertshaw was working up to his annual climax about the effect of brass bands on the intensity of the knee-jerk.[15]

The effect of brass bands upon the knee jerk! What a Dickensian flight of fancy! But Lombard had determined the effect of brass bands upon the knee jerk. One spring afternoon in 1887 when Lombard was measuring the intensity of his knee jerk a parade went past the College of Physicians and Surgeons. As the band played "My Maryland," or "O Tannenbaum" as Lombard would have remembered it from his days in Germany, his knee jerk was strongly reinforced.

Students who disliked Lombard, hell-raisers like Clif Clawson who mocked him in the lecture room, did not know that every so often Lombard would appeal to the rest of the faculty to reduce the burden on the students. He would appear at faculty meetings with charts showing that students were required to put in too many hours studying, and he would plead for a reduction in the schedule. No one ever paid attention. After Lombard died Reuben Peterson wrote to Dean Furstenberg: "He was a perfect gentleman and never spoke ill of anybody if he could help it. Always at the Faculty meetings, if there was a case of discipline, we knew that we should hear from Lombard on the side of the culprit."[16]

Lombard loved apparatus, and he expressed his love by developing a laboratory course in physiology (fig. 7–2). At first it was voluntary. A little later it was paired with pharmacology; a student could elect either one. Then it was required of all medical students. Occasionally a professor from another university took it in order to learn how to mount one like it in his own institution.

Lombard went to Europe in 1898 with five hundred dollars of university money to buy apparatus. He could attend the International Congress of Phys-

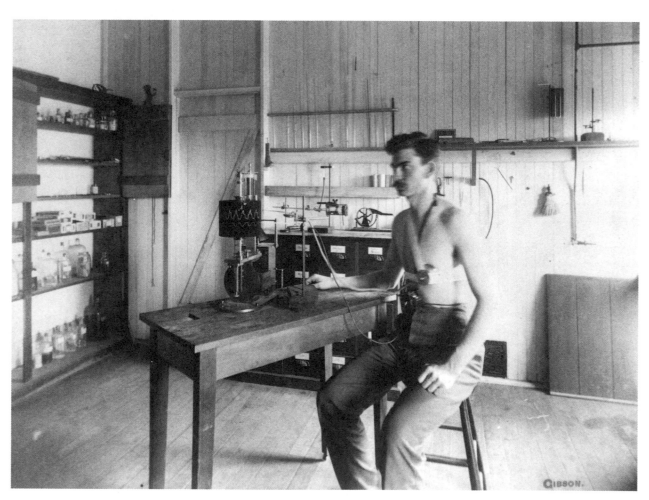

Fig. 7–2. Measuring heartbeat and respiratory movements on a kymograph. (Courtesy of the Bentley Historical Library, University of Michigan, Medical School Records, Box 136, "Gibson #3.")

Physiology

iologists at Cambridge on the trip, and he dined well in Trinity College in company with the Sherringtons, the Darwins, the Gaskells, the Wallers, Michael Foster, Sydney Ringer, and Willy Kühne. He spent the money in Leipzig and Berlin, and when the equipment arrived in Ann Arbor he could give a thorough laboratory course (fig. 7–3). In addition to the customary nerve-muscle and isolated heart experiments Lombard provided a surprising number of observations on the human subject, medical students themselves. There were determinations of the central nature of fatigue of voluntary muscle, identification of motor points, measurement of the apex beat, counting pulse rate and finding its form with a sphygmograph, measuring blood pressure, and, of course, demonstrating reinforcement of the knee jerk.

Carl Wiggers's Start in Physiology

Lombard always had student assistants in the teaching laboratory, as many as six medical students at a time who earned extra money helping other students. In addition he always had an instructor, a man who had previously been his student assistant and who stayed on for some years teaching in the student laboratory and quizzing dental students. Carl Wiggers, a member of the class of 1905, was horrified by Lombard's disregard for all pedagogical principles, and when he had the opportunity to take either physiology or pharmacology laboratory he signed up for pharmacology. The university registrar, doubtless guided by one of the invisible, interpenetrating Spirits Thomas Hardy described in *The Dynasts,* assigned Wiggers to physiology instead. Wiggers was fasci-

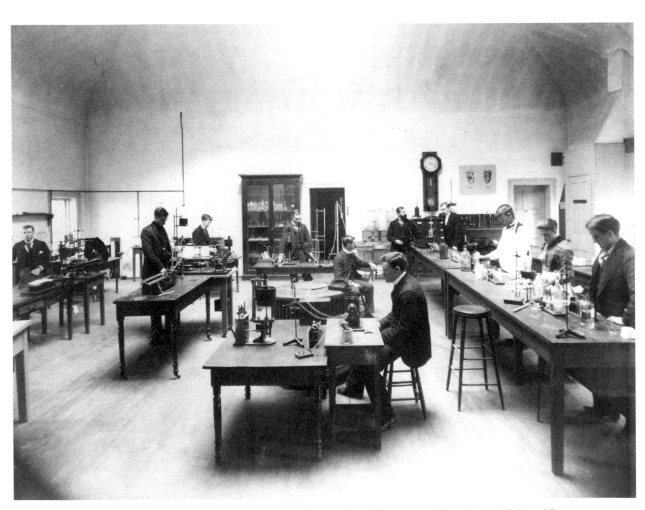

Fig. 7–3. Warren Plimpton Lombard *(left of clock)* in student laboratory, old Medical Building. (Courtesy of the Bentley Historical Library, University of Michigan, Medical School Records, Box 136, "Gibson #3.")

nated by experimental physiology and in particular with the research W. P. Bowen and G. O. Higley were doing in the corner of the laboratory. Wiggers gladly undertook a little research, and Lombard assigned him the problem of whether the knee jerk really is a reflex. Lombard offered Wiggers six hundred dollars a year if he would teach physiology to dental students while taking two years to complete his junior year. When Wiggers graduated in 1906 he became an instructor in physiology, and he remained such until he left for Cornell Medical School in 1911. From Cornell Wiggers went to be head of the Department of Physiology at Western Reserve, and for more than thirty years he was the most productive U.S. cardiovascular physiologist.

Wiggers had a deep affection for Lombard, but that did not stop him from realizing that Lombard was an ineffectual scientist who seldom carried a research project to completion. Wiggers, on the contrary, was then and remained a hard-driving scientist who published thirteen full-length papers while he was at Michigan. Because in those days there were no grants from the U.S. Public Health Service to pay summer salaries, four of those papers reported work done in the summers of 1909 and 1910 in the Detroit Research Laboratories of Parke, Davis and Company. Wiggers also practiced medicine for a while, but he said that because the patients got in the way of the experiments he took down his shingle.[17]

The Lombard Balance

Lombard's chief research accomplishment at Michigan grew out of his ability to encourage others as he had encouraged Wiggers. Two young men, George O. Higley and Wilbur P. Bowen, measured respiratory exchange during exercise. They set up a bicycle ergometer in a corner of Lombard's teaching laboratory, and they passed the subject's expired air through a sulfuric acid drying tube and then through a canister containing soda lime to absorb the carbon dioxide. Volume of the remaining gas was continuously measured by a gas meter. The cylinder in which carbon dioxide was absorbed continuously gained weight, and the rate of gain was a measure of the subject's metabolism. Higley and Bowen hung the canister on one beam of a torsion balance, and by opposing the mass of the canister with a helical spring they converted the beam balance into a tor-

sion balance. As the beam rotated, it inscribed a curve on a slowly rotating smoked drum, and the slope of the curve was proportional to the rate of expiration of carbon dioxide.

Lombard used the same principle in constructing a balance capable of measuring the rate of change of weight of a man to within five milligrams a minute. Lombard wrote in his description of his balance: "The loss of weight from the lungs is the algebraic sum of the carbon dioxid lost plus the water lost, minus the oxygen absorbed. If the subject should breath[e] through a train of tubes, the first containing sulphuric acid to take up the water of the breath, and a second containing soda lime, to absorb the carbon dioxid given off, the amount of the loss of water and carbon dioxid from the lungs could be determined by weighing the tubes before and after the experiment. Further, if this train of tubes was on the same side of the balance as the subject, so that what he gave off from the lungs was held beside him on the balance, any recorded change in weight would be due to the loss of water from the skin and gain of oxygen by the lungs."[18]

Lombard demonstrated that his balance could measure the changes in a man's weight, but he never used it for systematic measure of metabolism. Years later F. G. Benedict, who had collaborated with W. O. Atwater in constructing an enormous metabolism chamber and who had invented a much easier and more reliable method of measuring metabolism, copied Lombard's balance and used it for an elaborate analysis of the factors governing insensible perspiration. He also constructed a Lombard balance in the Deaconess Hospital in Boston to measure metabolism of diabetic patients. In his paper, written in German with his wife, Benedict pronounced Lombard's scientific epitaph.

Die Genauigkeit solcher Wägungen erreichte ihren Höhepunkt in der außerordentlich genialen Stoffwechselwage von *Lombard,* welche aber leider nur für wenige Beobachtungen angewendet wurde. [The possibility of such weighing reached its highpoint in *Lombard's* extraordinarily ingenious metabolic balance which was, however, used for only a few observations.][19]

When the American Physiological Society met in Ann Arbor in 1928 members were weighed on Lombard's freshly calibrated balance, but the memory of the event was the only trace of Lombard's ingenuity for the next sixty years.

Lombard's Measurement of Capillary Pressure

Lombard went to Europe every chance he had, and in 1910–11 he spent part of his sabbatical leave with Max von Frey in Würzburg while Carl Wiggers took care of things at home. In those days a professor on leave had to pay his substitute, and Lombard gave Wiggers two thousand dollars out of his salary of three thousand. In the course of attempting to identify cutaneous nerve endings mediating the sense of tickle, Lombard found that if the skin was wet with glycerin or a transparent oil, one could obtain, with the aid of a microscope, a beautiful picture of the papillae and of the superficial blood vessels. An ink fleck on the epithelium looked like a red scum floating on the surface of a clear pool and far above the loops of capillaries, which appeared like scarlet weeds on the yellow bottom of the pool.[20]

Lombard sat with his left hand resting palm down in a plaster of Paris mold one hundred millimeters below his second intercostal space. After clearing an area of skin with glycerin, he placed a carefully measured one-millimeter-square piece of cover glass on the skin and pressed it down with a known weight. Observing the area by means of a binocular microscope he determined the weight that was required to close one or another of the small vessels, and he converted the weight to millimeters of mercury by dividing by 0.01316. His results in millimeters of mercury were

Subpapillary venous plexus	10–15
Most superficial and smallest veins	15–20
Most compressible capillaries	15–25
Average capillaries	35–45
Most resisting capillaries and arterioles	60–70

These results confirm the pressures required if the Starling hypothesis is valid. That was a debated point for years, and August Krogh ignored Lombard's results in favor of Poul Rehberg's erroneous ones.[21] Sir Thomas Lewis referred to Lombard's method only in a single sentence and did not appear to understand the importance of Lombard's results.[22]

When Wiggers was a student he worked for Arthur Cushny as well as for Lombard, and he drew a contrast between Cushny, who employed relatively simple equipment but who had the vision to formulate research problems of signal value, and Lombard, who delighted in apparatus but who failed to make

use of the apparatus in experimental work. After Wiggers left Ann Arbor Lombard did carry several projects to completion, but like the capillary pressure work they had no impact on the course of physiology.

Lombard in Retirement

A few days after his wife's death in 1923 Lombard resigned as of the end of the 1922–23 academic year, and he received a Carnegie pension.[23] Arthur Curtis, president of the medical class of 1923, collected $226.85 to pay for a portrait of Lombard that hangs in the departmental library, to which Lombard bequeathed his journals and slightly over five thousand dollars.

Lombard inherited his wife's position as president of the Ann Arbor Art Association, and he was very enterprising in promoting appreciation of art in Ann Arbor. His wife had been a watercolorist, but Lombard found he could not handle the medium. He turned to etching, exhibiting often and even selling some etchings. Many are depictions of subjects such as *The Old Wharf*, made during his summers on Monhegan Island, but in old age he began a striking series of single flowers. When he died in 1939 he left his etchings to the university, and they are presently stored in the Collections Room of the Museum of Art on central campus.

In an entirely characteristic action Dean Furstenberg visited the dying Lombard. He wrote: "It was sad to see Doctor Lombard slowly sinking during the past few days. I went in to see him Monday night, and he shook my hand with a firm grip. He died this morning at five o'clock [13 July 1939], and I understand that he was to be cremated this afternoon or tomorrow morning. . . . I always felt that his charming personality was an inspiration to students, and that his staunch citizenship left an influence which will not fail of lasting recognition at Michigan."[24] Alas, it did fail.

Finding Lombard's Successor

On 9 January 1923, Dean Cabot appointed C. W. Edmunds, F. G. Novy, and H. B. Lewis as a committee to recommend Lombard's successor. By 5 February they had accumulated a long list of possible candidates, but only two, Robert Gesell and Walter

Meek, were invited to visit Ann Arbor. Gesell came on 26 March, and when he returned home he wrote that he preferred not to make any suggestions until he had time to think. Meek, who is remembered as the author, with J. A. E. Eyster, of a seemingly endless stream of papers describing electrical activity of the heart, came on 30 April, and he talked on his recent work in which he and Eyster timed X-ray photographs of the human heart with the beginning of the QRS complex and the end of the T wave, obtaining roentgenograms at the end of diastole and at the height of systole.[25] When he returned to Madison, Wisconsin, Meek wrote declining an offer from Michigan. The tone of his letter suggests that he had obtained concessions at home. Gesell accepted an offer on 7 May.

Robert Gesell's Background

Robert Gesell had completed the first two years of medical school at Wisconsin in 1910, and he had served as assistant to Joseph Erlanger, the professor of physiology. In that year Erlanger moved to Washington University in St. Louis, and he took Gesell with him as assistant and then as instructor in physiology.[26] After Gesell received his doctor of medicine degree in 1914, he rose quickly to become an associate professor. In 1919 Gesell was called to the University of California as professor of physiology, but he returned to Washington University as an associate professor in 1922.

When Gesell worked with him, Erlanger was still a cardiovascular physiologist, for he had not yet begun to make his own cathode ray oscilloscopes from distilling flasks. It was natural that Gesell at Erlanger's suggestion should undertake a cardiovascular problem as his first independent research project. Yandell Henderson at Yale had said that in the dog auricular fibrillation has no influence on ventricular filling.[27] Henderson had put the ventricles into a Roy-Adami cardiograph, a rigid chamber acting as a plethysmograph, and had recorded changes in ventricular volume during the cardiac cycle. He found no increase in diastolic volume at the time of auricular contraction. Gesell thought the device too insensitive to detect such changes, and he made no attempt to imitate Henderson. Instead he measured arterial pressure, saying that, after all, arterial pressure is the end result of ventricular function. He crushed the atrioventricular bundle with Erlanger's clamp so that auri-

cles and ventricles beat independently. In the cleverest part of the work Gesell drove the two pairs of chambers electrically at slightly different rates, the ventricles at sixteen beats per minute and the auricles at seventeen. Therefore, auricular contraction precessed through the ventricular cycle. As a result there were phasic increases and decreases in arterial pressure corresponding to the beats of two slightly different musical notes. Pressure was highest and ventricular filling greatest when the auricles contracted 0.008 to 0.02 second before the ventricles.[28]

When the war came Erlanger among many others turned to a study of shock, and Gesell worked with him.[29] The importance of this for Gesell is that it started him on a long study of the relation between blood flow and tissue function that he continued at Michigan. For one thing, he cannulated the duct of the submaxillary gland of a dog so that he could measure rate of secretion, and he simultaneously measured blood flow through the gland. There are no vasodilator nerves to the gland, Gesell thought; dilatation following stimulation is the result of increased tissue metabolism.[30] When the animal was shocked by abusive manipulation of the intestines or by hemorrhage, there were decreased secretion and blood flow. Even a small hemorrhage, less than 10 percent of blood volume, caused decreased function of the gland. Gesell concluded that the decrease in blood volume by "eliciting a vascular constriction reduces the flow of blood to a level below that essential for normal nutrition and far below that essential for deteriorated tissues. The condition [shock] is thus sustained by the disturbed nutrition and by the consequent inability on the part of the animal to recover the normal permeability of the vessels and therefore restore the normal blood volume that is so essential for an adequate flow of blood."[31]

These paragraphs summarize only a small part of Gesell's work before he came to Michigan. He published twenty-five full-dress papers between 1911 and 1921, some of them very long. Those describing work continued in Ann Arbor will be summarized later. The papers demonstrate that Gesell did a lot of hard work along classical physiological lines, using acute preparations or isolated tissues; that he was ingenious in devising experiments and constructing apparatus; and that he was fond of discussing his conclusions at length to demonstrate his invariable correctness.

The pages of many of Gesell's papers in the *American Journal of Physiology* preserved in the Taubman

Medical Library, alone among the papers in the same volumes, are worn to shreds. In many instances the pages are held together only by being pasted over with transparent cloth. The papers were so diligently read not on account of their exemplary merit but because Gesell required his students to read them.

East Medical Building

One reason Lombard retired when he did was that the university was preparing to construct the East Medical Building, now the C. C. Little Building, to house anatomy, physiology, and bacteriology. Lombard wanted his successor to plan physiology's space. Gesell did do the planning, and he was proud of his accomplishment. He had thirty-two thousand square feet, more than enough to provide laboratory space for each of his relatively small staff and to have rooms left over for storage, miscellaneous use, and teaching. Aside from the walnut-paneled Lombard Library and the office of the chairman, none of the rooms had finished walls. Gesell did not like paint, so the dingy terra-cotta walls were left mottled brown, not improved over the years by soot from the burners used to smoke kymograph paper. Gesell spent the summers at his farm near Manchester, Michigan, but one day he returned unexpectedly to find the Plant Department painting David Bohr's room. Gesell immediately went to the Personnel Office to demand that the secretary who had permitted the outrage be dismissed at once.

Gesell provided an aquarium room to house the innumerable frogs and turtles used in the student laboratory. The slate tanks with sloping floors had no covers, for it had not occurred to anyone that frogs can jump. As a result every cranny of the room was stuffed with desiccated frogs. Gesell was proudest of the animal quarters on the roof. There were rooms for birds, rabbits, and rats and for weighing and anesthetizing dogs, but most of the space was occupied by thirty-two kennels for dogs, each with a large, open pen in which the dogs could run. The kennels were heated by pipes along the ceiling so that in the winter the floor where the dogs lay was freezing cold. In addition, many of the dogs chewed off the canvas flap separating the kennels from the runs. The runs had one defect that was no fault of Gesell. The Plant Department in constructing the building had laid a layer of cement to be the ceiling of the fourth-floor rooms below. On this was a layer of felt and then

another layer of cement that was the floor of the kennels and runs. The cement cracked, and not only rainwater and melting snow but water with which the pens were washed down seeped through the cracks, saturated the felt, and then dripped through cracks in the lower layer upon the occupants of the fourth-floor rooms.

Animal Procurement and Animal Care

Gesell and his staff used a large number of dogs acutely in research and teaching. Those were the days before the advent of experts in laboratory animal medicine, and the animals were cared for by untrained men. Every so often one of the dieners (laboratory assistants) was sent by truck to Detroit where pound dogs were loaded, six at a time, into great iron cages to be brought back to Ann Arbor. When the dogs were loosed into their pens on the roof, each member of the staff ran to claim the best and biggest he could, leaving those with sniffles and enteritis to die in a few days. Surviving dogs were fed garbage collected from local boarding houses; they were unwashed; and they stank. As the dogs ran about their open pens they barked at any provocation. Neighbors objected, and at first dogs were debarked by having their vocal cords cut. That became too much of a bother; the neighbors had to put up with the barking and the dean with the neighbors' complaints.

Gesell's Staff

Gesell began by getting rid of Otis Cope, who had been Lombard's instructor for many years. In anticipation of moving into East Medical Building he brought Alrick Hertzman from Wisconsin, and in a move unusual at the time he hired Daniel McGinty, who had earned a doctor of philosophy degree in physiological chemistry under H. B. Lewis. McGinty was to supply biochemical expertise needed in Gesell's study of lactic acid production in hypoxia. In another unusual move Gesell brought Kenneth Franklin from Oxford. The record does not show whether the appointment was intended to be permanent, but Franklin soon returned to Oxford.

As soon as he had graduate students Gesell began the practice of appointing them as assistants and then as instructors as soon as they received the doctor of philosophy degree. The first of these was Detlev Bronk, an instructor in 1925. Bronk soon left to work with Edgar Adrian in Cambridge in a famous collaboration[32] and for a career that culminated in his receiving more than fifty honorary degrees as president of Johns Hopkins University, the Rockefeller University, and the National Academy of Sciences. The second was John Bean, who remained at Michigan as did others who rose slowly in academic rank. The slowness was not entirely Gesell's fault. He repeatedly proposed his men, Hayden Nicholson, Charles Brassfield, and others, for promotion, only to have the Executive Committee delay promotion on the grounds that the candidate had not yet displayed qualifications for higher rank. That was because they had been, in effect, merely Gesell's hand in research. Some graduate students in physiology, like Gesell before them, worked for the doctor of medicine degree while serving as assistants in the department. Of those, Theodore Bernthal and Hayden Nicholson became assistant professors before 1940 and carried much of the load of service teaching. The result of Gesell's habit of recruiting from within was that by the mid-1930s every member of the department was a Michigan product, having learned his physiology from Gesell and having learned to accept Gesell's domination.

Gesell, Bronk, and the Submaxillary Gland

When Detlev Bronk became Gesell's first Michigan graduate student Gesell enlisted Bronk in a collaborative effort to extend his earlier work on the submaxillary gland. Gesell had placed a wick electrode on the surface of the exposed gland and had measured the potential difference between it and an indifferent electrode with a Leeds and Northrup potentiometer. He found that when the gland was stimulated, either through its nerves or by injection of pilocarpine, there followed an elaborate variation in the potential. Although Gesell determined the effect of asphyxia, occluding the gland's blood supply, and so on, he could extract no meaning from the results. Because it was generally thought that a change in permeability underlies a change in potential, Gesell and Bronk set about measuring permeability of the exposed gland.[33]

Bronk had wandered into physiology from physics, and he was a master of the vacuum tube

technique of the day. He converted Gesell's direct current methods into alternating ones. Bronk built a vacuum tube amplifier leading to a string galvanometer or into a d'Arsonval galvanometer to measure the gland's potential changes. To measure conductivity he fed thousand-cycle alternating current into electrodes placed on either side of the gland and used a vacuum tube circuit to measure changes in resistance that could be converted into changes in conductivity. Gesell and Hertzman had devised a manganese dioxide electrode for measuring hydrogen ion concentration, or C_H, as it was called, of blood draining the gland, but Bronk replaced the potentiometer they used with a vacuum tube voltmeter. He even dispensed with the Du Bois-Reymond inductorium and replaced it with an alternating current device whose output he measured by means of a thermocouple. All these outputs were recorded on photographic film. These techniques disappeared with Bronk, and Gesell and his pupils for many years thereafter reverted to smoked paper and mechanical recording of direct current variations.

The names Bronk and Gesell do not appear in the section devoted to electrophysiology of the salivary glands in chapter 10 of Burgen and Emmelin's comprehensive *Physiology of the Salivary Glands*. After summarizing work similar to Bronk's, Burgen and Emmelin concluded: "Despite valiant attempts, analysis of the external salivary electrogram has not yielded results useful in explaining secretory activity but the presence of such electrical activity has encouraged the development of more sensitive methods of study."[34]

Chemical Control of Respiration

By the time he settled in Ann Arbor Gesell thought he knew how respiration is controlled. It had long been known that pulmonary ventilation is increased by breathing carbon dioxide, and Haldane and Priestley had demonstrated the precision with which respiration maintains the constancy of alveolar carbon dioxide.[35] Carbon dioxide is potentially an acid, and many physiologists believed that acid in the blood is the effective stimulus of the respiratory center.

When Gesell reviewed the evidence,[36] much of it his own, he found many circumstances in which there is no correlation between acidity of the blood and pulmonary ventilation. Chief among these is the hyperpnea occurring when an animal breathes oxygen at low pressure; the blood becomes alkaline and remains alkaline as hyperventilation is sustained. Gesell concluded that acidity of extracellular fluid bathing the respiratory center in the brain cannot be the controlling factor; it must be the acidity within the cells of the center themselves. That is governed by the acid metabolism of the cells and by the rate at which acid is removed from their environment by blood flow.

Cell membranes are permeable to carbon dioxide, and when the partial pressure of carbon dioxide in the blood rises, the molecule diffuses into the respiratory center's cells, becomes hydrated to carbonic acid, and thereby stimulates respiration. Gesell persuaded himself that a rise in plasma bicarbonate, by mass action, increases carbon dioxide concentration and thereby stimulates respiration. The center's cells themselves produce acid, either carbon dioxide as the result of their oxidative metabolism or lactic acid as the result of the Pasteur reaction when they are hypoxic. Metabolism rises when temperature rises; hence the hyperventilation of hyperthermia. Acid produced within the cells is carried away by the blood. If blood flow through the center is decreased, acid accumulates; hence the hyperventilation of hypovolemia. Hemoglobin is the major buffer of the blood, and when it is reduced by deoxygenation, it buffers some hydrogen ions with no change in their concentration in plasma. Although Gesell never made any quantitative estimate of the magnitude of the Haldane-Bohr effect, he was convinced that the dual function of hemoglobin, as he called it, also governs the rate of removal of acid from the respiratory center. If blood is hypoxic, metabolism decreases, less oxygen is removed from hemoglobin, the second half of the dual function of hemoglobin is missing, acid is removed less effectively, and respiration is stimulated. Likewise, if an animal is made to breathe oxygen at high pressure, the amount of oxygen dissolved in the blood is adequate for metabolism, and hemoglobin is not reduced in the tissues. This explains the toxicity of oxygen at high pressure.

Gesell worked out the implications of this theory, and he set himself, his staff, and fifteen or so students to demonstrate its correctness. His support came from generous grants from the dean for equipment, from the department's current account, and at first from the American Medical Association. Later he received thirty thousand dollars from the Rockefeller Foundation to be spent at the rate of five thousand a year. Between 1923 and 1941 the work produced

201 scientific papers, many of them very long. Gesell's name is on 108 of them, often first. Ten were on Gesell's old topic of salivary secretion, and about 20 were on miscellaneous topics not immediately related to respiration. A few were derived from respiratory problems such as John Bean's on the toxicity of oxygen at high pressure or John Haldi's on lactic acid formation by the liver. The rest described in great detail elaborate, difficult, and time-consuming experiments to prove Gesell was right, or so he said.

Gesell's Instrumentation

From the beginning Gesell displayed a talent for instrumentation, and at Michigan he had a full range of means for recording physiological variables. One early device was a bloodless way of estimating blood flow.[37] The vein draining an organ was occluded downstream by a lever. As the vein filled a plate resting upon it rose, and when the vein was full a contact on the plate activated a solenoid that lifted the lever to let the vein empty. As soon as the vein was empty, the solenoid was inactivated, and the lever fell to occlude the vein once more. After the instrument was calibrated the number of releases and occlusions, recorded on smoked paper of a long-paper kymograph, permitted calculation of the rate of blood flow. Later Gesell replaced the device with a thermal method.[38] Blood flowing through an exposed vessel warmed water flowing through a tube parallel with the blood vessel, and the extent of warming was detected by thermopiles whose potential difference was measured with a d'Arsonval galvanometer. Gesell followed the reflection of light from the galvanometer's mirror by means of a target moved along a track by a hand-driven windlass. Displacement of the target was relayed by threads over pulleys to a pen scratching a record on the smoked paper of a kymograph. Alternatively, potential difference was followed by a Leeds and Northrup potentiometer.[39] As the drum carrying the slide wire was rotated by hand to keep a galvanometer at its null position, threads wrapped around a spindle on the drum carried its displacement to a pen writing on smoked paper.

Gesell's devices generated or measured direct current. East Medical Building was poorly supplied with alternating current, but Gesell installed an elaborate direct current system. There was a battery room filled with 110 lead-plate batteries storing electricity and generating explosive hydrogen gas. A large AC-to-DC converter charged the batteries, and there was an enormous plug board from which any combination of direct current voltages could be sent to smaller plug boards throughout the department. Timing was provided by a pendulum clock sending impulses to the same plug boards. This instrumentation committed Gesell's department to direct current technology just at the time it was becoming obsolete.

Because Gesell's department was entirely devoted to the study of respiration, every research laboratory and one large student laboratory contained great stainless steel tanks in which gas mixtures could be made for delivery to the experimental animals breathing spontaneously or with forced ventilation. If the animal rebreathed from the tank after carbon dioxide was absorbed by soda lime, a spirometer on the tank recorded the rate of oxygen consumption on smoked paper. Some of the spirometers were sealed with mercury. Mercury was also used in devices to transfer gas samples and in the Haldane gas analysis apparatus. Mercury was inevitably spilled, and every crack in the floor of the department was filled with globules of mercury waiting to be dust borne.[40]

The Haldane apparatus gave spot analyses of gas samples, but Gesell needed continuous measurement of carbon dioxide and oxygen in expired air. For carbon dioxide he bathed a manganese dioxide or quinhydrone electrode in a poorly buffered solution and separated the solution from the gas phase by a permeable animal membrane. Carbon dioxide diffusing through the membrane determined the pH of the solution in contact with the electrode, and the electrode's potential permitted calculation of the partial pressure of the carbon dioxide. This was in 1926, long before commercial versions of the system were available. To measure oxygen Gesell mixed a continuous sample of expired air with illuminating gas and burned the gas in a small flame. The intensity of the flame varied with the partial pressure of oxygen, and Gesell measured the heat produced with a thermocouple.[41]

To build apparatus for research and teaching Gesell had a resource Lombard must have envied: a well-equipped machine shop manned by an expert machinist. Gesell had found Mr. Bryant in California, where he had made the first lie detector for August Volmer, the famous Berkeley chief of police. Earl Bryant (fig. 7–4) was a highly competent metalworker of the old school who designed and built apparatus: kymographs with elaborate gear systems, manometers, valves, spirometers, and all the rest. His work was beautifully finished, and he would let no brass part leave his shop until it had been nickel plated. He was equally precise in his habits. He arrived at exactly 7:30 each morning, left at exactly 12:00 for lunch to return at 12:30. At exactly 3:50 he blew the cuttings from his lathe with high-pressure air in order to leave at exactly 4:00. Every so often Gesell would open the door to the shop a crack in order to peek in to see if Mr. Bryant were really working.

The large student laboratory classes used much apparatus built by Mr. Bryant. Over the years a drawer in the stockroom was filled with elegantly designed Gaskell clamps used to crush a turtle's AV bundle. There was another drawer filled with Hürthle manometers for recording blood pressure. A Hürthle manometer consists of a shallow chamber covered with a thin rubber membrane, and the pres-

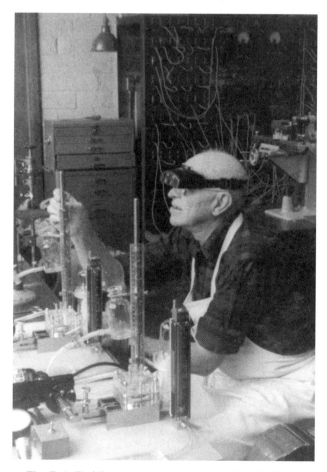

Fig. 7–4. Earl Bryant, instrument maker for the Department of Physiology. (Photographer: Horace W. Davenport, courtesy of Dr. Arthur J. Vander, University of Michigan.)

sure in a blood vessel is conducted to the chamber through rubber tubing. A metal foot resting on the membrane carries its movements to a light lever writing on smoked paper. The fidelity with which the manometer transcribed rapid pressure changes was not very good, but it was much better than a mercury manometer. Time out of mind the rubber membrane was made from a condom. The department had a standing order at a local drugstore for condoms, and Gesell had his secretary cut the tips from the condoms to prevent graduate students from using them for another purpose.

Hypoxic Stimulation of Pulmonary Ventilation

Hyperpnea of hypoxia provided a test of Gesell's ideas. The hyperpnea of exercise might have provided another, but because Gesell worked almost entirely with anesthetized or decerebrated animals, he never seriously considered the problem of exercise. Although he began his first long review of the control of respiration, published in *Ergebnisse der Physiologie*,[42] with a graph relating pulmonary ventilation to oxygen uptake, in the rest of the review and in an even longer one on the neurophysiological integration of the respiratory act,[43] he did not mention exercise.

Gesell believed hypoxia causes intracellular acidosis by promoting glycolysis. To demonstrate glycolysis in the brain Gesell beheaded a small dog with a T-shaped guillotine so arranged that one blow was sufficient to sever the head from the body and to split it in half. One half was frozen in liquid air to serve as a control, and the other half was incubated at room temperature. The biochemist, McGinty, found a rapid rise in the second's lactic acid content.[44]

Cyanide inhibits intracellular oxidation and upon combining with the iron of hemoglobin eliminates the Haldane-Bohr effect. Therefore, Gesell thought, the transitory stimulation of ventilation that follows intravenous injection of a small dose of cyanide is caused by rapid onset of glycolysis within the respiratory center and by failure of hemoglobin to remove acid from the cells' environment. The effect of cyanide is greatest when it is injected into the internal carotid artery, and since no stimulation is obtained when the internal carotid artery is clamped, it is assumed that peripheral chemical stimulation in the head region is of little significance in respiratory control.[45]

When J.-F. and C. Heymans began to demonstrate that peripheral chemical stimulation in the head is indeed significant,[46] Hertzman and Gesell on two occasions repeated the Heymans' experiment of perfusing the isolated head with blood from a donor dog, leaving the trunk connected with the head only by the vagus nerves. Suspending artificial respiration of the trunk almost invariably elicited increased respiratory movements of the isolated head, but when Hertzman and Gesell ventilated the lungs with nitrogen or injected cyanide intravenously there was only inconstant and delayed reflex stimulation of the head. They wrote: "Our experiments would, therefore, support the view of the significance of the peripheral mechanical factors of the control of pulmonary ventilation. While they can also be said to support the possibility of a normal mechanism of peripheral chemical control, they can hardly be considered by themselves to point to that probability."[47]

Gesell did not discover the carotid body reflexes, because he was not looking for them. Eventually he wrote: "No one had actually demonstrated that either excess of carbon dioxide or lack of oxygen, restricted solely to the medulla, is capable of augmenting pulmonary ventilation. Such central stimulation was simply taken for granted. . . . It was a shaky foundation upon which all of us worked. So when Heymans, *et al.,* produced hyperpnea by a lack of oxygen or an excess of carbon dioxide confined to the aortic and carotid chemoceptors, he gave to us a new outlook on respiration for which physiology is deeply indebted."[48]

Gesell extended his intracellular acid theory to the carotid body, and for many years thereafter he and his students assiduously investigated the exact relation between hypoxia and carbon dioxide excess in stimulating the carotid bodies. They studied reflex responses to distention of carotid sinus as well, and both lines of research brought them into conflict with Carl Schmidt and Julius Comroe.[49] Theodore Bernthal made the most lasting contribution in describing cardiovascular reflexes following carotid body stimulation, and his results are extensively cited in Heymans and Neil's *Reflexogenic Areas of the Cardiovascular System*,[50] whereas Gesell's work is barely mentioned "among others."

The Respiratory Center

About 1934 Gesell, using some of his Rockefeller money, bought a General Electric multiple oscillograph and began exploring the brain stem to find the respiratory center.[51] He used a pair of needle electrodes, bare at the tip and one millimeter apart, and he fed the signals they detected through amplifiers built by electrical engineering students he hired by the hour to a galvanometer in the oscillograph. The galvanometer had a reasonably high frequency response, and Gesell could record individual action potentials on photographic film. He used the machine's other two channels to record tracheal airflow and tracheal pressure.

Gesell exposed the brain stem and upper spinal cord, and with electrodes held in a micromanipulator allowing controlled movement in three directions, he sought action potentials related to the respiratory rhythm. He found inspiratory signals in the cuneate nucleus. Nerves near his electrodes began to fire as tidal air was drawn into the trachea and abruptly stopped firing at the end of inspiration. He made an electrolytic lesion so that later he could determine the locus of the active neurons. In experiments on eighty dogs Gesell found a main "center" in the reticular formation of the medulla and descending pathways in the cord. Although potentials within the center were associated with inspiration or expiration, Gesell found no anatomical grouping that indicated structural collections of cells. These results controverted those obtained by Lumsden in the early 1920s when, by sectioning the brain stem of, as he boasted, more than two hundred animals of several species, he identified four discrete centers: a gasping center, an inspiratory center, an apneustic center, and a pneumotaxic center.[52]

A little later Robert Pitts temporarily abandoned his study of the kidney in order to work at Northwestern University with S. W. Ranson, the premier U.S. neuroanatomist, and with H. W. Magoun, a coming man. Together they explored the brain stem of cats decerebrated under ether. They used bipolar electrodes separated by 0.2 millimeter and carrying stimuli of eight volts at 240 cycles per second. They did run up and down the scales of voltage and frequency, but they found those cited gave the clearest results. They repeated their observations on unanesthetized cats using electrodes sealed in place under anesthesia five hours earlier. The cats breathed into a Krogh recording spirometer. Pitts and his colleagues found centers in the reticular formation: an inspiroinhibitory center corresponding to the apneustic center of Lumsden and an expiratory center. These centers were within the limits described by Gesell, but

the anatomical evidence showed they were clearly discrete and not diffuse as Gesell had said.[53] Pitts, Magoun, and Ranson confirmed the existence of a pneumotaxic center, and they worked out the functional relations among the inspiratory center, the expiratory center, and the incoming vagal fibers.[54] Their scheme provided a very clear-cut and intelligible explanation of how the respiratory center accomplishes the periodic act of breathing, and it was immediately adopted by teachers of physiology.

The Pitts-Magoun-Ranson scheme was not accepted by Gesell. He set John Brookhart, his graduate student, to repeating the work on the dog. In more than one hundred observations Brookhart completely failed to confirm the existence of compact inspiratory and expiratory centers.[55] The decade ended with a characteristic controversy, Gesell asserting the superiority of Brookhart's work. Brookhart had used Gesell's needle electrodes, and they were superior to Pitts's. He had used lower voltages, 0.5 to 1.5 volts instead of 8, and he had taken precautions against current spread. His anatomical locations, Gesell said, were superior to those of Ranson.

Gesell's Teaching

Gesell's teaching was the despair of Dean Furstenberg, who said that for twenty-five years medical students lined up outside his door to tell him how bad physiology was. One of Gesell's graduate students said: "Gesell's lectures were pure catastrophe! Word eventually came back to him about the quality of his presentation so his secretary (a shy young woman whose name I have forgotten) was assigned the job of going to his lectures, taking notes and criticizing his presentation. His problem was an absolute monotone in his speaking—this was deadening. There was, however, complete organization and integration of materials."[56]

Unfortunately, the material however well integrated was largely Gesell's own interpretation of the control of respiration and circulation together with an exposition of his own quixotic notions about generation of trains of impulses by a nerve cell and its dendrites.[57] Class after class of medical students pleaded for something more than one or two lectures on the kidney and for something on the physiology of reproduction, and they repeatedly suggested that a clinician, emphatically not Gesell, be assigned to teach pathophysiology to insert some relevance into their study of physiology. Nothing helped, and the rest of the faculty resigned itself to saying that under the present circumstances, meaning during Gesell's tenure, physiology should not be assigned more time in the curriculum.[58]

Gesell illustrated his lectures with numerous demonstrations. There was Lillie's iron-wire model of nerve conduction, and there was a demonstration of chronaxy using a great motor-driven rotator that on its terminal use blew up, scattering fragments like shrapnel on the students. Here, as everywhere, Sherrington's law held: "The actual performance by the student of some few such main experiments gives him, I am convinced, a better insight into their general significance and into the problems they touch than does the mere inspection at a demonstration however skilfully conducted. Indeed, paradoxical though it may sound, *the more skilfully a demonstration experiment is performed the less from it do some students learn.*"[59]

Gesell did give students many experiments to do. Early in his time at Michigan he had a superbly equipped student laboratory for the study of human respiration with gas-mixing tanks, recording spirometers, and many Haldane gas analysis machines.[60] This turned out to be too much for the staff as well as the students, and it was abandoned. In an equally well-equipped mammalian laboratory students made the classical observations on salivary secretion, blood pressure, and shock in anesthetized dogs. Students had to write up the results in detail on 5½-by-22-inch paper, and it was the tedium of this they compared unfavorably with their experience in biochemistry.

Gesell's student laboratory contained sixty-nine benches at which students did numerous experiments using tissues of turtles and frogs, confirming Pflüger's law and the like. Those experiments were what the students remembered of the physiology laboratory, and one exclaimed in exasperation: "When the first frog walks into my office I will know exactly what is the matter with him!"

Some of Gesell's junior staff were better teachers. When Theodore Bernthal, who taught the service courses, left in 1940 for a not very much better job at Vanderbilt, the heads of the departments his courses served wrote long letters to Dean Furstenberg deploring Bernthal's departure and urging that some way be found to keep him. The dean took advantage of Hayden Nicholson's good reputation as a teacher when in 1940 he sent Nicholson on a six-month tour of other physiology departments, notably Harvard's, in the hope that Nicholson could bring back some improvements. That did not help, for Gesell continued to dominate teaching as well as research until one spring evening in 1954, when he was on a walk with his wife and a neighbor's dog was snapping at his heels, he fell over dead.

8
Materia Medica and Therapeutics, Pharmacology

From the beginning the professorship of materia medica and therapeutics was handed from one professor to another, and it was always combined with something else: pathology, physiology, ophthalmology, or whatever. Teaching, such as it was, consisted of lectures on the polypharmacy of the day (fig. 8–1). Because doctors dispensed drugs, medical students were taught practical pharmacy by Albert Benjamin Prescott in the Chemical Laboratory. Prescott, who started as assistant to Silas Douglas in 1863, had a particular interest in detecting adulteration of drugs. Under Prescott a program leading to a degree in pharmaceutical chemistry (Ph.C.) was instituted in 1868, and often a student earned that degree as well as a doctor of medicine.

In 1876 Henry Sylvester Cheever told President Angell that the university must promote the study of the actions of medicines as well as physiology by providing a separate chair for a qualified man and by giving him adequate support. Sometime in 1890 Victor Vaughan received a letter from John Jacob Abel in Europe, a graduate of Michigan's Literary Department, asking for a job as professor of pharmacology. Abel had been a student of Oswald Schmiedeberg, Europe's premier pharmacologist, and after consulting Schmiedeberg Vaughan offered Abel the job. Although Abel was alarmed by Michigan's practice of making the initial appointment for one year, he came to Ann Arbor as lecturer in January 1891. He was made professor of materia medica and therapeutics the next year. Abel and his successors were called professors of pharmacology, but "materia medica" remained the title of the chair until 1942.[1]

Abel's Preparation

Abel's bachelor of philosophy degree earned in Michigan's Literary Department in 1883 signified he had taken the new "scientific course" rather than the older classical one. Vaughan and Sewall had been among his teachers. After spending a year with Newell Martin at Johns Hopkins, Abel went to Europe determined to learn chemistry to be applied to medicine. He went first to Carl Ludwig's Leipzig Institute, where he was a fellow student with Lombard.

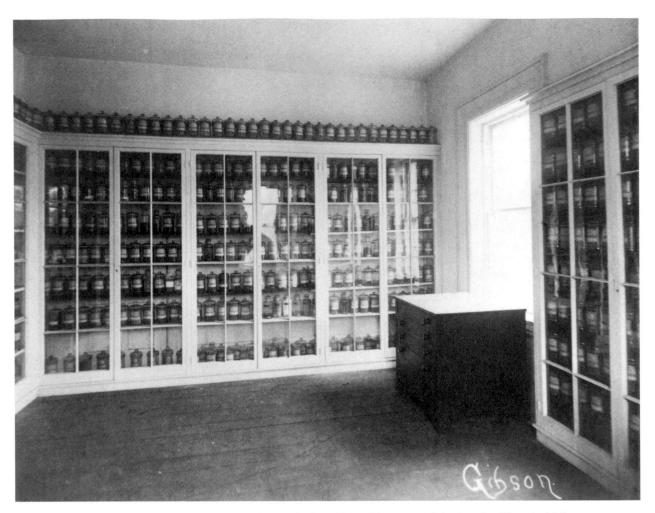

Fig. 8–1. Museum of materia medica, old Medical Building. (Courtesy of the Bentley Historical Library, University of Michigan, Medical School Records, Box 136, "Gibson #4.")

Ludwig set him to answering the question: How does the negative variation of nerves in the spinal cord of the frog behave during stimulation of the sensory and motor roots? That was a good Du Bois-Reymond problem, but it was hardly suitable for training in chemistry. Abel spent much effort making a capillary electrometer work, and he did detect potential differences between nerve roots when the skin of a frog was stimulated with Lombard's thermal stimulator. He wrote up his results in May 1885. Abel also took a course in pharmacology from Rudolf Boehm, and he made the acquaintance of Edmund Drechsel, Ludwig's physiological chemist. After two years in Leipzig and in the custom of the country, Abel wandered from one German university to another, and after passing through Heidelberg and Würzburg he stopped at Strassburg, where the new

German Empire was making the university a major intellectual center. Abel had intended to study biochemistry under Felix Hoppe-Seyler, but finding Hoppe-Seyler too busy to pay attention to students, Abel spent a year with Schmiedeberg. At the same time he qualified for his doctor of medicine degree, fishing his Leipzig work out of his suitcase and presenting it as his inaugural dissertation.[2] Professor Dr. Goltz accepted it on behalf of the medical faculty.

Abel studied clinical medicine in Vienna for a while, and then he went to Bern to work under Marcel von Nencki, who had been professor of chemical physiology there since 1877.[3] Nencki gave Abel one of his old problems: the composition of melanin and hemosiderin. Abel said: "Our knowledge of tissue coloring matters is poor,"[4] but he did little to enrich it. He also applied Raoult's method, determination

     Not Just Any Medical School

of freezing point depression by solutes, to measure the molecular weight of cholic acid, cholesterol, and bilirubin.[5] For cholesterol dissolved in phenol Abel got an average molecular weight of 401 in eight observations with a range of 343–431. The accepted formula weight then was 372. Abel thought the method could be used to determine whether the simplest formula weight of a large organic compound or some multiple of it is the correct one.

Nencki also gave Abel the problem of finding a water-insoluble compound of urea to be used in determination of urea in biological fluids. Abel reacted molten urea with benzyl chloride and obtained benzylidene biuret. The compound was of no use for quantitative estimation of urea or even, as Abel said, for qualitative purposes, but he described it and the corresponding thio- compound as chemical curiosities.[6]

Vaughan's offer reached Abel in Bern, and Nencki urged him to accept it. Although Abel was not then a pharmacologist he would find pharmacology one of the broadest fields of medicine. Instead of going directly to Ann Arbor Abel went back to Leipzig, where he worked a while with Edmund Drechsel. On standing in alkaline solution, urine of herbivorous animals deposits crystals, and Abel and Drechsel identified the crystals as calcium carbamate.[7]

Abel in Ann Arbor

At first Abel was given one small room in the old Medical Building (fig. 8–2), but eventually he moved into two rooms on the second floor that remained the home of pharmacology until 1910. The regents gave him nine hundred dollars for equipment and supplies and another six hundred dollars later. Considering the substantial amount of equipment Lombard could buy later with five hundred dollars, the appropriation was generous. The equipment was slow in coming from Europe, and Abel had to borrow apparatus for demonstrations and use easily available chemicals for research. Archibald Muirhead, a medical student, became his assistant.

Abel took over the old materia medica lectures in the first year of the curriculum, converting them into pharmacology lectures illustrated with demonstrations. He inherited the old lectures on toxicology and the laboratory teaching of pharmacognosy, but for lack of space, equipment, and time in the curriculum he could not give a laboratory course in pharma-

cology. The next year Abel's lectures were moved into the third year, where they remained for a long time. Abel organized a journal club for better students, and he offered them the opportunity to do research. Students were enthusiastic about his teaching, but there is no record that any did research with him or took the graduate course in therapeutics he offered.

Abel's Ann Arbor Research

Abel did not accomplish much research in his Ann Arbor years. The primitive conditions of his laboratory afforded one reason, but for another, he went back to Europe in May 1892 to work again with Drechsel, who had succeeded Nencki in Bern, and he did not come back until November. It was not until he moved to Johns Hopkins in 1893 that he began his only partially successful attempt to isolate the blood-pressure-raising principle of the adrenal gland, work for which he incorrectly gets credit for "isolating the first hormone."[8] His only research accomplishment at Michigan was described in a paper published once in German and once in English.[9]

Victor Vaughan had been consulted by a mother who gave her baby limewater "pretty freely." That treatment was then recommended for children suffering from chronic vomiting or diarrhea. She found the baby's diapers to smell of ammonia, and Vaughan, who had studied the reaction of the urine, found the child's urine to be alkaline. Because Abel and Drechsel had found carbamic acid in alkaline urine, Abel looked for it in the child's urine. In addition, he and Muirhead turned the normally acid urine of a dog alkaline by giving the dog capsules containing calcium hydrate. The dog's urine promptly turned alkaline, and it was full of crystals of calcium magnesium phosphate as well as calcium carbamate. Although the urine smelled strongly of ammonia, it contained much less ammonia than acid urine. On the basis of these findings Abel speculated that carbamic acid is an intermediary in the synthesis of urea.

When Johns Hopkins could finally open its medical school in 1893 Dean Welch offered the professorship of pharmacology to Abel, and Abel accepted it although he knew he would have to teach physiological chemistry as well. Vaughan consulted Oswald Schmiedeberg, and Schmiedeberg recommended another student, Arthur Cushny, who was then, as Abel had been, in Bern.

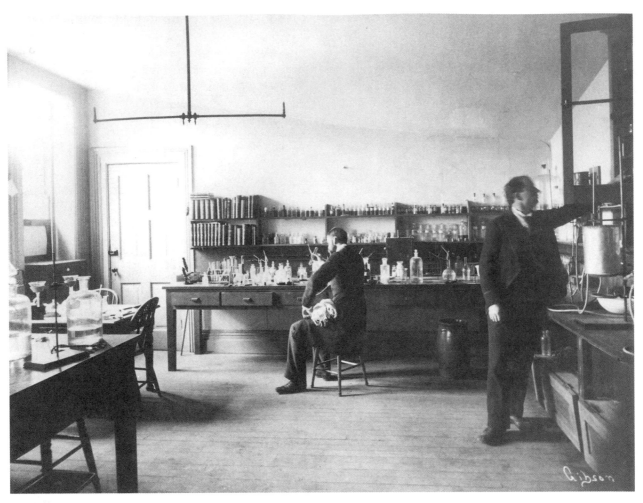

Fig. 8–2. John Jacob Abel *(seated)* and his assistant, Archibald Muirhead, in his laboratory. (Courtesy of the Bentley Historical Library, University of Michigan, Medical School Records, Box 136, "Gibson #3.")

Cushny's Preparation

After receiving his medical qualifications at Aberdeen, Arthur Robertson Cushny went to Strassburg, where Schmiedeberg gave him classical training in pharmacology. Cushny extracted and purified "gelseminine" from *Gelsemium sempervirens,* the yellow jasmine, and he concluded that the extract is poisonous and therapeutically worthless. He worked with muscarine and piperidine, and he found that the poisonous principle in an aqueous extract of the castor bean is a protein effective in minute doses when given intravenously. Cushny was able to make an animal immune to it by giving repeated small doses.[10]

From Strassburg Cushny went to the physiological institute in Bern, where Hugo Kronecker gave him the job of testing the conclusions of the Hyderabad Chloroform Commission. Since its introduction in 1847 chloroform anesthesia had caused numerous deaths. Scottish opinion was that death results from respiratory paralysis; London opinion was that chloroform paralyzes the heart. Neither the Scots nor the English observed liver damage. Chloroform, not ether, was used in India on account of the heat, and in the late 1880s a commission was appointed by the nizam of Hyderabad to determine the cause of chloroform death. It reported that in chloroformed dogs the heart's action never became affected until after cessation of respiration and that death from chloroform narcosis is absolutely avoidable so long as respiration is maintained. The report created such an uproar in London that Lauder Brunton was sent out to India in 1889 to head a second commission whose conclusions, after 571 dogs had been chloroformed, were the same as the first's. The second report was greeted in London with predictable comments: "My clinical experience is to the contrary" and "One observation on a patient is worth a thousand on dogs."[11]

Chloroform had always been given by dripping the fluid onto a cloth-covered mask. Cushny used a better quantitative method.[12] Air from a pump was split into two streams by a Y tube. One stream was saturated with chloroform by bubbling through the liquid. The other stream was saturated with water vapor. When the two streams were united Cushny could vary the percentage saturation of the gas by varying the proportion of the two streams. He found, as might have been expected, that the results depended upon the concentration of chloroform. With a highly saturated mixture the heart of a dog, rabbit, or guinea pig stopped before or at the same time as the respiration. With a weaker mixture death resulted from cessation of respiration.

Having determined the safe concentration of chloroform Cushny was allowed to give chloroform to seven patients in the operating room of the canton hospital and to compare the results with ether given eight times. Cushny found that a higher concentration of ether than of chloroform was required for complete narcosis, and he believed that anesthesia by ether was facilitated by asphyxia. This was Switzerland before the days of iodized salt, and six of the procedures were for struma (goiter). Five others were for complications of tuberculosis. Cushny concluded that the danger of respiratory paralysis or cardiac arrest could be avoided if chloroform were given properly diluted, and he prescribed the concentrations to be used for children and adults. Otherwise, if the anesthetist could not make an adequately defined chloroform mixture, respiration must be watched.

Cushny and Digitalis at Michigan

Cushny became professor of materia medica and therapeutics at Michigan in 1893, and the major problems he investigated while he was in Ann Arbor were the effects of digitalis on the mammalian heart, saline diuresis, and the function of the renal tubules.[13]

Cushny knew the literature on digitalis, for it had been reviewed by his teacher Schmiedeberg.[14] Cushny began his first paper with a long historical introduction.[15] Digitalis had been known to slow the

heart and to raise arterial blood pressure in its first, or therapeutic, stage and in its second stage to cause irregularities in the rhythm of the heart. In the third stage the ventricular rhythm is accelerated and very irregular. Most of the previous work on the effect of digitalis had been done with frogs; Cushny instead used the mammalian heart, those of cats, rabbits, and dogs, and he used the Roy cardiograph and cardiometer.[16] C. S. Roy was professor of pathology at Cambridge, but he was in actual fact an experimental physiologist who left "undertakers' pathology" to the hospital pathologists. His myocardiograph, extensively used in the last part of the nineteenth century, recorded the distance between two places on the heart's surface. His cardiometer was an oncometer or plethysmograph in which the whole heart or only the ventricles were enclosed and that, therefore, allowed measurement of diastolic, systolic, and stroke volume. With these Cushny was able to observe the effects of intravenously injected drugs over many hours.

Cushny found that the first stage of cardiac deceleration is the result of central stimulation of the vagus nerves. Its extent varies in different animals and with different members of the digitalis series. If slowing is extensive, the ventricles assume their own rhythm. Relaxation of the ventricles is lessened, and ventricular contraction is more complete. As the result of increased stroke volume and of arteriolar contraction, arterial blood pressure rises. Cushny found no difference in the action of drugs on either side of the heart. Pressure in the pulmonary artery is unaffected by some of the digitalis drugs and increased by others. In the second stage when the heart accelerates, irregularity of the beat is the result of increased excitability of the heart muscle. Cushny summarized the bearing of his work on therapeutics: the diuretic properties of digitalis result from increased arterial pressure, an action probably resulting from improved nutrition of the heart and a consequent increase in cardiac output.

Cushny, with his assistant S. A. Matthews, was led by the observed irregularities of the heart to determine the effects of electrical stimulation upon the mammalian heart. By this time, 1897 or thereabouts, the excitability of the amphibian heart was well known, and the famous "figure 19" of Marey[17] demonstrating the effects of weak electrical stimulation at different phases of the cardiac cycle of a frog was reproduced in every textbook of physiology (fig. 8-3). The mammalian heart had been studied as well,

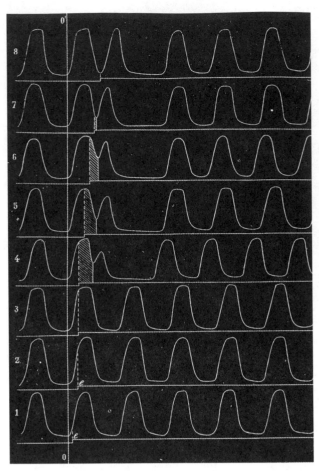

Fig. 8–3. Effects that produce weak electric stimulation applied to different stages of activity of the heart of a frog. Stimulation *(lines 1 to 3)* that happens at the beginning of the systolic stage is without effect; what happens at a more advanced stage of the systole *(lines 4 to 8)* is efficacious, and the accidental systole that it provokes retards so much the less in the instant of stimulation than in the one that happens more slowly. (0′, 0 mark for the superimposition of the curve.) (From E.-J. Marey, *La circulation du sang à l'état Physiologique et dans les maladies* [Paris: G. Masson, 1881], 42.)

by perfusing the coronary vessels by way of the aorta. Langendorff stated flatly and with emphasis: "The most important result of my research is that the mammalian heart behaves like the frog heart" [my translation].[21] Cushny and Matthews, using the dog's heart in situ, obtained the same results: an absolute refractory period occupies the whole time from a brief period before contraction begins until immediately before completion of systole. Thereafter is a period of relative refractoriness. Cushny concluded that the refractory period occurs because "the whole of the potential energy accumulated in the heart is expended whenever a contraction occurs."[22]

A premature systolic contraction occurring during the relative refractory period is followed by a long diastolic pause. Cushny gave the standard explanation: the next regular impulse arriving at the ventricles finds them absolutely refractory. On this basis Cushny attempted to "fill in one hiatus existing between clinical observation and physiological experiment" by publishing two papers on the irregular pulse.[23] One was in the *Journal of Experimental Medicine*, but the other was intended to reach the wider audience that read the *British Medical Journal*. An intermittent pulse occurs either when the ventricles fail to respond to an impulse arriving from the auricles or when the auricles fail to emit pulses at the ordinary intervals. In the first instance the ventricles are refractory because they have experienced a premature contraction whose feeble contribution to the radial pulse can be seen in the sphygmogram. A double sound can also be heard at the beginning of the intermission. Therefore, the ventricular pause should be two times the normal interval between contractions. When the impulse from the auricles is irregular, the interval between ventricular contractions is shorter than twice the normal interval.

for Gley had published in 1889 a figure showing the determination of the refractory period of the dog's heart that is almost identical with Marey's.[18] In the first paragraph of his paper, Cushny cited some related papers but dismissed them because "their accounts show a number of [unspecified] discrepancies."[19]

One of those papers, a long confused and confusing one,[20] was by J. A. MacWilliam, professor of physiology at Aberdeen and therefore well known to Cushny. Another was by Langendorff, describing his method of maintaining the isolated mammalian heart

The Explanation of Delirium Cordis

At the beginning of his 1899 paper Cushny compared his observations on the dog's heart undergoing auricular fibrillation with the clinical condition delirium cordis, in which the pulse is utterly irregular. He did "not wish to assert that the clinical delirium cordis is identical with the physiological delirium auriculae, but the resemblance is certainly striking."[24] He did make the assertion shortly thereafter. On 29 December 1901 Charles W. Edmunds, an intern in the University Hospital, observed that a woman who had been operated upon five days earlier by Reuben Peterson had bouts of irregular pulse, and he consulted Cushny.[25] Cushny saw the patient the same day, and he made the diagnosis of intermittent auricular fibrillation. On 12 March 1902 Edmunds reported the case at a meeting of the Ann Arbor Medical Club, and Cushny commented. Edmunds and Cushny did not publish their observations and conclusions until 1906, when they published in a Festschrift for the professor of pathology at Aberdeen. The next year they published essentially the same paper in the more widely distributed *American Journal of the Medical Sciences*. The paper clearly demonstrated the correspondence between the irregular ventricular pulse observed in the patient (fig. 8–4) and the similar pulse seen in a dog (fig. 8–5) when auricular fibrillation is either spontaneous or induced by electrical stimulation.

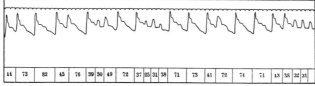

FIG 1.—Pulse tracing at 1.45 P.M. December 29.

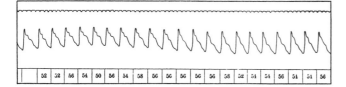

Fig. 8–4. Pulse tracings from Edmunds's patient taken with a sphygmochronograph. (From A. R. Cushny and C. W. Edmunds, "Paroxysmal Irregularity of the Heart and Auricular Fibrillation," *Am. J. Med. Sci.* 133 [1907]: 68.)

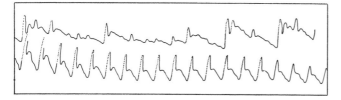

Fig. 8–5. Pulse tracing from dog's carotid taken with Hurthle's tonometer. The lower tracing is normal; the upper was taken during auricular fibrillation from rapid electrical stimulation of the auricle. (From A. R. Cushny and C. W. Edmunds, "Paroxysmal Irregularity of the Heart and Auricular Fibrillation," *Am. J. Med. Sci.* 133 [1907]: 75.)

Cushny and George Dock were good friends, and they sometimes "ran a century" by cycling the hundred miles to Detroit and back. Cushny was consulted by Dock on cardiological problems, but "Cushny fought, bled, and died trying to teach him [Dock] that delirium cordis was auricular fibrination,—he [Dock] made lots of polygraph tracings but couldn't convince himself, did not trust the dogs."[26]

James Mackenzie, the major authority on the pulse, could not know of Edmunds and Cushny's work when he published his book on the pulse in 1902.[27] He did cite Cushny's "admirable paper" of 1899 as confirming his conclusions of 1894.[28] Mackenzie failed to determine the cause of completely irregular pulse. When he found no auricular wave in his jugular sphygmogram he assumed the auricles were paralyzed. He wrote: "I have no clear idea of how the stimulus to contraction arises, and so cannot definitely say how the auricle modifies the ventricular rhythm. But as a matter of observation I can with confidence state that the heart has a very great tendency to irregular action when the auricles lose their power of contraction."[29]

Mackenzie eventually saw that the auricles were not paralyzed,[30] and he invented a condition called "nodal rhythm" to explain the supposed simultaneous contraction of auricles and ventricles. It was the recollection of Edmunds and Cushny's 1906 paper that convinced Thomas Lewis when he had the electrocardiographic evidence in hand that delirium cordis is caused by auricular fibrillation.[31]

Saline Catharsis

George Wallace was an instructor in pharmacology in 1897 after he had graduated from the University of Michigan Medical School.[32] At that time Cushny was writing his textbook of pharmacology,[33] and he had assembled a list of salts generally regarded as saline cathartics. When Wallace and Cushny looked over the list "it [was] apparent that the anion, or acid constituent of the salt, is generally the determining factor. Thus sodium sulphate, potassium sulphate, sodium phosphate, potassium tartrate, potassium-sodium tartrate, potassium citrate, potassium ferrocyanide, and sodium ferrocyanide, are all looked upon as cathartics, while sodium chloride, potassium chloride, sodium acetate, potassium acetate, etc., are believed to be indifferent so far as action on the bowel is concerned. . . . As regards the magnesium salts the basic constituent or cation would also seem to be involved."[34]

Wallace and Cushny used twenty-six salts of sodium, and they began by dissolving a salt in water and then diluting the solution until it had the same freezing point depression as a 1 percent solution of sodium chloride. Thus, all solutions were essentially isotonic to begin with. They injected fifteen to thirty-five milliliters into tied-off loops, thirty to forty-five centimeters long, of small intestine of anesthetized cats or dogs. As a control they tested the ability of each loop to absorb the 1 percent solution of sodium chloride quickly. At the end of thirty, forty, or sixty minutes they removed the residual solution and measured its volume. They calculated the rate of absorption of the solution, but they did not measure the rate of absorption of the solute. Some of their solutions, those of sodium fluoride and oxalate, were obviously toxic, and some, those of nitrate, were irritating. Setting aside results obtained with toxic or irritating solutions, Wallace and Cushny concluded that "[d]ilute solutions (isotonic) of the saline cathartics retard the absorption of fluid from the stomach and small intestine, and thus act by rendering the contents more watery and more easily moved through the lower parts of the alimentary canal."[35]

Renal Catharsis

If Cushny is remembered at all it is for his *Secretion of the Urine*.[36] When Ernest Starling persuaded Cushny to write that book Cushny had not worked on renal physiology for years, and in preparation for writing Cushny merely read and thought. His own two papers on the kidney had been written years before when he was still in Ann Arbor. Cushny's attention was first drawn to the subject by his observation that chloride excretion in the urine is greatly increased during phlorhizin glucosuria. This suggested to Cushny that when fluid is flowing rapidly through the renal tubules less time is available for reabsorption of chloride. To test this idea Cushny devised an experiment in which he could increase the time available for tubular reabsorption.[37]

Ludwig had proposed that an ultrafiltrate of plasma is expressed from the glomerular capillaries and that it is partially reabsorbed by osmosis in the tubules.[38] Because the composition of bladder urine is different from an ultrafiltrate of plasma, Cushny concluded that the tubules must be differentially per-meable to the constituents of the glomerular filtrate. Thus, the tubules share the property Wallace and Cushny had already demonstrated to be present in the intestine. Cushny tested the permeability of the tubules by partially obstructing the ureter, making the urine flow from it against a pressure of thirty millimeters of mercury. This, he thought, gave a longer time for reabsorption to occur within the renal tubules. The extent of reabsorption could be determined by comparing the composition of the urine from the obstructed ureter with that of the free-flowing urine caught from the unobstructed ureter of the other kidney. In order to make the flow particularly rapid, Cushny established diuresis by intravenous infusion of equimolar mixtures of sodium chloride and sodium sulfate or sodium chloride and urea. Thus, Cushny's experiment was a partial version of the stopped-flow experiment performed at Michigan fifty-four years later.[39]

Cushny found that when he infused sulfate, there was less chloride from the urine of the obstructed kidney than from the normal one. Therefore, there was differential reabsorption of the two anions, and sulfate was relatively less able to penetrate the renal tubules. More chloride was reabsorbed from the slowly flowing than from the rapidly flowing urine. Because sulfate and chloride are not reabsorbed at the same rates, reabsorption of ions from the tubular urine cannot be explained by the process of diffusion Ludwig had invoked. Cushny said: "Some unknown force causing a current from the lumen towards the blood must be assumed here exactly as in the intestine."[40]

Because sulfate is poorly reabsorbed from the renal tubule, just as it is poorly absorbed by the intestine, it retards absorption of water and promotes diuresis. Cushny found that when he infused urea intravenously less urea was reabsorbed than chloride. It too causes diuresis by osmotic retention of water.

Cushny turned his attention to reabsorption of cations as the means by which urine is acidified. This work was done just before Sørensen developed the concept of pH and before the theory of indicators was entirely worked out. Although Cushny did not use the pH terminology, he displayed a grasp of the way indicators reveal the acidity of a solution and the ionization of acids. The urine is never alkaline to phenolphthalein nor acid to methyl orange; the interval corresponds to the ionization of mono- and disodium phosphate. For the urine to be acidified there must be a salt in the glomerular filtrate that is capable of hydrolysis, the cation penetrating the tubular wall more readily than the anion. Hydrogen ions replace the cation removed from the tubular fluid, and the urine is thus acidified. Phosphate alone of all salts examined fulfills these conditions completely. Bicarbonate does not, because it is completely reabsorbed. Sulfate does not, because it fails to penetrate the tubule and it holds back sodium. Otherwise the urine would contain sulfuric acid. Had the concept of pK_a been presented to Cushny, he would have exclaimed: "That is what I am trying to say!"

Cushny's Teaching

The pharmacology Cushny taught can be recaptured from his laboratory manual and his textbook.

Cushny inherited Abel's schedule of lecturing five hours a week throughout the third year. In 1894 he was able to offer an optional course in practical pharmacology, four afternoons a week for six weeks. This was paired with the optional course in practical physiology, and it was the one Wiggers wanted to take. Wiggers, however, was employed by Cushny to smoke kymograph drums and to set up apparatus for other students to use.

By Cushny's last year at Michigan, 1904–5, there were the same lectures throughout the third year, but as college courses were being squeezed out of the earlier years of the medical curriculum there was room in the second year for two laboratory courses. One, a course in pharmacognosy and prescription writing, was given by C. W. Edmunds, and he was helped by Elija Houghton, a Michigan bachelor of pharmaceutical chemistry and doctor of medicine who was research director of Parke, Davis and Company. Students were examined:

Prescribe: a. Chloral and opium for sleeplessness
            b. An antipyretic
            c. . . .
            d. Iron in chlorosis

and so on.

The year after Cushny left Ann Arbor, Edmunds published *Laboratory Guide in Experimental Pharmacology,* derived from the course developed by Cushny.[41] The course contained a full set of experiments on frogs, dogs, and rabbits, demonstrating the actions of narcotics, diuretics, pilocarpine, muscarine, the belladonna series, and so forth, through a list

that might be studied today had pharmacology laboratory survived "curriculum reform." A notable feature was that students observed on themselves the action of amyl nitrite, strychnine, atropine, nitroglycerin, digitalis, and nicotine.

The content of Cushny's lectures is preserved in his *Textbook of Pharmacology and Therapeutics,* published in 1899.[42] This was the first of a long series of texts that would carry Michigan teaching of medical sciences worldwide, and it went through thirteen editions. Cushny said his object was "to show how far the clinical effects of remedies may be explained by their action on the normal body, and how these may in turn be correlated with physiological phenomena. It necessarily follows that the subject is treated from the experimental standpoint, and that the results of the laboratory investigator are made the basis of almost every statement."[43]

Cushny was not the first to make such an attempt in English. Lauder Brunton had been a student of Ludwig, and nearly half of his massive *Text-Book of Pharmacology, Therapeutics, and Materia Medica* was devoted to a description of the physiological action of drugs.[44] However, the second half was a compendium of outworn materia medica, and the book ended with a long list of drugs to be used in specific instances. Nymphomania, for example, was to be treated with bromide of potassium in large doses, with digitalis, or with sulfuric acid internally. The twenty-three remedies for peritonitis began with aconite and ended with *Veratrum viride.* Cushny cut this exposition of materia medica to a minimum, but he did not reach Osler's level of therapeutic nihilism.[45] His correlation with physiological phenomena was most successful in those instances in which science provided a firm foundation. His discussion of digitalis, based largely upon his own work, approached his ideal. So did that on ether and chloroform narcosis. On the other hand, in dealing with cod liver oil, he could only conclude that it "has not been shown to have any action apart from its being an easily digested food."[46]

Cushny's Successor

Late in 1904 Cushny was offered the professorship of pharmacology at University College London, and for some reason he was asked to begin on 1 May 1905. He resigned his Michigan job in March 1905. An anonymous editorial in the locally published *Physi-*

cian and Surgeon deplored his departure, its author stating that Cushny left in part because he was British but that he was also influenced by lack of facilities at the University of Michigan. He had not been given space in the new Medical Building; he had no fully equipped laboratory and no assistants; and he had too much teaching. Cushny stayed in London until 1918 when he, a Scot, was pleased to accept the professorship at Edinburgh, where he died at the age of sixty of heart disease.

Charles Wallis Edmunds, who had worked with Cushny since 1902, was put in charge of the department, and in 1907 he was made professor of materia medica and therapeutics. There is no evidence that Victor Vaughan looked for anyone else, but the evidence may be missing. Edmunds remained head of the department until his death in March 1941. He was secretary of the Medical School from 1911 to 1919, and in that position he carried on the routine business in Vaughan's frequent absences. One duty was to inform the numerous persons who wanted to sell their bodies to the Medical School that state law forbade such transactions.

Edmunds's Teaching and Staff

Pharmacology teaching remained much the same as it had been in Cushny's time throughout Edmunds's tenure. There were about ninety hours of lecture in the third year, and for many years these were supplemented by lectures on therapeutics in the fourth year. Mark Marshall, who was in charge of the Outpatient Clinic and whose primary appointment was in the Department of Internal Medicine, gave them. Eventually the subject was informally incorporated into the course, and the appointment of a clinician in pharmacology was dropped. Nevertheless, students complained in 1934 that they did not get enough on the treatment of pain, nausea, vomiting, diarrhea, and the like. There were introductory lectures in the second year to accompany the laboratory course. Work in the laboratory as demonstrated by successive editions of the Edmunds-Cushny laboratory manual remained much as Cushny had left it,[47] though by 1939 experiments on students themselves were reduced to their breathing three drops of amyl nitrite.

Edmunds always had a small staff, often no more than an instructor to handle pharmacy teaching and some medical students to help in the student labora-

tory. Over the years those assistants included A. C. Furstenberg, Arthur C. Curtis, Franklin Johnston, Perrin H. Long, and Carl Moyer. Some of them, Long and Moyer for instance, collaborated with Edmunds in research. Edmunds had a hard time recruiting staff, and he was not helped by Dean Cabot, who told President Burton in 1922 that pharmacology at Michigan had advanced very little in recent years and that its budget was too large. Edmunds did get a succession of undistinguished assistant professors who left after a few years for jobs in the Public Health Service or minor universities. The last was Ralph G. Smith, a doctor of philosophy from the University of Chicago, who helped Edmunds edit the *United States Pharmacopoeia*. In 1930 when Edmunds established a unit on drug addiction five or six persons were attached to the department in research capacities. There was no graduate program, perhaps because Edmunds believed pharmacologists should be doctors of medicine, not doctors of philosophy.[48] Until 1942 only one person earned a doctor's degree in materia medica.

In addition to the clinician who taught therapeutics, Edmunds's roster contained two others whose primary duties were elsewhere. One was H. W. Emerson, who ran the Pasteur Institute, and the other was Laura M. Davis, R.N., who was responsible for supervising administration of anesthesia in the hospital and for teaching anesthesia to medical students and nurse-anesthetists. After 1934 her appointment was transferred to the Department of Surgery, and her work will be described in connection with that department.

Edmunds as a Pharmacologist

At the time Edmunds became a pharmacologist T. R. Elliott had suggested that epinephrine, or adrenalin as almost everyone called it in disregard of the registered trademark status of the word, is a chemical transmitter at postganglionic sympathetic nerve endings.[49] No one knew that acetylcholine is the transmitter at the myoneural junction and at most parasympathetic effectors. Consequently, no one thought that a drug could act by blocking the action of a transmitter on the effector. Everyone thought atropine accelerates the heart by paralyzing the endings of vagal fibers to the myocardium, and Edmunds said: "For the last fifty years one of the first facts learned by students of physiology and pharmacology has been that curara caused a paralysis of the endings of the motor nerves."[50]

Physostigmine was a well-known drug, but the mechanism of its action, inhibition of choline esterase and prolongation of the life of acetylcholine, was yet to be discovered. The drug was said to increase excitability of muscle to slight stimuli or to slow the heart by rendering the vagus more excitable.[51] Consequently, Edmunds interpreted the action of other drugs in a similar manner.

When Edmunds became Cushny's assistant after finishing his internship, Cushny gave him the same training in pharmacology that Cushny had received from Schmiedeberg. *Lobelia inflata,* Indian tobacco, had been so extensively used by physicians of the Thompsonian sect that they had been called Lobelia doctors, and as Edmunds said some had stood trial for manslaughter resulting from fatal use of the drug. Edmunds prepared the active principle, some in crystalline form, from dried seeds given him by Parke, Davis, and Company, and he made a thorough pharmacological analysis of its action on frogs, turtles, cats, and dogs. In warm-blooded animals it was an emetic and a powerful respiratory stimulant. As for its action on the heart, Edmunds thought it first stimulated and then paralyzed sympathetic ganglia.[52]

Edmunds must have endeared himself to Victor Vaughan when he performed an elaborate analysis of Vaughan's protein poison.[53] Edmunds found the effects to be almost identical with those of anaphylactic shock. Because the poison caused a fall in blood pressure after the central nervous system had been completely destroyed and the sympathetic ganglia inactivated by large doses of nicotine, it must paralyze vasomotor endings on blood vessels.

Nevertheless, Edmunds reached a different kind of conclusion when he compared the effects of physostigmine on normally innervated and on denervated gastrocnemius muscle of Plymouth Rock hens. Innervated muscle began to contract ten to fifteen minutes after a large dose of physostigmine, and relaxation began at once if curare were given. However, denervated muscle also contracted in response to physostigmine, and it was far more sensitive than innervated muscle after the cut fibers had degenerated. Curare antagonized this action of physostigmine as well, and Edmunds concluded that both drugs act on the muscle substance itself.[54]

Edmunds did not follow up his new idea, nor could he quite free himself from the idea of nerve-ending paralysis. In October 1919 five persons died after a banquet in Grosse Pointe, Michigan, and H. W. Emerson identified botulism toxin in the ripe olives they had eaten.[55] This was only one episode in a nationwide epidemic of botulism resulting from consumption of improperly canned olives.[56] Edmunds, using toxin prepared by Emerson, found curare-like action on voluntary muscle, in particular the diaphragm. Poisoned animals died of asphyxiation, but a poisoned dog could be kept alive as long as three days by artificial respiration.[57] Likewise, the toxin blocked the action of parasympathetic nerves upon the heart, the salivary glands, and the eye. Therefore, botulinus toxin paralyzes the nerve endings to voluntary muscle and of the parasympathetic system. Edmunds had previously shown that epinephrine acts directly on smooth muscle,[58] and he found that muscle from the esophagus, stomach, and intestine of botulinus-poisoned animals reacts in normal fashion to physostigmine and epinephrine.[59]

Diphtheria

In the 1920s patients with diphtheria seldom died of suffocation; instead, some died suddenly of cardiovascular collapse. At that time Edmunds thought that continuous secretion of epinephrine by the adrenal medulla sustains arterial blood pressure, and he had worked extensively on what he called "adrenal exhaustion," by which he meant exhaustion of the adrenal medulla, not the cortex.[60] For example, when an animal was given injections of physostigmine, the epinephrine content of the adrenal glands fell to one-eighth the normal value, and the animal became lethargic and died.[61] However, in animals given diphtheria toxin, exhaustion of the adrenals occurred over several days, but collapse was sudden, a matter of an hour or two. Others thought digitalis would prevent collapse, but Edmunds found this not to be true.[62] In fact, dogs and cats became more sensitive to digitalis when they were poisoned by diphtheria toxin.[63] Strychnine and camphor were useless as well. Edmunds believed that collapse was the result of "distributive oligemia," pooling of blood in the large vascular bed of the abdomen caused by paralysis of the splanchnic nerves. Administration of isotonic saline solution did no good, and giving gum acacia suspension, gum acacia then being the only colloid available for such purposes, resulted in only temporary improvement. Instead, Edmunds gave a large volume of 10 percent dextrose, and he found the treatment lifesaving. His remedy was taken up at the Municipal Contagious Diseases Hospital in Chicago, where the expected mortality of patients with "malignant diphtheria" was 60 percent. Excluding two patients who died almost immediately after admission, mortality in eighty-one patients given dextrose was only 9.8 percent.

Morphine and Coffee

In the 1930s the National Research Council, supported first by the Bureau of Social Hygiene and then by the Rockefeller Foundation, began to search for a nonaddictive morphine substitute. Compounds were synthesized at the University of Virginia, assayed at the University of Michigan, and tested clinically by the Bureau of Narcotics. Work in Edmunds's department resulted in at least fifteen publications.[64] The first was a description of general methods, and subsequent papers described variations of the toxic effect of morphine, codeine, and seven derivatives with the age of the test animal. One paper reported results of 4,802 injections into 3,057 rabbits from 678 litters. The chief result of the program, discontinued in 1939, was to correlate chemical structure with physiological activity.

There was a slightly different motive behind another project occupying Edmunds's department in the 1930s. W. K. Kellogg's Seventh-Day Adventist brother, John Harvey Kellogg, the founder of the Battle Creek Sanatarium, believed that "[b]iologic living demanded total abstinence from alcohol, tea, coffee, chocolate, and tobacco." His biographer wrote that "if [J. H.] Kellogg did not succeed in converting all Americans to a vegetarian diet and in persuading them to discard coffee, tea, alcoholic beverages, and tobacco, it was not because he did not make a major effort in that direction."[65]

Although the brothers had quarreled bitterly by 1933, W. K. Kellogg, perhaps in the interest of promoting sale of his coffee substitute, gave the University of Michigan money to support a program of research on the physiological and psychological effects of coffee and caffeine. The result was a series of papers demonstrating that a dose of three to four milligrams per kilogram of caffeine or its equivalent in coffee caused an average increase of 8 to 9 percent in basal oxygen consumption of fourteen subjects, mostly medical students, an increase of five to ten

millimeters of mercury in arterial blood pressure, and a fall of five beats a minute in heart rate. The subjects' performance of a simple motor test improved, but there was a deleterious effect that lasted several days upon the performance of an acquired motor skill.[66] At least the program supported some deserving medical students, and William D. Robinson, later chair of the Department of Internal Medicine, and J. Robert Willson, later chair of the Department of Obstetrics and Gynecology, became coauthors of scientific papers early in their careers.

Edmunds as a Good Citizen of Pharmacology

When Edmunds died the heartiest tribute came from the Council on Pharmacy and Chemistry of the American Medical Association, praising his services to pharmacology.[67]

Medical students in Edmunds's early classes prepared and assayed extracts of digitalis. When Edmunds compared the students' extracts with those obtained from wholesale manufacturers and from retail druggists, he found potencies of sixteen preparations to differ by a factor of more than three.[68] The toxic dose of four samples from one supplier, one who did not himself assay his product, was 0.08, 0.19, 0.27, and 0.28 cubic centimeter. Another manufacturer, when confronted with discrepancies, admitted that he probably made mistakes in diluting his extracts. Still another said they "do not think it right to control the effect of their medicines on man by experiments on the lower animals."[69] Edmunds found the situation even worse when he assayed commercial preparations of ergot. An agreed method of assay was required, and Edmunds thought the U.S. Public Health Service might set the national standard. He wrote: "Perhaps the revisers of the next Pharmacopoeia may see their way clear to insert some such method [of assay], but for the present we are left helpless so far as they are concerned."[70]

Edmunds said that useless drugs were still listed in the Pharmacopoeia because general practitioners wanted to prescribe them.[71] Every time a drug was deleted there was a great outcry from both physicians and pharmaceutical manufacturers. The result was, as might be expected, that Edmunds himself set the standards of assay of digitalis and ergot for the Public Health Service, and eventually he supplied the standard preparations of digitalis for the entire country.[72] He became a member of the committee on assay and a member of the committee for revision of the Pharmacopoeia in 1910, chairman of the committee on assay and a member of the executive committee in 1920, and president just before his death. The trustees of the Pharmacopoeia gave him grants and sent fellows to work with him. Edmunds's meticulous comparisons of USP standard preparations with European standards brought him into conflict with J. H. Burn, J. H. Gaddum, and H. H. Dale, but he stood his ground.[73]

The Council on Pharmacy and Chemistry was founded by the American Medical Association in an effort "to rid therapeutics of the multitudinous so-called remedies which had been foisted upon it by commercial interests."[74] The council with Edmunds as a member from 1921 prepared *New and Non-official Remedies,* and in its work Edmunds was particularly valued because he could be depended upon and for his ability to bring harmony and compromise in a difficult situation.

Edmunds's Successor

Shortly after Edmunds's death in 1941 Dean Furstenberg appointed H. B. Lewis, Cyrus Sturgis, and Carl Weller as a committee to recommend a successor. Lewis reported on behalf of the committee on 22 July 1941. Maurice Seevers of Wisconsin, an expert on the pharmacology of anesthesia, was the best of a long list of candidates, but there were problems. Seevers had not made a favorable impression on some when he had visited Ann Arbor, and there was the possibility that he would display too-great aggressiveness in the question of management of anesthesia in the hospital. And there was the question of the position of Ralph G. Smith in the department if Seevers came. The committee had concluded that Smith was not good enough, and the school should find some way of compensating him for his disappointment.

The job was offered to Seevers. He accepted; Smith left for Tulane; and pharmacology at Michigan was off to a new start.

9
Anatomy

Corydon Ford (fig. 9–1) had been Michigan's professor of anatomy since 1854.[1] Lombard thought Ford was the best lecturer in anatomy the country had ever seen, and his opinion was shared by Will Mayo.[2] Ford had spent many hours preparing dissections to be demonstrated in his lectures, and he accumulated a notable collection of anatomical specimens that he gave to the university. However, he did no research. Vaughan changed that tradition by finding James Playfair McMurrich to be Ford's successor.

McMurrich's Preparation

Vaughan worked fast, for he was able to present McMurrich's name to the regents at their meeting on 11 June 1894. The appointment was approved by a vote of four to two. There were two reasons for the divided opinion. McMurrich was a zoologist who did not have the doctor of medicine degree, and some thought medical qualifications necessary for a teacher in a medical school. The second reason was that a local anatomist who wanted the job worked through a regent to oppose McMurrich's appointment. Here Vaughan's fine talent for academic intrigue prevailed, and the rival anatomist soon left to enter private practice. The struggle was not quite over, for the next year a regent proposed in the interest of economy to eliminate McMurrich's professorship by combining it with the chair of surgery. The proposal was defeated two to five.

J. Playfair McMurrich had been born in Toronto, the son of a Scottish businessman who had early emigrated to Canada and who attained enough success in Canadian politics to be known as the Honorable John McMurrich. Young McMurrich attended Upper Canada College, the Eton of the West, and he graduated from the University of Toronto in 1879. Consequently, he had a sound education in Greek and Latin. In the course of his professional life he became fluent in the modern European languages, and while he was in Ann Arbor he added Arabic so that he could follow the transmission of ancient anatomical knowledge through the Arabs to the Italians of the Renaissance.

McMurrich studied medicine for two years, but he did not complete his work for his doctor of medicine degree. Family tradition said the reason was "stomach trouble," but his record

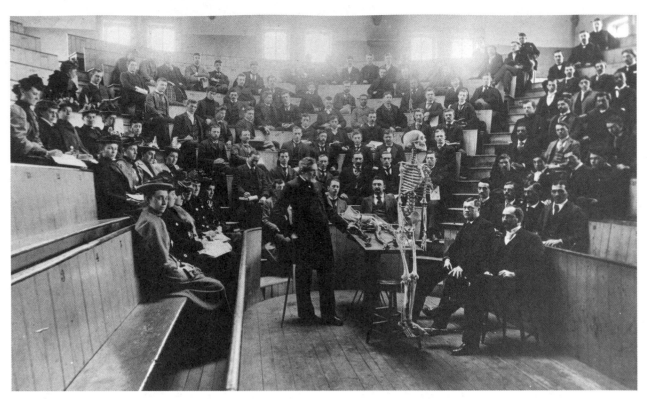

Fig. 9–1. Corydon Ford in the lecture room, old Medical Building. (Courtesy of the Department of Anatomy, University of Michigan.)

in medical school was undistinguished. In the second examination in the first year he was first in class I in physiology, but he placed ninth in class III in both anatomy and materia medica. The next year he placed first in class II in clinical medicine and clinical surgery, but he was third class in medicine, surgical anatomy, obstetrics, and pathology.[3] After briefly teaching biology at Guelph Agricultural College he moved to the more exciting intellectual atmosphere of the Johns Hopkins Graduate School. This was in 1884–85, long before the medical school opened with Franklin P. Mall as professor of anatomy. Since its founding in 1876 the Department of Biology had been directed by Newell Martin, who had enlisted William K. Brooks to be his second. Brooks, who had been trained at Harvard by Alexander Agassiz,[4] was an invertebrate zoologist, and he in turn trained many of the major U.S. biologists, E. B. Wilson, E. G. Conklin, and T. H. Morgan among them. McMurrich became familiar with the fauna of Chesapeake Bay, the North Carolina coast, and the Bahamas. In 1886, the year after receiving his doctor of philosophy degree,[5] he remained as instructor in

mammalian anatomy, and he wrote a note on the details of the hypoglossal nerve.[6] Then McMurrich taught at Haverford, being one of the few Johns Hopkins graduates in any field who did not serve for a while at Bryn Mawr. He was recruited by G. Stanley Hall to be a member of the initial faculty of Clark University, an institution Hall intended to be a "purer Hopkins."[7] There he was a colleague of Mall and Lombard. When the mass faculty resignations occurred in 1892 McMurrich had to find a job as professor of biology at the University of Cincinnati.

Although Alexander Agassiz's father, the great Louis Agassiz, had not believed in evolution, biology taught by Brooks was permeated with the doctrine. Consequently, McMurrich's work on invertebrate zoology, work he continued during his Michigan years by spending summers at Woods Hole, was no mere description of a few more species. His contributions to embryology and physiology of the actinozoa place the animals in the evolutionary sequence as they demonstrate the origin of the endoderm in the absence of gastrulation. The long papers are elegantly illustrated by foldout plates labeled *J.P.McM. del.*[8]

Not Just Any Medical School

Given McMurrich's industriousness, his zoological studies resulted in a 661-page *Text-Book of Invertebrate Morphology* written while he was teaching human anatomy at Michigan.[9]

McMurrich's Teaching at Michigan

At Michigan McMurrich displayed a mastery of gross anatomy that would meet any Scottish standard, and he quickly dispelled doubts about his competence. While he was in Ann Arbor he edited *Morris's Human Anatomy* and a three-volume translation of Johannes Sobotta's *Atlas der Anatomie des Menschen* (1906).[10] He was one of five contributors to Piersol's *Human Anatomy*,[11] and at the end of his time at Michigan he was president of the Association of American Anatomists. When he wrote his book on Leonardo's anatomy late in life he demonstrated utter familiarity with the details of human and comparative anatomy.

In his presidential address to the American Association of Anatomists[12] McMurrich said it was preposterous to expect medical students to master the details of human gross anatomy and that demonstrations in the manner of Corydon Ford and formal lectures on anatomy were medievalism rampant. The primary aim of elementary teaching should be to impart to students by observation and deduction the fundamental principles, leaving the details for later as the student encountered clinical problems. Nevertheless, under McMurrich the Michigan tradition of anatomical teaching was continued with ninety-six hours of lecture and eighty hours of recitation on osteology and descriptive anatomy in the first year. Students did, however, spend three hundred hours in seeing for themselves by dissection. McMurrich soon added a course in the anatomy of the nervous system, giving two lectures a week to accompany a laboratory course on the structure of the central and peripheral systems and special senses. Anatomy of the brain was taught from sheep, for human brains were hard to obtain. Gross anatomy spilled over into the second year, for medical students were given instruction in regional and surgical anatomy by the surgeon Cyrenus G. Darling. Second-year students were also offered an elective course in comparative anatomy. These courses were open to graduate students, but no doctor's degree in anatomy was earned at Michigan during McMurrich's tenure.

Although junior members of his department supervised much of the work in dissection, McMurrich displayed his interest in the minutiae of gross anatomy and his familiarity with the dissecting room by publishing notes on anomalies found in anatomical specimens: a case of crossed dystopia of the kidney, the occurrence of congenital adhesions in the iliac veins, and a pair of fully developed cervical ribs.[13]

McMurrich's Research and Medical History

McMurrich read at least two papers before the Catholepistemiad Club of the University of Michigan.[14] The first asserted his belief that Darwin had placed anatomy in relation to the other biological sciences and that anatomy was no longer tied to the apron strings of medicine. *The Origin of Species* was its Declaration of Independence. Anatomical problems were endless, and one was traced to the gradual increase in complexity in lower forms of life in order to understand the final complexity. To carry out this program McMurrich extended his phylogenetic studies to vertebrate forms. He collected early or embryonic specimens of amphibia and reptiles (including an iguana given him by Professor Reighard), and he studied them in hope of demonstrating "a detailed homology of the arm muscles in these groups and then to extend the homologies to the mammalian muscles."[15] Mammals he examined included the cat, the mouse, and the human. He cut and stained serial sections of the forearm of each, and he believed he had succeeded in "tracing with greater exactness the processes by which the final arrangement [of flexor muscles] has been acquired" (208). For example: "In the last or mammalian stage the flexores breves superficiales become transformed more or less completely into the tendons of the flexor sublimis, and as the scale is ascended, a gradually increasing amount of the superficial portion of the flexor communis separates to become continuous with these tendons, until, in man, the entire condylar portion of the muscle, except so much as is represented by the palmaris longus, is taken up into the flexor sublimis" (208). With equal thoroughness and in three equally massive papers McMurrich described the phylogeny of the palmar musculature, the flexors of the leg, and the plantar musculature.[16]

In his second Catholepistemiad Club paper McMurrich began his historical publications. Vesalius had been accused of plagiary by Estienne, and McMurrich cleared him of that ancient charge. More recently one E. Jackschath of Tilsit had tried to demonstrate that *De fabrica corporis humani* was, in fact, merely a transcription of a complete textbook of anatomy written by Leonardo da Vinci.[17] McMurrich's paper demolished the claim, and it was the seed from which his book on Leonardo grew. At the time of McMurrich's retirement George Sarton persuaded him to do a thorough job on the subject. McMurrich responded with a definitive analysis of Leonardo's drawings, showing what, for example, had been observed during dissection of a human subject and what had been interpolated from dissection of animals.[18]

G. L. Streeter's Background

In 1907 McMurrich was offered the professorship of anatomy at Toronto, and he resigned his Michigan job. Victor Vaughan turned once more to Johns Hopkins University for McMurrich's successor. Franklin P. Mall recommended George Linius Streeter, and Streeter, after a visit to Ann Arbor on which he made a favorable impression, was duly appointed professor of anatomy by the regents on 20 July 1907.

After graduating from Union College in 1895 Streeter became a medical student at the College of Physicians and Surgeons in New York City. "P & S," as it was usually called, had been nominally associated with Columbia University since 1861, but it had become an integral part of the university only in 1891. The medical curriculum had been lengthened to four years only the year before, and the faculty experienced considerable anguish over the decline in entering students, for the four-year curriculum drove students to less demanding schools.[19] In Streeter's time as a student at P & S, John G. Curtis, a gentleman and a scholar but an unproductive scientist, was professor of physiology. Reid Hunt and Frederic S. Lee were tutors in physiology, but Streeter was most deeply impressed by George S. Huntington, a surgeon who also taught anatomy.[20]

Streeter interned for a year at the Roosevelt Hospital, and then he returned to Albany to practice neurology. During the two years he was in Albany, Streeter demonstrated anatomy of the nervous system at the Albany Medical College. In 1901 he determined to improve his skill as a neurologist by

studying in Germany. He began, apparently at Mall's suggestion, to study with Ludwig Edinger in Frankfurt. Like many Americans who went to Europe for clinical training, Lombard and Mall among them, Streeter quickly abandoned the clinic for the scientific laboratory.

In Frankfurt Streeter found three ostrich spinal cords in the collection of Dr. Senkenberg's Anatomical Institute. He wrote at the beginning of a paper describing the cords: "It is related by Herodian how the Kaiser Commodus beheaded ostriches and then watched them with delight and wonder as they continued running about the amphitheater, apparently to no great extent inconvenienced by the loss of their heads. . . . What is, then, this arrangement of nervous elements of the spinal cord of a bird that enables it to functionate so completely after separation from the higher centers?"[21] Streeter found a great tumorlike enlargement, or locomotor brain, in the spinal cord corresponding to the massive leg musculature. Using other material from the same Frankfurt collection, Streeter tried to determine how much the surface anatomy that can be seen on the floor of the fourth ventricle reveals of the underlying structures. He made a careful drawing of the floor in an adult human brain hardened in formalin, and then he made serial sections two or four millimeters thick. As an example, he found that "[l]ying against the median line in the caudal half of the floor is an oval elevation, 5.2 × 1 mm. This represents the rounded frontal end of the hypoglossal nucleus, and may therefore be called the '*eminentia hypoglossi*.'"[22] And so on.

That was Streeter's last work with adult tissues, for when he went to Leipzig he fell under the influence of Wilhelm His, who had previously converted Mall into an embryologist. When Mall's work had contradicted the conclusions of His about the origin of the thymus gland His had written Mall's paper in German and had published it in his own journal. Later, convinced that Mall had been right, His published a retraction of his own views. That kind of generosity was passed on by Mall to Streeter. Streeter's interest in embryology was strengthened by subsequent work with Oscar Hertwig in Berlin. When Streeter returned to the United States in 1902 Mall made him first an assistant and then an instructor in Mall's department of anatomy at Johns Hopkins. There Streeter's young colleagues included Florence Sabin and Ross G. Harrison. With Mall's encouragement Streeter began work in experimental amphibian embryology and descriptive human embryology. After four years at Johns Hopkins Streeter became associate professor at the Wistar Institute in Philadelphia,[23] then directed by the Hopkins-trained neurologist H. H. Donaldson, who had been a colleague of Mall and Lombard at Clark University. Streeter seems to have taken the Wistar Institute job for the reason that there was no prospect of academic advancement at Johns Hopkins, and it may have been the same ambition that drove him to accept the job at Michigan the next year. At the age of thirty-four Streeter came to Ann Arbor to be responsible for gross anatomy as G. Carl Huber was responsible for microscopic anatomy.

Streeter's Michigan Teaching

Throughout Streeter's time at Michigan every hour of the morning, five days a week in the first year, was given over to lectures and dissection in gross anatomy. The only relief was provided by a few lectures at eleven o'clock on physiology in the second term. Streeter was a lucid lecturer, and he used many teaching aids of his own devising. He projected stained celloidin sections of tissues like lantern slides, and he thought extra sections might be exchanged with other medical schools. He also projected flat mounts of the semilunar valves, and he preserved and mounted laryngeal cartilage for demonstration.[24]

Streeter had a staff of seven to help him. There was always Cyrenus Darling to teach surgical anatomy. A demonstrator was responsible for preserving cadavers—often enlisting the help of the janitor to do so—and for supervising dissection. Until 1909 the demonstrator was Simon Yutzy, who held the job for many years. Several graduate physicians helped a year or so before moving on, and there were usually four or more medical students, often one a woman, who acted as assistants in the dissecting rooms. Over the years one medical student, Rollo McCotter, worked his way up to become a professor, and he eventually took charge of dissection. Graduate students in anatomy were something new at Michigan. At the end of Streeter's period one of the student teachers in gross anatomy was Wayne J. Atwell, who, instead of going on to earn a doctor of medicine degree, earned a doctor of philosophy and became professor of anatomy at Buffalo.

Streeter was not primarily a gross anatomist, but he took his job seriously. The first thing he did was

to clean up the Anatomical Laboratory, using plenty of soap and water, and the next thing he did was to permit men and women to work together at the same table.[25] In the early days Michigan, like every other medical school, had great trouble procuring cadavers,[26] but as the result of the legislature's 1909 revision of the Anatomical Act of 1875 Michigan legally and relatively cheaply received more than one hundred bodies a year. Streeter thought that "[t]he character of the dissection material together with a well lighted and well arranged dissection room are about the only factors for which the student is clearly dependent upon the teacher."[27] The dissection material should be fully saturated to the point of edema so that the areas not directly reached by the vascular system will be preserved by diffusion. This is particularly important, for a large number of bodies are those of elderly individuals with sclerotic arteries and frequent thromboses. Streeter devised a method of injecting twenty to thirty quarts of embalming fluid under pressure, and he thought the apparatus so foolproof that their janitor or "any ordinary janitor" could use it without assistance. Streeter agreed with Mall that the student, once provided with a suitable cadaver, should learn on his or her own. He reduced the number of lectures and increased the hours of dissection. He wrote a tiny manual of sixty-eight octavo pages[28] designed to guide the student through the dissection of three regions: extremities; abdomen and pelvis; and head, neck, and thorax. Each region was to be dissected in eight weeks. The manual admonished the student on almost every line: "Read . . . Study . . ." Students followed that advice, for the pages of the one surviving copy are covered with textbook page numbers written against the name of every part.

Having adequate anatomical material, Streeter assembled collections of bones to be lent to students. Fat was sweated out of the bones in a drying oven, and then, after they had been rinsed in gasoline, the bones were bleached in potassium permanganate followed by sulfurous acid. Durability of fragile bones was increased by immersion in melted paraffin. By the end of Streeter's tenure there were fifty half-skeletons in the loan collection.

Streeter's Amphibian Embryology

The frequency of Streeter's publications fell off when he was in Ann Arbor, but it is clear that he accomplished a great deal of research while he was a teacher and an administrator. A long paper published in 1914 describes the completion of a study begun at Johns Hopkins on the development of the ear of the tadpole.[29] The work was begun as an attempt to trace the central acoustic path after unilateral or bilateral extirpation of the auditory vesicle and ganglion. Streeter saw that extirpation produced definite abnormalities in behavior, and consequently he shifted for a while to a study of equilibration. In the tadpole the ear vesicles are essential for development of the power of equilibration, but in normal specimens well-developed equilibration is present before the completion of the semicircular canals that must, therefore, be inessential. When one ear vesicle is removed the remaining vesicle performs the work of both so that the casual observer would mistake the tadpole for a normal individual. If both vesicles are removed, the animal is completely unable to maintain equilibration.

Streeter transplanted ear vesicles. He wrote: "The experiments were carried out on larvae of Rana pipiens . . . at the end of the non-motile stage. . . . The ear consists of an invaginated saucer-shaped mass of cells just in the process of being pinched off from the deeper layer of the skin. . . . Two larvae are removed from their gelatinous capsules and placed side by side in distilled water, under a binocular microscope. With two no. 12 embroidery needles, a linear transverse incision is made through the ectoderm of one of the specimens over the site of the ear vesicle, . . . the right side of the animal always being used for the operation. The lips of the wound are [then] gently everted, . . . which discloses the thin lateral wall of the vesicle. . . . With the needles the vesicle is now loosened from its pocket and cast away. This leaves an empty pocket, free for the transplantation. The right vesicle of the second specimen is uncovered in a similar way, loosened from its pocket and then slipped into the empty right auditory pocket of the first specimen. . . . The lateral and median surfaces of the vesicle are easily recognized and therefore this transplantation in a reversed posture can be done with great accuracy. . . . The specimen is now set aside and in the course of three or four hours all traces of the wound have disappeared. The specimens are allowed to go on with their development for fourteen days, the period usually necessary for the formation of the canals, at the end of which time they are preserved in a chrome-acetic mixture and are ready for examination. . . . Wax-plate models after the Born method were made of them all."[30]

Wax models of more than thirty labyrinths showed Streeter that the primitive ear vesicle is specialized so that when it is removed from its natural relations and placed in a new environment it continues to differentiate into a structure resembling the normal labyrinth in a normal attitude in reference to the brain. If a left-sided vesicle is transplanted to the right, it develops with an anterior-posterior position as though it were rotated 180 degrees. A vesicle transplanted upside down ends as a labyrinth right side up. Streeter dismissed the possibility that the cells are undifferentiated at the time of the operation and that they subsequently differentiate in accordance with how they chance to lie. This cannot be the case, for they are already differentiated into left and right. Cells of the upside down vesicle actually rotate to achieve the correct ventral-dorsal relation. This movement cannot be influenced by gravity, for the embryo with its labyrinth removed always lies on its side. If gravity were the controlling force, all ear vesicles would turn into obliquely placed labyrinths, but they do not. Nerves and a ganglion grow from the transplanted vesicle and establish complete nervous connections between the labyrinth and brain at an abnormal place. There is no evidence that the labyrinth has any functional ability.

Streeter's Human Embryology

By the time Streeter arrived at Johns Hopkins, Mall's interest had shifted from the vasculature and lymphatic drainage of the stomach and from the functional ability of reversed segments of the small intestine to human embryology. A human embryologist has trouble obtaining accurately dated and well-preserved specimens. Mall was very proud of his "embryo no. 2," and he took it with him to Germany as a present for Wilhelm His. His refused to take it and instead gave Mall some of his own material. That must have been passed on to Streeter, for when Streeter published his first paper on human embryology he said the material was provided by Oscar Hertwig, His, and Mall.[31]

Streeter studied the development of the cranial and spinal nerves in the occipital region of thirteen embryos, 4.0 to 65 millimeters long. Their ages were estimated by Mall's rule: the age in days equals the square root of the greatest length in millimeters times ten.[32] They were, therefore, twenty to eighty-one days old. The nature of the work can be judged from a quotation: "In tracing out [the] early history [of the eleventh cranial nerve] it becomes more than ever apparent that it is absolutely similar and continuous with the tenth or vagus nerve. In the embryo these exist, not as two independent cranial nerves, but rather as parts of a single structure, each part possessing mixed motor and sensory roots with root ganglia derived from the same ganglion crest."[33]

For his next work Streeter went slightly anterior to study the development of the membranous labyrinth, acoustical nerve, and facial nerves in the human embryo.[34] This paper like all of Streeter's other publications was illustrated by his own drawings. His problem was to show the relations among three-dimensional objects. His outline drawings are crisp and dramatic, and others are so subtly shaded that they themselves appear three dimensional. The reader cannot possibly misunderstand Streeter. The drawings in Streeter's Johns Hopkins papers were prepared "under the guidance of Mr. Max Brödel," the greatest of medical illustrators, but Brödel obviously had an apt pupil.

At Michigan Carl Huber was collecting human embryos for his study of the development of the kidney, and he gave Streeter a particularly fine one 10.2 millimeters long. It had no clinical history, but Streeter estimated it to be thirty-one days old. He made five-micron serial sections and reconstructed the embryo and its parts by the wax plate method. His first brief publication demonstrated that the rhombic grooves on the floor of the fourth ventricle of that embryo and of embryos of other species of corresponding age are a reality and not an artifact of preservation.[35] Then Streeter published a detailed description of the embryo's brain and spinal cord, cranial nerves, nerves of the special sense organs, somatic muscle groups, spinal nerves, and sympathetic system (fig. 9–2).[36] All this was done with no grant support.

The German embryologist Franz Keibel together with Franklin P. Mall edited a massive two-volume *Manual of Human Embryology* that was published simultaneously in German and English.[37] Keibel translated the chapters originally written in German, and J. Playfair McMurrich translated the German ones into English. Streeter's contribution was a long chapter on the nervous system illustrated with drawings from his own publications and with fresh ones.

By 1911 Mall had accumulated 533 human embryos, 335 normal and 198 pathological.[38] Three

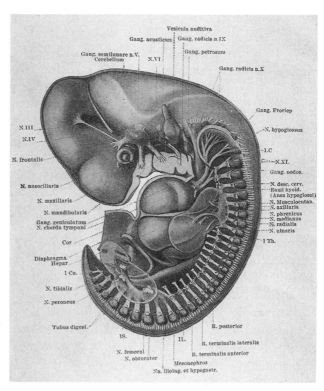

Fig. 9–2. Streeter's embryo. (From G. L. Streeter, "The Peripheral Nervous System in the Human Embryo at the End of the First Month (10 mm.)," *Am. J. Anat.* 8 [1908]: plate 1 following p. 301.)

hundred had been given him by Maryland doctors, but one had been sent from Denver by Henry Sewall. Mall said: "Gross anatomy as a science is bankrupt. It is made solvent through embryology, which alone illuminates it."[39] He made a plea for an institute of human embryology: "We should have anatomic institutes for research, not in a vague way, as in the universities, but for specific investigations which are beyond the reach of a single individual or university department."[40] The plea was heard by the Carnegie Institution of Washington, and the institution established in 1914 a laboratory of human embryology in Baltimore with Mall as director. Streeter accepted Mall's offer to become associate director, and he left Michigan, where teaching and administration conflicted with what he believed to be the highest human activity: scientific research. Three years later Mall died at the age of fifty-five following a cholecystectomy, and Streeter became director of the laboratory until 1941. During his tenure he built up the world's greatest collection of human embryological material, adequately preserved and accurately dated. His own work was so perfect that it superseded all others.[41]

Rollo McCotter

To replace Streeter the university made Carl Huber director of the Anatomical Laboratory as well as director of the Histological Laboratory. Thereafter until his death in 1934 Huber was in effect head of a single department of anatomy. Of the two divisions, that responsible for gross anatomy had the larger teaching load and the smaller intellectual interest. Huber depended upon Rollo Eugene McCotter to carry the burden of gross anatomy.

McCotter taught in the dissection room in both his junior and senior years as a medical student at Michigan, and because teaching prevented his attending surgical clinics, McCotter's degree was delayed until February 1910. After that McCotter was an instructor in anatomy for a while, and then he entered private practice in a small Michigan town. Finding practice unsatisfying, McCotter accepted a call from Vanderbilt University to improve its teaching of anatomy, histology, and embryology. He stayed at Vanderbilt only a year, for as soon as Huber became head of anatomy he brought McCotter back to Ann Arbor to supervise gross anatomy. McCotter did that until he died in 1946.

McCotter had begun teaching under Streeter, and Streeter encouraged him to do research. His first paper was on the connections of the vomeronasal nerves with the accessory olfactory bulb in the opossum.[42] It began with an exhaustive review of the literature, demonstrating that Michigan's library was good. McCotter made serial sections of the snouts of the opossum and rat, and he made fresh dissections by dividing the heads of those and nine other species to one side of the midsagittal plane. He examined the fresh specimens under water with a binocular microscope. He found that the accessory olfactory bulb is a ganglion mass receiving fibers from the vomeronasal organ and giving off fibers centrally to join the lateral olfactory tract. He thought that in addition to olfactory fibers and vomeronasal fibers there might be a third group of fibers in the olfactory nerve. That third group, the fibers of the nervus terminalis, was the chief subject of subsequent research.

McCotter found in the dog and cat "a slender ganglionated nerve which in its position and character corresponds completely with the nervus terminalis as described by previous authors in lower forms. . . . Connected with [the olfactory bulb] are several small bundles that usually unite into a single trunk which extends caudoventralward on the medial sur-

face of the olfactory peduncle where it appears to enter the brain substance some distance from the olfactory bulb."[43] In the other direction the filaments extend into the nasal cavity and terminate within or very close to the vomeronasal organ. McCotter found ganglion cells within this extension of the nervus terminalis.

A little later McCotter described what he found in several human fetuses and in two adult heads.[44] There the nervus terminalis is essentially the same as in other mammals. In the adult stage the human has no vomeronasal apparatus, and the fibers of the nervus terminalis, after passing through the cribriform plate, are distributed to the nasal mucosa.

McCotter's work stimulated Huber and his graduate student Stacey R. Guild.[45] On account of his extensive work on the sympathetic nervous system Huber was familiar with ganglion cells, and he concluded that "[i]f we consider only the peripheral distribution of the [nervus terminalis], the size of the component fibers, its arrangement in loose plexus, character, number and disposition of associated ganglion cell groups, we should favor ascribing to it an autonomic function."[46]

During McCotter's and Huber's lifetimes the central connections and the messages the nervus terminalis carries were not identified, but they have been worked out by means of techniques unavailable to McCotter and Huber.[47]

McCotter's Teaching

Huber preempted the nervus terminalis, and during World War I he took away all McCotter's glassware for his own research on regeneration of nerves.[48] McCotter never returned to research, and he contented himself with diligent teaching of gross anatomy for the next twenty-eight years.[49]

By the time McCotter returned from Vanderbilt, teaching of bacteriology in the first year had expanded to occupy afternoons from March to the end of the academic year. Gross anatomy filled the afternoons from September to March and then shifted to the mornings. It was followed by regional, topographic, and surgical anatomy in the second year. Throughout McCotter's tenure there were between 78 and 90 hours of lecture on gross anatomy and 225 to 320 hours in the dissection room. Regional and topographic anatomy used 40 to 64 hours of lecture and 66 to 80 hours for laboratory. In addition McCotter had the responsibility for teaching gross anatomy to dental students although junior members of the department usually did much of that work. Eventually he provided short courses for students of nursing and physical education. He gave even shorter courses for students of speech and sculpture. One result of the latter was that the Mormon sculptor Avard Fairbanks presented a doctor of philosophy thesis, "Anatomical Design," in 1936, illustrated in his romantic-realist style. Fairbanks also made a bust of Huber and numerous plaster illustrations of dissections that littered the department until the 1980s. McCotter shared teaching of surgical anatomy first with Darling and then with Cabot and Coller. One can imagine that busy surgeons left much of the work to McCotter, who also taught residents in ophthalmology.[50] Then there was always the summer session with forty or more students of gross anatomy. In 1936–37 McCotter's students totaled 578, and in the 1930s between four hundred and five hundred bodies were used each year. By this time Streeter's janitor had been replaced by a full-time embalmer, but McCotter had the task of keeping accurate records, supervising the cremation of remains, such as they were, and seeing to it that the ashes had Christian burial in the university's graveyard plot. All in all, McCotter was responsible for more than fourteen thousand cadavers.

Like McMurrich, McCotter reported dissection room findings. His first paper, written while he was still a medical student, described the occurrence of a pulmonary artery arising from the thoracic aorta.[51] The paper contains a characteristically thorough review of the literature, citing cases of accessory pulmonary arteries in man and lower vertebrates, including reptiles and amphibians, and it analyzed the possible causes of the anomaly on the basis of embryological development. McCotter's method of dissecting the back made it easy to determine the relations between the neural segments of the spinal medulla and the vertebrae, and McCotter published measurements found in 234 dissections, thereby dotting quantitatively an anatomical *i*.[52] McCotter reviewed fifty-seven references in a paper describing two cases of persistence of the left superior vena cava he had found in the dissecting room at Vanderbilt set aside for African American students and another he had found at Michigan. "In the first case, there is a persistence of the primitive venous system—the cardinal veins—without an apparent attempt at the metamorphosis to the adult condition. In the second case the left superior vena cava not only has the usual origin, course, and termination of this vein but also communicates by a large oval foramen with the left atrium. The left superior vena cava in case three terminates in the left superior pulmonary vein."[53]

McCotter pointed out that two superior venae cavae are the rule in ruminants and rodents. When he told the story to the Clinical Society of the University of Michigan someone asked if the anomaly caused murmurs. McCotter had not heard any in his subjects.

10
Microscopic Anatomy
and Neuroanatomy

Howell and Lombard each had the title professor of histology as well as professor of physiology, but after 1887 G. Carl Huber carried the burden of histology. Huber was appointed assistant demonstrator of anatomy immediately after graduation from medical school in 1887, and he was made instructor in histology in 1889 (fig. 10–1). Thereafter until his death in 1934 Huber taught microscopic anatomy.

Before Howell came to Ann Arbor, Huber had published only one short paper on the vexed question of the identity of phthisis or consumption with tuberculosis.[1] For generations there had been a controversy whether they are one or two diseases. In Huber's student days the official Michigan doctrine as expressed by Professor Palmer was "[t]hat pulmonary phthisis is a perversion of nutrition in the lungs, . . . but in a majority of cases, though probably not in all, during the progress of this inflammation and caseation, true tubercle is developed, invading the lung tissue, becoming itself caseous, and aiding in producing destructive changes in the organs."[2] Huber worked under the direction of Heneage Gibbes, the pathologist who did not believe the tubercle bacillus causes tuberculosis, and he found that caseous degeneration and tubercle formation were never intermixed in sixteen cases of lung disease.

Howell and Huber

Howell and Huber must have hit it off at once, for they were able to publish a short paper together in 1891 on the physiology of the communicating branch between the superior and inferior laryngeal nerves.[3] The paper is short, but it is packed with information derived from acute and chronic experiments. Howell and Huber found that the sensory fibers from the trachea travel and then branch upward into the communicating branch.

While they were doing that work Howell and Huber embarked on an elaborate piece of research on nerve degeneration and regeneration in competition for a prize of $250 offered by the American Physiological Society. The money was donated by the society's president, the neurologist S. Weir Mitchell. Using dogs under ether anesthesia Howell and Huber cut,

101

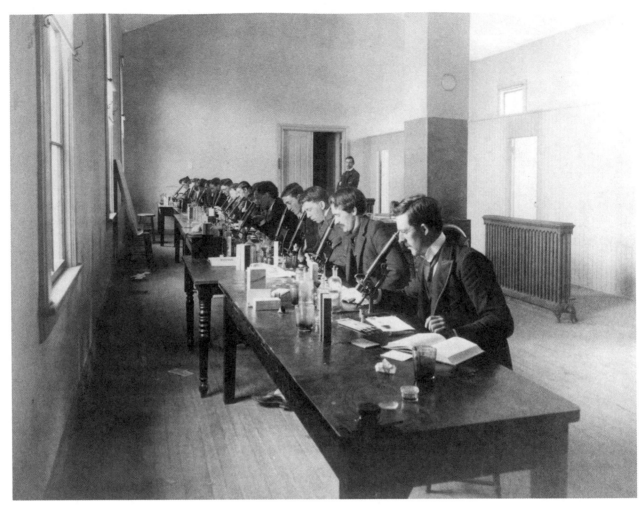

Fig. 10–1. Instructor in histology, probably Carl Huber, and students using the microscopes purchased by Stowell. Histology was variously associated with pathology, physiology, and anatomy. (Courtesy of the Bentley Historical Library, University of Michigan, Medical School Records, Box 136, "Gibson #2.")

crushed, or coagulated the ulnar nerve on one side. After a certain time the animals were examined. Howell and Huber found that healing never occurred by first intention, that the nerve below the lesion completely lost its function in four days, that regeneration is evident first at twenty-one days, that it spreads centrifugally with great slowness, and that sensory nerves recover before motor ones.[4] Though they did not know they were working with cholinergic nerves, they were able to get union with return of function when they anastomosed the central portion of the ulnar nerve with the distal portion of the median nerve, both cholinergic. They won the prize.

Their papers are illustrated with numerous drawings of degenerating and regenerating nerves. Those must have been made by Howell. Huber fixed,

embedded, and sectioned the specimens, but he left for Berlin before they could have been studied. Perhaps it was this experience of working with a first-class scientist, fresh from the heady atmosphere of Johns Hopkins, that determined Huber to get some real training as a neuroanatomist. In any event, he spent the academic year 1891–92 in the Microscopic Division of the Physiological Institute in Berlin.

Huber's Berlin Training

Huber settled into lodgings in Berlin in the early autumn, and to occupy his time before the term began he saw at least forty postmortem examinations, finding German methods to be different from those at home.[5] At first Wilhelm Waldeyer, one of the greatest anatomists of the day, refused Huber a place in his laboratory, and Huber arranged to study microscopic anatomy under Privatdozent Carl Benda. At a second meeting Waldeyer treated Huber most cordially and invited him to work in his private laboratory on the microanatomy of the inner ear. Thereafter for the first semester Huber was at the institute from 8 A.M. to 6 P.M. six days a week. He attended lectures by many anatomists, but most of his time was spent in the laboratories of Benda and Waldeyer. He must have done well, for at the end of his stay Benda's chief diener (laboratory man-of-all-work), always the one best informed about a student's performance, told Huber that there was hardly another as good as he. The next term he rose even earlier, beginning his university work at 7 A.M. He continued with Benda and Waldeyer, but he was also given places in the laboratories of Oscar Hertwig and Paul Ehrlich. When he returned to Ann Arbor in the late summer of 1892 Huber had been thoroughly immersed in the best microscopic anatomy and embryology Berlin had to offer.

Huber's Early Research at Michigan

In Ann Arbor Huber began work on the structure of the autonomic nervous system, and he continued it for years. His favorite dye was methylene blue. He either soaked freshly excised tissue in a solution of methylene blue or injected it intravenously before he killed the animal. He also used the Golgi silver precipitation method. Cells of the spinal or dorsal roots and ganglia had been found to be round or oval with a single process that divides into two branches. The cells of sympathetic ganglia were known to be multipolar, having one axis cylinder and numerous protoplasmic branches. Huber said the two types were not to be confused. He found the latter type in the numerous small ganglia innervating the sublingual and submaxillary glands, and he traced the axis cylinders to their endings in the perialveolar plexus and onto the ducts. Huber found a basketlike plexus surrounding the ganglion cells, and he thought it was the ending of fibers running in the chorda tympani.[6] He did not see cell bodies of fibers innervating blood vessels in the glands.

From 1896 to 1910 Huber had the collaboration of Lydia De Witt, a Michigan medical graduate (1898) who eventually became a pathologist of dis-

tinction. Together they matched McMurrich's effort in gross anatomy, for De Witt translated and Huber annotated Sobotta's *Atlas and Epitome of Human Histology and Microscopic Anatomy.*[7] They published papers on nerve terminals, each paper containing an exhaustive review of the literature.[8] The first was on motor nerve endings and those in muscle spindles. All the work was done using Huber's favorite methylene blue technique, and the endings in striated, cardiac, and involuntary muscle of many species were surveyed. They found that the motor endings in striated muscle lie under the sarcolemma, and their colored figures illustrate the structure of the end plate. They saw varicose cardiac nerves terminate in a bulb with no characteristic terminal structure. Fibers in involuntary muscle were found to be similar to those in cardiac muscle. Huber and De Witt's description of the muscle spindle was largely a gloss on Sherrington.[9] They agreed with him that there are sensory nerves from the spindles, but unlike Sherrington they did no conclusive physiological experiments. Huber himself did observe degeneration and regeneration after he crushed the rabbit's posterior tibial nerve, but his description contained nothing new.[10] In a definitive review of the innervation of the muscle spindle, Huber and De Witt appear "among others."[11]

In 1913 Huber was invited to give a lecture on the morphology of the sympathetic nervous system to the Seventeenth International Congress of Medicine in London, and the invitation signaled Huber's mastery of the subject.[12] He told the assembled physicians essentially what he had told Michigan medical students in four special lectures delivered in May 1897[13] when Langley's own authoritative summary had not yet been published.[14] Huber's account in 1897 was at the time the best general exposition of the organization of the sympathetic nervous system. Huber himself had worked on the minute anatomy of sympathetic ganglia,[15] and his long paper on that subject was illustrated with twenty-six beautiful figures. He also studied the endings of sympathetic nerves on cerebral blood vessels.[16] He found sympathetic nerves forming a perivascular plexus in the brain and medullary sensory nerves terminating in the dura. He said: "A knowledge of the existence of vaso-motor nerves on the intra-cranial vessels must of necessity weaken the position of physiologists, who . . . deny the existence of such nerves."[17] In his lecture Huber repeated a great deal of the detail of nerve cell structure discovered by himself, Dogiel, and other neuroanatomists, but if the tedious detail were removed the rest is what any beginning student is expected to know today. Huber ended with a three-color diagram of the arrangement of sympathetic nerves that the same student should be able to reproduce on an examination.

Huber had used the Golgi method, but he asserted many times that the method, depending as it does on precipitation of silver on the outside of cell bodies and their processes, is a priori incapable of revealing intracellular structure. When Huber turned to a study of neuroglia he used a very elaborate differential staining method devised by Benda, his teacher in Berlin. He may have been deceived by what he saw. When he edited Böhm and Davidoff's textbook[18] before 1900, Huber stated that although a large number of neuroglia fibers are processes of neuroglia cells, there are many neuroglia fibers that appear to have no connection with cells. Huber could see the cytoplasm of neuroglia cells in addition to their processes and fibers. He found that "neuroglia fibers are . . . in permanent relation with the protoplasm of neuroglia cells, either in close contact with it or embedded in the peripheral layer of the protoplasm of these cells."[19] His numerous illustrations show fibers passing through the cells.

Huber's Teaching

Huber and his junior staff taught microscopic anatomy in a course that included embryology and the anatomy of the nervous system. The course occupied 130 hours of lecture and 270 hours of laboratory work, October through February in the afternoons of the first year. Later it was switched to mornings, but it remained much the same with a few hours' difference here and there throughout Huber's tenure. Huber wrote a laboratory manual,[20] and he described how he and his technicians rapidly prepared the large number of slides required.[21] Fixed, stained, and embedded tissues in large numbers were supplied to the students, who were expected to mount sections they cut with a razor. Other sections of fresh tissues were cut on a freezing microtome. Huber's own preparations of motor end plates, tactile corpuscles, and brain tissue stained by Golgi's method were demonstrated, and students teased tubules and glomeruli from macerated kidneys. Huber moved through the

class, commenting on a student's sketches and helping each one observe and identify structures seen under the microscope. Thirty years after Huber's death a student remembered him as a "wonderful teacher."

Huber edited "with extensive revisions" an English translation of Böhm and Davidoff's *Text-Book of Histology*,[22] making it available for medical students. The most inquisitive students could consult Sobotta's *Atlas*. Although Huber remained in charge of teaching students of dentistry, nursing, and physical education, his own advanced students, beginning with Lydia De Witt, taught the service courses. After 1911 there were graduate students working for the doctor of philosophy degree who gradually advanced in rank as they advanced in teaching and research experience. When a summer course in microscopic anatomy was introduced in 1916 they gained more experience as they earned a summer salary.

Immediately after he returned from Germany Huber began a course in embryology. The course remained under Huber's direction, but it must have been supported by McMurrich, who published in 1902 a 527-page elementary textbook, *The Development of the Human Body*.[23] The book was "an attempt to present a concise statement of the development of the human body and a foundation for the proper understanding of the facts of anatomy" (iii). It was by no means an encyclopedic research production, and it relied heavily on publications of His, Hertwig, and Kollmann. There is no way of knowing how many students found a "concise" 527-page book useful.

The preclinical departments were then, as they remained, firmly in the grip of the medical faculty, but they had the responsibility to provide instruction in their disciplines for the rest of the university. In 1899 Huber told the dentists that the central laboratories of the Medical School gave dental students far better opportunities for instruction and postgraduate work than they could get in the School of Dentistry.[24] He thought the current program of postgraduate study in the dental school was not up to standard; dental students with the capacity should be better advanced in work in the medical departments. It was a long time before dental students took advantage of the opportunity, but Huber's offer was the germ of a notable program in which Michigan dentists earned the doctor of philosophy in anatomy.

Huber's Students

Lydia De Witt was a medical student who became an anatomist and then a colleague of Huber. She was only one of many doctors of medicine of the time who like Huber himself became a preclinical scientist without bothering to get the doctor of philosophy. She began by working on Huber's problems with Huber's methods, but she eventually became an independent scientist and a pathologist of enough distinction to be starred in the 1921 edition of *American Men of Science*.[25] At the time Huber was studying the structure of the renal tubules, De Witt, on her own, made an elaborate investigation of the islets of Langerhans and their blood supply using the wax plate method.[26] Huber never did anything more physiological than to test a nerve's ability to conduct, but De Witt, using cats, attempted to determine the function as well as the structure of the pancreatic islets. She tied off the pancreatic ducts, sparing their blood supply, and in those animals that survived long enough she found that the acinar cells had completely degenerated, leaving the islets alone embedded in connective tissue.[27] There was no sugar in the cats' urine. De Witt extracted the degenerated pancreas with glycerin or water, and she tested the extracts for enzymatic activity. Absence of proteolytic and lipolytic action showed that the exocrine cells had disappeared and that her extracts were derived from the islets. De Witt thought she had found evidence that the extracts had an "activator" action on glycolysis. She concluded that the islets must pour some secretion into the blood that affects carbohydrate metabolism, but she did not inject any of her extracts into a diabetic animal.

Over the years many medical students worked for a while with Huber before graduating and going on to clinical careers. One was E. W. Adamson, a graduate of 1904 who became a surgeon in Arizona. When Adamson was a medical student Huber was constructing models of renal tubules, and he put Adamson to work doing the same thing for sweat glands in embryonic and adult human subjects.[28] The wax models showed that in some instances the sweat glands are highly convoluted. At the same time, their colleague Arthur Cushny was demonstrating differential reabsorption in renal tubules, and Huber and Adamson thought there might be an analogy between coiled sweat glands and equally coiled renal tubules. In the next year another student, by training a chemist and bacteriologist, studied some dyes related to Huber's methylene blue.[29] Much later another studied the origin of the sensory root of the trigeminal nerve in the rat.[30] Some graduate students simply earned a master's degree and no other.

George Morris Curtis, the first to earn a doctor of philosophy rather than a doctor of medicine while working in anatomy, was studying under Huber when McCotter went to Vanderbilt in 1913. McCotter took Curtis with him to Nashville to handle histology and embryology although Curtis had not yet received his degree. When McCotter returned to Ann Arbor Curtis stayed behind, first as acting head and then as head of the department at Vanderbilt. He was the first Michigan product to become a chairman of anatomy elsewhere.[31] Curtis did manage to get back to Ann Arbor in the summer of 1914 to finish his research and qualify for his doctor of philosophy degree. Tubules were a favorite subject with Huber, and Curtis's thesis reported a study of the structure of the seminiferous tubules in the adult mouse and rabbit, again with the wax plate method.[32]

Huber's next doctor of philosophy students were Wayne J. Atwell and Stacey R. Guild. Atwell used the wax plate method to determine the development of the hypophysis in the rabbit, frog, and toad,[33] and he found a clever way to derive a line drawing from a wax model.[34] Guild worked with Huber on the problem of collateral buds of neurones in peripheral ganglia.[35] Huber wrote that much earlier he had described fine recurrent collateral branches but that their existence had been forgotten until Cajal "practically rediscovered" them. He and Guild demonstrated that the cells had three types of processes, some from the primary axon and some from the cell body itself, that ended on the cell of origin. When World War I came along Guild shifted to a study of war deafness and its prevention.[36] He fired a 44-caliber revolver near a hill that could stop the bullets. He tested the effects of various devices, some patented and some "sent by Major V. C. Vaughan of the National Research Council," in preventing injury to the middle ear. Later, in the Physiological Laboratory and with the help of Otis Cope, he attached a rubber tambour with a lever writing on a kymograph drum to the meatus of an artificial ear. He fired 22-, 38-, and 44-caliber pistols, this time using blank cartridges, and measured the excursion of the lever. He found that stuffing the ear with cotton saturated with oil was more effective in damping the lever's excursions than were two of the patented devices.

Huber published frequently with his students, but

when they matured he did not put his name on their papers. All along he was working on his own problems, and while he was on sabbatical leave at the Wistar Institute, of whose advisory board he was a member, he returned to embryology, describing the origin of the chorda dorsalis in the pig and human embryos from his own and Mall's collection.[37] He concluded that the head process—chordal canal, chordal plate, and chorda dorsalis—is "a derivative of the ectoderm in the sense that the mesoderm is derived from the ectoderm of the primitive streak region of the embryonic shield."[38] Using H. H. Donaldson's rat colony, Huber studied the development of the normal and abnormal ovum of rats from the first to the ninth day. The result was a 142-page monograph.[39]

Embryology of the Kidney

Huber began to study the embryology of the kidney in the spring of 1902. This work, summarized by Huber in a Harvey Lecture delivered 18 December 1909,[40] is the definitive work that could be supplemented only by electron microscopy.

Huber used Born's wax plate method to construct models of nephrons.[41] Others had used it too for the same problem, but Huber believed their sections, ten to twenty microns thick, did not allow them to distinguish one tubule from another. Huber cut sections five microns thick.

In addition to sectioning animal embryos, Huber used some human specimens. One human embryo ten millimeters long was sent him by Dr. Steiner of Lima, Ohio. David Steiner as a student had helped Henry Sewall settle the problem of the effective stimulus of the depressor nerve twenty years before.

Huber used a sliding microtome instead of an automatic one, and he floated his sections one by one onto albumin-coated slides. He might accumulate an unbroken series of three hundred to six hundred sections. He made camera lucida drawings of known magnification, and using a drawing as a template he cut a corresponding section from a wax plate. It was necessary to maintain an equal ratio between the lateral dimensions of the section and those of the drawing with the thickness of the section and that of the wax plate. After assembling the plates in order of the sections, Huber smoothed their edges. Failure to smooth, Huber said, had misled earlier workers. He found it relatively easy to construct models of earlier stages, but he had trouble with mature kidneys. With

them he was sometimes able to follow a loop of Henle its entire length and, using the loop as a starting point, to trace out the rest of the tubule. His paper is illustrated with drawings of forty-two models ranging from those of tissues found in a cat embryo thirteen millimeters in length to a kidney from a fully developed cat embryo.

For one thing, Huber solved the problem of the relation between the ascending tubule and the glomerulus. The uriniferous tubule, after leaving the glomerulus and wandering as the proximal tubule, the long loop of Henle, and the distal convoluted tubule, returns to the renal corpuscle of its own nephron and attaches itself to the vascular pole. The question is how the ascending tubule finds its own glomerulus and no other. The answer is that in the very earliest embryological stages the cells that are to become the most distal part of the distal tubule make permanent contact with the cells that are going to be the most proximal part of the proximal tubule. Then the tubules elongate, and the loop of Henle forms between them. The distal tubule need not find its way back, for it had never left.

Huber injected the renal artery of a freshly exsanguinated animal with a solution of celloidin stained with a red dye. When the celloidin had set he macerated the kidney in 75 percent hydrochloric acid and stained fragments with hematoxylin and eosin. Pieces two to five millimeters thick mounted in balsam showed the arrangement of the vascular units, and Huber reproduced three elegant drawings of such preparations. He found that with the rarest exception, all blood flowing to the peritubular capillaries first flows through the glomeruli. The exceptional vessels appear to be nutrient ones for the renal pelvis.

Huber found the wax plate method satisfactory for determining the relatively, but only relatively, simple structure of the embryonic renal tubules and those of the adult amphibians, but he despaired of using it for the long and complex tubules of the higher vertebrates. Instead, he developed a method of teasing out whole tubules from macerated kidneys, and consequently he was able to describe in detail and to illustrate with drawings the tubules of many species of vertebrates. He demonstrated, for example, the difference between the length of the medullary loop of tubules from renal corpuscles on the cortex and those from deeper corpuscles, and he speculated on the significance of the difference.[42] Toward the end of his life Huber wrote a definitive summary of the morphology of renal tubules of vertebrates, carrying the description as far as it could go until electron microscopy appeared.[43] His figures have been reproduced in many textbooks.

Huber said little about the relevance of his findings to understanding the function of the nephron, but at the end of his Harvey Lecture he rather plaintively expressed the hope that in "future experimental work on the mammalian kidney, due recognition be given to the structural and morphological characteristics of the mammalian renal tubule."[44] He had particularly in mind that he had demonstrated at least four kinds of epithelium in the tubule, and he was sure they must have different functions other than the simple reabsorption postulated by Ludwig long before.

Nerve Regeneration Again

On 9 December 1893, a year after he returned from Europe, Huber took up the problem of nerve regeneration where he and Howell had left off. In their prize-winning work they had studied the regeneration of peripheral nerves whose severed ends could be brought together. Now Huber addressed himself to the problem of regeneration when a segment of nerve was lost and the two ends could not be apposed. He performed fifty experiments in which he removed a portion of the left or right ulnar nerve of a dog, and after the segment had been replaced and the wound closed, he followed the process of regeneration for as long as 182 days. In twenty-six experiments Huber replaced the missing segment with another piece of dog nerve, and in twenty-five instances he found satisfactory repair. Surgeons had tried other methods in patients without, as Huber said, bothering to test their methods experimentally. Huber did the experiments. He replaced the segment with a tube of decalcified bone or with a bundle of catgut; he used nerve flaps; and he cross sutured two severed nerves. After the animals had been killed Huber made a histological examination of the nerves.

Huber published a 112-page paper on his work in the *Journal of Morphology*.[45] In those days editors were generous with their heavy paper stock, and Huber was allowed to begin his paper with an utterly detailed review of the experimental and clinical literature and to print a 14-page table summarizing surgeons' reports of twenty-three cases. He gave his histological methods in detail, and he concluded with the protocol of each of his experiments. The paper

ends with twenty-one colored figures of nerves in various states of regeneration. When he finished, the reader could agree with Huber that "the operation of implanting a segment taken from another nerve [in the same animal] promises the most favorable results."[46] Huber was under the impression that "surgeons as a rule have a somewhat vague and imperfect idea as to what the processes of repair in injured nerves are, and as to what conditions favor, retard or prevent such repair."[47] He could not rely on their reading the *Journal of Morphology*, so he gave a long description of his work and its results before a meeting of the Michigan State Medical Society in 1896. Huber read the surgeons an elementary lecture on the anatomy of the peripheral nervous system; he explained the newly confirmed neuron doctrine; and he described the process of peripheral degeneration before giving his own results.[48] To reach a wider audience Huber published essentially the same paper in the *International Journal of Surgery*.[49]

Reuben Peterson was not yet on the Michigan faculty, but he heard Huber and read Huber's paper. While he was still in Chicago Peterson published a long report of the results he had obtained when he successfully transplanted the sciatic nerve of a dog between the severed ends of the median and ulnar nerves of a young man, the brother of a medical colleague.[50] The patient's wrist had been cut by a buzz saw. There was complete loss of function and sensation, but both returned slowly after the transplantation. Huber examined the amputation neuroma Peterson had removed, and Peterson said: "If the present paper shall prove to be of any scientific value I feel that it will be due largely to the assistance of my friend, Professor G. Carl Huber of the University of Michigan, whose splendid work on nerve degeneration and regeneration is so well known."[51]

During World War I the Office of the Surgeon General detailed five neurosurgeons in succession to work with Huber on the same problem: the case in which severed nerves cannot be brought together to bridge the gap left by the wound. From February 1918 to March 1919 the surgeons performed 279 operations, chiefly on rabbits, in a series of twenty-one types of experiments. The animals were kept after the operation for a few days up to nearly a year, and at the end of the period the nerves were exposed, tested for function, and fixed for histological examination. More than seventy thousand sections were made and stained by the pyridine-silver method. It took the Medical Department of the Army another eight years to get around to publishing the results,[52] but Huber saw to it that they were quickly known. He told the Chicago Neurological and Pathological Societies what he had found on 19 April 1919, and he published the same summary in two major journals[53] and in a textbook[54] written by one of the neurosurgeons, who expressed his "distinct pleasure to have had the opportunity to work with [G. Carl Huber] during part of his latter experimental work."[55]

The first problem was prevention of an amputation neuroma, which "indicates an attempt which is thwarted or blocked by scar tissue on the part of the neuraxes of a divided nerve to seek the distal segment and thus complete nerve repair."[56] Neuroma formation could be prevented by injection of absolute alcohol into the nerve about an inch above the plane of section. At the end of the fourth or fifth week there was downgrowth of the central neuraxis, not in a very regular fashion but not crisscross as in a neuroma.

Huber and the surgeons, repeating Huber's work of more than twenty years earlier, found that an autotransplant is the most satisfactory means of bridging a gap. A less important nerve could be sacrificed for a more important one, and four segments of a small nerve could be sewn together as a cable. Connective tissue eventually formed an epineural sheath around the autotransplant. Downgrowth was good in six experiments using homotransplants, nerves from another animal of the same species. Huber's team used guinea pig or dog nerves in rabbits, but they found the outcome less certain and less satisfactory than with homotransplants. Downgrowth of the neuraxes tended to pass outside instead of growing through the heterotransplant. If homotransplants are better than heterotransplants, homologous tissue might be salvaged and stored. Nerves kept in petroleum jelly (Vaseline) at three degrees centigrade were just as good as fresh ones, and so were homologous transplants stored five weeks in liquid petrolatum. Regeneration even occurred through homotransplants that had been stored at room temperature in 50 percent alcohol, but there was no successful regeneration through stored heterotransplants. The surgeons tried wrapping the transplants in a sheath, ox peritoneum treated with alcohol, fascia from the same animal, or a length of formalized carotid artery. None helped. A tension suture was no good at all. Whatever the method the surgeons used, accurate end-to-end suturing, careful technique, and a dry field were essential for success.

Elizabeth Crosby's Background

When Elizabeth Crosby walked into Huber's office in 1920 (fig. 10–2) to ask for an opportunity to work on the anatomy of the nervous system, Huber had read her one publication, a long paper on the forebrain of the alligator,[57] and he soon received a letter of recommendation from her former mentor, Charles Judson Herrick of the University of Chicago.[58] Huber could not know that she would change the direction of his own research and add luster to the department.

Elizabeth Crosby had just resigned as superintendent of schools in Petersburg, a tiny town in southeastern Michigan, and she was willing to support her-

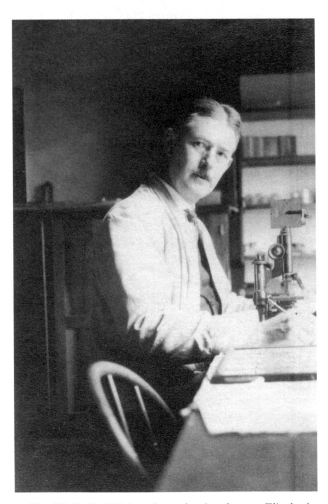

Fig. 10–2. Carl Huber about the time he met Elizabeth Crosby. (Courtesy of the Department of Surgery, University of Michigan.)

Not Just Any Medical School

self with her savings for a while. She had grown up in Petersburg, and her father had promised to give her four years of college education. When she graduated from nearby Adrian College in three years, she took the fourth year as a graduate student at the University of Chicago. Although she had majored in Latin and mathematics at Adrian, she was determined to begin advanced work in biology under Herrick, the comparative neuroanatomist who had replaced H. H. Donaldson at the University of Chicago. Refusing to begin with the introductory courses she had missed at Adrian, she was reluctantly permitted to begin with gross anatomy and neuroanatomy as taught to medical students. She did so well that she was given an assistantship in anatomy and allowed to begin research. She earned a master of science in 1912 and a doctor of philosophy in 1915.[59]

Herrick had earned his own doctor of philosophy at Columbia with a thesis that established the central connections and peripheral ramifications of the cranial nerves of a bony fish, and since then he had distinguished himself by publishing on the organization of the medulla of fish, showing that the great variation occurring in closely related species correlated with the equal variation in sensory organs sending afferent fibers to the medulla. By the time Crosby came to him, Herrick was a major authority on the anatomy of the amphibian brain. He was an inspiring teacher of graduate students, and he set Crosby to work on the forebrain of the alligator, a step up the evolutionary scale.

Elizabeth Crosby's Early Comparative Neuroanatomy

For her thesis work Crosby made serial sections in three planes of the brains of alligators thirty to fifty-five centimeters long, and she stained the sections with toluidine blue or by the silver method of Golgi. She identified the cellular structures of the forebrain, and she traced the fiber pathways in detail, illustrating her findings with forty-six figures drawn in a meticulous and easily identified style.

At that time neuroanatomists recognized two major problems of development: what directs individual neurons during the course of ontological development to make their specific connections? And what directs the phylogenetic differentiation of the nervous system? Both questions had been answered by Cornelius Ariëns Kappers, the Dutch comparative neuroanatomist, in his law of neurobiotaxis: cell bodies tend to migrate along their dendrites toward the source of their stimulation.[60] Ariëns Kappers had justified the application of his law to ontogeny with much naive neurophysiology and biochemistry. Crosby's interpretation of the structure of the alligator's forebrain was explicitly along Ariëns Kappers's lines.

The olfactory system is highly developed in the reptilian forebrain, and the alligator is distinguished by having particularly large olfactory lobes. Crosby traced the fiber connections from the olfactory mucosa through the lobes and into the nuclei of the forebrain, because "[t]he specific distribution of the olfactory and the non-olfactory fibers, the positions and the relations of the various centers and, finally, an analysis of these data in terms of their functional significance, these are all essential to the adequate understanding of the morphology and the evolution of the forebrain." She concluded that "[o]ne of the causes at least, for the outward migration of cells of the dorso-medial area to form the hippocampal cortex is probably to be found in the operation of the law of neurobiotaxis. . . . The medial olfactory tracts and other tracts bearing afferent impulses to the hippocampus are on the medial surface of the hemispheres and the cells of the developing cortical layers move out toward the surface of the hemisphere in order that they may come into closer relationship with the incoming impulses." Although the forebrain is largely dominated by the olfactory system, "its differentiation into basal and cortical centers is due, directly or indirectly, to the entrance of non-olfactory, diencephalic impulses. . . . A variety in the type of incoming diencephalic impulses has led to the differentiation of a number of different basal nuclei, for it has not been the number of synapses through which an impulse has passed, nor the number of fibers coming into a nucleus, but the variety in the types of stimulation received which has led to the differentiation of the telencephalic centers."[61] Crosby's paper was at once recognized as a masterpiece of descriptive neuroanatomy.

Crosby's Early Teaching

While she was working with exemplary diligence on the forebrain of the alligator Crosby was also teaching neuroanatomy. Herrick had never taught medical students before he arrived in Chicago, but at once he began a comprehensive course in neuroanatomy suitable for a wide range of students. He wrote an elementary textbook for the course.[62] His lectures were accompanied by a laboratory course to which Crosby made substantial contributions, particularly concerning human neuroanatomy. Her name was coupled with Herrick's in *A Laboratory Outline of Neurology*.[63] The book was designed to be used in a shorter or longer course of comparative anatomy of the nervous system. If medical students actually followed the directions, they worked hard. Neuroanatomy was presented as the basis of function, and the brief section on the spinal cord is an example. Students were asked to fill in outline sketches of the cervical, thoracic, lumbar, and sacral cord by observing cell bodies in Nissl-stained sections, and they were directed to consult nine reference books.

With the aid of your reference books build up a clear picture of the mode of connection of these neurones in typical spinal reflexes. See Herrick ('15), Figs. 60, 61; Herrick and Coghill ('15); Howell ('15), Chapters VII, VIII; Morris ('14), Fig. 610, p. 767; Quain ('09), p. 99; Sherrington ('06), Chapters I to IV, especially the diagram on p. 46; Starr, Strong, and Leaming ('96).[64]

The Howell chapters are "Reflex Actions" and "The Spinal Cord and Paths of Conduction" in *A Text-Book of Physiology for Medical Students and Physicians*, 6th ed. (Philadelphia: W. B. Saunders, 1915). The Sherrington reference is *The Integrative Action of the Nervous System* (New York: C. Scribner's Sons, 1906), and the diagram illustrates the dog's receptive fields and the spinal arcs involved in the scratch reflex.

When the laboratory manual was published in 1918 Crosby was listed on the title page as "Principal of the High School in Petersburg, Michigan." Upon receiving her doctor of philosophy she had returned to Petersburg to take care of her elderly, infirm parents. She taught Latin, mathematics, and zoology, and she coached a basketball team. By 1920 her mother had died, and she brought her father to Ann Arbor. Huber gave her an assistantship in gross anatomy, and he appointed her to teach the next summer at a salary of $425. She rose slowly through the ranks, being promoted to a full professorship in 1936. Not until the Rackham grants from the Graduate School became available in the mid-1930s did she have any support for her research other than departmental funds administered by Huber. The

Rackham grants were for $1,500 or $2,000 a year, the larger part paying the salary of an assistant. Crosby took several leaves of absence without pay to work abroad, and in 1939–40, the end of the period considered in this book, she went to Aberdeen to reorganize Marischal College's teaching program in neuroanatomy and to institute a research program. Correspondence in the dean's file in the Bentley Historical Library indicates that at the end of her Aberdeen appointment she was negotiating with the University of Manchester for a permanent job. Perhaps she found Michigan under Huber's successor distasteful. The war forced her to return to the United States.

Crosby's Early Research at Michigan

When Herrick wrote Huber he said he regarded Crosby's thesis research "as an exceptional piece of work for thoroughness, accuracy, and grasp of the morphological problems involved. Though of course, it was done under close supervision; it is thoroughly her own work and she is fully qualified to prosecute further research independently; in fact, she has a second paper on the thalamus of Alligator well under way."[65]

Much of the work that would eventually be published had been done during summers at Chicago, but when it was published six years after Crosby came to Michigan Huber's name appeared ahead of Crosby's as it did on all subsequent joint publications. The justification was that "[t]he major portion of the work has been done at the Anatomical Laboratory of the University of Michigan where Dr. Huber has become associated with the work and in this contribution assumes joint responsibility for the descriptions and interpretations of the tracts and nuclei."[66] This kind of work was new for Huber, and one wonders whether the magnitude and quality of his contributions justified his assumption of priority.

The first of two long papers published by Huber and Crosby described the thalamic and tectal nuclei and their fiber tracts in the alligator, and the second described the optic tectum in turtles, lizards, and snakes as well as in the alligator.[67] In parallel work they described the nuclei of the avian diencephalon and their connections with the telencephalon.[68] They had much of the material on hand for an extension to the human thalamus, but that work was not separately published. Their reasons for doing all that work were to compare the structure of the brain with the behavior of animals, to contribute to understanding of phylogenetic development, and to provide the exact knowledge of neuroanatomy they thought vital for experimental work. Lesions, they said, must be accurately placed in well-defined structures, for subsequent observations on degenerated tracts give only partial information. They themselves never made behavioral or experimental studies, but others were doing so at the time.[69] In a long review of somatic and visceral connections of the diencephalon, they ventured some psychological interpretations.[70] They thought the thalamus is much more than a gateway to the cortex; it is an important reflex center and a center involved in affective tone. Except for olfactory impulses, the vast majority of nerve impulses reaches the cortex only after relay in the dorsal parts of the diencephalon. Hence, there are no pure sensations in normal human psychology.

Crosby's Graduate Teaching

As soon as Elizabeth Crosby was well established in what Huber designated as the Laboratory of Comparative Neurology she began to attract graduate students. Of the more than forty who eventually earned the doctor of philosophy under her, twelve completed their thesis work before 1941. Postdoctoral fellows came to work with her as well. All eventually expressed their thanks to Dr. Elizabeth Crosby for her untiring energy in helping them, and they called her an unfailing source of inspiration and assistance in the accumulation, organization, and presentation of their work.

Crosby's first doctor of philosophy student, Elisha Gurdjian, struck a new note by selecting the albino rat.[71] He thereby laid the foundations for collaborative association of neuroanatomists with the growing number of behavioral and neurophysiological scientists in the United States who were employing mammals in their research. It was a step neurophysiologists thought long overdue. Crosby's first postdoctoral fellow, David Rioch, continued with three long papers on the diencephalon of the dog and cat.[72] Rioch selected the dog because it was a commonly used laboratory animal. His work on the cat turned out to be more useful, for adult cats, in contrast with dogs, have a relatively uniform head and are suitable for stereotaxic work. Thereafter Crosby and her students worked on

the nervous systems of higher rather than of lower forms.

Crosby, Huber, and Ariëns Kappers

When Crosby was young the foremost comparative neuroanatomist was Cornelius Ariëns Kappers,[73] who had published his two-volume *Die vergleichende Anatomie des Nervensystems der Wirbeltiere und des Menschen* in 1920–21.[74] In 1926 Crosby took a leave from Michigan, and after stopping for a while in London she worked with Ariëns Kappers in his Central Institute for Brain Research in Amsterdam. Ariëns Kappers suggested that she and Huber translate his book into English, and they agreed. In the ten years required to produce *The Comparative Anatomy of the Nervous System of Vertebrates, Including Man*[75] the major burden fell upon Crosby. Huber, in addition to his teaching, had other things to do. He had to administer what was now a substantial department with a large teaching load and other research programs; he was dean of the Graduate School; and he was on national committees and editorial boards. He was growing old, and he was ill. Huber died the day after Christmas in 1934, and Crosby with the help of students spent much of the next two years seeing the manuscript through the press. The result was an essentially new book, not a mere translation. For example, the chapter on the telencephalon occupies 149 pages with 87 figures in the German edition. It occupies 277 pages of the same size with 107 figures in English. That chapter has 284 references in German but 785 in English, each reference carefully considered and woven into the text. When Ariëns Kappers produced a shorter French edition in 1947, he simply referred readers eager for detail to the English work.[76]

Crosby, the Clinicians, and the Medical Students

Michigan's preclinical and clinical departments were separated by nearly a half mile of Ann Arbor streets, but there was a wider intellectual gap seldom bridged. Of course, the pathologists always and bacteriologists sometimes worked with the clinicians, but Cushny's frequent consultation with George Dock is one of the few identifiable examples of cooperation between basic scientists and clinicians until the practical value of Crosby's knowledge of human neuro-anatomy was recognized. Apparently the first to enlist Elizabeth Crosby's cooperation was A. C. Furstenberg, an otorhinolaryngologist and dean of the Medical School after 1935. The result was four joint publications on hypertensive deafness, neuro-logical lesions affecting the sense of smell, distur-bances in the function of salivary glands, and respira-tory distress following suppuration of paranasal sinuses.[77] Eventually neurologists and neurosurgeons attended Crosby's postgraduate course, and one oph-thalmologist earned a doctor of philosophy working with her on pathways concerned with automatic eye movements.[78] Max Peet, the neurosurgeon, fre-quently consulted Elizabeth Crosby, but more formal and extensive collaboration began sometime around 1950 when Crosby began regularly to spend at least three hours a week in rounds and consultation with Edgar Kahn and his neurosurgical staff (fig. 10-3). For the first edition of Kahn's *Correlative Neuro-surgery*[79] Crosby contributed sections on anatomical considerations to chapters on gliomas and on tumors of the sellar region, the third ventricle, and the poste-rior fossa. By the time the book had reached a two-volume third edition Crosby was a full-fledged coau-thor. Eventually her *Correlative Anatomy of the Nervous System* was studied by neurologists and neu-rosurgeons as well as by anatomists and physiologists.[80]

Crosby always taught neuroanatomy for medical students, and after Huber died she was in full charge of a course occupying 36 hours of lecture and between 86 and 120 hours of laboratory. Her course was pitched at a high level, and it was never easy. Her clear, forceful lectures helped students attain a com-prehensive view of the subject. In the laboratory stu-dents were expected to master detail precisely. What she taught is revealed by examination questions she posed. Some were perfectly straightforward.

Explain, by diagrams of the paths involved, why a hemisec-tion of the cord results in the loss of pain and temperature on the contralateral side of the body but leaving general tactile sensibility intact.

Another question demonstrated Crosby's conception of neuroanatomy as the basis for understanding func-tion.

Explain the path by which a pain impulse from a tooth pro-duced dilation of the pupil.

Students loved it; they loved Elizabeth Crosby; and they loved the certainty she brought amid the confu-sion of neurology.

Choosing Huber's Successor

Soon after Huber died Dean Furstenberg appointed Edmunds, Coller, and Weller as a committee to find Huber's successor, and the committee quickly accu-mulated a list of almost every senior anatomist in the country. Most were not interested in the job, and when the committee reported on 26 June 1935 it put Bradley Patten, who had been recommended by G. L. Streeter, first. Patten visited Ann Arbor in early July, and he spelled out his requirements in detail to Dean Furstenberg and President Ruthven. Patten was assistant director for medical sciences of the Rocke-feller Foundation at the time, and when President Ruthven telegraphed him on 15 July that the regents would meet his demand, Patten was on his way to Europe on behalf of the foundation. Patten would

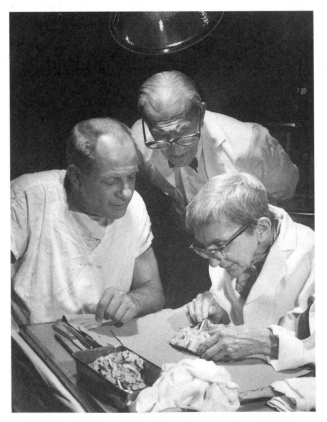

Fig. 10–3. Richard Schneider *(in surgical garb)*, Edgar Kahn, and Elizabeth Crosby. As a team they described the anatomical bases for neurosurgery. (Courtesy of the Department of Anatomy, University of Michigan.)

Not Just Any Medical School

not be free until February. In the meantime McCotter was made acting head of the department, and Dean Furstenberg found Patten a house he could rent when he came.[81]

Bradley Patten's Background

Bradley Merrill Patten had earned his bachelor's degree at Dartmouth, where his father was professor of biology. After receiving his doctor of philosophy from Harvard in 1914 Patten became a member of the faculty of Western Reserve University Medical School in Cleveland, Ohio, and he remained in its Laboratory of Histology and Embryology until 1934. The Great Depression hit Western Reserve hard, and in 1934 Patten, together with other long-serving members of the faculty, was firmly encouraged to find another job. The Rockefeller Foundation made him responsible for its international fellowship program.

When Patten was a graduate student under G. H. Parker, Jacques Loeb was a major intellectual force in U.S. biology, and his doctrine of tropisms purported to explain behavior.[82] Loeb had found, for example, that when "two sources of light of equal intensity and distance act simultaneously upon a [*negatively*] heliotropic animal, the animal puts its median plane at right angles to the line connecting the two sources of light."[83] The behavior of a horseshoe crab can be completely controlled by the relative intensities of light falling on each of its sides, and Loeb wrote: "I consider a complete knowledge and control of these agencies (which determine behavior) the biological solution of the metaphysical problem of animal instinct and will."[84] Patten confirmed Loeb in a series of studies of the response of the larva of the blowfly to symmetrical and asymmetrical illumination. The work was elaborate and well done, but it merely confirmed Jacques Loeb.[85]

Embryology of the Heart

Patten's research on the normal and abnormal development of the heart continued through his period at Michigan. He began at Western Reserve by making clay models of twelve chick embryos from twenty-nine to one hundred hours old to show the development of the cardiac loop, and he published drawings of ventral, dextral, and dorsal views of the models,

saying that "[s]ince these phases of heart development all involve complex changes in configuration and relations, the figures constitute a graphic summary much more satisfactory than a written résumé."[86]

Patten was able to study the development of the interatrial septum and closure of the foramen ovale in the chick heart by making wax models, but when he took sabbatical leave at the Pathological Institute in Vienna he could study the process in seventy-four fetal and newborn human hearts in first-class condition.[87] Early in embryonic life the development of the partition between left and right atria is interrupted by establishment of communicating openings in that part of the septum already formed. "Instead of a few circular openings which look as if they had been cut out with a punch, the openings are numerous and irregular."[88] The septum is flaccid, and when the right atrium fills, the septum balloons into the left atrium. The openings are stretched, allowing blood to flow from right to left. When pressure in the two atria becomes equal, the septum is forced back to the median position with consequent reduction in size of the apertures. At the same time overlapping strands of interforaminal septal tissue partly obliterate the small foramina and effectively bar backflow.[89] In the development of the human heart the valvula foraminis ovalis on the left side of the interatrial septum partially covers the foramen ovale, reducing its functional size and limiting flow from left to right. Finally, in the last third of the first year after birth the valvula becomes an integral part of the interatrial septum.

Patten found an opening in the interatrial septum through which he could pass a probe in about 20 to 25 percent of adult human hearts, but that opening had no functional significance. He thought there is a gradual change, not a radical upheaval, at the time of birth. Blood is circulating through the lungs at the end of fetal life, and in the neonatal period the volume in the pulmonary circuit gradually increases. With rising left atrial pressure there is progressive functional closure of the foramen ovale as in the chick heart. Anatomical closure follows in most but not all adult hearts.

Patten's Textbooks

Patten confirmed the rule that often the most effective textbook for beginners is written by one who is also beginning. Shortly after joining the embryology laboratory at Western Reserve Patten began to write his *Early Embryology of the Chick,* and the first edition was published in 1920.[90] Patten said: "This book has been written in an effort to set forth for [the beginning student] in brief and simple form the basic facts of development. It does not purport to be a reference work. . . . Because of my conviction that so-called elementary texts too frequently overreach their avowed scope, the ground covered by this book has been rigidly restricted."[91] Patten might have been comparing his little book with McMurrich's 527-page volume. Patten's 167 pages contain eighty-seven illustrations, many drawn by Patten himself, and the three-color frontispiece, also by Patten, shows a wax plate reconstruction of a four-day-old embryo.

Patten had written a pedagogical classic, and generations of U.S. students began their study of embryology with Patten's *Chick* in hand. By 1927 Patten had begun to master mammalian embryology, in part by working with G. L. Streeter. Streeter allowed Patten free use of young embryos, and C. S. Minot's widow turned over part of Minot's collection for Patten's use. The result was an equally classical elementary textbook, *Embryology of the Pig.*[92] It reached a third edition in 1948 and was repeatedly reprinted.

The Beating Embryonic Heart

Patten went on to an even more dramatic representation of the developing heart. Sometime in the 1920s he showed living chick embryos to a fellow ornithologist, S. Prentiss Baldwin, who was a pioneer in bird banding and the proprietor of the Baldwin Research Laboratory at Gates Mills, Ohio. Baldwin had graduated from Dartmouth, where he had known Patten's father. He earned a law degree from Western Reserve in 1895, and he entered practice in Cleveland. He discontinued practice in 1902, and he spent the rest of his long life in his bird research laboratory. Baldwin had money of his own, but his marriage to the daughter of Mark Hanna, who was an industrialist, adviser to William McKinley, and U.S. senator, further facilitated his substitution of wrens for writs at the age of thirty-four. He had made motion pictures of birds in the field, and he asked Patten if he could make a motion picture of the beating embryonic heart. He offered to pay for construction of the apparatus.[93]

After five unsuccessful attempts Patten and Theodore Kramer, Baldwin's former assistant, did build a motion picture apparatus for microscopic work that could operate at as many as sixteen frames a second. Patten said of Kramer: "His genius for devising and successfully operating intricate apparatus has been indispensable in securing the micromoving pictures of the embryonic heart."[94]

The most important aspect of the apparatus was complete separation of its major parts, for otherwise vibration of the camera was inevitably transmitted to the microscope. The microscope with side viewer and an incubator system in which the embryo could be mounted on a cover glass in a hollow-ground slide was supported on one five-hundred-pound concrete pier, and the camera with its drive mechanism was mounted on another independent five-hundred-pound pier. Separately mounted arc and incandescent lights provided illumination. The whole cost five hundred dollars, including one hundred dollars for shop work.[95] Patten intended to continue the work at Michigan, and a concrete foundation for the camera was poured in the back entrance of East Medical Building. It was never used.

There is inevitably a certain gee-whiz aspect to cinemicrophotography, but Patten's films showing the embryology of the chick heart provided a particularly dramatic view of the development of the heart, of the assumption of regular contraction, and of the initiation of the circulation. The views of the embryo freely floating within the periodically contracting amnion are memorable. When Patten was at Michigan he regularly showed the silent films to his embryology class, and he made tapes of the narrative with which he accompanied them.[96]

The original thirty-five-millimeter nitrate prints were transferred to sixteen-millimeter acetate stock, and for a while they, or parts of them, were widely distributed through Michigan Media, an office of the university. They were eventually "retired," a polite term for "destroyed." Theodore Kramer kept one copy, and when he retired after a long career as assistant professor of anatomy at Michigan he took it with him to his farm. When I was writing this section I asked Ted Kramer if I could see the film. He brought it to the Department of Physiology, where we projected it for the last time. Kramer moved to a nursing home, and when he died at more than ninety years of age knowledge of the film and tape died with him.

Rehabilitation of the Department of Anatomy at Michigan

Patten, like many newly appointed chairs, was dismayed by the condition of the department he inherited. Gross anatomy was adequate and neuroanatomy was very good, but histology and embryology, he said, were, deficient.[97] Equipment was obsolete and unsuitable for experimental work. The faculty was overburdened with teaching, and there were courses that must be eliminated. The staff was inbred, and some members were unproductive in research.

Patten used some of the $15,000 allotted him for rehabilitation to replace microscopes he found old and out of order. He immediately discarded 25 microscopes bought before 1890, and in the next two years he got rid of 12 acquired about 1895. By 1939 he had 180 satisfactory microscopes. Only 39 were more than twenty-five years old, and 37 were newly purchased. Students were given loan collections of slides instead of being required to make their own. Patten spent $4,500 for 30,000 slides: 130 sets of 150 slides each for medical students, an additional 130 sets of 30 neuroanatomical slides, 60 sets of 100 slides for dental students and 600 special slides for demonstration. However, Shirley Smith, the secretary of the university and the officious watchdog of the budget, would not allow Patten to buy additional equipment, saying four epidiascopes were enough. Patten bought an embryological collection at the cost of $5,140, and he continued to collect human embryos. He converted space formerly used for descriptive work, Huber's wax plate room, for example, to space for experimental studies, and he installed an operating room.

Patten found the staff, particularly the junior members, underpaid, and over the first three years he devoted 83 percent of the money available for raises to the instructors. Raises were selective; three instructors were given none to indicate Patten's opinion of their weakness. He did, however, recommend a substantial salary increase for Elizabeth Crosby when he put her up for promotion, but she quixotically refused the raise. One day Patten was astonished when McCotter burst out, displaying great bitterness over the way he had been treated by "someone." During the depression his salary had been reduced, but "someone" had never restored the cut. Patten immediately wrote a holograph letter to Dean Furstenberg asking if something could be done for McCotter at once.

McCotter and Crosby were the only senior staff when Patten came to Ann Arbor. There was an assistant professor whom President Ruthven had called unfit for permanent appointment. Five instructors and all of the assistants had been trained by Huber. Patten quickly got rid of four instructors. One left in a great cloud of acrimony, accusing Patten in a long and bitter letter of lying and of deliberately trying to destroy neuroanatomy at Michigan. At the time Patten told one of the instructors, a woman and friend of Elizabeth Crosby, that she should find another job, Crosby resigned in a letter to the dean that gave no reason for her action. Dean Furstenberg talked Crosby into withdrawing her resignation. Patten made a strong but unsuccessful effort to recruit Donald Barron, an American who was then teaching anatomy at Cambridge University and working with Joseph Barcroft on fetal circulation.

Patten did bring in new staff from the outside, but their productive period was after the war and beyond the scope of this book. Two long books, *Human Embryology* and *The Foundations of Embryology,* were Patten's chief scholarly accomplishments before he retired in 1959.[98]

11
Pathology

In Michigan's early days the professorship of pathology was combined with whatever other professorship happened to be handy: physiology, materia medica, or physic. Alonzo B. Palmer was made professor of pathology as well as of medicine in 1861, but Palmer admitted he had never studied morbid anatomy. Henry Sylvester Cheever, when he assisted Palmer in private practice, did a few autopsies,[1] and from the late 1870s Palmer had several assistants responsible for practical pathology.[2]

On 18 October 1887, a few months before Palmer's death, the medical faculty made this entry in its minutes.

> Whereas the Science of Pathology is at present regarded as one of the most important branches, and, whereas, instruction in Pathology should be largely given as laboratory work, and whereas the Department of Medicine and Surgery is greatly deficient in this branch, Resolved that this Faculty earnestly petitino [*sic*] the Board of Regents to establish and fill a chair of Pathology during the present school year.
>
> After discussion the following rerolution [*sic*] was made and carried: Moved that the Faculty ask the Board of Regents to appoint Mr. N. H. Gibbs [*sic*] of London, as Professor of Pathology.[3]

Nothing in the minutes or in any contemporary account answers the two questions, Why did Michigan pick Heneage Gibbes to be its professor of pathology? and Why did Gibbes leave London for Ann Arbor?

Experience of Heneage Gibbes

In his old age Aldred Scott Warthin wrote of his predecessor: "The then Professor of Pathology was a Britisher, lately retired from the command of a gunboat, chasing pirates in the China Sea, and had been picked up in London and brought to Ann Arbor by one of the members of the medical faculty."[4]

The sparse biographical notices of Gibbes say nothing about gunboats or pirates,[5] but it is quite possible that Gibbes had an adventurous naval career before qualifying in medicine. Gibbes earned his bachelor of medicine and master of surgery degrees from Aberdeen in 1879 and his licentiate of the Royal College of Physicians in the same year. In the custom of the country he proceeded to his Aberdeen doctor of medicine in 1881. The entry for Gibbes in *Who Was Who in America* does not give his birth date, but his brief obituary notice in the *Journal of the American Medical Association* says he died in 1912 of senile decay, aged eighty. If the age is correct, he was born in 1832 and would have been forty-seven years old when he graduated from Aberdeen.

Warthin did not identify the Michigan faculty member who brought Gibbes to Ann Arbor, but Palmer had spent considerable time in London preparing his textbook. Palmer's commanding position at Michigan would have made it easy to persuade his colleagues that Gibbes should be made professor of pathology.

Gibbes and Cholera

When cholera began to invade Europe from India and Egypt in 1883 the German government appointed Robert Koch head of a commission to investigate the disease. Koch quickly established that a bacillus he discovered and named the comma-bacillus is the cause of cholera and that the disease is spread chiefly through contaminated water supplies.

In 1884 the British government appointed Emanuel Klein as cholera commissioner and sent him to India to make an independent investigation. Klein was lecturer on advanced bacteriology at St. Bartholomew's Hospital, and he had published a manual on bacteriological technique.[6] He took Gibbes, lecturer on normal and morbid anatomy at the Westminster Medical School, with him to India. On returning from India Klein and Gibbes presented their official report.[7] Klein published the same report under his name alone in a popular medical journal,[8] and he participated in discussions that were summarized in the 1885 issues of the *British Medical Journal*. Klein, with Gibbes tagging along, concluded that Koch's statement that the comma-bacillus occurs in rice-water stools of cholera patients is correct, but he could not agree with Koch that "the lower part of the ileum contains an almost pure cultivation of the comma-bacilli."[9] The organism is not found in the patient's blood and tissues, and therefore it cannot be responsible for the systemic manifestations of cholera. Furthermore, the intestinal mucosa does not contain the comma-bacillus, and Koch's theory as to the comma-bacillus present in the mucous membrane secreting a chemical inducing the disease cannot,

therefore, be correct. Neither Koch's experiments nor those of Klein and Gibbes themselves prove that the comma-bacillus is capable of producing cholera or any other disease in animals. Finally, comma-bacilli occur in the mouths of healthy persons and even in common articles of food, and in India water grossly contaminated did not produce an epidemic of cholera. Consequently, "it is quite clear from all this that the statement of Koch and his adherents as to the importance of the comma-bacillus in the water in producing cholera is in direct opposition to known facts."[10]

A distinguished committee of medical men assembled by the secretary of state for India in Council to review the report agreed wholeheartedly with Klein and Gibbes that Koch had been wrong and that there was no need whatever for quarantine or a cordon sanitaire. Sir William Gull, for example, said: "It appears to be abundantly proved that cholera is not an infectious or contagious disease. The soil and other local conditions of the place in which it prevails are responsible for it, and not the sick who suffer and die of it."[11]

Victor Vaughan wrote that when he was learning bacteriological techniques in Koch's laboratory in the summer of 1888

Professor Koch summoned me to a conference in his private room. I felt highly honored to be thus distinguished, but the burden of his talk was the condemnation of the University of Michigan for retaining as its professor of pathology a man who did not accept the well established fact that bacteria cause disease, referring to Professor Gibbes, whose name Koch pronounced with bitterness, biting it into two syllables.[12]

Gibbes at Michigan

Gibbes taught a class in pathology that was squeezed into the third year of the four-year curriculum. He gave sixty-four hours of lecture and a laboratory course occupying fifty hours, in which students followed directions in Gibbes's laboratory manual.[13] Warthin said: "The only pathology given to students was a crude course, chiefly histologic, of thick sections cut with a razor on an ice-and-salt freezing microtome, and stained with log wood, usually so black that no details could be recognized."[14] A student was expected to perform one autopsy in the senior year.

Gibbes quickly came into conflict with Vaughan, and the battleground was tuberculosis. Are phthisis and tuberculosis one disease or two? If they are one disease, is Koch's bacillus the cause? Gibbes firmly and repeatedly stated his belief at medical meetings that there are two diseases.[15] Vaughan tried to rebut him.

Gibbes declared that one of the diseases begins with an inflammatory process followed by tissue breakdown and eventual tubercle formation. The tubercles never contain tubercle bacilli. There are no bacilli in the patient's sputum, even in long-continued cases. In the other disease tubercle bacilli are in the center of the lesion, but their presence is the result rather than the cause of tissue breakdown. In hundreds of instances, Gibbes had never seen bacillus-free lesions in the same lung. Transmission of tuberculosis in animals proves nothing. In the first place, the disease in animals is different from the disease in humans. In the second, no one has ever demonstrated that cultures of Koch's tubercle bacillus are totally free from morbid products taken from a diseased lung. The morbid product, Gibbes thought, is probably the cause of the disease.

Vaughan used George Dock's skill as a pathologist to get rid of Gibbes. At the meeting of the regents on 6 February 1895, Regent Kiefer moved that the chair of pathology be combined with that of internal medicine, thereby eliminating Gibbes's job. The excuse was economy, and at the same time for the same reason another regent moved that the chair of anatomy be combined with that of surgery. This game of medical musical chairs unseated Gibbes but not McMurrich. Because Vaughan had worked in harmony with Kiefer for more than five years, it is impossible to believe Vaughan was not a party to the game.[16]

Aldred Scott Warthin

George Dock had become a competent pathologist as a disciple of William Osler. After finishing his internship in Philadelphia, he had worked under Karl Huber in Leipzig, hardening and staining tissues handed him at the autopsy table. Then Dock had studied both gross and microscopic pathology under Virchow in Berlin and Weigert in Frankfurt. He had been professor of pathology at the University of Texas in Galveston for two years (1889–91) before coming to Ann Arbor, and at Michigan he did his own autopsies at first.

Throughout his time at Michigan Dock practiced what would now be called clinical pathology in the chemical laboratory he had installed in the hospital. There he, his assistants, and his students examined sputum, vomitus, stool, exudates, and puncture fluids.[17] Consequently, when Gibbes was dismissed it was rational to look to Dock, but it was irrational to expect him to be the school's pathologist as well as its internist. Fortunately for Michigan, his demonstrator in medicine, Aldred Scott Warthin, was in training to become a pathologist.

Warthin had been an undergraduate at Indiana University when David Starr Jordan was the university's professor of zoology and president, but before graduating in 1888 Warthin earned a diploma in music teaching from the Cincinnati Conservatory. After graduating doctor of medicine from Michigan in 1891 he immediately became Dock's assistant. Warthin went to Europe in the summers of 1893, 1894, and 1895 to study pathology, for in those days the University Hospital was closed in the summer. He studied first under Ernst Ziegler in Freiburg im Breisgau and then in Vienna. As soon as he attained competence he did Dock's autopsies, and after 1895 he was Dock's deputy as university pathologist, examining all surgical specimens and doing all autopsies. Warthin was promoted rapidly, and in 1903 his status was recognized by his appointment as professor of pathology.

Warthin, Dürer, and Wagner

On his way through Nuremberg in 1893 Warthin saw Dürer's *Ritter, Tod und Teufel* in a shop window. He bought it as the first of his collection that eventually contained 685 books, etchings and other prints, and drawings of death.[18] Near the end of his life he published a handsome volume, *The Physician of the Dance of Death,* of which he said: "This study of man's changing psychical reactions to the concept of Death, throughout six centuries, has occupied the writer, in his scattered hours of leisure, affording him much stimulating interest and mental recreation."[19] Warthin was carrying on the Osler-Dock tradition of historical scholarship, and he dedicated the book to George Dock. Warthin inscribed a copy with a shaky hand:

George Dock from Aldred Scott Warthin, in memory of the good times we had together in the early 1890s.

As a musician Warthin quite naturally attended concerts and the opera when he went to Europe early in the 1890s. He was particularly struck in Munich and Vienna by the thought that the musical *Schwärmer* (enthusiasts) in their state of rapport with Wagnerian music were self-hypnotized.

In giving themselves up to the emotional effect of the music, these people were putting forward their subjective natures at the expense of their objective relations to the world; for the time, being in a state exactly analogous to the hypnotic state, if not really the same. From this it was but a quick passage to the thought that the power of music . . . might . . . be displayed and felt in its greatest and purest force . . . in a complete hypnotic state.[20]

Accordingly, Warthin did the obvious experiment.

Warthin's subjects were five men and two women who were "healthy and passed for normal individuals."[21] None was a musician, and in the usual state music produced no great emotional effect or apparent physiological action. Each was hypnotized in a room containing a piano, and when the hypnotic state had been induced the subject was told: "You are dead to everything else in the world except the music which is now to be played, and you will feel and know nothing but this music. Moreover, when awakened, you will remember what effect it has had upon you."[22] When Wagner's *Ride of the Walküre*[23] was played to a forty-year-old physician his pulse rate rose from 60 to 120, and his respiratory rate increased from 18 to 30 a minute. His face showed great mental excitement; his whole body was thrown into motion; his legs were drawn up; his arms tossed in the air; and he was bathed with profuse sweat. On awakening he said he had been riding furiously through the air.

Warthin continued:

The effect of single chords in certain relations produced wonderful effects. If during the height of excitement caused by the "Ride of the Walküre," in the key of B major, the chord of B minor was suddenly and loudly played, a most remarkable change was produced in the subject. In the case of the physician all excitement suddenly ceased, the subject's face became ashy pale, and covered with cold sweat; the pulse-rate dropped from 120 to 40 per minute, and became very irregular, soft, and small; the respirations decreased in number, and became sighing in character. The whole picture presented was one of complete collapse, so that all who saw it were alarmed. On being awakened the subject said that he had been oppressed by a horrible fear, because "everything had suddenly seemed to come to an end."[24]

Warthin encountered other curious effects. One subject was thrown into a state of hyperesthesia by the overture to *Tannhäuser.* The blunt end of a needle was pressed against his arm, but he was told the needle was running into his skin. He shrieked loudly. Another subject went into the hypnotic state whenever he heard the "Pilgrims' Chorus," and he had to be released from this influence by word suggestion during hypnosis.

Warthin had heard that sexual orgasms had been produced by some orchestral performances, and he tried to discover whether a similar effect could be caused by music popularly thought to be particularly suggestive. Notorious passages from *Die Walküre* and *Tristan und Isolde* aroused feelings of frenzy or longing in Warthin's hypnotized subjects but not sexual desire. That could, however, be produced by coupling word suggestion with the music.

Warthin thought the experiments dangerous, and he warned others against repeating them.

Warthin's Teaching

Gibbes had taught pathology by lecture and laboratory in both halves of the junior year, but when stiffer entrance requirements permitted elimination of nonmedical subjects from the first year pathology was moved a semester earlier. Until 1899 Dock gave sixty-four lectures while Warthin supervised the laboratory, but thereafter Warthin was in full command. Warthin always had a succession of assistants, some paid by the university and some volunteer. Peyton Rous, fresh from his Johns Hopkins training with William Welch, was an instructor for two years. Many years later Warthin dedicated his book *Old Age*[25] to Rous as a "One-time Assistant of Mine, and Ever Since a Dearly Beloved Friend." Medical students worked for Warthin without pay, but one of them, Carl Vernon Weller, was employed as an instructor from 1911 to 1913. After Weller received his doctor of medicine degree in 1913 he was Warthin's right-hand man until Warthin's death in 1931. The small staff had a lot to do, for in addition to teaching it had to make diagnoses for the clinical departments.

At first the student laboratory was held five afternoons a week for five weeks, but it was soon extended to nine weeks. The work was so intensive that students came Saturday mornings and had little time to study for other courses.[26] Warthin established the Michigan tradition of rigorous laboratory teaching in pathology by providing each student with 175 unknown slides for observation and discussion. Some of the material had been collected in Freiburg and Vienna, and Warthin himself prepared 30,000 slides. "Sections were given out as unknowns, studied and analyzed by the student, and the final diagnosis rounded off by student and teacher together. It was hard teaching, but I do not regret it."[27] Students were required to hand in written reports and fifty drawings. The best two sets of drawings earned prizes of fifteen dollars and five dollars. Students used Warthin's 134-page laboratory manual,[28] and after 1903 they could study Warthin's translation of Ziegler's *General Pathology*.[29] Students were required to attend and report on twenty autopsies in their junior and senior years, and they were excused from other classes when an autopsy occurred, much to the annoyance of other professors. To make sure they did a thorough job, Warthin required each student to use a blank book of autopsy protocols.[30] The ten pages for each autopsy were to be filled in from dictation during the process of examination, and the report was to be completed several days later when the results of microscopic and bacteriologic examinations came through.

Warthin drove the students hard, and Weller said that those who had little personal contact with him generally disliked him.[31] Warthin knew of "the resultant bad reputation which my courses came to have among the unintelligent student majority of that period. But student popularity was neither a thing desired nor sought by me, unless it came as an unasked appreciation from my best students. And this it has always been."[32] Malcolm Soule said Warthin was positive and dogmatic,[33] and reading Warthin's harsh, boastful criticism of others[34] it is clear why he had enemies among the faculty as well. Nevertheless, as Weller continued: "To the individual student, however, he was always ready to give sympathetic encouragement, and his friendly and understanding attitude toward the individual was in sharp contrast to the pedagogical pressure which he put upon his students en masse."[35] Students did respond, and many attended a journal club he organized. The club studied medical history as well as pathology, and in some years fifteen students reported on their original research. An impressive list of fifty-four former students, including Alice Hamilton and Carl Wig-

gers, contributed to a Festschrift assembled for Warthin's sixtieth birthday.[36]

Warthin's Pathological Material and Staff

Dock said that in the early days gross pathological anatomy had to be pursued in the back rooms of undertakers' establishments or bedrooms of lodging houses, but little was missed even under those difficult conditions. While Gibbes was still professor of pathology, Dock and Warthin did their pathological diagnostic studies sub rosa, but after 1895 Warthin could practice pathology in the old Pavilion Hospital. There he began to assemble a museum that was praised by William Osler when he came to Ann Arbor to visit George Dock. In 1903 space became available in the new Medical Building, and the headquarters of the department remained there for fifty years. Adequate accommodations for gross pathology, including a museum and a handsome theater with an autopsy table, were provided when the new hospital was occupied in 1925 (fig. 11–1).

In the first year after Gibbes left, Warthin performed 12 autopsies and reported on 158 diagnostic specimens. The number of autopsies grew very slowly, and there were only 22 in 1910–11. Warthin persuaded the regents to rule that all surgical specimens removed in the University Hospital must be turned over to the Pathological Laboratory, so the number of diagnostic cases had grown to 1,820 in the same year. By 1920–21 there were 131 autopsies and 5,419 diagnostic cases. After 1925 and until Warthin's death in 1931 there were between 350 and 400 autopsies performed each year, representing just over 50 percent of hospital deaths. In Warthin's last year the department handled 18,194 diagnostic cases.

Warthin and Weller after him always had a small professional staff to carry the teaching and service load. From 1900 Warthin had an assistant or an instructor, such as Peyton Rous,[37] and from 1913 to 1921 Weller was all Warthin had to help him. Promotion came slowly for Weller until he began to receive offers from the outside, and on 5 March 1924, Warthin recommended Weller's promotion to a full professorship to head off a bid from the University of Iowa. After 1921 the two occasionally had an additional instructor, and for a while Harriet Taylor was an assistant professor handling dental pathology. In the 1920s Ruth Wanstrom

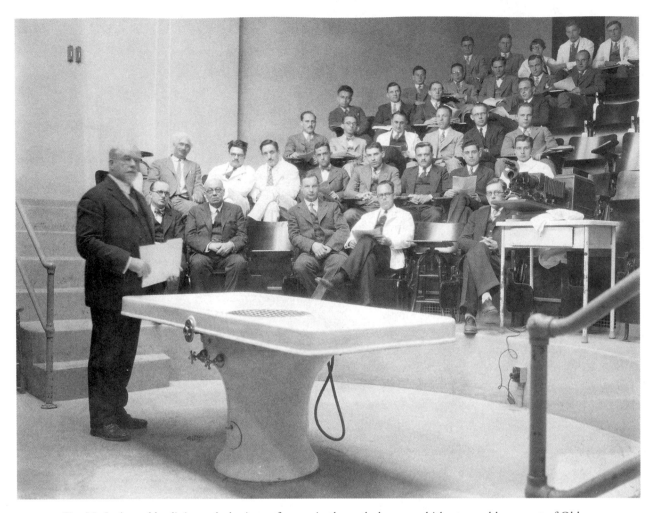

Fig. 11–1. A weekly clinicopathologic conference in the pathology amphitheater, subbasement of Old Main, 1926–27, with pathologist Aldred Warthin *(standing)*, roentgenologist Preston Hickey, and surgeon Max Peet *(seated in front row, second and third from left)*. (Courtesy of the Department of Pathology, University of Michigan.)

became an instructor after serving as a research associate. Dean Cabot antagonized Warthin by refusing to support Wanstrom's promotion to an assistant professorship on the ground that she had not given enough evidence of professional accomplishment. Warthin prevailed; Wanstrom was promoted in 1925 after a period of study in Vienna. Occasionally there was an intern in pathology, and after 1920 there were always one or two teaching assistants.

Clinicians were not always pleased by Warthin's reports. When he told Nancrede that a giant cell sarcoma was relatively benign and should be treated by local excision rather than by amputation, Nancrede furiously informed him that the only diagnosis he

wanted was that of sarcoma. When Warthin told the gynecologist Martin that the pus tubes he had sent were gonococcal,

[Martin] shouted, "What do you mean, young man, by saying that these tubes are infected with gonococci? These are all decent, married women." . . . Still more reluctantly [Warthin said] were diagnoses of syphilis in operative material received. Often at first they roused active dissent. When cases of gummatous lesions of the skin, bone, and lymph nodes had been clinically demonstrated as neoplasms and operated upon as such, it was but natural that the clinician should object to a returned diagnosis of syphilis. Even after the demonstration of the spirochete had been made possible, this same reluctance to accept a pathologic diagnosis of syphilis persisted for some time.[38]

Not Just Any Medical School

Eventually the clinician accepted the law laid down by Warthin, or so Warthin said, and sometimes cases were referred to him before operation.

The Pathology Diagnostic Fund

Warthin was also a private practitioner of pathology, and he handled hundreds of slides referred to him each year. He charged for his services. After he died in 1931 the Pathology Service in the University Hospital was put on a full-time basis, and there was a prolonged debate on what to do with outside referrals. At first it was suggested that Weller continue the service, keeping half the fees and giving the rest to the university. Eventually the Pathology Diagnostic Fund was created. Weller could continue to do outside, routine diagnostic work. He would collect the fees and keep the books. Each month receipts were to be transmitted to the treasurer of the university for deposit in the diagnostic fund, and a report would be submitted to the Executive Committee of the Medical School. Money in the fund would reimburse the university for services of its staff, an early version of overhead, and $4,000 would be added to Weller's salary. The substantial residue would be used for the benefit of the Medical School, but it was made clear that there would be special attention to the needs of the Pathology Department. In the year 1935–36, 6,042 specimens arrived from fifteen hospitals, and in 1939–40 the cash receipts were $14,182.50. In later years the report to the Executive Committee often said receipts were falling, the reason being that community hospitals were acquiring competent pathologists, some trained by Warthin and Weller.

Warthin's Research Accomplishments

When, near the end of his life, Warthin surveyed the slides and records of 150,000 cases he had collected over nearly forty years, he said: "This collection, which has taken a whole lifetime to assemble, could now be utilized for a lifetime of research and study."[39] He had, in fact, used it for a lifetime of research as he conceived research, and he was proud of his accomplishments. He had demonstrated tuberculosis of the placenta in over a dozen cases, and with a collection of 50,000 tonsils the complete pathology of the tonsil had been described in his laboratory. Warthin had refuted the concept of "sarcoma of the breast" and of the "adenomatous prostate." He had shown that the broad tapeworm had become endemic in the Great Lakes region although no one had believed his prediction that it would. He had demonstrated the tissue lesions produced by irradiation and the pathology of mustard gas poisoning.[40] He had proved the importance of fat embolism, the existence of hemolymph glands in humans, the nonexistence of Banti's syndrome, and, contrary to the opinion at the Mayo Clinic, the rarity of the conversion of gastric ulcer to gastric cancer. He was particularly proud of his work on the thymicolymphatic constitution, the heredity of cancer, and the prevalence of syphilis.

The Thymicolymphatic Constitution

As early as 1614 the sudden death of a five-month-old child had been blamed on compression of the great vessels in the chest by a mass subsequently identified as the thymus.[41] From then on some pathologists asserted and some denied that an abnormally large thymus is the cause of strident breathing, cyanosis, and sudden death until the literature, as Edith Boyd said in 1927, was utter chaos.[42] Warthin believed that death from compression of the trachea by the thymus had been demonstrated beyond a doubt.[43] He gave clinical evidence that stridor could be relieved only by passing a tube deep enough into the trachea to reach beyond the thymus, and he gave explicit directions for demonstrating compression of the trachea at autopsy. The trouble, he thought, is that the great vessels, the trachea, the esophagus, and the thymus are contained in a space no more than two centimeters deep between the sternum and the vertebral column. Any enlargement, either absolute as the result of primary hyperplasia or relative as the result of persistence of the thymus, can compress the trachea. This is particularly important in a child with constitutional status lymphaticus, and Warthin showed how to diagnose an enlarged thymus. The child with an enlarged thymus must be guarded with extreme care.

Status lymphaticus had been defined in 1889 and 1890 by the Viennese forensic pathologist Arnold Paltauf.[44] In the first half of his paper Paltauf had described autopsy findings in five infants who had died suddenly. The enlarged thymus gland, whose dimensions he gave, was clearly the cause of death. In the second half of his paper Paltauf described his findings at autopsy of five men in their twenties who had died suddenly, three while swimming in the Danube, one while playing cards, and one while walking in the Prater. Paltauf had said that the hyperplasia or long persistence of the thymus was not the primary cause of death but the thymicolymphatic constitution was. The enlarged thymus is but a sign of that constitution. Warthin agreed with Osler, who said that the thymicolymphatic constitution is "a combination of constitutional anomalies among which are hyperplasia of the lymphoid tissues and of the thymus, hypoplasia of the cardiovascular system and peculiarities of configuration with frequent sudden death."[45]

Soma Weiss pointed out that none of the sudden deaths had been observed by a doctor or nurse qualified to determine the nature of the death, and he thought that "asystole of various types and ventricular fibrillation are the usual causes."[46] However, at Michigan A. C. Furstenberg, a thoroughly competent observer, did see sudden death in a child while he was bronchoscoping her, looking for a foreign object. The mucous membrane of the bronchi became swollen and edematous, giving the appearance of a sudden allergic reaction. At autopsy the membrane was perfectly normal. Furstenberg in his diplomatic fashion said he did not believe an enlarged thymus could cause sudden death by compressing the trachea, the great vessels, or the nerves, and he gave cogent evidence for his belief. Nevertheless, Warthin continued to blame the thymicolymphatic constitution for such occurrences.

In addition to predisposing to sudden death the thymicolymphatic constitution included psychical instability leading to drug addiction and suicide. To protect the child the enlarged thymus must be removed surgically, or, more easily, it could be destroyed by roentgen irradiation. With the latter treatment the child ran the risk of developing thyroid cancer, but the Michigan experience was not bad.[47] Results of irradiation of the thymus before 1931 have not been collected, but from 1932 through 1938, about 80 to 160 children were treated with X rays to the thymic region each year. The number fell off to about 60 in 1939 and 1940, and it decreased steadily until the treatment was stopped altogether in 1952. A follow-up study in 1958 found that 754 patients aged zero to twelve months and 175 aged one to twelve years, 8 more than twelve years, and 21 of uncertain age had

received radiation in the thymic region in those years, and 867 could be traced. In 15,130 patient-years five patients had died of malignant neoplasms that developed after irradiation. Two had a lymphoblastoma—one leukemia and one lymphosarcoma—and that was a bit but not significantly higher than expected on the basis of vital statistic rates for the United States in 1950. The one instance of carcinoma of the thyroid was definitely more than the one-twentieth of a case expected.

During Warthin's lifetime the most devastating criticism of his concept of thymic death came from Edith Boyd, a University of Minnesota pathologist. She had not seen a single instance in which death had been caused by pressure on the trachea. She found that the anatomical picture described by Paltauf as status thymicolymphaticus represented the normal thymus and lymphatic tissue of a well-nourished child.[48] She demonstrated this point with great thoroughness in a long paper containing twenty-seven closely printed tables.

When illness has lasted longer than twenty-four hours, the weight of the thymus is reduced regardless of the cause of death. . . . The concept of a pathologic state arose from misconstruing the normal prominent thymus and lymphoid tissue for a constitutional abnormality and vice versa, the involuted, inconspicuous thymus of inanition being misconstrued for the normal.[49]

The thymicolymphatic constitution lingered on as official doctrine at Michigan throughout Warthin's time and into Weller's. In an introductory lecture Weller gave in 1955 in the last course he taught, he described the thymicolymphatic type. He did admit that it was the subject of legitimate controversy. The type was very rare in Europe and in the eastern United States, but it was seen along the Pacific Coast and in the Great Lakes region. It was once thought that if the thymus is enlarged it could compress the trachea and cause death by asphyxiation, but this is now known to be very rare. More commonly, children in status lymphaticus die of circulatory collapse, which may be brought on by minor surgery, anesthesia, immersion in cold water, or any minor traumatic event. Although roentgenologists in the University Hospital had stopped irradiating the thymic region three years before, Weller said that in the case of elective surgery the enlarged thymus of a child scheduled for operation could be reduced by three hundred to four hundred rads.[50]

The Heredity of Cancer

For Warthin the thymicolymphatic constitution was only one of many inheritable susceptibilities to disease. Pernicious anemia results from intrinsic weakness of the red-blood-cell forming tissue, and many causes may lead to excessive hemolysis and anemia. He cited examples of food faddists, the floating semiinvalid sanatarium class, who develop pernicious anemia. There is also Graves' constitution associated with the lymphatic constitution, for hyperplasia of the thymus is found in every case of exophthalmic goiter. "Basedow's or Graves' disease, 'toxic goiter' and 'toxic adenoma' are *pathological reactions* [the emphasis is Warthin's] potentially predetermined in the individual at birth by virtue of his constitutional anomaly."[51]

Very early in his career as a pathologist Warthin became convinced that there are hereditary immunity to cancer and hereditary susceptibility. As a pathologist in a university hospital in a small town in the center of a rural area Warthin had an advantage over a pathologist in a city hospital, for he could work up the histories of several generations of a stable family. For hereditary immunity he cited his own family. An eighth great-grandfather had nine thousand blood descendants in whom cancer was one of the rarest occurrences. Warthin, however, was the fourth generation male in direct line to have Dupuytren's contracture.[52]

By 1913 Warthin had found twenty-nine cancer kindreds in Michigan. In one the grandfather, five of his ten children, and twelve of twenty-four grandchildren had cancer. This illustrated Warthin's belief that multiple occurrences in one generation always mean occurrence in the preceding generation. In cancer families cancer tends to occur earlier in younger generations and to be more malignant. Furthermore, cancer is associated with marked susceptibility to tuberculosis.[53] In 1925 Warthin was able to extend one of his genealogical tables, finding twenty-seven instances of carcinoma in 144 descendants of a cancerous progenitor.[54] He also had three sets of identical twins, one pair of sisters with malignant teratoma of the ovary, one pair with cancer of the breast, and a pair of brothers with malignant teratoma of the testicle. In all instances the tumors were in mirror image locations. Warthin thought the cancer tendency was probably dominant, in some cases rising and in some cases not rising above a clinical horizon.

Warthin believed in the inheritance of acquired characteristics,[55] and he knew one of the mechanisms of transmission: blastophthoria, the degeneration of the germ plasm from poisoning by lead, alcohol, or syphilis. Weller had found that in male guinea pigs chronically poisoned with lead there were instances of sterility, a reduction of the offspring's birth weight by 20 percent, an increased number of deaths in the first week of life, and retardation of development.[56] In a limited group of males there was complete aspermatogenesis with atrophy and vacuolar degeneration of the germinal epithelium. Weller found blastophthoria to result from acute alcoholic intoxication as well.[57] Warthin extended the concept generally, saying that a person should not marry soon after recovering from a debilitating disease such as typhoid fever. The eugenic implications were obvious. Although physicians and medical students no longer took religion seriously, the Ten Commandments could be derived from evolution, and biology had substituted race immortality for personal immortality.

The voluntary exposure of the individual to any form of infection or intoxication that may affect the vitality of his germ-plasm must be placed in the same category of biologic sin. . . . The State should require eugenic marriages, and prevent non-eugenic ones. No individual should be allowed to produce children, who possesses a germ-plasm so seriously below par as to make of him an undesirable citizen.[58]

Marriage should last twenty-five years in the interest of the children, and trial marriage and divorce should be discouraged.

Syphilis

Warthin was surprised to learn that in 4,880 autopsies at Bellevue Hospital in New York City a pathologist had found syphilis in only 314 instances.[59] He himself had found syphilis in 300 of 750 autopsies by 1919. The populations were different. Warthin thought the depraved poor of New York City would have syphilis much more frequently than the better elements of the virtuous middle class living in the semirural Midwest and coming to the University Hospital in Ann Arbor. The difference lay in the method of diagnosis. The New York pathologist had relied entirely upon gross evidence of syphilis; Warthin demonstrated the presence of *Spirochaeta pallida* in microscopic sections. At first Warthin used the silver-reduction method of Constantin Levaditi that required seven to ten days to give results, but by 1920 he and his research assistant, Allen Starry, had improved the method so that it could show spirochetes in a single tissue section within a few hours. The section on a cover glass was soaked for thirty minutes to an hour in silver nitrate, and then the silver was reduced with hydroquinone. The organisms appeared dark reddish brown to jet black against a very light background.[60] With continued modifications the Warthin-Starry method became standard.[61] Eventually Warthin had a single technician who specialized in the method. Consequently, Warthin could demonstrate syphilis in pathological specimens others thought free of the disease. He continued to publish abundantly on the subject until his death.[62]

In patients dying with obvious syphilis Warthin found perivascular infiltration of lymphocytes and plasma cells. Consequent fibrosis obliterated arterioles. In the skin thrombosis in the corium and epidermis caused sharply circumscribed ulcerative lesions.[63] In the heart the vascular lesions resulted in diffuse myocarditis. In such cases Warthin was usually able to find spirochetes in the walls of the small blood vessels and in the surrounding interstitial fluid, but the lesions were so characteristic that Warthin was able to diagnose latent or congenital syphilis even when he completely failed to find spirochetes.

Before the discovery of *S. pallida* Warthin had learned to diagnose latent syphilis when he stood beside Alexander Kolisko at a Viennese autopsy table in 1893.[64] The patient being examined had no gumma, but Kolisko showed Warthin the tough body tissue resulting from fibrosis and the focal thickening of the meninges. Warthin continued to diagnose latent syphilis in the absence of gumma by the same criteria. Between 1910 and 1929, 494 instances of latent syphilis were found at the University Hospital in 1,675 autopsies of persons dying over the age of twenty-five. Spirochetes had actually been demonstrated in only "about 50%" of the cases. Warthin saw sharply focal lesions in the meninges by oblique light or by floating the membrane on water. At microscopic examination he saw perivascular infiltration and proliferation.[65] Myocarditis was frequently present, and Warthin believed that persons with latent syphilis usually die of acute myocardial insufficiency and dilatation.[66] He concluded that a little over 25 percent of patients from the middle and

lower classes coming to the University Hospital had latent syphilis. He also believed that treatment never cured syphilis; it only made the disease latent.

Unsuspected congenital syphilis produced similar lesions, and Warthin found syphilitic myocarditis in twelve young patients who had died of cardiac disease, only one of whom had been known before death to have congenital syphilis. He also found syphilis in the stillbirths of women with negative Wassermann reactions who, along with their husbands, had no history of syphilis whatever. The women must all unknowingly have had congenital syphilis, and Warthin found reason to believe their fathers had been infected.

Warthin's Successor

When Carl Vernon Weller (fig. 11–2) turned down an offer from another university the dean congratulated Michigan on having such strong backup for Warthin. Consequently, when Warthin died it was to be expected that Weller would immediately become director of the Pathological Laboratory, and because

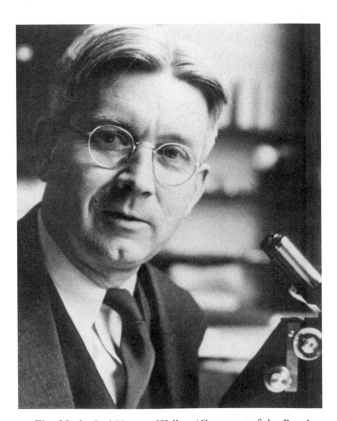

Fig. 11–2. Carl Vernon Weller. (Courtesy of the Bentley Historical Library, University of Michigan, Medical School Records, Box 136, "Pathology Department.")

Weller had worked in harmony with Warthin for more than twenty years, it was also to be expected that Weller would display many of Warthin's characteristics.

In the first place, Weller followed Warthin's strict morphological approach to disease. His material was provided by thirteen thousand necropsies and more than a half million surgical specimens. With such a large pathology service Weller turned up a few oddities. He added two more to the seventy known cases of endometriosis of the umbilicus,[67] and he described a teratological case as a "diprosopus diotus diophthalmus distomus dignathus with anencephalia and rhachischisis lumbo-sacralis."[68] Not content with local material, Weller examined tissues from the Naval Hospital in Port-au-Prince. The question was whether yaws and syphilis are one or two diseases. Weller could not decide, but he concluded that if they are two diseases they produce the same aortic pathology.[69] He went on to describe the lesions in the heart, adrenals, liver, brain, meninges, and testes, reaching the same conclusion.[70] Years before, Weller had fed graded doses of white lead to guinea pigs,[71] and he had participated in the mustard gas experiments, but when he became director there was no experimental laboratory work in his department as there was in that of the roughly contemporary pathologist, George H. Whipple. Weller was "one of the few remaining classicists and perfectionists in medicine and pathology."[72] When he was within a year or so of retirement he saw to it that the new pathology building being planned would have no wet laboratories where experimental work could be done.

As a master of all topics in pathology Weller always gave nearly all the lectures in pathology for sophomore medical students, and each year he spent as much time preparing his lectures as though he had never given them before. He continued the student laboratory as an exhausting exercise in identification of unknowns, and teachers in courses given at the same time had difficulty competing for the students' attention. At his weekly clinical pathological conferences he had senior medical students present the cases, and approximately one hundred cases were examined each year. The student report on the curriculum made in 1934 said the conferences were not intellectually stimulating. Weller was firm but fair with his students, and, in the Austro-German *Herr Professor* tradition he had inherited, he demanded strict adherence to the rules. Weller's rigid devotion to duty never permitted his outside work as editor or

officer of national organizations to interfere with his work at home: he did not even take time off to see his son receive the Nobel Prize in 1954.[73]

Intrinsic and Extrinsic Factors in Cancer

At first Weller accepted Warthin's opinion that susceptibility is inherited, and he extended research on Warthin's cancer family to another generation.[74] He also accepted Warthin's eugenic stance, and he said: "[S]terilization of any child surviving retinoblastoma and the interdiction of further progeny to the parents of a child with this disease appear to be justifiable measures."[75] John Bugher reinforced Weller's belief in hereditary susceptibility by demonstrating that the actual incidence of multiple malignant neoplasms exceeds that expected by chance alone.[76] Perhaps as the result of Weller's study of occupational diseases, he came to appreciate the importance of extrinsic as well as of intrinsic factors.[77] When he surveyed the incidence of bronchiogenic carcinoma, at first Weller thought it impossible that the apparent increase in the disease was something new. It might result from increasing age of the population, the advent of radiography, increased clinical awareness, or better diagnostic methods. However, as early as 1929 he began to think the disease is caused by smoking. He said: "If this be the true explanation, there should be an alteration of the present ratio of the incidence in men to that in women within the next decade or two."[78] Eventually, he gave up his opinion that chromosomes are stable, and in his Beaumont Lecture he said: "As of today [1955], I must agree with many of the specialists in statistical analysis and in the epidemiology of cancer, that this association [of bronchiogenic carcinoma with smoking] has been established."[79]

Weller's Staff and Students

At the time of Warthin's death there were twenty-four members of the Department of Pathology, counting the technical staff. Under Weller the professional staff expanded. Ruth Wanstrom slowly climbed the academic ladder, and in the 1930s she was joined by John Bugher and Lloyd Catron. The flood of interns and residents began to reach full tide, so that by the end of Weller's life he had trained hundreds. More than fifty became professional pathologists. Many earned a master's degree or a doctor of philosophy in pathology, chiefly by working up the abundant necropsy and surgical material in the department's files. The numerous papers from the department were no longer by Warthin or Weller alone. Before 1941 Weller's students published on such topics as the incidence of trichinosis in the Detroit area, a study based on five hundred consecutive autopsies; the relative sizes of the liver and spleen, based on one thousand autopsies; and the occurrence of periappendicitis without appendicitis, based on 26,051 surgical specimens. Weller meticulously organized his students' manuscripts as he did his own.

Weller trained his successor as Warthin had trained him, but until 1941 the only persons from the department who remained in academic life were Peyton Rous, Ruth Wanstrom, Weller himself, and John Bugher. In Warthin and Weller's fifty years, Michigan was not the source of professors of pathology and deans as Welch's department at Johns Hopkins was.

12
Internal Medicine, 1891–1918

When George Dock arrived in Ann Arbor in 1891 he found that medical patients were seldom admitted to the old Pavilion Hospital on North University, and he had to give his first clinic with a patient borrowed from the dermatologist William Breakey.[1] Dock and his demonstrator, Aldred Scott Warthin, sent notices to local physicians and clergy, saying they would see indigent patients, and they quickly accumulated cases to be used in teaching. At that time the new hospital was being constructed, and Dock was soon able to move his medical service to Catherine Street.

The Catherine Street Hospitals in George Dock's Time

The legislature had impartially provided one building on Catherine Street for the "regular" Department of Medicine and Surgery and another for its rival, the Homeopathic Department.[2] The buildings had been designed by an architectural firm with little experience in hospital construction. The open wards of the eastern building, the new University Hospital, had originally been planned for two rows of beds, but an extra row was squeezed in at the last minute. There were five beds in obstetrical wards and twelve single rooms, provided not for privacy but for care of seriously ill patients. The building had no classrooms and no laboratories of any kind. Patients were prepared for operation in a bathroom. Students were taught and patients were demonstrated and operated upon in a small pit from which rose a semicircular array of uncomfortable wooden benches.[3]

In 1901 the Homeopathic Department acquired a new hospital of its own off North University, and the Departments of Internal Medicine, Neurology, and Dermatology moved into the vacated Homeopathic Hospital then called the West Ward. The East Ward was left to the Department of Surgery and the surgical specialties. The University Hospital then had 114 beds in wards, 20 beds in single rooms, 14 beds in small wards, and 3 isolation beds in a former laundry.[4] By 1906, with the Palmer Ward and the Psychopathic Hospital, bed capacity was more than 200.

In theory only indigent patients were admitted to the University Hospital, and their charges were borne by the county of residence or by the state of Michigan. Some patients who

129

could afford to pay were admitted for one reason or another, and Dock sometimes admitted one of his few private patients to be used for teaching. Consequently, there were occasionally great uproars in medical circles over the admission of patients who could afford to pay for medical services. The regents received memorials and deputations, and newspapers asserted that soon after "free medicine" the university would provide "free law." One regent from the Upper Peninsula, however, demanded to be taken care of in the University Hospital, and Dock, to discourage such a practice, had senior medical students practice gastric lavage on him twice a day. The regent was pleased by the constant attention he received.

Eventually a committee of which Reuben Peterson was a member drew up regulations to solve the problem, and they were approved by the State Medical Society. The faculty asked the regents to restrict admission to the University Hospital to the following.

1. Those whose admission is provided for by special statutes,
2. Emergency cases,
3. All students in attendance at the university,
4. All persons bringing letters recommending their admission from their regular medical attendant, and
5. All persons applying for admission and not coming under the classes mentioned above who make an affidavit that they are financially unable to pay the usual minimum fees of the profession for such treatment as required.[5]

Later the Board of Regents declared that the hospital should be self-supporting, and fees were adjusted to meet expenses. In Dock's time and ever afterward there was conflict between the professional staff, who wanted better maintenance and more equipment and supplies, and the director of the hospital, whose duty it was to keep expenses less than income. The conflict was exacerbated by the fact that the medical staff had no control over the director, who reported directly to the regents.

George Dock's Medical Service

Throughout his tenure as professor of internal medicine at Michigan, 1891–1908, George Dock had only a small staff. When Warthin became responsible for pathology he was succeeded by Theodore L. Chadbourne, James Arneill, and Roger Morris as instructors. David Murray Cowie began to assist

Dock in 1896 and then gradually assumed responsibility for pediatric patients. From 1891 there was a house physician to the University Hospital, and after 1899 there were also interns, sometimes as many as six. Those interns were supplemented by senior medical students acting as interns, and near the end of Dock's time in Ann Arbor they were allowed free lodging and meals in return for their services. In 1892–93 Alice Hamilton was one of those special students. Dock followed Osler's practice of inviting his staff to his home to discuss medicine.

As his clinical notes show, Dock kept himself thoroughly informed about everything occurring in the hospital, and he seems to have had a talent for organization. Some sixteen years after Dock left Michigan, George Herrmann, then an instructor in medicine at Michigan but previously on Dock's staff at Barnes Hospital in St. Louis, published a 521-page book, *Methods in Medicine: The Manual of the Medical Service of George Dock, M.D., Sc.D.*[6] The book describes in detail the duties of every member of the medical staff, special clinical and laboratory methods of investigation, therapeutic and dietetic methods, ways of recording case histories, and methods of referral. Of course, Barnes Hospital in 1924 was larger and more complex than the University of Michigan hospital in Dock's time, but the administrative skills displayed at Barnes must have been used earlier in Ann Arbor.

Dock let his staff know exactly what he expected of them, and his sharp tongue and blunt expression of opinions often offended others. His vocabulary was uncensored, and sometimes he shocked the prim Warthin.

Teaching Third-Year Medical Students

One or another of Dock's assistants did most of the teaching of internal medicine in the third year. Class size ranged from 71 to 120 students, and the class was divided into sections for practical work in physical diagnosis: inspection, palpation, percussion, and auscultation, first on healthy persons and then on patients. Students were taught chemical, microscopic, and bacteriologic manipulations, for they were expected to use common laboratory methods in the fourth year. There were lectures as well, and what the students were expected to learn can be seen in a few representative examination questions posed in the third year.

1. Draw temperature curves for typhoid fever, scarlet fever, measles, smallpox, yellow fever with the characteristic pulse in each disease.

2. Give cause, physical signs, symptoms and pathological anatomy of chronic emphysema of the lungs.

3. Give causes, physical signs and course of aortic insufficiency.

Dock himself read the examination papers, and he corrected mistakes in spelling.[7] He did not care whether there was one or two ells in *traveler,* nor did he object to a slip of the pen when *crysis* followed *lysis,* but he thought systematic misspellings of medical terms or of proper names previously written on the blackboard were inexcusable. Among the dozen ways of spelling *Koplik* (Dr. Henry Koplik)[8] he found *Coplic, Caplex,* and *Poplick. Gastritis of the stomach* or *lied down*[9] reflected, he thought, on the preliminary training of the writers.

George Dock's Fourth-Year Teaching

Dock's major teaching, like Osler's, was done at the bedside or in his demonstration clinics (fig. 12–1).

In the fourth year all students attended diagnostic clinics lasting one and a half hours each Tuesday and Friday afternoon. From 3 October 1899 until 16 May 1908 a typewritten stenographic transcript, occupying sixteen enormous volumes, each containing about 400 pages, is preserved in the Bentley Historical Library (fig. 12–2).

At the first session of each year Dock told the students what he expected of them. The fourth-year class, now numbering fifty-eight to ninety-six students, was divided into sections of six to nine students each, and a section was responsible for patients presented in four consecutive sessions. Cases were assigned in order, and students were to work them up and to submit a written report on both the patient and the disease. Students were to follow their patients to autopsy, and they were questioned on autopsy findings. To encourage thorough work Dock exempted students who had handed in the best reports from the final examination.

Dock gave explicit directions on how to take a history, how to do a physical examination, and how to write a report. Dock reviewed the histories in class. The advice was at first reinforced by mimeographed handouts, the first of thousands given Michigan medical students, and then by a little book that went

through three editions.[10] A student was to see his or her patient every day at least and to record changes in the patient's condition. Dock required students and staff to keep complete notes, and if some incident were not recorded, Dock considered that it had not existed. When a student said he did not have time, Dock told him, "Remember that time was made for slaves, and you being a slave take your time."[11] A student should see the patient in the patient's home if necessary.

Throughout the year Dock gave many demonstrations: how to sterilize needles and a syringe, how to give injections, and how to tap a chest to remove pus. The students in the current section helped him, and they were expected to learn the procedures. Dock once drew 123 milliliters of fluid from a cystic goiter in front of the class. He showed how to evacuate a joint, how to do a rectal examination, and how to use a proctoscope. A tumor of the stomach was found by palpation after the stomach had been inflated, and Dock debated whether it was worthwhile to refer the patient to a surgeon. Likewise, tumors of the spleen or kidney were differentiated by inflating the colon with air. He advised using a syringe bulb, but he added that a simple rubber tube could be used to inflate the colon by mouth. "I advise you to get the first blow."[12] Dock gave much practical advice: how to deal tactfully with a pregnant unmarried girl and how to examine a child. "Don't stare at a child. Observe him without letting him know it."[13] At the end of each year most of the students would go directly into practice, and Dock told them what equipment they would need, how to keep records, and how to deal with colleagues.

A Clinical Demonstration

Two or three patients were studied each Tuesday or Friday. Dock did not believe in false modesty, and he made sure each patient was adequately exposed. He questioned a student, often not the one responsible for the patient, and he was sometimes rough with the student whom he led step-by-step through the examination. Here is the first page describing the examination of the first of three patients on 5 March 1907.

Dock: Miss Berry, have you seen this lady before? What do you think about her.
Student: (Couldn't hear.)
Dock: Why?

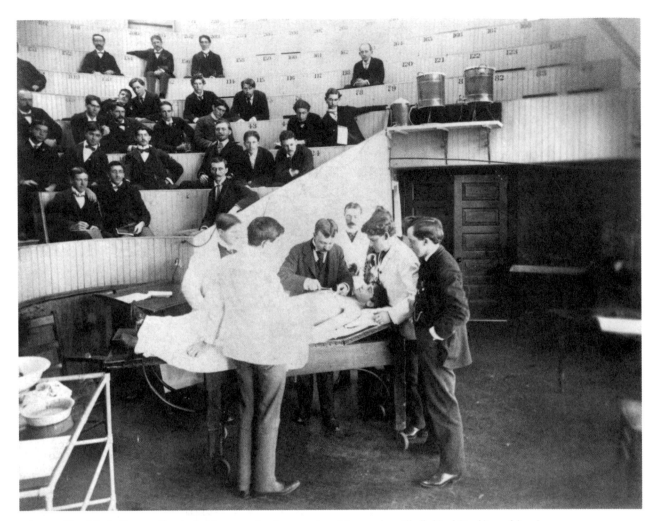

Fig. 12–1. George Dock *(with percussion hammer)* and James Arneill *(behind Dock)* teaching in amphitheater of Catherine Street Hospital. The "patient" is probably a student. (Courtesy of the Bentley Historical Library, University of Michigan, Medical School Records, Box 136, "Classes by Subject, Surgery and Anatomy Amphitheater Views.")

Student: She has dyspnœa; her mouth is drawn.

Dock: What else do you see, Miss Humphrey?

Student: Her lips look purple but then—

Dock: She is not distinctly cyanotic, though, is she? What else can you see?

Student: She has some pulsations in her neck.

Dock: And what else?

Student: A marked dyspnœa.

Dock: What is the character of her dyspnœa? Yes, the expiration is prolonged and labored. What else? Yes, there is an epigastric pulsation. What do you suppose is the matter with her?

Student: I suppose there is some heart lesion.

Dock: What would you do next in order to see?

Student: I would percuss the heart and auscult.

Dock: Suppose you go ahead and examine the heart.

Student: There is a strong apex beat.

Dock: Can you localize it? Where?

Student: It is in the nipple line.

Dock: Where is the upper border? Do you think that is dull there? Where is the absolute dulness? Suppose you go a little bit lower and see what you get. Where is the beginning of absolute dulness? Why do you have such a fear of going lower down? One must always allow the percussion to develop itself and not force it. Where is the left side? That gives you the lower border, doesn't it? Now how are you going to get the left side? You can't percuss through the mammary gland, can you? What we do is push the mammary gland away and percuss over the chest wall.[14]

Not Just Any Medical School

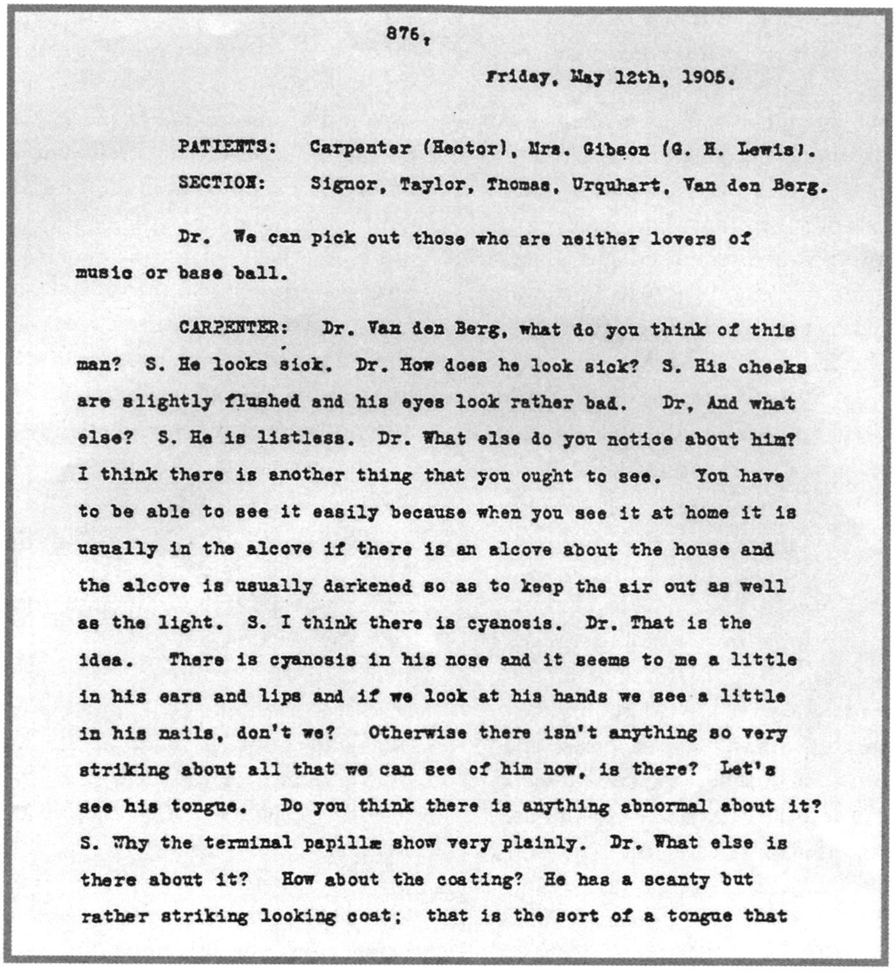

876,

Friday, May 12th, 1905.

PATIENTS: Carpenter (Hector), Mrs. Gibson (G. H. Lewis).
SECTION: Signor, Taylor, Thomas, Urquhart, Van den Berg.

Dr. We can pick out those who are neither lovers of music or base ball.

CARPENTER: Dr. Van den Berg, what do you think of this man? S. He looks sick. Dr. How does he look sick? S. His cheeks are slightly flushed and his eyes look rather bad. Dr. And what else? S. He is listless. Dr. What else do you notice about him? I think there is another thing that you ought to see. You have to be able to see it easily because when you see it at home it is usually in the alcove if there is an alcove about the house and the alcove is usually darkened so as to keep the air out as well as the light. S. I think there is cyanosis. Dr. That is the idea. There is cyanosis in his nose and it seems to me a little in his ears and lips and if we look at his hands we see a little in his nails, don't we? Otherwise there isn't anything so very striking about all that we can see of him now, is there? Let's see his tongue. Do you think there is anything abnormal about it? S. Why the terminal papillæ show very plainly. Dr. What else is there about it? How about the coating? He has a scanty but rather striking looking coat; that is the sort of a tongue that

Fig. 12–2. A page from the stenographic typescript of George Dock's fourth-year diagnostic clinics, illustrating Dock's methods and his habit of giving offhand practical advice. The line about music and baseball refers to the fact that on that afternoon Theodore Thomas's orchestra under the direction of Frederick Stock gave the second of that year's May Festival concerts and that Michigan played Wisconsin, winning four to three. (Courtesy of the Bentley Historical Library, University of Michigan, George Dock Notebooks.)

There are eight more pages of typescript before the second patient is reached.

George Dock's Clinical Laboratory

Dock said that at Michigan he had cramped space for his clinical laboratory but good equipment.[15] Immediately after arriving in Ann Arbor he solicited equipment from the regents. After he had talked for an hour on the merits and needs of a laboratory one regent said: "Now, Dr. Dock, you have talked for quite a while about this laboratory. Can you tell me in a few words what it's for?" Dock replied: "Mr. Regent, a clinical laboratory is a place where you smoke cigarettes and piss in the sink."[16] Appropriately, Dock's first clinical laboratory was in a ten-by-ten-foot water closet. The administrative office of the hospital was moved in 1896 to a small building of its own, and the space vacated was devoted to the clinical laboratories. Dock's office was in the laboratory, and he did his own analyses. Dock and his staff examined sputum, vomitus, urine, and stool. Dock regretted that the laboratory was too small to allow the students to use it, but sometimes a student did special work there such as following urinary excretion of sugar by a diabetic patient being evaluated. Dock did not use the laboratory for prolonged and systematic study of a particular problem, and, in fact, he was not a scientist at all.[17]

Dock used the microscope both for routine clinical observation and for investigations resulting in publications. There were always microscopes available in the demonstration clinics, and students used them under Dock's direction. Dock regularly made both red and white blood cell counts, and he told his students that in practice they must have access to a microscope, a hemocytometer, and red and white cell pipettes. He searched the blood for malaria parasites in cases of myocarditis that had been diagnosed as malaria by local physicians.[18] Dr. McMurrich helped Dock to identify the *Trichomonas* parasite.[19] Dock found leuckocyte counts useful in diagnosis of appendicitis, and when the diagnosis was made he at once referred the patient to Dr. Nancrede. The days of expectant treatment of appendicitis were over. Dock examined cells found in ascitic and pleural fluids.[20] He found mitotic figures in leukemic blood as well.[21]

Dock said he had done thousands of gastric analyses,[22] but the number seems a bit exaggerated. Results of gastric analysis were considered by the class, and Dock thought them most useful in functional disorders of the stomach, for excessive secretion might result in severe neurasthenia or impotence in the male. He found achlorhydria in cancer of the stomach and in pernicious anemia. Blood hemoglobin concentration was estimated by means of the Tallqvist scale, in which the tint of a drop of blood on white blotting paper is compared with that of a standard. Dock thought it more accurate than other commercially available methods. Of the few other clinical tests used, one was Ehrlich's diazo reaction that was supposed to detect something in the urine diagnostic of typhoid fever, tuberculosis, or measles. Dock did the Widal test, agglutination of typhoid bacilli by the patient's serum, but when Warthin did the autopsy on a patient whom Dock had diagnosed with endocarditis, the cultures from the heart were made under the direction of Dr. Novy.

Clinical Problems

There was the inevitable typhoid fever, and Dock drilled his students on its characteristics as Osler had.[23] He gave directions on how to tub a patient who must be made to void before being abruptly plunged into water at sixty degrees Farenheit. He dressed down a student who did not participate in tubbing his patients. There was some malaria in Michigan, but not so much as in the South. A Michigan patient never had a malaria chill in the winter unless he had one the previous summer. During the smallpox epidemic of 1904 Dock used Dr. Huber's little girl as an example of the technique of vaccination. He thought that the current methods of haphazard vaccination resulted in high morbidity, and he wrote that systematic vaccination should be carried out by public officials, using vaccine manufactured under controlled conditions.[24] There was diabetes mellitus whose prognosis was grave, particularly in a child. Dock advised his students to perfect their ability to measure sugar in the urine while they were still in school, for they would need to know how to use Fehling's solution when they were in practice. There was rickets, and there was scurvy. Dock showed skiagrams of a scorbutic child who had recovered quickly when given orange juice. He was not sure whether scurvy was the result of quantitative or qualitative defect in the diet or action of some toxic substance.[25] Dock was surprised to see more goiters in a year in Michigan than he had seen in many years in Philadelphia and Texas. He made a careful study of the distribution of goiters in Michigan, and he associated their occurrence with the use of well water rather than lake water. He found large goiters, but he said that "even the largest native goitre I have seen would excite little interest in Savoy."[26] He also said he had seen no myxedema in Michigan, and he treated some of his goitrous patients with dried thyroid with equivocal results.

Dock had a special interest in cardiovascular diseases, and while he was in Ann Arbor he edited with numerous additions Jürgensen, Schrötter, and Krehl's *Diseases of the Heart*.[27] The additions ranged from a few sentences here and there, one gently correcting the Germans on the distribution of the bundle of His, to more than two pages on recent advances in the knowledge of heart block made by Joseph Erlanger. Diagnosis of valvular disease was emphasized in Dock's clinics. Sometimes the diagnosis was corrected when Warthin reported autopsy findings.[28] Blood pressure was first estimated by feeling the pulse, but by 1904 systolic blood pressure was determined by Riva-Rocci's method.[29] Korotkoff sounds were not heard in Ann Arbor until after Dock left in 1908.

With his knowledge of medical history Dock was well aware of the correlation between John Hunter's anginal attacks and his coronary occlusion, but he said: "On the whole, such cases were not common enough to soon make an impression on the profession as a whole, and it is not surprising that later writers allowed the subject to escape them."[30] Dock himself saw three cases in which coronary occlusion found at autopsy had been responsible for anginal attacks, "asthma," or dropsy, but he did not follow up his observations while he was in Ann Arbor, leaving it to J. B. Herrick to establish firmly the clinical features of obstruction of a coronary artery in 1912.[31]

In 1898 there were 2,728 reported deaths from tuberculosis in Michigan with a death rate of 114.2 per one hundred thousand. One person in eight would die of the disease. Tuberculous patients seen in the University Hospital were usually in an advanced stage of the disease, for incompetent physicians had failed to diagnose it early when it might still be curable. Dock made a particular point in drilling his students in the early diagnosis of tuberculosis by both laboratory and physical findings. X-ray diagnosis was not used until 1902. Each student who had a tuberculous patient was enrolled as a member of that year's Tuberculosis Club, and at the end of the year one or more of the diagnostic clinic sessions was devoted to hearing the club members read reports on their patients. One reason for failure to diagnose early was that tuberculosis was thought to be hereditary, and physicians and family alike adopted a fatalistic attitude. Dock himself refuted the idea by a neat epidemiological study in the countryside around Ann Arbor clearly showing the role of contagion. There was no tuberculosis ward in the University Hospital, and Dock thought there should be one in every community hospital. The first state sanatorium was not opened until 1907, and that was in Howell, a few miles from Ann Arbor. Although some of Dock's patients had done well by going west he taught his students the principles and practice of home treatment. A patient could do as well in Podunk as in Arizona.

The Medical Library

By 1860 the University of Michigan medical library subscribed to twenty-four of the best English and Continental medical journals, and Abram Sager, the professor of diseases of women and children, could display familiarity with current European medical literature by writing reviews to keep his colleagues up-to-date.[32] Each professor had an annual budget of two hundred dollars for books, and in the 1880s Vic-

tor Vaughan persuaded them all to consolidate the money in his hands as a regular appropriation for the library. By 1892 the library contained sixty-one medical periodicals, but only one, *Archiv für Anatomie und Physiologie,* was complete.[33] There were always textbooks, many of them out-of-date.

George Dock had Osler's love of books, and he encouraged medical students to improve their education by a systematic reading of foreign journals in German, French, and Italian. He thought they should read medical classics and that when they were in practice they should combine with other doctors in the town to form a medical library.[34] Consequently, Vaughan was glad to make Dock chairman of the library committee in 1892. Dock worked quickly, and by 1895 he had completed from volume 1 all journals already taken. When he instituted new subscriptions he bought full sets of back numbers. The result was that by 1905 the library contained 13,455 bound volumes and 226 journals of which 89 were complete.

When Dock left in 1908 he was succeeded as chairman of the library committee by Warthin, also a confirmed bibliophile. The Medical Library Association met in Ann Arbor in 1916, and Warthin was proud to describe Michigan's medical library. The library, he said, was part of a relatively young state university, and it had no special endowment or gifts of any magnitude. Yet with 30,000 volumes it outranked libraries in some great eastern private universities. Yale had the same number of medical volumes as Michigan, and Pennsylvania had only 28,315. Before the interruption of the European war Michigan received 370 journals, 151 in the German language, 130 in English, 10 in Italian, and 14 in Dutch, Spanish, and the Scandinavian languages. This was on an annual appropriation of four thousand dollars. No attempt was made to get or keep minor provincial journals, but Warthin confessed the library was weak in Spanish-American publications. The library was housed as part of the university's General Library, and consequently it was reinforced by chemistry and natural science collections. The Psychopathic Hospital had its own library, but Warthin thought departmental libraries a nuisance. Clinical departments, far away from the library on the central campus, repeatedly asked permission to subscribe to journals or to buy books from their current accounts. Lombard had set them an example by paying the subscriptions for physiological journals out of his own pocket. Textbooks, chiefly in English, were bought with five hundred dollars from student fees, and these were kept in a small reading room reserved for students.

The Clinical Summer Session

The Medical School *Annual Announcement* of 1893–94 said:

The rapid development of medical science has necessitated the introduction of many new subjects into the curriculum, and this leads practitioners, who wish to keep abreast of the times, to return to the University in order to take special courses in the newer subjects.[35]

At that time there were still many schools whose standards were far below Michigan's, and the announcement stated that graduates of such schools might upgrade themselves by taking graduate courses in Ann Arbor. Accordingly, the university admitted medical graduates to any of the courses in the undergraduate curriculum, and in addition it provided a few special courses in hygiene and bacteriology, pathology, physiology and histology, neuroanatomy, and therapeutics. These special courses all included laboratory work, and students were given the opportunity to do research. The course in hygiene and bacteriology, for example, was open only to those who had completed the undergraduate course in bacteriology, and the part arranged for public health officers included chemical and bacteriological examination of food, water, soil, and air. The course in physiology was particularly designed to instruct teachers with a modern course amply illustrated with demonstrations and laboratory exercises.

Only a few students enrolled in these courses. In the next twenty years the announcement listed between three and fourteen "resident graduates." The thirteen who attended in 1894–95 were representative. Eleven had the doctor of medicine degree, and two had the doctor of dental surgery degree. All but two were graduates of Michigan. Ten of the thirteen took bacteriology, and seven took more than one course. Four attended clinics; three, including Alice Hamilton, studied histology; and one took ophthalmology.

After 1902 physicians could attend the university's summer session for six weeks to learn methods that would contribute to their success in practice. In the summer of 1906 courses were offered in medicine,

surgery, gynecology and obstetrics, and otolaryngology. We know exactly what those students did, for those who taught it published a full report.[36] The work in clinical subjects in addition to internal medicine is described here to show what was going on in the University Hospital in George Dock's time.

Eight of the sixteen students had earned their doctor of medicine degrees at Michigan. Four were graduates of the two Detroit medical schools, and one each was from Jefferson, Queen's, Hahnemann in Chicago, and the Cincinnati Medical Institute.

The course in internal medicine and diseases of the stomach began with some introductory lectures by Dock on modern diagnostic instruments, but Murray Cowie and Hugo Freund carried the major burden. They taught laboratory methods for examining blood, urine, sputum, gastric contents, stool, and milk, and their sections lasted from 8 A.M. to 11 A.M. five days a week for six weeks. Students were expected to turn up in the afternoons to perfect their technique, and they assisted in the routine work of the service. Eighty-eight patients were admitted to the medical service in those six weeks, and their problems covered essentially the whole range of internal medicine. Fifty-three were discharged "recovered" or "improved." The five who died had mitral regurgitation, intestinal obstruction, acute meningitis, or miliary tuberculosis.

Cowie and Freund chose one of the two cases of pernicious anemia for intensive study. Students examined her blood, and they found her hemoglobin to be only 19 percent of an unstated normal standard and her erythrocyte count to be less than a million. The patient had an uncontrollable desire to sleep. In this case "[t]he improvement . . . was rapid and marked. In four weeks the hemoglobin had risen to fifty-two per cent and the red corpuscles to two million one hundred thousand."[37] Treatment was not described, but at that time Osler's textbook, recommended to the students, prescribed bed rest, open air, good food, and arsenic in increasing doses.[38] A patient with myelogenous leukemia and an enormously enlarged spleen gave the students the opportunity to make white cell counts before and after the patient was treated with X rays and arsenic. In two instances the students examined biopsy specimens obtained from patients with Hodgkin's disease. The students were taught the method of gastric analysis, and they found that the patient with pernicious anemia had achylia gastrica. The students were taught about hypersecretion and peptic ulcer.

Cyrenus Darling taught the surgical part of the summer course, and he listed what had been done on the service in the six weeks from 23 June to 3 August.[39]

Total number of patients treated	130
Total number of operations performed	107
Total number of anesthetics	67

Ether	58
Chloroform	1
Local	8

Total number of urine analyses	278
Total number of blood examinations	171
Total number of pathological specimens examined	39

The operations ranged, alphabetically, from nineteen treatments of abscesses to one of venous ligation of a varicocele. There were three deaths, two from long-standing infection, and one from shock following a devastating railroad accident.

Reuben Peterson also tabulated the work done on his gynecological service in the same period.[40]

Patients admitted	80
Operations performed	94

1 per patient (1 anesthetic)	24
2 per patient (1 anesthetic)	13
3 per patient (1 anesthetic)	9
4 or more per patient (1 anesthetic)	4

Laparotomies	22
General anesthetic for operation	49
General anesthetic for examination	2
Local anesthetic for operation	1
Urine examinations	160
Blood examinations	50

The complete tabulation of procedures occupied two-and-one-half pages.

Reuben Peterson said:

[T]he student could examine and follow every case from the time of entrance to the hospital until the patient was discharged. He was privileged to see her not only once, but many times during her stay in the hospital. He was able to verify his diagnoses by what he saw at the operations. Above all, he could follow the postoperative course of the patient and judge whether primarily the operation was or was not successful. . . . Amphitheatre teaching, with the

benches filled with students who could see and hear but not touch, was conspicuous by its absence.[41]

The newly appointed professor of otolaryngology, R. Bishop Canfield, described the three divisions of his summer course.[42]

1. Examination and diagnosis of the common forms of ear, nose, and throat conditions with special reference to treatment. Hearing tests were made, and students were given the opportunity to become proficient in all methods of diagnosis and treatment.

2. Demonstrations of the anatomy of the ear and of operative techniques were given in the clinical laboratory, and students had abundant material for practice.

3. Transillumination and X-ray diagnosis of the nasal accessory sinuses were demonstrated, and students performed operations upon the cadaver.

The clinical material used was as follows.

Patients presented	94
Conditions presented	171
Operations performed	62

The Move to Detroit

The report on the clinical summer session of 1906 was published in *The Physician and Surgeon*, a medical journal widely read in Michigan, and it constituted an ostentatious display of clinical opportunities in Ann Arbor. The authors had an ulterior motive. Darling began his report by saying:

So many disparaging statements have been made in medical society and daily newspaper by interested persons that medical men not acquainted with the University hospital clinics might believe that the facilities for teaching medicine and surgery at the University of Michigan are seriously hampered because of lack of material. This report is presented for the purpose of placing before the medical profession a few facts which should refute the charges of inadequate clinics. No other hospital in this country gives to its students such an opportunity for studying disease.[43]

Peterson was even more emphatic.

Not infrequently the clinical teacher in the University of Michigan is asked, "How large is Ann Arbor?" When told that it is a town of less than twenty thousand inhabitants, the next query is, "What do you do for clinical material?" . . . Having given the matter but small thought, he assumes that the hospital material is drawn largely from the town in which the University is situated. But when he once grasps the idea that only a very small proportion of the material comes from the town, and that loyal alumni of the medical school, located not only in Michigan but in three or four surrounding states, refer their patients to the hospital for treatment, his eyes are opened to the possibilities of an institution so situated. He is no longer amazed when informed that there are over two hundred beds in the University Hospital usually filled and patients waiting their turn for admission. His eyes are opened, unless for reasons of his own, he keeps them tightly closed and refuses to be convinced. . . . [T]hose who know the facts, yet still keep up the cry of "no material" . . . would . . . [say] the same if a thousand major operations were to be performed daily in the hospital.[44]

At that time Dean Vaughan was once more attempting to move the clinical years to Detroit. The Detroit Medical College was in financial trouble, and Detroiters proposed that the university take over the school. Vaughan thought the entire university should have been built on Belle Isle in Detroit, and he regretted that the Medical School was in Ann Arbor.[45] He even opened an office in Detroit, but that was apparently to give his sons a leg up in the practice of medicine. Vaughan was supported by those who thought practice in Detroit would be more lucrative. Dock believed the two-hundred-bed University Hospital, in which he had about one hundred beds, had an adequate and diversified patient population and that a student who was familiar with all the patients in the hospital was far better off than one in a great metropolitan hospital where he might see only a restricted number of patients on a particular service.[46] Reuben Peterson was even more vehement in his opposition to the move, and he persuaded seven of the physicians who had taken the 1906 summer course to sign a summary of the work done and the operations performed that summer, concluding: "We feel that we have made no mistake in choosing Ann Arbor for our postgraduate work and that she needs no amalgamation [with the Detroit school]."[47]

George Dock's Departure

In the spring of 1908 President Angell wrote Dock saying he had heard rumors that Dock was thinking of accepting a job at Tulane. Michigan would be sorry to see Dock go, but if he were going, would he

please make up his mind in a hurry so that Michigan could get on with the job of finding his successor.[48]

Peterson said that Dock impulsively accepted the offer from Tulane in a fit of pique with Victor Vaughan.[49] Dock and other members of the faculty had just defeated Vaughan's effort to move the clinical years to Detroit. Vaughan had been disingenuous, and Dock did not trust Vaughan not to try again. Dock had another reason as well. Starting from nothing, he had built up an adequate clinical laboratory for himself and his staff. However, it was too small for medical students to use it routinely. For years Dock had tried to persuade the university to provide a central clinical laboratory in the hospital for student use, and on 8 January 1908 he had written a round-robin letter to the clinical faculty asking for help. Dock wanted a central laboratory in which every fourth-year student could have a desk and a microscope. There should be a laboratory director and a servant to look after equipment and supplies. He did not get the laboratory, but there was one in New Orleans. At that time Tulane was more primitive than Michigan; it had, for example, only the year before required that entering students have completed four years of high school. However, it did have access to the nine-hundred-bed Charity Hospital in which "an excellent teaching laboratory of clinical pathology" had been installed by Dr. C. C. Bass, "who had a remarkable gift for his work."[50] Dock's move to Tulane was a mere stopgap. After two years in New Orleans he went to Washington University in St. Louis when that school was being reorganized with the help of Abraham Flexner and Rockefeller money.

Finding Dock's Successor

Michigan offered Dock's job to Rufus Cole, and Cole would have been a splendid catch. He had graduated from Michigan's Literary Department in 1896, and he had attended Michigan's Medical School for one year before transferring to Johns Hopkins. After graduating from Johns Hopkins he stayed on under Osler and Lewellys Barker, applying bacteriological methods to clinical problems. Cole admired Osler's careful clinical observations, but he thought Osler was utterly superficial in making no attempt to understand the fundamental nature of disease by application of the biological sciences. On the contrary, Cole believed with Barker that the primary function of a university department of medicine should be the encouragement of just such research.[51] Cole accepted the directorship of the hospital of the Rockefeller Institute. He took Donald D. Van Slyke, a Michigan Ph.D., with him to the hospital, thereby helping to lay the foundations of modern clinical chemistry, and his own work on lobar pneumonia, continued by Dochez and Avery, was a masterpiece of scientific clinical investigation. For Michigan, Cole recommended Walter Hewlett, who was thirty-three years of age when he came to Ann Arbor to be professor of internal medicine.[52]

Walter Hewlett's Background

Albion Walter Hewlett had grown up in San Francisco as a boyhood friend of Joseph Erlanger.[53] Together they obtained early admission to the University of California at Berkeley. When they graduated in 1895 Erlanger went to Johns Hopkins as a medical student, but Hewlett entered Cooper Medical College in San Francisco. At that time Cooper was still a private affair, for it did not become a part of Stanford University until 1908. Hewlett discovered that Cooper really was not satisfactory, and in his second year at Cooper he frantically applied for admission to the second-year class at Johns Hopkins. In his letter to Dean Welch he compared himself favorably with Erlanger, who was doing well at Hopkins. Hewlett was reluctantly admitted on the condition that he pass examinations in normal histology and physiological chemistry and demonstrate that his knowledge of physiology and anatomy was reasonably up to Hopkins standards. Hewlett repeated the second year and graduated in 1900, a year behind Erlanger.

Erlanger and Hewlett completed a long study of the metabolism of dogs with shortened intestines while they were medical students.[54] They used dogs left over from experiments by other medical students. One dog had intractable diarrhea and died, but the other two with bowels shortened by 70 and 83 percent survived. Erlanger and Hewlett fed each dog each day 150 grams of a carefully standardized mixture of lean beef and soda biscuit to which they added from 10 to 100 grams of olive oil. They collected and analyzed the urine and feces, and they compared the results with those obtained on one normal dog and with those gathered from the literature. The dogs with shortened intestines behaved like normal dogs so long as the diet contained a small

amount of fat. When fat was increased, fat lost in the stool rose to 25 percent of that fed. Erlanger and Hewlett observed an important fact seldom emphasized: when steatorrhea occurs, loss of nitrogen in the stool parallels loss of fat.

Hewlett interned for two years at the New York Hospital and then spent eighteen months with Ludolf Krehl in Tübingen. Krehl had worked in Carl Ludwig's Leipzig Institute, and Ludwig's name was not on Krehl's two papers, one on the mechanism of closure of the tricuspid valve and one on the results of cutting the vagus nerve.[55] Krehl moved from one German university to another developing expertise in diseases of the circulation, and he was one of the authors of the book on heart disease edited by George Dock. Hewlett's one paper from Tübingen was on the properties of blood after injection of Witte's peptone,[56] but he must have studied the circulation under Krehl. Thereafter Hewlett's publications were on that subject.

Hewlett's Early Cardiovascular Research

Hewlett returned to Cooper Medical College, where he rose from assistant to associate professor of medicine. Almost immediately he translated Krehl's *Pathologische Physiologie* into English.[57] The book, famous in its day, is an elementary, not to say superficial, description of the physiological bases of clinical findings, and it is almost totally devoid of quantitative information. Hewlett added a little on Cannon's work on the mechanical factors of digestion, something about blood pressure, and something on cardiac arrhythmias. The only illustrations are those inserted by Hewlett, a couple of tracings from Cushny and a few of his own.

The tracings are those in which the sphygmogram of the radial pulse is compared with the jugular venous pulse. In those days the only method of timing events in the cardiac cycle was the use of Mackenzie's polygraph. Three waves were usually found in the jugular pulse. Allowing 0.13–0.15 second for transmission from the heart, the A wave probably timed contraction of the auricles, and the C wave timed the ventricular contraction and coincided with the carotid pulse. The V wave occurred as the auricles filled while the ventricles were still contracted. There were frequent disagreements among experts about the meaning of the waves. Their timing, not their magnitude, was important. The apex beat recorded from the chest wall timed ventricular contraction. Hewlett listened to the heart while making his records; if there was an apparently dropped ventricular beat he could tell by the presence or absence of a first sound whether the ventricle contracted feebly or not at all.

At first Hewlett measured systolic blood pressure by palpation. After 1904 he estimated systolic and diastolic pressure by means of the apparatus devised by his friend Joseph Erlanger.[58] That device recorded on smoked paper the abrupt beginning of oscillations in a Riva-Rocci cuff as the pressure in the cuff was lowered and then the maximum oscillations as pressure was lowered further. A mercury manometer in parallel with the recording lever was read at the moment oscillations began, and that was taken to be the systolic pressure. The reading when oscillations were at their maximum was taken to be the diastolic pressure. Experts thought Erlanger's method the best available,[59] but the apparatus was too delicate and bulky for general use. By 1909 Hewlett was hearing Korotkoff sounds.[60]

Throughout his time at Cooper Hewlett analyzed cardiac arrhythmias by means of sphygmograms and pulse tracings. On one occasion he deduced that digitalis had produced a block between the great veins and the auricles. The description of the sinoauricular node had not yet reached San Francisco.[61] On another occasion he thought there were conduction blocks in the ventricular wall.[62] Other papers were little more than glosses on Cushny and Edmunds's explanation of irregular pulse. Immediately after Hewlett read Minkowski's papers,[63] he tried to detect movements of the left auricle by recording pressures from a small balloon in the esophagus.[64] At Michigan Hewlett and two assistants, J. G. Van Zwaluwenburg and J. H. Agnew, used Frank capsules and optical recording on bromide paper to make careful measurements of pressures in the carotid artery, jugular vein, and the chambers of a dog's heart.[65]

Hewlett at Michigan

Hewlett had a small staff at Michigan. There was always David Murray Cowie to look after pediatrics in the Palmer Ward, and Cowie usually had an instructor to help him. Hewlett himself had only one or two assistants, at first J. G. Van Zwaluwenburg, then Luther F. Warren, Harry B. Schmidt, Quinter

O. Gilbert, James H. Agnew, and finally Frank Wilson. Two became professors of medicine elsewhere, Warren at Long Island and Agnew at Alabama, where he was disappointed by the quality of the school. When there were two instructors one was designated instructor in clinical microscopy. There were assistants and interns, never more than three. All of Hewlett's staff except one were Michigan graduates. After 1911 there were also laboratory assistants. As in Dock's time some medical students lived in the hospital and helped on the wards.

Hewlett's teaching schedule, with a few exceptions, was much the same as Dock's. He began a course in pathological physiology in the second year, and sophomore students were taught the elements of physical diagnosis. Third-year students had further training in auscultation and percussion. After 1910 there was a course in clinical microscopy for third-year students that required an instructor and a laboratory assistant. There was the inevitable didactic course in which the textbook was read to third-year students. Fourth-year students were assigned cases in rotation. They had to work up their patients as they were admitted, and they presented their findings at twice weekly clinics. Hewlett identified the best of the fourth-year students, and he called them his "medical staff." Those students were assigned ward work throughout the year, and Hewlett made rounds with them on Sunday mornings. Times had changed a bit. When a rumor spread that Dock required students to appear at the hospital on Sundays, pious citizens had complained. Dock ironically declared that if students wanted to see him on Sunday, they would have to see him in church.[66]

Shortly after Hewlett came to Ann Arbor he issued a manifesto in the form of an address to a local medical society.[67] The most important factor in medical education, he said, is that the medical school must control the clinical material used for teaching, and it must have an adequate hospital of its own near the rest of the medical school. A large hospital has advantages; the minimum number is 100 to 200 beds. The medical school must also control all other departments of the hospital: nursing, special forms of treatment, diet kitchen, and so on. In controlling the hospital, the medical school also controls the professional appointments; its professors are the attending staff, and it does not have to accept the attending staff of a privately or municipally controlled hospital as its professors. In this respect Michigan is of particular interest: its medical school is in a town of only twenty thousand, yet it has a hospital now being enlarged to 270 beds. There are 4,250 patient visits a year and nearly 2,000 inpatients. This compares with Johns Hopkins having 353 beds of which 288 are teaching and Jefferson with 346 total and 286 teaching beds. Michigan thus follows the pattern common in Germany but rare in the United States. At present [1909] the preclinical departments are fully professional, and that is the case at Michigan. The clinical departments are moving that way, and, again, Michigan has a professional clinical staff. Michigan, like the best schools, looks for those who will devote themselves fully to a career of research as well as teaching and not to private practice. The search for professors must be a national and not a local competition. Pathological anatomy has served as the foundation for surgery; pathological physiology will serve as the foundation for academic internal medicine. The new breed of internists must be themselves capable biochemists and physiologists, for although professional biochemists and physiologists have made important contributions, their interests, quite naturally, are elsewhere. Such an internist must be chiefly a hospital man with little or no private practice. However, medical students need to be exposed to men in private practice; this can be met by clinical appointments. Students, of course, must work on the wards, and it is good for the staff to have them there. Hewlett quoted the Philadelphia surgeon W. W. Keen: "I always feel at the Jefferson Hospital as if I were on the run with a pack of lively dogs at my heels."[68]

Hewlett published a lot while he was at Michigan; in fact, he sometimes published the same paper twice.[69] One early paper demonstrated the value of X rays in proving the diagnosis of thoracic aneurysm.[70] Other papers were case reports: extreme cyanosis[71] or infantilism in pituitary disease.[72] The AMA Council on Pharmacy and Chemistry asked Hewlett to evaluate the results of a blind trial of natural versus synthetic salicylic acid. Hewlett reported that the differences were not statistically significant, but he used no statistical method to reach his conclusion.[73] Once a patient in the hospital was carelessly given ten times the fatal dose of strychnine. Hewlett recounted the heroic measures by which the patient was saved, but he did not say what the patient thought of the episode.[74] To determine whether the symptoms of uremia are the result of high levels of urea, Hewlett swallowed 125 grams although his three collaborators took only 100 grams each. Hewlett and the others were nauseated. Otherwise, the symptoms

appeared to be like those seen in the asthenic type of uremia.[75]

Plethysmography

Hewlett in his one last endeavor at Cooper attempted to determine the effect of amyl nitrite inhalation upon blood vessels, and he used a plethysmograph to measure changes in the volume of the patient's arm.[76] In those days the arm was thrust to or beyond the elbow into a long glass jar having a small hole at the far end. Such jars were readily obtainable, for they were "percolation vessels" used by pharmaceutical chemists in the extraction of simples. A cuff at the large end sealed the subject's arm, and some kind of sensitive volume detector attached to the other end recorded changes in the volume of the subject's arm confined within the jar. Pulse volume changes coincident with each heartbeat were seen as jiggles in the record. Plethysmography was a common tool of physiological research. Bowditch used it at Harvard, Lombard had recorded changes in the volume of Franklin P. Mall's arm when the two were at Clark University together, and in Ann Arbor Lombard worked with a psychologist to study the effects of emotional stress upon pulse volume. Lombard had even made plethysmography a class exercise for Michigan medical students.

Soon after coming to Michigan Hewlett resumed plethysmography, but he made a profoundly important change in technique. T. G. Brodie, the physician-superintendent of the Brown Institution of the University of London, had wanted to measure blood flow so that arterial-venous differences in oxygen content could be used to calculate oxygen consumption.[77] He had observed that ordinarily renal veins are not full; they can accommodate extra blood without blocking flow through the capillaries. Consequently, if an organ such as the kidney is enclosed in an oncometer, or plethysmograph, and if the veins draining that organ are briefly occluded, the initial rate of increase in volume of the organ confined within the plethysmograph is equal to the rate of arterial inflow.[78] Hewlett put a Riva-Rocci cuff around his subject's arm just outside the plethysmograph (fig. 12–3). When the cuff was suddenly inflated to a pressure that blocked the venous outflow but not the arterial inflow, the rate of change of volume of the arm within the plethysmograph measured the rate of arterial inflow. Hewlett reduced his values to flow per one hundred cubic centimeters of arm by measuring the volume of water it displaced.[79]

After giving a preliminary report Hewlett and Van Zwaluwenburg published their first full-dress paper on plethysmography in the new English journal *Heart*.[80] The title page of volume 1 read:

Edited by Thomas Lewis, M.D.
Aided in the selection of papers by
Dr. W. H. Gaskell

Prof. A. R. Cushny   Prof. A. W. Hewlett
(London)   (Ann Arbor)
Dr. Leonard Hill   Prof. G. N. Stewart
(London)   (Cleveland)
Dr. J. Mackenzie (London)

Hewlett was in good company.

Hewlett and his junior associates found that venous occlusion pressures between forty and eighty millimeters of mercury were satisfactory and that, depending upon the rate of blood flow, the slope of the line initially inscribed after venous occlusion gave a reliable estimate of the rate of blood flow. They determined the normal resting values when the subject was in a comfortable thermal environment, and they found variations up to 100 percent with the Traube-Hering waves. Exercise of the other arm had no effect, but exercise of the arm in the plethysmograph raised blood flow from 4.5 cubic centimeters per 100 cubic centimeters of arm to 27.3 (fig. 12–4). They had to compare blood flow in the hand alone with flow in the whole arm, for G. N. Stewart, using a thermal method for the hand,[81] had obtained values different from theirs. Flow per 100 cubic centimeters of hand was higher than flow in the whole

arm. Raising the room temperature until the subject perspired increased flow about five times, and chilling the room lowered it again. Flow was exceptionally slow in a feverish subject as his body temperature rose and moderately accelerated as his temperature fell. Hot water in contact with the arm increased flow four to eight times. It must have been very hot water, for Hewlett thought he had seen vascular paralysis. Cold water reduced flow to one-fourth or one-half control values, and Hewlett detected reactive hyperemia.

Hewlett himself was one of the subjects used to test the effects of hydrotherapeutic measures. A hot bath followed by a cold shower raised and then lowered arm blood flow. When Hewlett reported these results before the Association of American Physicians he agreed that mouth temperature was an inaccurate measure of core temperature, but he said measuring rectal temperature while in a tub was impractical. Henry Sewall was the first to comment on the paper; he suggested that the authors had measured flow through the skin and not through deeper structures.

The Pulse Wave

The plethysmograph showed an elevation at each heartbeat, and there was often a dicrotic notch. Hewlett became fascinated by this pulse wave, and to record it more accurately he increased the sensitivity of his instrument by replacing the bellows recorder, first by a soap bubble whose surface could be photographed and then with a Frank capsule, a stiff membrane on which a mirror is mounted.[82] He found that if he gave a subject nitroglycerin the wave became peaked; in other circumstances it was clearly

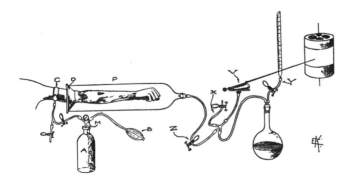

Fig. 12–3. Hewlett's plethysmograph. (From A. W. Hewlett and J. G. Van Zwaluwenburg, "The Rate of Blood Flow in the Arm," *Heart* 1 [1909]: 88.)

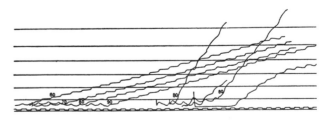

Fig. 12–4. Plethysmographic records obtained with the arm at rest *(first 4)* and after resistance exercises of the hand. The numbers are pressures (millimeters of mercury) to which the cuff was inflated. (From A. W. Hewlett and J. G. Van Zwaluwenburg, "The Rate of Blood Flow in the Arm," *Heart* 1 [1909]: 92.)

dicrotic. Hewlett attempted to explain his findings by postulating reversed flow in the artery during diastole, changes in the elasticity of the arterial wall, and reflection of waves from the arterioles. The physical problem is far too complicated to be solved by Hewlett's methods, and despite his enthusiasm and persistence he accomplished nothing.

The Beginning of Electrocardiography at Michigan

The first electrocardiograph used in the United States was manufactured by Edelmann in Munich and brought to this country in 1909 by A. E. Cohn, then at Mt. Sinai Hospital in New York.[83] Edelmann instruments were soon installed at Johns Hopkins and at the Presbyterian Hospital in New York City, but Michigan did not get an electrocardiograph until 1914, when Hewlett was able to raise the money to buy one manufactured by the Cambridge Instrument Company, Horace Darwin's shop in England. Hewlett put it in his private office, and Frank Wilson, Hewlett's newest assistant and a medical graduate of 1913, had the machine working by 11 March 1914, when he recorded the electrocardiogram of a seventy-two-year-old farmer.[84] In one instance the QRS complex was normal, but the PR interval was only 0.11 second, and the P wave was inverted (fig. 12–5). Wilson deduced that the impulse had started in the conducting system of the ventricle and had spread into the auricles as well as into the ventricles. In another instance the normal QRS complex was preceded by no P wave. Wilson had arranged to record the venous pulse together with the shadow of the quartz fiber, as Thomas Lewis had been doing for several years, and he found the auricular wave of the venous pulse occurred at the normal time. He deduced that an ectopic beat had originated in the junctional tissue at the same time as an impulse originated in the sinus region and that the electrical effects of the two in the auricles had neutralized each other. The odd shape of the QRS complexes in other records convinced Wilson that premature contractions had originated at different levels of the conducting system. The next month Hewlett and Wilson studied another farmer with auricular fibrillation. Normal P waves were absent from the electrical records, but there were vibrations of the string at about 450 a minute during diastole.[85]

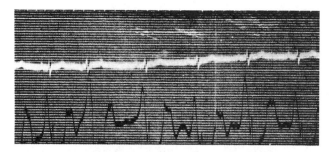

Fig. 12–5. The first electrocardiogram published by Frank Wilson. (From F. N. Wilson, "Report of a Case Showing Premature Beats Arising in the Junctional Tissues," *Heart* 6 [1915]: fig. 1.)

In the next few months Wilson obtained enough experience to allow him to write three research papers, a survey of ectopic rhythms for Vaughan's journal, and a review explaining the significance of the electrocardiogram to pediatricians.[86]

The End of Hewlett at Michigan

At the end of Hewlett's tenure at Michigan he had completed the manuscript of his *Functional Pathology of Internal Diseases*.[87] In the preface to the students' edition he said:

The gap between physiology and biochemistry, on the one hand, and clinical medicine, on the other, is felt by students as well as by teachers. The present work helps to bridge this gap, because the manifestations of disease are discussed as alterations in normal physiology.[88]

Because the book was thoroughly up-to-date, it demonstrates an internist's comprehension of the basic sciences in 1916 as well as how medicine was taught at Michigan in Hewlett's time.

The longest section, 130 pages of 686, is, of course, devoted to the circulation. Starling's experiments and Starling's curves are used to illustrate the normal and abnormal function of the heart, and the effects of valvular lesions are presented in detail. The long section on cardiac rate and rhythm is illustrated by twenty-three figures of the electrocardiogram, often in three leads, "kindly furnished by Dr. F. N. Wilson."[89] All Wilson's electrocardiograms are accompanied by tracings of the venous or carotid pulse. In the section on gastrointestinal motility the results and diagrams of Cannon are freely used, and there are tracings of X-ray photographs made by

Holzknecht and Hertz. Pavlov is extensively cited on the nervous control of secretion, but in the paragraph on chemical control Edkins is credited with having shown that "substances which are formed or absorbed at the pyloric end of the stomach or the duodenum may stimulate the fundus cells to increased activity" (139). Popielski's concurrent discovery that histamine stimulates acid secretion would not be published for another four years.[90] Haldane's results figure largely in the section on respiration, but Hewlett did not believe that oxygen is secreted into the blood by the pulmonary epithelium. Diabetes occupies much of the section on metabolism. Hewlett described the D:N ratio as proof that glucose can be derived from protein, but he could not decide whether overproduction or underutilization of glucose is the cause of hyperglycemia. In considering the chemical regulation of body functions, Hewlett described the role of the thyroid gland in myxedema and sporadic cretinism, but he could not be sure that Graves' disease is equivalent to thyrotoxicosis. He knew that scurvy and beriberi are deficiency diseases, and he thought rickets and pellagra might be too.

In 1916 Ray Lyman Wilbur, who had been professor of medicine at Stanford, became president of the university, and Hewlett was summoned to San Francisco to succeed him. In a farewell address Hewlett said that the decision not to move the clinical years to Detroit had been amply justified.[91] In 1915–16 there had been 11,000 patient visits to the hospital. The medical wards had been crowded with 740 inpatients. This was because the legislature had provided that indigent patients from all over the state could be sent at public expense to the University Hospital for expert attention. Consequently, the very rich and the very poor had the best medical service. The hospital must be enlarged, and outpatient facilities must be improved. Microscopic and chemical examinations of the blood, gastric contents, and excreta were now routine, and so were cardiographic, bacteriological, and serological studies. Means for research on cardiovascular diseases were good, but there was only a beginning in other lines. Hewlett hoped that his successor would be able to apply biochemistry to the study of disease. Finally, as Dock had done, Hewlett said there should be a clinical laboratory in the hospital.

Hewlett worked as vigorously and effectively at Stanford as he had at Michigan until he died of a brain tumor shortly before his fifty-first birthday.

Nellis B. Foster, Hewlett's Successor

Hewlett announced his impending resignation in December 1915, and Vaughan, who was busy with a dozen other things beside the deanship, began to look for a successor. He found time to interview Nellis B. Foster in New York, and after considering one or two others he decided that Foster was the man for the job.

Nellis Barnes Foster, then forty years old, was the metabolically oriented physician Hewlett thought Michigan needed. He had graduated from Johns Hopkins in 1902, and he had postgraduate training in Europe. From 1906 he was in practice in New York City with an appointment at the New York Hospital, and he had a faculty appointment at Cornell. At the same time he taught biological chemistry at Columbia's College of Physicians and Surgeons. His specialty was diabetes mellitus, and he wrote a practical textbook on the subject for the use of practitioners.[92] The book has 240 octavo pages of large print, and it is an accurate and judicious summary of what was known about diabetes mellitus at the time. It begins with an elementary review of carbohydrate, fat, and protein metabolism as known in 1915. Glycosuria results when blood sugar increases over the power of the kidney to retain it, and Foster distinguished between diabetes mellitus and renal diabetes. In the latter the blood sugar is not over 0.1 percent, but the permeability of the kidney is increased. Acidosis results from incomplete oxidation of fat, and it is the cause of death in the great majority of cases. In diabetic coma the amount of bicarbonate required is enormous. Foster ended his book with a long chapter describing his experience with dietetic control of diabetes. The object is to free the urine of sugar, or at least to reduce glycosuria to a minimum. At first the diet is carbohydrate free, and then the patient is carefully titrated with increasing amounts of carbohydrate until sugar appears in the urine. The threshold quantity of carbohydrate is the amount of sugar the patient can burn, and it is the maximum to be eaten.

When Foster and his wife visited Ann Arbor in 1916 to look for a house Vaughan was away. Peterson took charge of Foster. Hewlett had not had a downtown office for private practice, but Peterson told Foster he would need an office and some beds in a private hospital for patients he would see in consultation. Peterson offered Foster an office and four beds in his own private hospital at sixty-five dollars a month. Foster wrote to Vaughan asking Vaughan's advice, but Vaughan cagily refused to give any. Foster did use some of Peterson's beds.

Foster arrived in Ann Arbor in September, and he quickly made himself popular with staff and students alike. He had made it a condition of employment that the university provide him with a laboratory for his metabolic studies, and the regents spent two thousand dollars fitting up the top floor of the old laundry building for him. Foster had published frequently before he came to Ann Arbor, chiefly on diabetes and uremia, but he could do little laboratory work or publishing in the year he was at Michigan. He was busy with administrative work, with teaching, and with managing patients. He did, however, regularly present cases before the Clinical Society of the University of Michigan.[93]

Foster joined the Medical Reserve Corps at the end of the 1916–17 academic year, and he was given leave of absence for the next year. Part of his military duties was to run a training course for young physicians joining the service, and he was horrified to discover that, despite the reforms of the past decade, only the graduates of a very few high-quality, class A schools were capable of making a correct diagnosis.[94] In other schools bedside teaching had been farcical, and a graduate of those schools, who might have had an internship, could not differentiate between a diastolic murmur and a systolic one, could not tell the difference between pleural effusion and pneumonia, had never done a thoracentesis, could not recognize meningitis, and had never even seen a lumbar puncture. The graduate could not recognize diphtheria or give antiserum.

On 12 August 1917 Foster wrote to President Hutchins that the Red Cross had asked him to go on a medical mission to Serbia, and four days later he wrote to the same effect to Victor Vaughan. In neither letter was there any hint he might not eventually return to Ann Arbor, but on 20 November he abruptly resigned, giving the reason that he would be on extended military service. Frank Wilson wrote that Foster "left the University, as a result of a misunderstanding with Dr. Vaughan, who was then Dean. . . . The differences with Dr. Vaughan probably were not initiated by Dr. Foster, and apologies were offered to him later."[95] After the war Foster returned to practice in New York City and to teach at Cornell.

Before Foster arrived in Ann Arbor he told Victor Vaughan that he wanted an experienced person added to his staff, and on 5 October 1916 Foster nominated L. H. Newburgh for the post. When Newburgh arrived Foster gave him charge of the metabolic ward, and he gave Mark Marshall, a Michigan medical graduate of 1908, charge of another ward. When Foster left Newburgh was made acting head of the Department of Internal Medicine with no authority over the budget or appointments, and he was made chairman of a committee to find Foster's successor.

13
Internal Medicine: Frank N. Wilson and L. H. Newburgh

———

Frank Wilson and L. H. Newburgh were not on speaking terms for much of their lives, but they share this chapter just as they shared the ground floor of the surgical wing of the University Hospital and the distinction of being two great men of Michigan medicine.

Frank Wilson away from Ann Arbor

Frank Norman Wilson was away from Ann Arbor between 1916 and 1920. When Hewlett left, George Dock took Wilson to Washington University in St. Louis, where Wilson was in charge of the heart station of Barnes Hospital. Dock himself was not in favor of the full-time system in force then at Washington University, but he recognized that a full-time appointment was appropriate for a dedicated scientist such as Wilson. Wilson's stay in St. Louis was interrupted when the United States entered World War I, for he accepted a commission in the Medical Reserve Corps and was assigned to the Military Heart Hospital in Colchester, England. Dock wrote a letter to William Osler at Oxford to introduce Wilson.

Thomas Lewis commanded the Heart Hospital's British and U.S. staff. Lewis and Wilson became friends, and Lewis introduced Wilson to his hobby: bird-watching, a suitable avocation for an electrocardiographer. Lewis, by the time Wilson met him, was firmly established as the premier electrocardiographer in the English-speaking world. He was known to the general medical profession as the author of a handbook on electrocardiography that went through many editions.[1] He was known to experts like Wilson for his numerous fundamental papers on the subject, many published in *Heart* and others in the *Philosophical Transactions of the Royal Society*. Lewis and Wilson published nothing together on electrocardiography while they were at Colchester, but they talked over the subject in the hospital and while they were stalking birds on the Essex coast.

Some seventy thousand men had been classified as cardiovascular casualties since the war began, and many were sent to Colchester for study by Lewis and his staff and for eventual rehabilitation. Lewis divided the problem into two parts: VDH, or valvular disease of the heart, and DAH, or disordered action of the heart. The nature of the first was obvious enough, but the latter, which included the effort syndrome, dyspnea on exertion, and the inability to perform the hard physical work required of a soldier, was more puzzling. Lewis pointed out that a large number of soldiers affected by the effort syndrome were simply constitutionally inadequate,[2] and anyone who remembers the physical differences between the British upper and lower classes before World War II will understand what Lewis meant. Otherwise DAH was more a disorder of the nervous system than of the heart. Its victims had been through the battles in Flanders, and many had been buried for unknown hours after being blown up by a shell. Wilson and his fellow officers, including Samuel Levine, found that soldiers with the effort syndrome had only slightly reduced vital capacity and normal carbon dioxide combining power.[3] Alan Drury, in related work, found that the patients had entirely normal alveolar partial pressure of carbon dioxide at rest and during exercise and normal response to inspired carbon dioxide.[4]

Some patients with VDH had a musical diastolic murmur audible five feet away. Wilson made phonocardiograms, finding one murmur beginning with an abrupt crescendo at 170 cycles a second followed by gradual decrescendo at 140 cycles.[5] Someone had said that the pistol-shot sound heard over the femoral artery is a heart sound. Wilson showed it to be produced where it is heard, and he wondered: "Indeed it seems strange that anyone could have thought otherwise."[6]

Wilson at Barnes Again

After the war Wilson returned to Barnes Hospital, and he became immersed in his research in his notoriously absentminded way, sometimes forgetting to meet his classes. George Dock was angry; it was just as bad to fail in one's duties on account of research as on account of private practice. Wilson and George Herrmann, who was completing his training in Dock's department, obtained electrocardiograms on fifty-one patients that subsequently went to autopsy. They carefully measured every quantity of the cardiograms. When the patient died Wilson or Herrmann trimmed the heart handed them by the pathologist, examined and removed the valves, and then measured the size of the ventricles by filling them with

mercury. With the mercury in place they immersed the heart in formalin, and when the heart had hardened Wilson or Herrmann separated and then weighed the left and right ventricles. At first they made the mistake of sectioning the heart, having misunderstood Lewis's brief description, but later they were able to obtain weights and left to right ratios that could be compared with Lewis's. They described their results in a paper containing twenty-four pages of detailed tables.[7] If the ventricular weight was less than 250 grams, the relative weights of the two ventricles had no influence upon the electrocardiogram, whose characteristics were determined chiefly by the position of the heart in the chest, by the arrangement of the ventricular conducting system, and by disturbances in intraventricular conduction. With equal diligence they produced two massive papers on bundle branch block, one in patients and one in experimental animals.[8] In the introduction Wilson said that the conclusions of Lewis "are so fortified on every side that it is improbable that they will need material revision."[9] Wilson himself eventually revised Lewis's concept of left and right bundle branch block.[10]

Wilson's Return to Michigan

Wilson returned to Michigan in 1920. He had been promised space for a heart station in the new hospital and money to buy an Einthoven string galvanometer. Completion of the hospital was delayed until 1925, and Wilson found his old galvanometer unusable. He spent much of the next two years writing up his research work at Barnes. In 1922 a Cambridge-Hindle galvanometer was delivered, and Wilson installed it in a sort of closet under the stairs leading to the theater in the old hospital. He was regarded as a harmless eccentric wasting his time on something utterly impractical.

In January 1924 Wilson went to see Dean Cabot with a request for a double-string galvanometer. There were several in this country, one at the Rockefeller Institute and one at Columbia. The apparatus would have to be made to order in Einthoven's shop, and Carl Zeiss would make the special lenses. It would cost between thirty-five hundred and four thousand dollars. Wilson asked for an additional fifteen hundred to two thousand dollars for spirometers and other equipment for the study of respiration and blood flow; those could be obtained later. Wilson used the one form of blackmail available to an academic: he had been offered a professorship at Vanderbilt, and he was obliged to decide by early March. Cabot was sympathetic, and he took the matter up with President Burton. Burton received favorable assurances from Dr. Sawyer, the medical member of the Board of Regents, who always had the deciding vote on medical matters. The result was that in February Wilson was promoted to a full professorship and given an immediate increase in salary. Wilson was pleased, but he remained anxious about his equipment.

In November Wilson tackled Cabot again. The room on the ground floor in the new hospital intended for the heart station had been plastered, and it would be ready as soon as any other part of the building. Furthermore, Professor Einthoven would soon be in Ann Arbor for a few days, and if Wilson had the money in hand he could place the order then. On 21 November Cabot officially asked the regents for not quite so much money as Wilson wanted. Wilson did order the apparatus, but it was not delivered for another three years. Thereafter Wilson had ample instrumentation, a place to see patients, and a laboratory for experimental work. His electrocardiograph was far from portable, so the hospital was wired to bring the impulses from a bedridden patient to Wilson's laboratory. Wilson trained a nurse to apply the electrodes.[11] When Cyrus Sturgis became head of the Department of Internal Medicine in 1928 he relieved Wilson of many routine responsibilities, and Wilson could see patients as he liked.

Wilson as an Electrocardiographer

Wilson had more than twenty disciples and junior collaborators, and he was generous and open with them. Each in turn had a master key to the heart station and a desk in Wilson's own office (fig. 13–1). Wilson's name was never on a paper unless he had done much of the work and usually most of the thinking, the thinking often many years before.

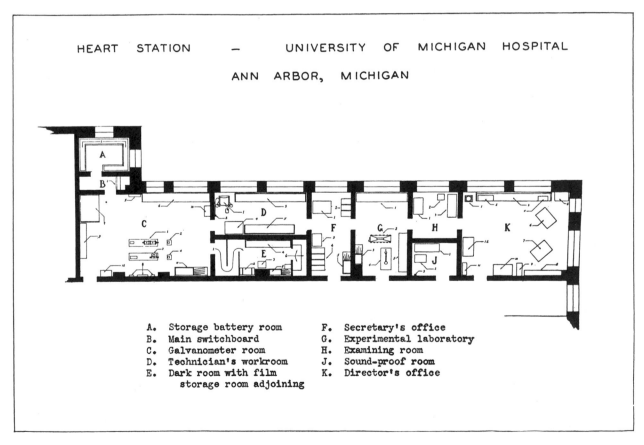

Fig. 13–1. The heart station floor plan, Old Main. (From F. N. Wilson and P. S. Barker, "The Heart Station of the University of Michigan Hospital," in *Methods and Problems of Medical Education*, 18th ser. [New York: Rockefeller Foundation, 1930], 90.)

Despite his commanding position as an electrocardiographer, Wilson thought that an electrocardiogram was only a small part of the examination of a patient. Near the end of his life he wrote a fundamental paper on the interpretation of the ventricular complex in which he said:

We shall not attempt a long discussion of the present wretched state of electrocardiographic diagnosis or the misery attributable to it. . . . Electrocardiography is one of the most exact diagnostic methods. Its potential value is great, but it is not being used to the best advantage. Electrocardiographic abnormalities are not diseases. They have no important bearing upon the life expectancy of the patient, or the extent to which his mode of life should be altered.[12] . . . [I]nverted T waves do not, of themselves, call for any kind of therapy.[13]

To illustrate the condition of electrocardiographic diagnosis, Wilson said he had recently seen a sixty-cycle artifact called evidence of auricular fibrillation.

Wilson's *Selected Papers* fill a volume of 1,090 pages, and his total accomplishment cannot be summarized. These three examples are presented to show something of the nature of his work.

Distribution of Cardiac Action Potentials

Wilson made a simple observation. He exposed the heart of an anesthetized dog. He attached one electrode to the dog's left hind leg. This was the indifferent electrode whose potential was supposed not to vary during the cardiac cycle. He placed the other electrode on the surface of the right auricle, and he recorded an auricular curve that "begins with a very gradual descent, which becomes steeper and steeper until a sharp inverted peak [of relative positivity] is reached. Then there is a very sudden shift to a peak similar in all respects to the first, except that it is above the base line [showing relative negativity]. The succeeding descent of the curve begins with a steep slope which becomes more and more gradual until the zero position is attained."[14] This is the beginning of the wave of excitation; the end of the wave is buried in the following ventricular complex.

At that time the wave of excitation of an excitable tissue, an axon or a small muscle, was usually measured when the tissue was surrounded by air, a dielectric. One electrode was on the tissue, and the other was placed on an injured region whose poten-

tial was thought to be that of the inside of the cell. When a wave of excitation passed over the tissue, the measuring electrode first saw a wave of negativity and then a return to the baseline, a record very different from that Wilson obtained from the heart. As early as 1920 Wilson began to worry about what potential the exploring electrode would see if the tissue were in a conducting medium as is the heart. The reference electrode would be far away in the same medium, not in contact with the interior of the cell. Wilson frequently emphasized the difference between his problem and that of an axonologist.

Wilson and Garrard MacLeod, his student in the mid-1920s, consulted mathematicians and physicists, but the experts did not understand the problem and, characteristically, were not interested in hearing about it. Wilson and MacLeod had to learn the mathematics and physics on their own. By the time Wilson had recovered from a long illness in 1927–29 he had mastered the relatively simple calculus necessary for handling the problem. His equations look more horrendous than they really are, for they are full of trigonometric functions. Wilson showed off a bit when he frequently said in his mathematical expositions: "It obviously follows that . . ."

Wilson began by considering current flowing between two points close together in an infinite plane of homogeneous specific conductivity. He deduced the potential in any point in the plane, and then he began introducing restrictions by considering the potential if the plane were a circular disc. Next, he considered the homogeneous medium to be an infinite volume in which current flows between two small adjacent spheres, and he found the potential at any point in the medium. Then he derived the equation for the potential on the surface of a sphere whose center is equidistant between the source and the sink. Finally, Wilson derived the equation relating the potential to a line of positive charges followed closely by a parallel line of negative charges over a conducting sheet when the exploring electrode is some distance above the sheet. This last is the potential his electrode on the auricle would see as the wave of excitation moved over the auricle, and its equation should describe the curve Wilson had recorded.

Time was not a variable in Wilson's equations. Instead he related the potential V to the distance x between the detecting electrode and the source and sink of current. Changes in relative distance substituted for changes in time. When Wilson plotted the calculated potential against the distance he obtained the same diphasic curve he had recorded when the auricle was excited. Wilson concluded:

The curves obtained from certain auricular regions . . . are, with respect to their general outline, of relatively simple form. The shape of these curves indicates that the electrical phenomena associated with the spread of the excitatory process are similar to those that would occur if the crest of the wave of excitation were immediately preceded by a positive pole, or source, and immediately followed by a negative pole, or sink.[15]

In all this Wilson did not postulate or even consider that the action potential begins with an abrupt reversal of membrane polarity or overshoot. Overshoot was not demonstrated in heart muscle until much later and then in collaboration with one of Wilson's last pupils.[16] What is new is that Wilson considered the consequences of an action potential whose front consisted of a dipole moving in a conducting medium and not in a dielectric. While he was thinking along those lines William Hofmeyr Craib, the South African classicist-mathematician-physician-soldier who was working in the heart station at Johns Hopkins, was having similar thoughts. Craib measured the action potential of a strip of cardiac muscle in 0.9 percent sodium chloride and of curarized frog sartorius muscle in the same solution.[17] He found the same initial positive deflections that Wilson found. Using the same reasoning Craib concluded that when a tissue is in a conducting medium there is

a three-fold change in the level of potential at the surface of the muscle, namely, first a rise (positivity), then a fall (negativity), and finally a further rise (positivity), the terms positivity and negativity being employed in relation to the level of the potential obtaining at the surface of the quiescent tissue.[18]

Wilson heard Craib describe his ideas at a meeting, and he said to him:

Craib, may I say that I am the unhappiest man in America today. You see, I know you are right and that I have missed the bus. I have been working for years on the same problem.[19]

Later Wilson wrote:

Between Craib and ourselves there is complete agreement. . . . In stating that work on the general subject of this monograph was begun in this laboratory a number of years before Craib's first paper was published [reference given]

and that many of the facts to which he has called attention were known to one of us [Wilson himself] long before that paper appeared, we do not wish to raise any question of priority or in any way to claim any share of the credit due Craib for the fine work he has done.[20]

The Central Terminal and Precordial Leads

Wilson had to brush aside some limitations in order to apply his knowledge of the distribution of potentials associated with the cardiac cycle to the conventionally recorded electrocardiogram. The body is really not a homogeneous regular polygon, but irregularities of current flow through lungs and bone are negligible. The irregular shape of the body is of less consequence than might be supposed, for there is no measurable potential difference along any extremity at any time. Wilson assumed current flow is steady, and he was sure that the influence of inductance could be neglected. Finally, K. C. Cole, the one axonologist who would listen to him, assured Wilson that changes in conductivity with frequency could be safely disregarded at frequencies below 1,000 cycles per second.

Wilson used the Einthoven triangle in 1915, and he satisfied himself that there is little or no potential gradient along the limbs. Therefore, limb leads allow measurement of the trunk potential in a plane. Wilson attempted to turn the triangle into a tetrahedron by placing one electrode on the chest over the heart, measuring the potential difference between it and a limb lead. He thought that so long as the limb lead is far from the heart, its own potential variations are negligible, and consequently the potential difference represents chiefly the potential of the chest electrode.

About 1920 Wilson began to reexamine the problem of the potential at a distant lead. He knew the assumptions underlying the use of the Einthoven triangle: that the three leads are at the apices of a flat plate of homogeneous conducting material, that the potential difference is generated by a small dipole lying close to the center of the plate, and that the electromotive force of the dipole is perpendicular to the plane of the plate. Wilson used these assumptions to derive the expression for the difference between the leads. Wilson's method was simply to determine trigonometrically the projection of the cardiac vector on each of the sides of the triangle. If the differences are e_1, e_2, and e_3, respectively, for leads I, II, and III, then

Potential at the foot $V_F = (e_2 + e_3)/3$,
Potential at the right arm $V_R = -(e_1 + e_2)/3$, and
Potential at the left arm $V_L = (e_1 - e_3)/3$.

As Wilson would say: "It is obvious that" if these potentials are added, the sum is zero. Therefore, if the three leads are connected through equal resistances, and *if the Einthoven assumptions are valid*, the potential at the point of connection does not vary throughout the cardiac cycle. Thus, Wilson invented the central terminal as a point of reference for the exploring electrode. Wilson and his colleagues made central terminals for their friends from 5,000-ohm resistors and some wire until electrocardiograph manufacturers caught on. With this zero reference electrode Wilson demonstrated the usefulness of precordial leads.

The Use of Precordial Leads

Thomas Lewis had identified electrocardiographic changes when right or left bundle branch block had been produced in dogs. Diagnosis of bundle branch block in humans was based on Lewis's criteria of the characteristics of the QRS complex in the three standard leads. There were two problems in transferring Lewis's concepts to humans. First, the position of the heart in the chest of a dog is different from its position in the human chest with consequent differences in the flow of current to the limb leads. Second, in attempting to crush one of the bundle branches, Lewis had apparently injured both so that he had a mixture of blocks.

Wilson and Herrmann had studied bundle branch block in humans and in exposed hearts of anesthetized dogs as early as 1919–20, but Wilson's interest in the problem of human bundle branch block was revived in 1929 by observations made by his colleagues, Paul Barker and Garrard MacLeod, while Wilson was on his farm recovering from his illness. Barker had a patient with purulent pericarditis, and John Alexander, the thoracic surgeon, performed an extrapleural pericardostomy under local anesthesia on 12 March 1928. With the patient's consent, Alexander placed a hastily made electrode on various parts of the patient's heart and carefully noted the coordinates of the positions of the electrode. At the same time Barker and MacLeod recorded the conventional lead II. They then caused premature ventricular systoles while recording both leads I and II. The patient con-

veniently died of disseminated pneumonia a little later so that the exact positions of the electrodes on the heart could be determined at autopsy by means of Alexander's coordinates. When the records were taken to Wilson he immediately recognized their importance in providing the foundation for interpretation of curves obtained during bundle branch block. He could tell by means of a direct lead from the heart through which ventricle the impulse spread more slowly as the result of the interruption of its usual pathway. A "semidirect lead," one separated from the heart by a short path of conducting medium, would give similar results. Wilson at once wrote a theoretical paper on the subject, and shortly after he returned to work he, Barker, and MacLeod reexamined the order of ventricular excitation in dogs and compared their results with observations made on patients with conduction block.

Wilson could not put leads directly on the heart of every patient, but he could use precordial leads. Those to the right of the heart recorded electrical events occurring primarily on the right ventricle, and those to the left recorded left ventricular activity.

Later, when Wilson had the central terminal, he could write of unipolar leads, and he said that

[e]xperiments upon dogs demonstrated that unipolar precordial leads from the extreme right side of the precordium . . . yield QRS deflections like those inscribed in unipolar leads from the anterior surface of the exposed right ventricle, and that unipolar leads from the extreme left side of the precordium . . . yield QRS deflections like those inscribed in unipolar leads from the antero-lateral surface of the exposed left ventricle. By means of multiple precordial leads it is, therefore, almost always possible to determine whether the epicardial surface of the human right ventricle is activated earlier or later than the epicardial surface of the left, and thus to differentiate right from left branch block with an accuracy which far surpasses that achieved by the use of limb leads alone.[21]

His conclusion was that, contrary to opinion based on Lewis's work, the common type of bundle branch block is left; the rare type is right bundle branch block. "Had precordial leads been employed at the start no mistake would have been made" (861).

At the beginning of his career the audience walked out when Wilson began to give a paper on electrocardiography. Toward the end of his career the audience that came to Ann Arbor to hear him teach was so large that his lectures had to be given in a hall far from the hospital. Wilson received most of the hon-

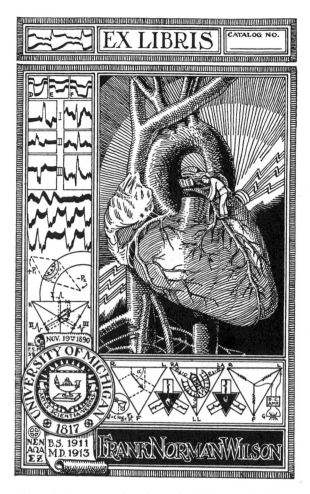

Fig. 13–2. Dr. Frank Wilson's bookplate was highly personal and reflects his more important achievements using illustrations from his scientific publications. *Left side, starting at the top:* ST elevation (current of injury) from margin of injured turtle ventricle; ST depression caused by subendocardial injury (turtle heart); three left and right bundle branch block patterns; recordings from an intramyocardial stab electrode in dog; and diagrammatic representation of the electrical field produced by an injured section of myocardium; computing the mean electrical axis of QRS. *Bottom row, from left:* Laws that govern the distribution of electric currents in volume conductors; vector cardiography; the course of ventricular excitation from within outward; and the circuit diagram from the Wilson central terminal that made unipolar electrocardiography possible and is still used in most electrocardiographic machines today. (Courtesy of Dr. Richard Judge.)

ors he might have expected, but he did not receive all. He was not, for example, elected to the National Academy of Sciences, whereas both Vaughan and Novy were elected. However, Wilson did know that he had made a substantial contribution to science and to medicine (fig. 13–2), and at the end of his life he wrote:

It may be pointed out also that such advances as have been made have come about not as the result of organized attacks aimed at the solution of specific problems, nor by the expenditure of large sums of money for elaborate apparatus, technical assistants, fellowships and the like, but by individual men who have been permitted to work on problems of their own choosing in their own way, under no pressure to make progress reports to justify the expenditure of the small sums at their disposal, or to present or publish the results of their efforts before they are ready.[22]

L. H. Newburgh's Background

Frank Wilson carried on Hewlett's tradition of cardiovascular teaching, research, and service. Had Foster returned in 1919 he would have provided the metabolic leadership Hewlett thought Michigan needed, but Foster could not have done better than L. H. Newburgh, the man Foster brought to Ann Arbor in 1916.

L. H. Newburgh, Louis but usually known as Harry Newburgh, had graduated from Harvard College in 1905 and from Harvard Medical School in 1908. He interned at the Massachusetts General Hospital for sixteen months, and then he spent a year in the Allegemeines Krankenhaus in Vienna in Carl von Noorden's First Medical Clinic, studying metabolic diseases under Hans Eppinger and Wilhelm Falta. Newburgh along with Falta became one of the authors of an enormous paper reporting the effects of various combinations of atropine, pilocarpine, and epinephrine upon seventy-one patients whose diseases ranged from scleroderma to diabetes mellitus to multiple sclerosis.[23] Despite the prestige of Viennese medicine at the time, the work reported in the paper was totally disorganized, and the results were worthless. It was poor training for Newburgh, who said later that he admired the scientific excellence of the Viennese doctors but despised their callous attitude toward their patients.

Newburgh spent an unhappy year practicing medicine in Cincinnati, his hometown, unhappy because "research was the first and lasting love of his professional life."[24] Newburgh returned to the Massachusetts General Hospital, where he was encouraged by David Edsall, the new Jackson Professor of Medicine brought from Philadelphia to dilute the Back Bay influence at Harvard. Edsall made Newburgh a Dalton Fellow, but he earned most of his meager living as assistant visiting physician. Among his patients were many constipated immigrants. Newburgh knew Cannon's work on the mechanical factors of digestion, and he decided nothing was wrong with the motor mechanism of his patients' colons. They had abandoned the rough diet of their homeland, and Newburgh cured their constipation by putting them on a high-fiber diet.[25]

Newburgh's Early Research

Martin Fischer, a student of Jacques Loeb, said that edema is the result of the increased affinity of tissue colloids for water caused by the accumulation of acids. The treatment, therefore, is to give alkali to neutralize the acid and salt to shrink the colloids. Newburgh had the temerity to put the idea to direct test. His patients with cardiac decompensation did not have diuresis when he gave them sixteen grams of sodium bicarbonate, and ingestion of sodium chloride made them worse.[26] At this point Newburgh turned to the laboratory, where he worked under the direction of L. J. Henderson, who did not like to do laboratory work himself. Henderson had been working at the Massachusetts General Hospital since 1911, when he had been forced out of the Department of Biochemistry at Harvard Medical School by Otto Folin, the newly appointed professor of biological chemistry. Folin had insisted Henderson give up his connection with Harvard College, where he had been teaching the history of science, and devote himself full time to the medical school. Henderson refused.[27] Henderson had already worked out the theory of acid-base regulation, and along with W. W. Palmer, another young student, he had devised a colorimetric method for determining the acidity or alkalinity of a solution.[28] Henderson and Palmer explained that they expressed the hydrogen ion concentration of a solution as the logarithm to the base 10 and omitted the minus sign. This is the now-familiar pH notation that had recently been proposed by S. P. L. Sørensen. Henderson, Palmer, and Newburgh measured the swelling of dried fibrin in solutions of various hydrogen ion concentrations, and they found no differential effect within the range known to occur in the body or in the urine. They said: "These theories, to any one acquainted with the facts, are clearly without foundation in quantitative experiment,"[29] and stated that it is utterly fallacious to assume that acidity is the cause of edema. The three also found there was no relation between hydrogen ion concentration of the urine and the magnitude of edema.[30] Newburgh in this collaboration learned about acid-base balance and the relation between the body's content of sodium and the volume of extracellular fluid.

In a long period of research beginning in 1915 Newburgh blasted another clinical superstition by careful study of patients and by work with animals in the laboratory of W. T. Porter at Harvard Medical School. Clinicians thought that death from pneumonia is the result of collapse of the circulation and that the proper treatment is to stimulate the heart with strychnine. Newburgh wrote: "For decades many physicians have relied, with unquestioning faith, on strychnin [sic] in the treatment of certain grave symptoms occurring in pneumonia, typhoid fever and other acute infectious disease."[31] Newburgh worked with George Minot, a house officer in the hospital who twice a day measured the systolic and diastolic pressure of fifteen patients with pneumonia. Five of the patients died. Systolic blood pressure was actually higher in the fatal cases than in those who survived.[32] Newburgh concluded that "[s]trychnin sulphate, in medicinal doses, does not increase the output from the heart, slow the pulse or materially raise the blood-pressure. There is no logical basis for its use as a cardiovascular stimulant."[33]

Newburgh and W. T. Porter cannulated the circumflex branch of the coronary artery of an anesthetized dog, cut out the piece of the ventricle served by the artery, and perfused the fragment with warm defibrinated dog blood. Muscle from ten normal dogs contracted on the average for 181 minutes whereas muscle from ten dogs that had died of pneumonia induced by intrapulmonic injection of Friedländer's bacillus contracted 200 minutes.[34] In nine papers that might well have been condensed into one or two Newburgh and Porter reported that the blood pressure in cats, dogs, and rabbits on the point of death from pneumonia is not low enough to endanger life and that vasomotor reflexes are normal. Any fall in pressure can be attributed to hyperthermia, not to exhaustion of the vasomotor center. Newburgh and Porter found that in experimental pneumonia the respiratory response to inspired carbon dioxide is far less than normal. If, however, the animal is vagotomized, the response is the same as in a normal animal.[35] They did not know the alveolar pressure of carbon dioxide in their sick animals, and they made no attempt to measure it.

J. Howard Means, Newburgh's slightly younger

colleague at the Massachusetts General Hospital, had learned the Krogh-Lindhard method for measuring cardiac output in humans when he worked in Krogh's Copenhagen laboratory.[36] The subject takes one breath of a gas mixture containing 10 to 20 percent nitrous oxide, a gas highly soluble in blood. A sample of alveolar air is taken, and after the subject has held his or her breath for a measured interval another sample is taken. Both samples are analyzed for nitrous oxide. The total volume of nitrous oxide in the lungs at the beginning and end of breath holding is calculated from the total lung volume measured as vital capacity and residual volume. The difference is the amount of nitrous oxide leaving the lungs in the interval between the two alveolar air samples. Knowing the solubility of nitrous oxide in blood and assuming the blood is saturated with the gas, the cardiac output is calculated. In six observations Newburgh and Means found that Newburgh's cardiac output while he was lying flat on his back averaged 4.52 liters a minute with a range of 3.75 to 5.56. Means's cardiac output under the same conditions averaged 3.97 liters a minute. Newburgh was slightly smaller than Means, 5 feet 6 inches and 134 pounds against 5 feet 9 inches and 161 pounds. When Means was exercising on a bicycle ergometer his cardiac output rose to 15.68 liters a minute.[37] They repeated the nitrous oxide measurements on a patient with both aortic and mitral murmurs, and they found that it rose to a maximum of 12.81 liters a minute. Like their cardiac output, an increase was first met by an increase in stroke volume and then by an increase in pulse rate.[38]

Newburgh at Michigan

Michigan was unable to find a head for its Department of Internal Medicine until 1922, and during the interregnum Newburgh carried on as acting head with a small staff. When Louis M. Warfield was finally appointed in 1922 Newburgh was rewarded by being made professor of clinical investigation. Perhaps because Newburgh had no real authority his actions as head are poorly documented, and there is only a slight trace of his teaching in that time. Professors were then as now supposed to send copies of their examinations to the dean's office. Once Newburgh did not send any, and McCotter as assistant in the office nagged Newburgh about it. On 12 November 1921 Newburgh replied that he had nothing to send.

Students on his wards were given case records of patients with well-marked pathology. Then they examined the patients and discussed the diagnosis, treatment, and prognosis with Newburgh.

When Newburgh came to Michigan in 1916 there were no animal quarters at the hospital and few facilities for chemical work. At first he was allowed to use space assigned to the Hygienic Laboratory in the basement of the building on East University Avenue. Vaughan was away most of the time, and the laboratory was unused. Eventually when the new hospital was completed in 1925 Newburgh had adequate laboratories at one end of the ground floor of the surgical wing. A small room for animals was supplemented by an animal house built in back of the hospital in 1924 at a cost of twenty thousand dollars. The fundamental problem was ignorant, untrained help in the absence of professionally competent supervision. For years Newburgh plagued the dean, demanding improvement. A faculty committee in 1938 found the place filthy and the animals in wretched condition. The committee said that there was an imperative need for five thousand dollars to replace urine-soaked, vermin-infested cages, and it recommended that James T. Bradbury, an endocrinologist working in the Department of Obstetrics and Gynecology, be placed in charge. Thereafter Bradbury pestered the dean on behalf of animal care.

Wilson's heart station was at the other end of the hall from Newburgh, and the proximity created some problems for themselves and others. There is no record of the origin of Wilson and Newburgh's quarrel, but they ignored each other as they walked down the hall side by side. Franklin Johnston, whose life had been saved by Newburgh, was married to Newburgh's chief assistant, but he was Wilson's devoted disciple and succeeded him as chief of cardiology. Relations between Newburgh and Wilson were not improved by the egalitarian attitude of the Medical School administration. In 1931–32 Newburgh received a salary of six thousand dollars from the university and two thousand dollars from the hospital for a total of eight thousand dollars. Wilson received seven thousand dollars, five thousand from the university and two thousand from the hospital. The Executive Committee with Novy as chairman thought they should receive the same amount, and on 10 May 1932 it voted that five hundred dollars should be deducted from Newburgh's salary and added to Wilson's. Otherwise, Newburgh's salary should be reduced by one thousand dollars. Those were the years of the Great Depression, and in 1932–33 Newburgh and Wilson were each paid forty-six hundred dollars by the university and two thousand dollars by the hospital.

Nephritis

Newburgh began to investigate the cause of nephritis. He wrote:

The chief business of the kidneys is to rid the organism of the end products of protein metabolism. This task is accomplished to a considerable extent by active secretion on the part of certain portions of the tubular epithelium.[39] Might not an excessive effort in this direction sufficiently prolonged end in a scar?[40]

Later he might have called into question all three assertions in that quotation.

Newburgh used rabbits, and he performed elaborate controls to demonstrate that his results were not the results of intercurrent infection, age, absorption of whole proteins, or the way the animals were housed. He had a frightful time getting the rabbits to eat a high protein diet. They died almost at once when fed coagulated egg white, and they refused to eat meat. Eventually Newburgh settled on a soybean diet or one of crumbled flour-and-bran cake baked with dried meat or casein. Rabbits fed soybeans having 40 percent protein had albuminuria and casts after four or five weeks, and their blood urea nitrogen averaged 100 milligrams percent compared with a control value of 31 milligrams percent. On histological examination the kidneys showed evidence of progressive chronic or subacute nephritis. Newburgh rebutted criticism of his work, but in his last paper on renal injury in rabbits he climbed down a bit.[41] He presented photomicrographs of the cortex of the kidney of a rabbit fed 36 percent protein for more than six months. There were dilatation of the tubules and flattening of their lining. Sometimes red blood cells were in the lumen, and casts were numerous. He summarized:

At least the initial lesion was caused by the products of the diet. . . . The evidence at hand suggests that the injury caused by the diet is either solely attributable to the excessive excretion of some amino acids or in part to the amino acids and in part to the acid character of the urine. . . . There is no intention on our part of claiming that this nephropathy is the anatomic analogue of human chronic nephritis.[42]

But Newburgh could not resist pointing out that red blood cells had appeared in the urine of normal men he had fed "enormous steaks."[43]

The rabbit is susceptible to atherosclerosis, and Newburgh found many discrete and confluent raised yellow patches in the root, ascending limb, and arch of the aorta in rabbits that had eaten his high protein diet for three weeks to a year. Only two of fifty-nine rabbits left over from the pharmacology and internal medicine laboratories examined as controls had atherosclerosis. Age, infection, or the laboratory environment was not responsible for the lesions.[44]

More Nephrotoxicity

Newburgh's work was criticized on the grounds that the rabbit, an herbivore eating a low protein, alkaline ash diet, is the wrong experimental animal. When the white rat became a common laboratory animal in the 1920s, Newburgh fed weanling rats one of nineteen different diets for as long as 480 days. All high protein diets caused albuminuria and the appearance of up to twenty times the normal number of casts. Liver and muscle proteins were the most damaging. In attempts to sort out the factors responsible Newburgh infused amino acids into puppies; 5.7 grams of tryptophan given intravenously to a dog weighing 5,600 grams caused fatal necrosis of the convoluted tubules.[45] Newburgh found cystine to be toxic as well.[46] A diet containing 20 percent sodium nucleate caused abundant invasion of the rat's kidneys by fibroblastic tissue, but the lesions were not the same as Newburgh had produced in rabbits.[47] Newburgh attempted to reproduce damage in human subjects, one a thirty-two-year-old member of his staff.[48] In a preliminary period of thirty-five days the man ate a diet containing less than 100 grams of protein a day, only 50 grams of it of animal origin. Then for six months he ate a special diet containing 338 grams of protein, 271 grams of fat, and 96 grams of carbohydrate for a total of 7,177 calories. The protein was from beef liver, veal round, beef tenderloin, and dried beef. The subject's blood pressure remained unaffected, but he had mild albuminuria after six weeks and casts up to 3,450 per hour. When given a free choice, he avoided meat, and albuminuria and excessive casts disappeared in two weeks.

Money and Fellows

All Newburgh's early work was done with little or no outside support, but he did have laboratory assistants paid from the Medical School's budget. As early as 1920 several gifts of one thousand dollars each came from persons in Jackson, Detroit, and New York City. Newburgh and Warfield appealed to President Ruthven for fellowships, but nothing came of it. Dean Cabot asked W. K. Kellogg of Battle Creek for money, appealing to Kellogg's interest in diets, and eventually Newburgh received support from Kellogg as well as from Parke, Davis and Company and grateful patients. When Parke, Davis gave the Medical School six thousand dollars to be used for a fellowship at the rate of two thousand dollars a year, Dean Cabot wrote to Walter Bauer at the Massachusetts General Hospital offering him an assistantship in clinical medicine to work with Newburgh. Bauer replied that the offer made him the happiest man in Boston, but in the end he did not come to Ann Arbor.

When a bright young student went to Newburgh with an idea, Newburgh would tell him that he had no technical help to offer but he did have three feet of laboratory bench the student could use. As a result many students had opportunities that led to careers in academic medicine. Rackham grants of seven thousand dollars, coming in the 1930s, provided salaries for a long list of professional associates, young men and women whose names Newburgh put, often first, on papers describing work done in his laboratory. Newburgh urged such collaborators to move on to independent careers after four to six years. Some went into practice, and some had careers at Michigan in other specialties: R. H. Freyberg in rheumatology, Arthur Curtis in dermatology, and John Sheldon in allergy. In the decade before World War II Jerome Conn became Newburgh's disciple, and Alexander Leaf was one immediately after the war. In addition, there were many laboratory assistants who measured total nitrogen in hundreds of twenty-four-hour urine specimens or who dried an equal number of stools on a water bath. Two groups of women made essential contributions. There were the dieticians, Frances MacKinnon, Anna Light, and Dorothy Waller among them. Then there were the women with chemical and physiological qualifications who saw that things were done properly in the laboratory and who were collaborators rather than assistants. Chief among them for more than twenty years was Margaret Woodwell, who married Franklin Johnston and whose name was usually first on Newburgh's papers and sometimes alone on others.[49]

In the following summary of Newburgh's work between 1926 and 1942 Newburgh's name must be understood to encompass those of his fellow workers.

Counting Calories

Newburgh had to measure energy balance for his study of diabetes and obesity. Energy intake is the sum of calories in the diet, and many of Newburgh's subjects were on a fixed diet of known composition for months at a time. Franklin Johnston was on one for years. Newburgh and his dieticians did not rely exclusively upon published data in calculating calories in their diets; in crucial instances they analyzed them themselves or had Thorne Carpenter in F. G. Benedict's laboratory in Boston measure the calories in a bomb calorimeter. Newburgh found that total calories of diets actually consumed ran some 3 percent below the sum derived from dietetic tables, probably as the result of losses during preparation.

Indirect Calorimetry

The most precise means of measuring energy output over days or one or two weeks is direct calorimetry, in which the subject's heat production is measured. W. O. Atwater had built such a calorimeter for men at Wesleyan University,[50] and Newburgh used an unprepossessing portrait of Atwater, "whose name should mean much to every American," as the frontispiece for one of his books.[51] Newburgh himself never used such a calorimeter, and he made do with three other methods: short-term indirect calorimetry, long-term indirect calorimetry, or calculations based on insensible water loss.

For short-term indirect calorimetry a subject breathes room air through a valve and discharges expired air into a Tissot spirometer. Margaret Woodwell Johnston supervised this. The volume and composition of the expired air are measured, and the rates of carbon dioxide production and of oxygen consumption are calculated. Their ratio is the respiratory quotient, RQ. The rate of nitrogen output in the urine is measured, and because proteins contain 16 percent nitrogen, nitrogen excretion times 6.25 is the rate of protein oxidation. From known values of calories per gram of protein the protein heat production is calculated. The amounts of carbon dioxide produced and oxygen consumed in protein oxidation are subtracted from the measured values to give the nonprotein quantities, and the nonprotein RQ is calculated. The RQ when carbohydrate is oxidized is 1.00, and the RQ for fat combustion is 0.707. Therefore, the amounts of carbohydrate and fat oxidized can be calculated from the nonprotein RQ and the nonprotein oxygen consumption. The amounts burned are multiplied by the caloric value of carbohydrate and fat to give the heat production attributable to each, and the sum of heat from protein, carbohydrate, and fat is finally calculated. Newburgh's team made hundreds of such calculations.

The calculation is valid only for the period in which the gas exchange is measured. Newburgh made several attempts to extrapolate to longer periods,[52] but for more accurate long-term measurement he sealed his subject into a metal chamber (fig. 13–3) whose dimensions were 10 feet 2 inches by 6 feet 8 inches by 6 feet 5 inches.[53] Dried room air was pulled through the chamber at a constant measured rate. Samples of air leaving the chamber were drawn continuously into spirometers and were analyzed for carbon dioxide and oxygen. Water evaporating from the subject was collected and measured as well. Calculations of heat production were made as for short-term indirect calorimetry. Newburgh went to considerable trouble to demonstrate that his method was accurate.

When a subject (male) entered the chamber for a long stay of a day or more he was accompanied by carefully prepared meals, each sealed in an airtight container. He discharged his urine and feces into separate cans, and those were designed with lids so that the smell did not continuously pervade the chamber. The protocols said nothing about toilet paper.

Insensible Water Loss

Energy exchange can be measured by these methods for an hour, a day, or a week, but Newburgh wanted a method he could use for the really long run, months or years. He spent an enormous amount of effort devising and validating a method based on measurement of insensible evaporation of water from the lungs and skin.[54] Every gram of water evaporating takes with it 0.58 calorie. If the rate of evaporation can be measured and if the fraction of total

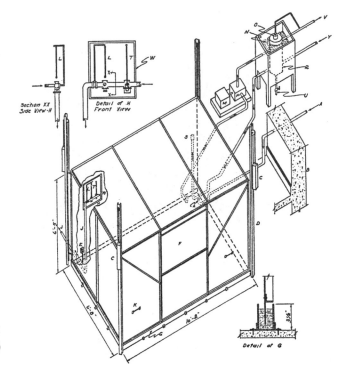

Fig. 13–3. Newburgh's chamber for long-term indirect calorimetry. (From L. H. Newburgh et al., "A Respiration Chamber for Use with Human Subjects," *J. Nutr.* 13 [1937]: 195. Reprinted by permission of the Wistar Institute, Philadelphia, Penn.)

energy dissipated through insensible evaporation is known, the total energy production can be calculated.

Newburgh based his method on the accurate measurement of the subject's weight by means of a balance used for weighing silk. If the intake of food and drink and output of urine and feces are taken into account, the subject's loss of weight in a given period is then known. That loss is the insensible water loss, provided sweating is avoided, plus the weight of carbon dioxide exhaled minus the weight of oxygen used. To know the weights of the gases, one must know the metabolic mixture, and that can be calculated without knowing the respiratory quotient. Oxidation of 1 gram of carbohydrate produces an amount of carbon dioxide weighing 0.41 gram more than the oxygen consumed. For 1 gram of protein the excess weight of carbon dioxide is 0.09 gram. For fat the weight of carbon dioxide produced is 0.08 gram less than the weight of oxygen used. Newburgh demonstrated that on a rigidly fixed diet adequate in carbohydrate the subject oxidizes all the carbohydrate eaten. Therefore, the carbohydrate correction for gas exchange can be calculated from the composition of the diet. Measurement of nitrogen excretion permits calculation of the contribution of protein to gaseous weight change. If the subject is in a steady state, fat oxidation is also the fat of the diet, and its contribution to gaseous weight change can also be calculated. Finally, the measured weight loss corrected for the various weight changes is the insensible evaporation of water, and that value times 0.58 is the calories lost by evaporation.

Newburgh determined the fraction of heat lost by vaporization using subjects on a known diet, comfortably clothed in a neutral thermal environment, not sweating, and not engaged in more than the usual activities of physicians and laboratory workers. Franklin Johnston was one such subject. He had been on a fixed, weighed diet in the hospital for five years with no long-term change in body weight. His diet was 57.7 grams of protein, 63.4 grams of carbohydrate, and 273.6 grams of fat, yielding 2,947 calories. The oxygen used to burn this in a day was 932 grams, and the carbon dioxide released was 1,235 grams. His heat loss by evaporation corrected for oxygen and carbon dioxide was 711 calories, or 0.242 of his total heat loss. Similar values for seven other subjects ranged from 0.238 to 0.280, and from these Newburgh chose 0.240 as his standard value for the fraction. An interesting point is that the paper describing this work presents masses of detailed data but it contains not a single calculation of error or statistical significance.

Frederick Allen's Starvation Diet for Diabetes Mellitus

Frederick M. Allen, who worked at the Rockefeller Institute, introduced his starvation diet for patients with diabetes mellitus in 1914. Allen said:

Briefly, then, diabetes mellitus is a weakness of assimilation of food, due to deficiency of the internal secretion of the islands of Langerhans. The treatment thus far is purely functional, and is successful in proportion to the efficiency with which the weakened function is spared.[55] . . . [L]ightening the total load upon the weakened assimilative function is the only present means by which it may be hoped actually to halt the diabetic process.[56]

Accordingly, Allen's patients were starved until sugar disappeared from their urine, and then they were maintained on a diet of about one thousand calories a day. Fat was forbidden in fear of producing dangerous acidosis. Diabetic coma was avoided, but on one thousand calories they were unfit for ordinary activities of life. Allen's diet was widely used in absence of anything better.

The Newburgh-Marsh High Fat Diet

Newburgh thought Allen's diet had improved the treatment of diabetic patients but that its failure to provide adequate calories was its fatal flaw. Carbohydrate could not be increased to provide the calories, for an increase would be followed by glycosuria. Neither could protein be increased, for about half of the protein is converted to glucose. That left fat. Beginning on 1 March 1918 Newburgh provided calories for his diabetic patients by increasing the fat in their diet. That had been specifically interdicted by Allen, who had said: "Fat unbalanced by adequate quantities of other foods is a poison."[57] Newburgh was soon joined by Phil Marsh, who had had a stormy time with the Promotions Committee before receiving his doctor of medicine degree in 1919.

A diabetic patient who entered the University Hospital was started on nine hundred to one thousand calories: 90 grams of fat, 90 grams of protein, and 14 grams of carbohydrate. After two weeks the calories were increased to as much as twenty-five hundred by raising the fat intake to as much as 180 grams. Newburgh and Marsh's patients could lead a moderately active life without glycosuria or ketonuria.[58] A little later Newburgh and Marsh defined the nitrogen requirements of their patients on a high fat diet.[59] They selected intelligent male patients who could be relied upon to collect total urinary and stool outputs and who would adhere to the diet prescribed. Newburgh's assistants did hundreds of Kjeldahl analyses for nitrogen, a tiresome task. Fat spared protein. Nitrogen balance could be established on about 20 to 30 grams of protein a day provided total calorie requirement was satisfied by fat.

By 1923 Newburgh and Marsh could report that in the years 1918–22 inclusive they had treated 190 patients with diabetes.[60] Of the 176 that could be traced, 15 had died in the hospital, and 6 were dead after being discharged untreated. Twenty-four had died though treated. That left 131 alive, and they did not have glycosuria, ketosis, or hyperlipemia. They were in nitrogen balance and avoided the evils of undernourishment.

Elliott Joslin, the Boston expert on diabetes,

harshly criticized the high fat diet on the grounds that it caused arteriosclerosis, but his evidence was an anecdotal account of a diabetic who had been starved on the Allen diet and then had regained 76.5 pounds on a high fat diet.[61] Joslin expanded his criticism in the 1924 edition of *Treatment of Diabetes Mellitus*,[62] the first edition to be published after insulin became available. Joslin praised Newburgh and Marsh for their courage, but he said their diet was really a low protein rather than a high fat diet, that Newburgh and Marsh did not stick to their diet, and that their results were really not so good as they said. Newburgh responded by asserting that Joslin's criticism was "an unjustified interference with a method that is working well"[63] and that there was no evidence that arteriosclerosis is the result of the high fat diet. Allen agreed with Newburgh on this point.[64] Newburgh once more showed that patients on his high fat diet did not have lipemia. In twenty-one patients the blood cholesterol concentration averaged 176 milligrams percent with a range of 126–223, whereas in the same number of controls the average was 156 with a range of 139–186.[65]

Obesity

Newburgh applied both short-term and long-term measurements of metabolism to the problem of obesity. His major accomplishment was to demonstrate once more the validity of the law of conservation of energy: energy output equals energy input minus energy stored. Despite Karl von Voit's and Max Rubner's findings in metabolic studies, there were some notions current that obesity results from violation of the law.[66] There is no specific metabolic abnormality in obesity.[67] An obese person actually has a higher than normal basal metabolism corresponding to the greater than normal surface area, and the obese individual uses more energy to accomplish a given task. An obese person's account of what he or she eats can be wildly misleading. Newburgh also showed that the average values for energy output in various occupations given in published tables are too low.[68]

The Oxidation of Glucose and Glucose Tolerance

Newburgh used his respiration chamber to measure the oxidation of glucose in normal and diabetic men

and to answer in part the vexed question whether hyperglycemia in diabetics is the consequence of underutilization or overproduction of glucose.[69] His subjects, normal or diabetic, were given a fixed diet some days before entering the chamber. In the chamber they were given various amounts of glucose ranging from zero to one hundred grams. Their respiratory exchanges were measured, and glucose oxidation was calculated. In normal persons the amount of glucose oxidized increased with the amount of glucose in the preparatory diet and with increasing amounts of glucose consumed in the chamber. The two types of increase were additive. Diabetics were qualitatively similar in their oxidation of glucose but quantitatively inferior. Underutilization is at least part of the diabetic condition.

These observations have an important bearing on how glucose tolerance tests are performed. Because previous restriction of dietary carbohydrate results in a decrease in the rate of glucose utilization, during the test the blood glucose concentration of a person on a restricted carbohydrate diet rises higher than that of one on a high carbohydrate diet. Therefore, the proper technique requires that the subject be fed a high carbohydrate diet before the test is performed.

Diabetes and Obesity

Newburgh distinguished between insulin-dependent juvenile diabetes and one form of adult diabetes. Among his obese patients were many who had been diagnosed as having diabetes and who had been treated with insulin and a diet restricted in carbohydrate. All had characteristically high blood sugar curves when given the glucose tolerance test. Most of the patients were fat but not grossly obese. Newburgh knew that restriction of carbohydrate results in delayed utilization of glucose, and he thought the liver of an obese person might not be able to handle glucose in an ordinary way. In a group of sixty-two such patients, forty-seven adhered to Newburgh's reducing diet and returned to an ideal weight.[70] In them, fasting blood sugar had been as high as 325 milligrams percent, but after weight reduction none was above 125 milligrams percent. In all, glucose tolerance returned to normal. Newburgh estimated that over 60 percent of "diabetics" of middle age and 44 percent of all diabetics were like those he had cured of "diabetes" by weight reduction.[71]

Treatment of Diabetes with Insulin

When insulin became available Newburgh asked whether insulin increases tolerance. He found that insulin does, of course, increase a patient's ability to use glucose but that, in a patient on a regimen of insulin, it does not increase the patient's glucose tolerance, the ability to use glucose in the absence of insulin.[72] The paper describing these results contains the case history of Franklin Johnston, who was working as an instructor in electrical engineering at the university and had not yet entered medical school.

Newburgh thought that the availability of insulin increases the physician's responsibility to adhere strictly to dietetic principles. Insulin "should only be used to aid the patient in obtaining sufficient energy for maintenance when a diet containing his caloric requirement causes glycosuria."[73] When a new diabetic patient arrived, provided he or she was not in coma, Newburgh sharply reduced the calories in the patient's diet, providing about fifteen hundred calories in 50 grams of protein, 135 grams of fat, and 20 grams of carbohydrate. Available glucose, counting that derived from protein, was 59 grams. Newburgh gave the patient insulin only if it was necessary to stop glycosuria. After the patient had been free of glycosuria for several days the patient was fed enough to meet his or her energy requirements, not more than twenty-two hundred calories in a diet containing 75 grams total glucose. Insulin administration, if any, was reduced. Every fifth or sixth day carbohydrate was substituted isocalorically for fat until sugar appeared in the urine. The amount of glucose just below that causing glycosuria was the patient's glucose tolerance, and the patient was discharged on a diet containing 20 or 30 grams less carbohydrate but enough calories to maintain a normal way of life. Newburgh found that 80 percent of his patients so managed could get along without insulin. In 1928 Newburgh treated 347 patients of whom 256 were on a diet of twenty-two hundred calories or more without insulin.

Teaching Dietetics

Newburgh, alone or together with dieticians, wrote some short, elementary books to explain his ideas to a wide audience.[74] *The Exchange of Energy between Man and the Environment* was intended for third-year medical students at Michigan.[75] Newburgh

agreed with the students that it is cruel to introduce another course into the already crowded curriculum, and he found a way to teach nutrition to the juniors while they were on the wards three hours a day for eight weeks. The dietician selected patients "whose illnesses are of such a nature that their successful management depends chiefly on an appropriate diet."[76] These were usually patients with diabetes mellitus, obesity, chronic nephritis, peptic ulcer, ulcerative colitis, or nutritional anemia. A student was assigned one of these patients to present before the class, and when the student did so Newburgh had the patient describe his or her diet before coming to the hospital. A diabetic patient might say that he had been forbidden white bread but allowed brown bread. A patient with polyneuritis as a complication of ulcerative colitis would describe her practically vitamin-free diet. There were no formal lectures, but Newburgh would outline the appropriate diet for the patient's illness, age group, and occupation. At the end the dietician described the technique of converting the prescribed diet into three palatable meals. Newburgh thought that with real patients, students were not on a paper chase.

Salt and Water

Newburgh's early observation that administration of sodium chloride does not relieve cardiac edema focused his attention on the relation between salt and water, and he clearly understood that the volume of extracellular fluid is determined by the quantity of sodium retained. A flame photometer was not available throughout most of Newburgh's life, and he emphasized solids rather than sodium itself. He became fascinated by the problem of osmotic work done by the kidneys, and he showed that a patient with nephritis cannot concentrate urine to the extent a normal person can. On this basis Newburgh devised a concentration test of kidney function. A patient is placed on a fixed diet for three days. Then at 6 P.M. the patient is deprived of food and drink until after 10 A.M. the next day. The specific gravity of the urine put out between 8 A.M. and 10 A.M. is measured. A normal person can form urine having a specific gravity as high as 1.026, but a person with nephritis cannot.[77] Later Newburgh shortened the period of preparation, and he declared that this concentration test is much more sensitive than the phenolsulfonphthalein test and far simpler than the measurement of urea clearance.[78] He concluded that the nephritic patient is edematous because he does not have enough urinary water to contain the solids at low concentration. The logical conclusion is to supply water, and physicians of the Newburgh school successfully treated edematous patients by forcing water at the rate of five or six liters a day.[79]

Newburgh emphasized the importance of dealing quantitatively with water in the study of disease.[80] He said that in the clinical literature "water balance" usually meant water in the food and drink versus water in the urine. Sometimes stool water was measured. Such a balance does not consider water evaporated from the lungs and skin, water formed by oxidation, or water freed when tissue components are burned. Newburgh calculated water formed from the metabolic mixture, and he said 3 grams of water are released for every gram of tissue protein oxidized. In fat oxidation the figure is 1 gram of water liberated for 10 grams of fat. One of his junior colleagues had previously shown that 2.4 grams of

water are released when 1 gram of glycogen is broken down. Newburgh demonstrated the importance of this calculation in one often reproduced graph in which he compared the observed weight of an obese patient on a low calorie diet with her theoretical weight. For weeks she maintained an almost constant weight despite a large negative calorie balance. Eventually a sudden diuresis brought the observed weight down to the theoretical one. These considerations of water and salt are those Newburgh taught Frederick Coller.

The coming of World War II closed this part of Newburgh's career. He was given leave to work at the Naval Medical Research Institute, and his salary of seven thousand dollars was paid by the Office of Scientific Research and Development through the university. When he returned to Ann Arbor he found that his respiration chamber had been destroyed to make room for other work, but Newburgh was able to resume his research with the help of Alexander Leaf.

Not Just Any Medical School

14
Internal Medicine, 1918–41

When Foster resigned as professor of medicine in 1917 the two major clinical departments were without effective leadership, for C. B. Nancrede had resigned as professor of surgery in the same year. Hugh Cabot would become professor of surgery in 1920, but the chair of medicine would remain vacant until 1922. At the same time there was no effective leadership in the dean's office, for Victor Vaughan was absent in Washington, D.C., as a member of the Executive Committee of the General Medical Board with responsibility for health in all army camps (fig. 14–1). Charles W. Edmunds as assistant dean dealt with routine matters. When Vaughan thought about the school at all he took a gloomy view. The university, he said, was in a bad way with no intellectual aims, and the poor old ship of medicine was so leaky that it might not weather the storm.

Vaughan had been a very busy man the last ten years. He had traveled a lot, spending many days in Boston, Chicago, and elsewhere conducting long written and practical examinations for the newly instituted National Board of Medical Examiners. He was president and trustee of the American Medical Association (AMA), and he went to Chicago and Chattanooga to help defend the AMA in a long trial of a suit brought by a patent medicine company. He testified as an expert witness in murder trials. Vaughan was president of the Michigan State Board of Health, and that involved trips to Lansing and an enormous correspondence about many things including the high-handed actions of the board's executive secretary. There were health problems all over Michigan to be looked into, one being a typhoid fever epidemic in Ann Arbor in which fifty-eight of fifty-nine cases, one fatal, were traced to a single milk supply. Working with the C. V. Mosby Company of St. Louis, Vaughan founded and edited the *Journal of Laboratory and Clinical Medicine* (fig. 14–2). That meant finding, reviewing, and rejecting papers, the last including one by a man who had proved that silica cures pellagra. Vaughan did not reply to the man's heated and ironical denunciation of Vaughan's invincible ignorance, but he had a large and miscellaneous correspondence about cancer cures, about cremation, which he favored, about the transfer of the Mayo Foundation to the University of Minnesota, about antituberculosis campaigns, and about the problems of the Board of Arabian Missions. He told a man from Texas that he thought there was no test to determine whether blood had Negro "contamination"; someone in Texas might know. Vaughan was

163

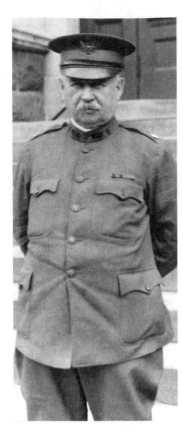

Fig. 14–1. Victor Vaughan during World War I. (Courtesy of the Bentley Historical Library, University of Michigan, Medical School Records, Box 136, "Photographs, General, Faculty, from Album of 1918.")

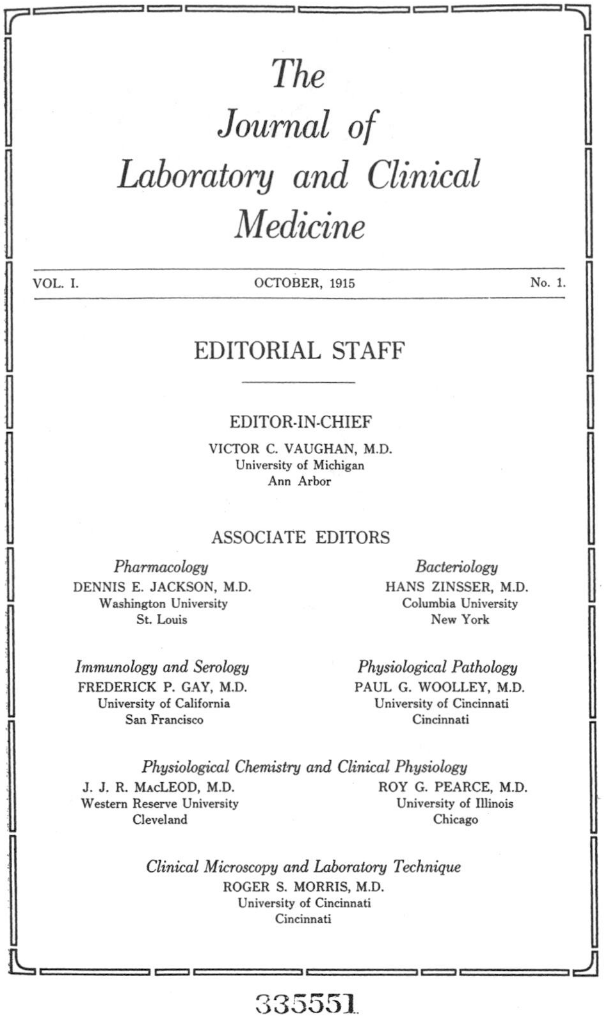

The Journal of Laboratory and Clinical Medicine

VOL. I. OCTOBER, 1915 No. 1.

EDITORIAL STAFF

EDITOR-IN-CHIEF
VICTOR C. VAUGHAN, M.D.
University of Michigan
Ann Arbor

ASSOCIATE EDITORS

Pharmacology
DENNIS E. JACKSON, M.D.
Washington University
St. Louis

Bacteriology
HANS ZINSSER, M.D.
Columbia University
New York

Immunology and Serology
FREDERICK P. GAY, M.D.
University of California
San Francisco

Physiological Pathology
PAUL G. WOOLLEY, M.D.
University of Cincinnati
Cincinnati

Physiological Chemistry and Clinical Physiology
J. J. R. MacLEOD, M.D.
Western Reserve University
Cleveland

ROY G. PEARCE, M.D.
University of Illinois
Chicago

Clinical Microscopy and Laboratory Technique
ROGER S. MORRIS, M.D.
University of Cincinnati
Cincinnati

335551

Fig. 14–2. Front cover of volume 1 of the *Journal of Laboratory and Clinical Medicine*

elected to the National Academy of Sciences, and with U.S. involvement in World War I coming on he became a member of the National Research Council. In refusing a charitable contribution Vaughan pleaded poverty because he had to pay for frequent trips to council meetings out of his own pocket. The university eventually reimbursed him. Nevertheless, Vaughan did find time to look for Foster's successor. The medical school's files are filled with letters from almost every eligible internist in the country, including George Dock, declining the job. Eventually someone in authority decided to let the matter drop until Vaughan retired in June 1921.

Money

One reason Michigan had trouble finding a successor to Foster was that in 1919 the faculty had voted for a full-time plan. Hitherto all clinicians supplemented their salaries by private practice, some like Nancrede's

small and some like Palmer's large. Private practice took clinicians away from the University Hospital. James Lynds, Murray Cowie, and Reuben Peterson each owned private hospitals, and Peterson ran his own nursing school. Other clinicians, Udo Wile, for example, had offices on State Street or downtown, and after 1911 they admitted private patients and operated at St. Joseph Mercy Hospital.

The full-time plan provided that a clinician with a private practice had time to withdraw from it, but none did. Some, like Mark Marshall, withdrew from the university instead. Every newly appointed clinician would confine his work to the University Hospital where he would have no private patients. Michigan, unlike Johns Hopkins, adopted the plan without the help of Rockefeller money. Vaughan and later Cabot had extensive correspondence with Abraham

Flexner, and Vaughan once sent Flexner the school's budget. Nothing came of it. All those declining Michigan clinical appointments cited the two stock objections to full time: a physician on full time is denied contact with the great world of medicine outside the University Hospital walls, and a physician with a private practice can make more money than one without. With surgeons the latter was particularly cogent. The school attempted to meet it by giving a clinician two salaries, one from the university and one from the hospital. Thus, when Hugh Cabot came to Ann Arbor after asserting that his Boston income was in the neighborhood of thirty thousand dollars, his professorial salary was five thousand dollars and his clinical salary was seven thousand dollars, soon raised to ten thousand. When Michigan finally secured Louis M. Warfield in 1923 to be professor of medicine, Warfield accepted a total of twelve thousand dollars for the academic year.

Trouble in the Hospital

The hospital had been poorly planned and was inadequately maintained. In July 1915 the clinical heads asked an architect to begin drawing plans, and in December 1916 the regents asked the legislature for a million dollars to be appropriated at the rate of $250,000 a year. The next February Vaughan and Peterson appeared before a legislative committee, but money was not appropriated until after the war. On 20 May 1920 a contract for the shell of the hospital was let at $1.5 million, but there was no money to fill the shell. Consequently, when the school was looking for new professors it could not assure candidates that they would have an adequate hospital. With returning prosperity the legislature did give money to finish the hospital, and it was occupied in the summer of 1925 (fig. 14–3). Will Mayo, a Michigan medical graduate of 1883, gave one of the dedicatory addresses on Thursday, 19 November. Earlier he had telegraphed Dean Cabot that he would stay over until Saturday if Cabot could get him tickets to the Michigan-Minnesota football game. Michigan won, thirty-five to nothing.

There was perennial conflict between the medical staff and the superintendent of the hospital. Tension was partially eased by formation of a hospital committee consisting of clinical heads, and the committee spent endless hours on housekeeping functions:

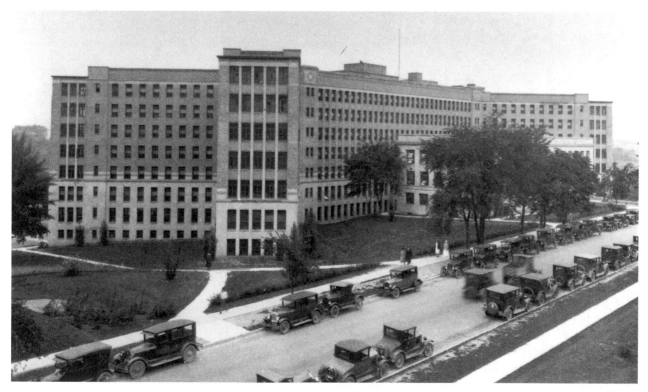

Fig. 14–3. University Hospital on Ann Street, 1927 (Old Main). (Courtesy of the Department of Surgery, University of Michigan.)

screens for the windows and toilets for the nurses. Peterson was appointed medical director of the hospital, and he repeatedly complained about his administrative burden. He said that when he died he wanted to be buried near the hospital so that he could continue to keep an eye on it.

At this time internships were not required, and Vaughan had extensive discussions with other medical deans about whether a compulsory fifth year should be added to the curriculum. Perhaps Detroit hospitals could be used for that year. Vaughan was despondent, so he wrote, because Chicago, Boston, and Baltimore were ahead of the University of Michigan. Michigan could not have a great school or a graduate program in medicine without Detroit clinical facilities. He sounded out Peterson, Barrett, Canfield, and Warthin, and he thought they were less hostile to the use of Detroit hospitals than before. He immediately wrote his son, J. Walter Vaughan, a surgeon in Detroit and a member of the Detroit College of Medicine, telling him to stir up those in Detroit who favored connection with the university. In 1916 the city of Detroit offered to turn over its new Receiving Hospital to be run by the regents of the university. The regents did not have to decide, for on Peterson's motion the faculty voted the proposal down. In 1917 Vaughan was told that Henry Ford might turn over the Henry Ford Hospital to the university, but of course he did not.

Louis M. Warfield at Michigan

Hugh Cabot began looking for a professor of medicine soon after he became dean in 1921, and in 1922 he recommended the appointment of Louis Marshall Warfield.

Warfield had been an undergraduate and a medical student at Johns Hopkins, where he played the airy flute and did well enough to be appointed an intern on Osler's service in 1901.[1] As one of Osler's disciples Warfield was 1 of 152 authors of a Festschrift presented to Osler on his seventieth birthday.[2] From 1904 to 1909 he practiced in St. Louis, where he founded the Missouri Anti-Tuberculosis Association. He moved to Milwaukee in 1909 to become pathologist and chief of the medical service of the County Hospital, and he was made professor of medicine when the Marquette Medical School was reorganized in 1911. Warfield published a large number of mis-

cellaneous case reports arising from his practice as a pathologist, but his chief interest, aside from tuberculosis, was cardiovascular diseases. He wrote an elementary textbook on arteriosclerosis, on the order of Foster's book on diabetes, that went through three editions.[3] Warfield made considerable effort to demonstrate that the fourth and not the fifth Korotkoff sound occurs at diastolic pressure, and he even went to the physiology department at Madison, where Walter Meek helped him to determine diastolic pressure in three dogs.[4] The reason for this interest in diastolic pressure was that Warfield thought that the pulse pressure is the driving force that keeps blood in motion.

At Michigan Warfield was particularly interested in the early detection of tuberculosis, and he practiced intradermal tuberculin testing. He had difficulty convincing his colleagues of the value of the test.[5] He published more case reports, and he gave practitioners advice at state medical meetings.[6] Sweat baths are useless in uremic coma, he said; instead place large mustard plasters over the kidneys. In diagnosing pernicious anemia, do not pay too much attention to the blood picture; detection of achlorhydria is more important. Transfusion is useless, but splenectomy is a logical procedure. Give Fowler's solution [arsenous acid], and have the patient sip dilute hydrochloric acid throughout a meal.

Warfield and Newburgh

Frank Wilson, in his account of the Department of Medicine in the *Encyclopedic Survey,* said that Warfield was unhappy at Michigan and on account of various controversies resigned in 1925.[7] Documentary evidence concerning Warfield's unhappiness is all one sided, consisting of Cabot's correspondence and two affidavits prepared by Warfield after he had quarreled with Newburgh and Cabot and was too excited to be quite rational. Judgment of Warfield might be more sympathetic had other documents survived.

After he had quarreled with Warfield, Cabot wrote that as a teacher Warfield was dictatorial and unreasonable. What was worse, Warfield did not know enough medicine, and he was often at a disadvantage compared with his colleagues. Furthermore, he could not obtain the loyalty of his staff, and he annoyed them by appearing to interfere with their work.[8]

When Warfield came to Ann Arbor he promised there would be no change in the status of Wilson and Newburgh, the two rising stars of Michigan medicine. He agreed to allow Newburgh a metabolic ward of his own and time for research. Wilson wanted similar privileges, and his position was consolidated by his negotiations with Vanderbilt. Sometime in 1923–24 Warfield quarreled with Newburgh, and when Warfield posted the assignments at the beginning of the 1924–25 academic year Newburgh found he had been assigned to the Outpatient Department in the mornings, where he would work under the supervision of an instructor, and to teaching clinics in the afternoons. Newburgh protested, and there was a meeting of Warfield, Cabot, Newburgh, and Wilson in President Burton's office. Warfield could give no justification for his action. On 25 September 1924 Cabot had a stormy meeting with Warfield. In reply to Warfield's assertion that his agreement with Newburgh was canceled, Cabot said that on the contrary what Warfield said was false and that the agreement remained binding. Cabot told Warfield that assigning Newburgh to the Outpatient Department was an extraordinary action. It was designed to interfere with Newburgh's work, and Newburgh had reacted in a quite human way in assuming that it was Warfield's intention to interfere. To top it off, Cabot dressed down Warfield for having hired a secretary when Cabot had told him not to.

On 28 September Cabot sent a long letter to Warfield summarizing the conversation. He also sent a copy to President Burton, who merely replied he had read the letter with great interest. Six days later Warfield presented Burton with two short letters, one resigning his job at the end of the academic year and the other asking for a leave of absence to begin at once. Burton accepted the resignation, gave Warfield leave, and notified Cabot.

On 8 October Warfield came to Burton brandishing a patient's record and two notarized affidavits. The first affidavit was signed by Warfield, and it accused Newburgh of gross neglect of duty. At Newburgh's request, Warfield had assigned Newburgh the care of diabetic patients. The previous spring, on 26 May 1924, while Warfield was out of town, a woman had been admitted to the surgical ward and was first seen by Mr. Hume. Mr. Hume was not, as an American might think, a medical student. He was a bachelor of science, fellow of the Royal College of Surgeons of England, a young man from St.

Bartholomew's Hospital who was in Ann Arbor as the result of contacts made by Cabot during the war.[9] The woman was diagnosed as having severe hyperthyroidism and at once transferred to Newburgh's metabolic ward, where she was first seen by Dr. Marsh. On 6 June her condition was so bad that she was moved to a private room on the women's medical ward. She was under the care of an intern who thought she was also diabetic. The intern sought Dr. Marsh, who had, with Newburgh, responsibility for the care of diabetic patients. The intern could not find Marsh. He found Newburgh in Warfield's office grading examination papers. Newburgh gave the intern advice and said he knew what to do. The intern panicked and looked for other staff members. He found an instructor who had not treated diabetic patients in the University Hospital. The instructor saw the patient and suggested she be given more insulin and glucose. The woman died on the afternoon of the next day in what Warfield said was diabetic coma, and it was on the basis of Newburgh's failure to see the patient that Warfield accused Newburgh of unprofessional conduct. The second affidavit was written by Warfield but signed by the intern. It recited the facts but omitted the accusation.

Burton sent the patient's record back to the hospital and gave copies of the affidavits to Cabot, asking Cabot's comments. Cabot interviewed everyone involved, studied the hospital record, and concluded that the patient had been overtreated rather than undertreated. He said it was clear the patient had acute hyperthyroidism and that her being approximately two months pregnant contributed to the severity of her symptoms. Her urine did contain varying amounts of glucose, but Marsh thought she did not have diabetes in the true sense. The sugar was referred primarily to disease of the thyroid. At the end of a very long letter to Burton, Cabot pointed out that Warfield, if he thought the patient had been neglected, had not mentioned that to Newburgh or Marsh in five months. If such accusations were to be made on such grounds it would be impossible to maintain a staff of self-respecting people. Warfield's judgment was unsound, and he was unfit to manage a department of medicine. However, Cabot hoped the regents would be generous in continuing Warfield's salary, for Warfield would have more expenses in leaving Ann Arbor in October than if he had resigned in July.

Interim Management of the Department of Medicine

Cabot made Preston Hickey, who was professor of roentgenology, head of internal medicine. Hickey had been a pathologist and an internist before he taught himself roentgenology, and he was liked and trusted. Then Cabot, who did not have much use for internists, including his brother Richard, brought James D. Bruce from Saginaw to be director of the Department of Medicine and chief of the medical service in the hospital. Bruce had graduated from the Detroit College of Medicine and Surgery and, except for a year under George Dock in 1904–5 and service in the Canadian army during the war, had been in general practice. He was hired to manage the department and to improve the university's relations with physicians throughout the state. With his own consent he was specifically not given a professorial title; he was not to be the department's intellectual leader. Occasionally he was described in print as professor of medicine, and Cabot thought the description was not without encouragement from Bruce.

The Simpson Memorial Institute

The problem of internal medicine was solved in a roundabout way by the death of Thomas Henry Simpson, a Detroit ironmaster, of pernicious anemia in 1923. His widow, acting through her attorney, gave the university $488,943.78 to build and endow a hematological research institute as a memorial to her husband. Mrs. Simpson, like Mrs. Leland Stanford, had definite ideas how the bequest should be spent, and she picked Albert Kahn to be the architect. The building he designed had sufficient walnut paneling to satisfy Mrs. Simpson, research laboratories, and on the third floor beds for patients to be studied.[10] The building was ready by 29 June 1926 (fig. 14–4), but there was no staff to fill it. An advisory committee with Cabot as chairman collected the usual vast list of prospects for the directorship. One eminent and well-connected Boston hematologist, after writing a four-page letter naming everyone who had ever seen a reticulocyte, said that Raphael Isaacs, although a good laboratory man, was unsuitable for the job; he was Jewish. Eventually the committee

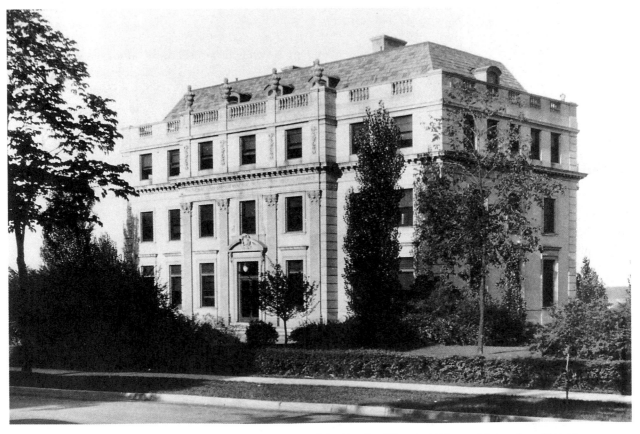

Fig. 14–4. Simpson Memorial Institute. (Courtesy of the Bentley Historical Library, University of Michigan, Photographs Vertical File, D13).

settled on Cyrus Sturgis, then at the Peter Bent Brigham Hospital in Boston, and Sturgis was invited to lecture in Ann Arbor and to be inspected. Later in that month Cabot wrote Sturgis telling him that he was definitely not making an offer but outlining the terms of an offer should there be one. Late in December President C. C. Little cleared the terms with Cabot and interviewed Sturgis in Boston in January. Sturgis was offered the job. He was to come to Michigan as director of the Simpson Memorial Institute with responsibility for organizing a research program in hematology. The next year, 1928, he would be made head of the Department of Internal Medicine while Bruce would be gracefully shelved in a new Department of Postgraduate Medicine. Little, Cabot, Bruce, and Sturgis were to keep this arrangement to themselves. Sturgis accepted, and he sent a junior colleague, Raphael Isaacs, ahead to begin organizing the institute. Sturgis himself moved to Ann Arbor in the summer of 1927.

Sturgis's Background

Joseph Wearn said that Sturgis had a warm personality with human understanding and compassion and that he was a gifted clinician and a natural teacher.[11]

Sturgis interned at the Peter Bent Brigham Hospital under Henry Christian after graduating from Johns Hopkins in 1917. During the war he was a member of Francis Peabody's unit at the U.S. General Hospital in Lakewood, New Jersey, inevitably studying disordered action of the heart. Sturgis returned to Brigham, and in the course of rising to be physician to the hospital he continued working with Peabody on respiration tests.[12] In the early 1920s measurement of metabolism by some version of Benedict's rebreathing apparatus was not yet a routine procedure.[13] Someone had suggested that it is easier to diagnose hyperthyroidism by giving an intramuscular injection of 0.5 milliliter of 1:1,000 epinephrine. In hyperthyroid patients the blood pressure and heart rate were said to rise more than in normal persons. Sturgis, working with Peabody and Wearn, found the test unreliable.[14] This experience started Sturgis measuring basal metabolism in hyperthyroidism, a study he continued until he came to Michigan. Sturgis followed the course of the disease and assessed the results of various forms of treatment: ligation of the thyroid arteries, roentgen irradiation of the gland, and partial thyroidectomy.[15] The

work was purely descriptive. The one exception was an experimental test of the possibility there might be some direct action of iodine upon the circulating product of the thyroid gland. Administration of iodine in the form of Lugol's solution was known to be a valuable preoperative measure, for it caused basal metabolism to fall for a while. Sturgis gave rabbits daily intravenous injections of one milligram of thyroxin and measured the animals' body weight, pulse rate, and oxygen consumption. Giving iodine by mouth did not alter the effects of thyroxin, and Sturgis concluded that iodine acts on the gland, not on the periphery.[16]

Raphael Isaacs in Boston

While Sturgis was advancing to an assistant professorship at Harvard, Raphael Isaacs was working at the Huntington Hospital down the street from the Brigham. He was a member of a group of Boston hematologists whose leader was George R. Minot, and when he came to Michigan he was a far more experienced hematologist than Sturgis.[17] Isaacs had been born in Cincinnati, Ohio, in the same year Sturgis had been born in Oregon—1891. He graduated from the University of Cincinnati College of Medicine in 1918. There he was an instructor in clinical medicine for a while, and he published the first of more than 250 papers. The subject of one paper was how to inject tapeworms with India ink to aid identification.[18] Another reported a large number of hydrogen ion concentrations and carbon dioxide combining powers of cerebrospinal fluid collected from patients with a wide variety of diseases.[19] Still another paper described a patient with polycythemia vera whose red cell count rose to 15,940,000.[20] In 1923 Isaacs got to Boston, where he was supported by a Bradford Fellowship and then by an instructorship in the full-time service at the Huntington Hospital. There Isaacs's research was entirely hematological. Isaacs obtained capillary blood from seventeen men before and after they ran in the Boston Marathon.[21] He found a relative and absolute increase in the number of polymorphonuclear neutrophile leukocytes, and he attributed the increase to stirring up of the blood during the race. Isaacs studied resistance of erythrocytes to heat,[22] and he found that young erythrocytes do not agglutinate. Young cells contained four types of intracellular granules. The first were "brilliant, highly refractile large granules," in some respects resembling Howell-Jolly bodies.[23] These "Isaacs bodies" have disappeared from the index of textbooks of hematology.

Isaacs was junior author with Minot of papers reporting Minot's large experience with leukemias.[24] One described the distribution by age and sex of 166 patients with acute myelogenous leukemia. Irradiation had little effect on the duration of life, those irradiated living an average of 3.50 years after irradiation and those not irradiated living an average of 3.04 years. In 477 patients with lymphoblastoma, irradiation slightly prolonged the lives of those destined to die within 2.5 years, but it did not influence the course of the disease in those living longer. Minot and Isaacs found that on average the nature of acute lymphatic leukemia was not recognized by the primary physician until the disease had run two-thirds of its course. In 57 such patients and in 98 with the chronic form irradiation likewise had no detectable effect on the length of life, and its other beneficial effects were slight and evanescent. This experience prompted Isaacs to submit an essay, "On the Nature and Action of the Roentgen Rays on Living Tissue," to the College of Physicians of Philadelphia, and the college awarded him the Alvarenga Prize. In Ann Arbor Isaacs continued to treat leukemic patients with X rays, and he found himself in controversy over dose schedules and efficacy. One discussant of a paper said: "Dr. Isaacs speaks with more assurance than I can bring to bear on the problem. I feel doubtful upon practically every point concerning which he speaks rather dogmatically."[25]

Treatment of Pernicious Anemia

Between the death of Thomas Henry Simpson from pernicious anemia in 1923 and the opening of the Simpson Memorial Institute in 1927 Minot and Murphy had discovered the efficacy of a diet of one-half pound of cooked liver a day in causing remission of the disease.[26] Because the institute was specifically dedicated to the study of pernicious anemia, Sturgis and Isaacs at once began to diagnose and to treat patients with the disease. At first they used the liver diet, but as liver extracts made by E. J. Cohn[27] became available from Eli Lilly and Company and Parke, Davis and Company they demonstrated, for example, that a massive dose of thirty vials of extract by stomach tube was as good as or better than a dose

of three vials a day for ten days.[28] This and the fact that all livers do not contain the active principle convinced them that it is stored in the liver and is not part of the liver substance.[29] Sturgis and Isaacs did not prepare liver extract on their own, but they did clean up commercial extracts by passing them through a column packed with permutit (zeolite). That treatment removed contaminants that caused headache, chills, and a fall in blood pressure.[30] Sturgis and Isaacs found the purified preparation, given intravenously, to be about forty times as effective as a corresponding amount of extract given by mouth. By the mid-1930s Sturgis had accumulated experience in treating over 600 patients with pernicious anemia.[31] In an article unaccountably entitled "An Analysis of the Causes of Death in 150 Fatal Cases of Pernicious Anemia Observed since 1927," Sturgis analyzed the cause of death in 147 fatal cases.[32] Exactly one-third had died as the result of their disease, seven because they discontinued treatment and forty-four of complications resulting from involvement of the spinal cord. Sturgis said that with modern treatment a patient may live to advanced age but will probably not attain normal life expectancy. As a result of this experience, together or alone, Sturgis and Isaacs were invited to give many talks before medical societies and to write reviews.[33]

Ventriculin

As Sturgis and Isaacs were beginning their work in Ann Arbor, William Castle in Boston was doing what Sturgis called his "classical experiments."[34] The cure of pernicious anemia by a liver diet suggests that it is a deficiency disease, but it cannot be one of the usual kind. Pernicious anemia patients have achylia gastrica, and Castle thought achylia may have an intermediate role. There could be deficiency in gastric secretion. Castle ate three hundred grams of raw ground beef, and one hour later he recovered his gastric contents and incubated them for six hours at pH 2. The product, neutralized with sodium hydroxide, was given by stomach tube to patients in relapse, and eight of ten such patients had a reticulocyte response. Castle and everyone else for a long time thought that the intrinsic factor secreted by the stomach is an enzyme. Sturgis and Isaacs wrote that

the gastric secretion of a patient with pernicious anemia is defective, as it is unable to liberate from protein a substance which prevents the development of pernicious anemia. . . . [We have] reasoned that the administration of desiccated normal stomach should have the capacity to remedy the fundamental defect in pernicious anemia either by supplying a sufficient amount of effective preformed material [the extrinsic factor], or possibly by introducing an unknown enzyme-like substance which could liberate the effective material from protein [the intrinsic factor].[35]

Accordingly, Sturgis and Isaacs worked with Elwood A. Sharp, director of the Department of Experimental Medicine at Parke, Davis, to produce such an extract of the stomach that would replace both the intrinsic factor and the extrinsic factor contained in a rival pharmaceutical company's liver extract.

Sturgis and Isaacs, or some technician working for them, removed the fat and surrounding mesentery from hog stomachs and chopped the stomachs very fine. After the tissue had been dried at low temperature, fat was extracted by repeated washing with petroleum benzin. One hundred grams of fresh stomach yielded 11.7 to 15 grams of powder that, because it was insoluble in water, was given to patients in tomato juice. Sturgis and Isaacs reported complete success in three patients, and they eventually obtained satisfactory results with more than one hundred patients with a dose equivalent to 60–70 grams of fresh stomach.

Sturgis and Isaacs found no response to stomach muscle alone, and of four patients fed mucosa three gave no response at all and one a questionable one. They concluded that the muscle alone does not contain the active principle, but when ground in the fresh state with mucosa an enzymelike substance acts on muscle protein to liberate the active principle.

Sharp, Sturgis, and Isaacs called their product Ventriculin, and they applied for a patent. The regents made a contract with Parke, Davis, and the profits were to be used for research in hematology. Isaacs, who told Dean Furstenberg that he had invented Ventriculin while Sturgis was on vacation, estimated that the university received ten thousand dollars in royalties.

Isaacs left Michigan in 1940 boiling with resentment. For some reason his salary had been reduced, and he told the dean that he could not bear this last insult or Sturgis's insane antipathy without protest. He went to Chicago, where he practiced hematology at the Michael Reese Hospital. The next year Sturgis took a half-time appointment and was permitted to admit private patients to the University Hospital.

Transformation of the Department

The Department of Internal Medicine headed by Sturgis was very different from that headed by Dock or Hewlett. For one thing, it was much larger. Dock or Hewlett had only one or two assistants and two or three interns. By 1930 there were three full professors, three associate professors, four assistant professors, and eleven instructors in addition to a large corps of house officers, each serving four years. In 1941 the department was half again as large. Dock and Hewlett had come from elsewhere, but the junior members of their department were invariably Michigan graduates. By 1930 the department was staffed by individuals from Harvard, Pennsylvania, Washington in St. Louis, Cincinnati, and McGill. Even the interns began to be outsiders: John Sheldon, for example, interned at Michigan after graduating from Nebraska.

Wilson had taken cardiology as his specialty, Newburgh endocrinology and metabolism, and Sturgis hematology. In Sturgis's time every member of the department began to have a particular interest, and subspecialties differentiated. John Barnwell, who had come from Trudeau's Adirondack Cottage Hospital, managed a tuberculosis service that was part of the state sanatorium system. Marvin Pollard bought a gastroscope, learned to use it, and established a gastroenterology service. A Rackham grant supported a new arthritis unit directed by Richard Freyberg. These and others were poised to become semiautonomous units when the disturbance of the war subsided.

15
Surgery to 1920

In 1889 Victor Vaughan brought the forty-two-year-old Charles B. Nancrede to Michigan to be professor of surgery. Nancrede remained in charge of surgery until 1914, when, on account of illness and age, he relinquished his administrative duties to Cyrenus Darling. Nancrede retired for good in 1917, and he died in 1921.

Nancrede's Ancestry and Name

Nancrede's grandfather, Paul Joseph Guérard de Nancrède, had been a lieutenant in Rochambeau's army before Yorktown. He returned to the United States after being discharged in France, taught French at Harvard, and published books in Boston. He married an American woman, and in 1797 he took his family to France so that his children could have a proper French education. Eight years later he brought his family back to the United States. Being a staunch republican, he dropped the aristocratic particle, and he and his son, a wholesale merchant in Philadelphia, bore the simple surname Nancrede. His grandson, the surgeon, remained "Charles B. Nancrede" for a few years in Ann Arbor, but in 1908 he appeared as "Charles B. G. de Nancrède" in a surgical textbook.[1] In 1906 he had changed his name legally to Charles Beylard Guérard de Nancrède, giving his reason that as the oldest surviving male member of his family he had the duty to resume the ancient and aristocratic patronymic. The patronymic was not, in fact, either ancient or aristocratic.[2] That he added the grave accent to the antepenultimate letter shows that he probably pronounced his name "Nan-cred" and not "Nan-creed."

Nancrede's Education

Young Nancrede received a classical and military education in private schools near Philadelphia, and thereafter he loved the military life. When he returned to Ann Arbor after his brief service in the Spanish-American War he wore his broad-brimmed officer's hat while riding his warhorse to the hospital, and he bitterly resented that when he was seventy years old, Victor Vaughan, then an important person in the War Office in Washington, D.C., would not allow him to be called to active duty in World War I.

Nancrede attended the University of Pennsylvania, but he went to Penn's medical school without completing his undergraduate education. He was sensitive on this point, and when he accepted his appointment at Michigan he apologized to President Angell for not having full academic credentials. Michigan repaired the fault by giving Nancrede an honorary master of arts degree and eventually a doctor of laws. Pennsylvania gave him an honorary bachelor of arts in 1892 as of the class of 1866. Nancrede earned his doctor of medicine in 1869 from Pennsylvania, and while he was attending surgeon at Jefferson Medical College that school gave him still another doctor of medicine as of the class of 1883.

Nancrede in Philadelphia

Nancrede acquired a profound knowledge of gross anatomy when he taught the subject for many years at Pennsylvania, and he demonstrated his knowledge by producing an anatomy crammer, *Essentials of Anatomy and Manual of Practical Dissection,* which went through seven editions.[3] Nancrede was an artist, and the book is illustrated with thirty elegant colored lithographs. W. B. Saunders, the publisher, used the same plates thirty years later in Keen and White's *An American Text-Book of Surgery.*[4] Nancrede condensed the book as *Questions and Answers on the Essentials of Anatomy.*[5]

Nancrede entered the practice of surgery after interning at the Episcopal Hospital in Philadelphia, and he performed operations covering the whole range available to a surgeon in 1870–90. The breadth of his practice can be observed in his numerous publications, often as many as six a year and mostly in local journals.[6] Nancrede's only nonsurgical paper was written with an internist colleague, F. P. Henry, and it was published in the widely distributed *Boston Medical and Surgical Journal.* The paper reported hundreds of red and white blood cell counts made with the newly available hemocytometer. Henry and Nancrede found commercial models to be inaccurately constructed and to give results differing by 14.7 percent. With an especially made hemocytometer Henry and Nancrede found that accuracy might be reached "through an amount of labor of which, so far, we have seen no detailed account."[7]

Nancrede's delicate hands and light touch served him in cataract extractions at Pennsylvania's Eye Clinic, but he also did major bone and joint, vascular,

abdominal, and brain surgery at the Jefferson and Episcopal Hospitals. He was orthopaedic surgeon to the Crippled Children's Hospital. He was a bold operator, but he was conservative in his attitude.[8] Nancrede's success could in part be attributed to his early conversion to the belief that microorganisms cause surgical infection.

Antisepsis and Asepsis

Nancrede was a junior colleague of the great Samuel D. Gross at the Jefferson Hospital. Gross concluded his lectures on listerism by telling the students he had given the lectures only because the trustees had required him to. In his opinion listerism "t'ain't worth a damn."[9] It is all the more remarkable that Nancrede and W. W. Keen, another junior colleague of Gross, were among the first to adopt antiseptic surgery in Philadelphia and a little later to be converted to aseptic surgery. Nancrede in his own lectures to students described in detail the technique of scrubbing one's hands and preparing the patient for aseptic operation.[10] If asepsis were accidentally broken during the operation, the hands could be rubbed with mustard powder mixed with sterile water. That was particularly good for combating the odor of feces.

Water for scrubbing, as hot as could be borne, was dipped with a sterile ladle into a sterile basin. Scrubbing began with ten minutes' vigorous brushing with soft soap containing 5 percent hydronaphthol or thymol. It concluded with dipping the arms to the elbows in saturated potassium permanganate solution and then with soaking the hands for five minutes in a 1:2,000 solution of corrosive sublimate (mercuric chloride). Nancrede recommended further brushing of the skin while the hands were in that solution. Mercuric chloride and then carbolic acid, in which the instruments were kept before being handed to the surgeon, ruined the nurses' skin, and before 1891 Halsted at Johns Hopkins had introduced rubber gloves for the instrument nurse as well as for the surgeon.[11] Soon the whole team was wearing rubber gloves, and Halsted said that "rubber gloves must, of course, be worn by all concerned with the operation." Some conservative surgeons condemned them for interfering with the surgeon's touch, but McBurney agreed with Halsted.[12] Nancrede did not mention rubber gloves in his lectures, his textbook, or his chapters on surgical technique. Pictures taken in Ann Arbor in the 1890s show him operating bare handed and bareheaded, but Michigan surgeons wore gloves after 1901.

There was another contrast with Halsted. Nancrede created no school of surgery. His students and assistants eventually practiced surgery, but none attained distinction. When Nancrede died the tributes came from members of the faculty but not from a band of disciples.[13]

Nancrede's Early Surgery

Nancrede's promptness in accepting antisepsis and then asepsis was matched in other aspects of surgery. Reginald Fitz demonstrated the imperative need for prompt diagnosis of appendicitis and speedy surgical intervention in 1886.[14] Within two years Nancrede performed what was said to be the first appendectomy in Philadelphia. After Hughlings Jackson described the focal nature of some forms of epilepsy Nancrede operated at the Jefferson Hospital upon a patient who had had seizures for eighteen years. The locus had been incorrectly diagnosed by someone, but Nancrede, working from the fact that the seizure began with movement of the right thumb, exposed the brain on the left side. He identified the motor area for the thumb by electrical stimulation, causing a typical paroxysm despite deep general anesthesia.[15] He removed the center and found no response to electrical stimulation at its former site. Nancrede reported three more similar operations done in Ann Arbor before 1893. In one he found nothing abnormal when he tested the brain with electric current, and he closed the skull without attacking the brain. He thought the operations to be only palliative, for seizures eventually returned in all patients.

After Nancrede came to Ann Arbor he quoted the remark that surgery of the biliary tract was in the same position surgery of the appendix had been ten years earlier. Cholelithiasis and cholestasis should no longer be considered medical affections. In reporting forty-four of his own cases Nancrede attempted to induce his "readers to recognize the existence of many serious hepatic and biliary conditions, which can only be properly met by use of the knife."[16]

Nancrede Comes to Ann Arbor

In 1889 Nancrede left his appointments in three well-equipped Philadelphia hospitals to accept the professorship of surgery in a small Midwestern town. The new University Hospital had been planned, but it was not completed until three years later. Nancrede's first operating room was in a wooden barracks (fig. 15–1). The university furnished no surgical instruments, no assistants, and no nurses. Reuben Peterson, who knew Nancrede well, said Nancrede accepted the job because in Philadelphia he had a small practice and a large family.[17] He needed the security of his university salary to support his wife and nine children. Everyone who knew Nancrede emphasized the difficulty of getting along with him, and according to Peterson the roughness of Nancrede's behavior prevented his acquiring an adequate surgical practice in Philadelphia. Despite all Nancrede's teaching and his hospital appointments he had no professorship that a man of his age, skill, and experience might expect.

From the earliest days when Moses Gunn professed surgery in Ann Arbor but practiced in Detroit, clinical faculty lived where lucrative practices were available. Maclean had left the university because he could not take the medical school with him to Detroit. When Nancrede learned that as a condition of his appointment the regents required him to live in Ann Arbor, he replied that he had no thought of doing otherwise. Throughout his time at Michigan Nancrede found his salary and the returns of occasional consulting almost adequate. For a while he supplemented his Michigan salary by teaching at Dartmouth in the summer months. Peterson said Nancrede was totally devoid of commercialism, and he made no attempt to build up a private practice. He never opened an office downtown.

Nancrede's Characteristics

Nancrede's colleagues admired him, but they did not like him. He was brusque to the point of rudeness and quick to take offense. He was extremely sensitive, and when he was clearly at fault he could not bring himself to acknowledge his error. His subordinates saw a different man, for he was kind and considerate to his junior staff and students. When he rode off to the Spanish-American War he was astride a fully caparisoned horse his students gave him. Later they gave him a silver loving cup to mark the fortieth anniversary of his doctorate. His enthusiastic support of athletics made him popular with the undergraduates, and for many years he was a member of the

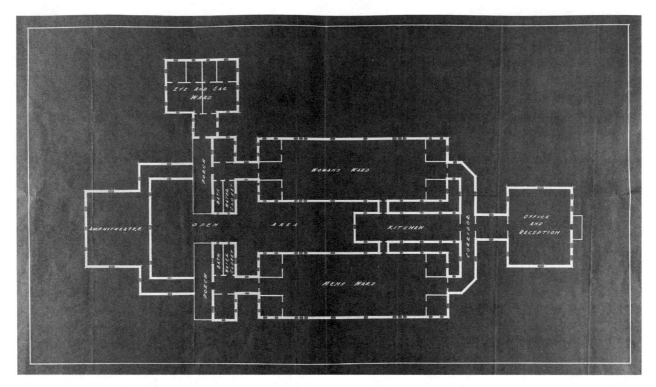

Fig. 15–1. Floor plan of the Pavilion Hospital on campus. Redrawn by the Building and Grounds Department from the Report of the Michigan State Board of Health on the Sanitary Condition of the Hospital at Ann Arbor, 1882. (Courtesy of the Bentley Historical Library, University of Michigan, Reuben Peterson Papers, Box 2.)

Committee on Athletics. In those days women did not attend athletic contests, but Nancrede's appearance at football games with his wife and daughters broke the sex barrier.

Nancrede was musical; he sang in the choir of St. Andrew's Episcopal Church; and he was a faithful member of the Choral Union. He painted, and he thought he might have been a successful painter had he not turned to surgery.

Nancrede's Department

Starting from almost nothing Nancrede built a university department of surgery. Almost from the start he had Cyrenus Darling as his assistant, and Darling remained his second until Nancrede retired. By 1896 Nancrede regularly had another assistant in surgery who served for two years. The number of assistants grew to four in 1901, and in that year the first intern was appointed at $125 a year. By the end of his tenure Nancrede had a staff of ten: Darling and Ira Loree as clinical professors, six assistants of various

seniority, an intern in the University Hospital and another in the Palmer Ward to look after children. In addition, there was a technician in the surgical laboratory and until 1911 a technician and photographer in charge of X-ray equipment.

Nancrede as a Surgeon

Nancrede was willing to undertake any kind of operation, and many were radical.[18] When he collected statistics it was to estimate the benefits to the patients. In his presidential address to the American Surgical Association he reviewed sixty-five cases of excision of the scapula, and to his surprise he discovered that a radical operation was the only one to be done. "I shall set my face absolutely against any partial resections of the shoulder-blade for malignant disease."[19] Nevertheless, he was often conservative. He would, for example, do no exploratory laparotomy, and often he and George Dock decided that a palliative operation, such as one for cancer of the stomach, was not to be done. Nancrede asked:

Not Just Any Medical School

"[D]oes the operation contemplate the cure or only the palliation of the disease; and secondly, in the latter event, is the knife especially dangerous to life?"[20] He worked as quickly as the condition of the patient would permit. He kept the patient warm, and he tried to avoid shock by keeping the patient's head low. If shock threatened, he gave one to three liters of sterile isotonic saline by vein. Sometimes he gave the solution by rectum or by hypodermoclysis. He was particularly solicitous in his aftercare, and he frequently stayed in the hospital all night to observe a patient. He changed the dressings himself.

Anesthesia

Nancrede preferred ether to chloroform. The anesthetic was given by one of his assistants who had learned by observing another assistant. If ether were used, unconsciousness was sometimes first induced by 98 percent nitrous oxide and 2 percent oxygen, and Nancrede did not realize that unconsciousness was then caused by severe hypoxia. If chloroform were used, strong men held the patient down until he or she passed through the stage of excitement.

Until 1911 there was no formal clinical training in anesthesia at Michigan. Medical students heard lectures on the subject in pharmacology, but there were no laboratory exercises with ether or chloroform until 1918.[21] Reuben Peterson, the gynecological surgeon, tried to give each senior medical student the opportunity of administering one anesthetic under the supervision of an assistant, but he thought that a medical student who spent extra time in the operating theater learned little about anesthesia by watching an intern give one.[22]

William Breakey on his trip to Europe in 1908 found that the hospital of the University of London had six anesthetists and had applied for two more. Guy's Hospital had seven, but Michigan had none. At that time Nancrede said that Michigan was criminal in not having an expert anesthetist in an institution where medical students were trained. The Michigan clinical faculty repeatedly asked the regents to provide for an anesthetist, but it was not until 1911 that Allen Richardson, a graduate of the medical class of 1910, was appointed demonstrator in anesthesia. The next year he disappeared into practice in Detroit, and his place was taken by a registered nurse, Laura M. Davis, later Laura Davis Dunstone, who remained solely responsible for teaching anesthesia to medical students and nurses until 1938.

The medical faculty did not treat Davis generously, for in 1913 it denied her one hundred dollars for a trip to New York to study anesthesia. Nevertheless, by 1915 she was providing instruction for medical students, who were excused from class when they were scheduled to give an anesthetic. She regularly listed medical students by name in her annual report to the faculty. Each student had given seven or eight anesthetics, and some had given more by being present at extra hours or during the summer session in which she taught a course.

Davis conducted a training program for nurse-anesthetists, and every year she presented the names of five or so nurses to the faculty to be given certificates in anesthesia. Once there was a squabble with the director of the hospital, who wanted to give the certificates in the hospital's name. He was overruled on the grounds that such training was an academic affair.

Nancrede's Teaching

Early in Nancrede's time in Ann Arbor third-year students heard three hours of lecture a week on surgery and attended a clinical course for two hours. Fourth-year students heard another three hours of lecture and went to surgical clinics two afternoons a week where they watched Nancrede operate (fig. 15–2). Whether they could see anything he did was in question. Fourth-year students also worked in the surgical laboratory practicing amputations on a cadaver under the eye of a demonstrator (fig. 15–3) and operating on animals under aseptic and antiseptic precautions. Students practiced bandaging and fracture dressing (fig. 15–4). As medical subjects gradually pushed nonmedical subjects out of the curriculum, students had more practical experience in surgery. In 1896 the class was divided into two sections for dressing patients and for bedside instruction. In 1900 students began to assist Cyrenus Darling in minor operations on Saturday mornings. Nancrede, like George Dock, had senior medical students living in the hospital and permanently attached to his service. Those students assisted at operations.

Nancrede's most successful teaching was at the operating table or at the bedside (fig. 15–5). His lectures were confused and rambling, and they consisted of readings from his textbook and tirades against the

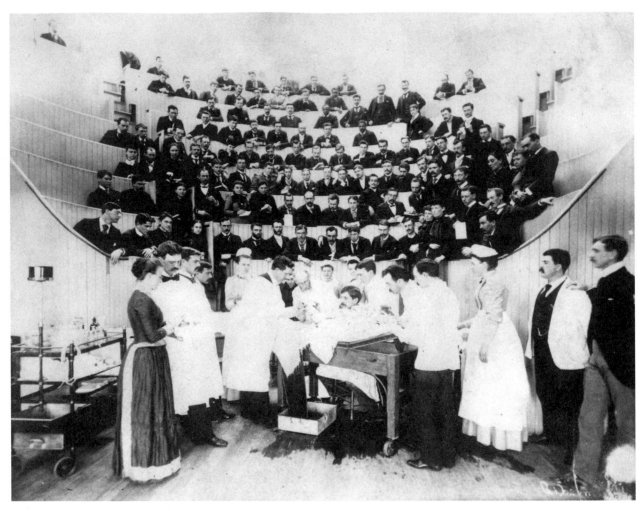

Fig. 15–2. Dr. Nancrede's clinic, Catherine Street Hospital, 1893. Alice Hamilton is seated in the front row of the benches *(fourth from left)*. (Courtesy of the Bentley Historical Library, University of Michigan, Medical School Records, Box 136, "Gibson #2.")

practices of other surgeons.[23] The textbook, *Lectures upon the Principles of Surgery*,[24] had been published in 1899 and reprinted in 1905. A large part is devoted to inflammation, and Nancrede has been accused of holding the untenable position that inflammation and infection are synonymous. A careful reading of the book demonstrates this to be a semantic confusion. Nancrede defined *inflammation* as infection, and any other kind of hyperemia—for example, that caused by a closed sprain—was not inflammation by definition. Nancrede's "Senior Lecture Notes," preserved in the Bentley Historical Library, consist of a well-worn packet of pages cut from his textbook and liberally underlined. They are supplemented by thirty-three pages of handwritten notes on various forms of hernia, and at their end

Nancrede penciled "8 hours." Students must have been bored.

The Specialties: Oral Surgery

Nancrede gave up surgical specialties as others developed skills. He relinquished gynecological surgery to James Martin in 1892, and although he occasionally did maxillofacial surgery,[25] he encouraged Cyrenus Darling to take over oral surgery. Darling had an office downtown and a large and miscellaneous general surgical practice. In addition to teaching elements of surgery to medical students in the dog laboratory and in minor clinics he taught physical diagnosis for George Dock as well. Nevertheless,

Not Just Any Medical School

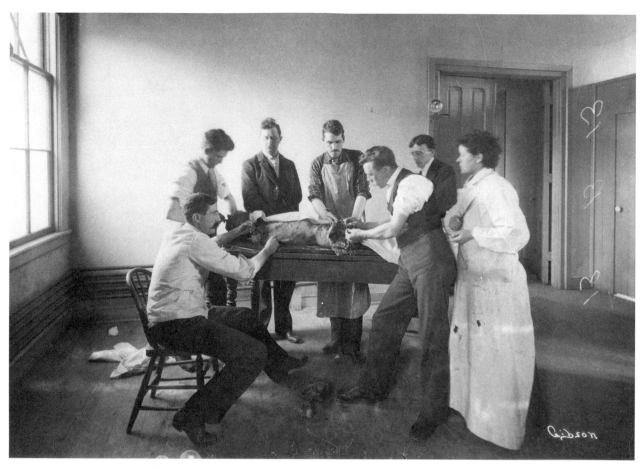

Fig. 15–3. Operating course in the surgical laboratory. Trephining and amputation at the hip and shoulder joints of a cadaver. Cyrenus Darling is the instructor standing second from left. (Courtesy of the Dean's Office, Medical School, University of Michigan.)

Darling was appointed to the faculty of the School of Dentistry as lecturer in oral pathology and oral surgery in 1892. Chalmers Lyons considered Darling to be one of the four founders of modern oral surgery.[26]

Lyons, an 1898 graduate of the School of Dentistry, had been in general practice of dentistry in Adrian, Michigan, until 1908, when he had some training in oral surgery under Truman Brophy in Chicago. He followed this by working as a nonresident instructor in dentistry at the University Hospital with Nancrede and Darling. Lyons moved to Ann Arbor in 1915, and the Medical School gave him a dental chair in the hospital so that he did not have to take his patients to the dental school for treatment. The state legislature provided that children with harelip and cleft palate were to be treated at the University Hospital at public expense, but the legislature craftily provided that the expense was to be borne by the county of residence, not the state. The result was that Darling and Lyons operated upon as many as two hundred patients a year, and there was a waiting list.

The Specialties: Genitourinary Surgery

In 1906 Ira D. Loree, a graduate of 1901, took over genitourinary surgery from Cyrenus Darling, who had been teaching it Saturday mornings. Loree's practice was confined to men, for Reuben Peterson dealt with corresponding problems in women. Loree remained in charge of that specialty until 1920. After 1908 he was clinical professor on account of his substantial private practice.

In 1916 Loree and R. W. Kraft described the prostatectomies they had done at the University Hospital in the year 1914–15.[27] The fact that R. W.

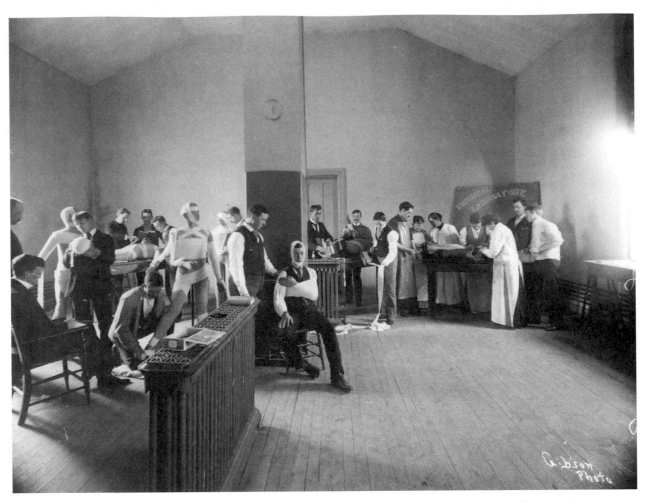

Fig. 15–4. Bandaging and fracture dressing. (Courtesy of the Dean's Office, Medical School, University of Michigan.)

Kraft was a senior medical student at the time the work was done illuminates the surgical training of medical students during Nancrede's later years.

A large number of men with senile hypertrophic prostates were now coming to the University Hospital. Most were poor farmers who had let the condition go, and they had to be kept in the hospital for weeks, hence a crowded hospital with low patient turnover. One patient with extreme dilatation of the bladder refused operation. His phenolsulfonphthalein (PSP) test was too low to be read, and his blood urea nitrogen was 3.50, units as usual being unspecified. He died five days later in uremic convulsions. Twenty-five men received preliminary cystostomy under 2 percent novocaine local anesthesia, and the rate of improvement of their PSP test determined when the second stage, suprapubic prostatectomy, was to be done under nitrous oxide–oxygen anesthe-

sia. One patient died of pneumonia, but twenty-four survived. Two other patients were operated upon after a previous perineal prostatectomy.

Loree's service was busy. In 1917 he told the dean there had been 3,304 outpatient visits in the first six months of the year, and he presented a long list of complaints and demands. The cystoscope room should be moved next to the X-ray department so that patients prepared for cystoscopy need not be wheeled from one building to another for X-ray examination. Loree needed two assistants, an intern, and fifteen beds permanently assigned to him. He said that students intending to become genitourinary surgeons should be excused from long training in general surgery. By 1920 his demands were more insistent. Loree now wanted to be made head of an independent department, and when he was denied that he abruptly resigned on 9 March 1920. The

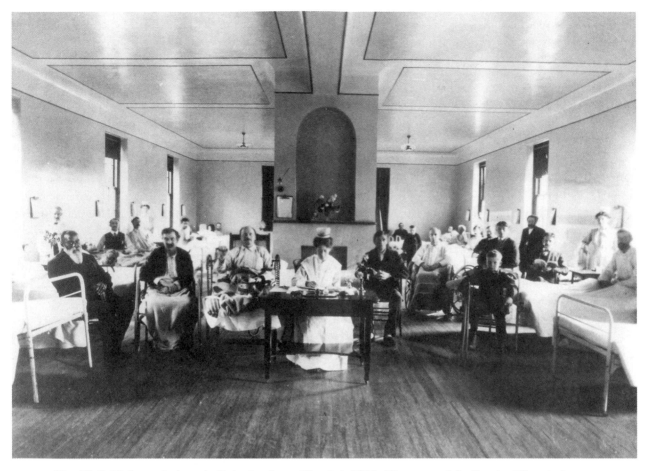

Fig. 15–5. Male surgical ward, Catherine Street Hospital, 1893. (Courtesy of the Bentley Historical Library, University of Michigan, Medical School Records, Box 136, "Gibson #2.")

arrival of Hugh Cabot, a genitourinary surgeon, to be head of the Department of Surgery may have had something to do with Loree's resignation.

The Specialties: Orthopaedic Surgery

Charles Washburne graduated from the Medical School in 1908, and he was intern and assistant surgeon under Nancrede and Darling, who both did bone and joint surgery. By 1911 he began to specialize in orthopaedic surgery by participating in closed reduction of congenital dislocation of the hip. He used the bloodless method introduced by Adolf Lorenz in Germany and popularized in the United States by a visit by Lorenz in 1902. Washburne's first patient was a girl of ten, and when she was under ether anesthesia Washburne stretched the structures around her hip joint by forcing the head of the femur downward and forward. Washburne used a padded

wedge under her thigh as a fulcrum. He gave up the attempt after two hours when X-ray examination showed that the head of the femur was not in the acetabulum. A second attempt reduced the joint in thirty minutes, and Washburne applied a plaster cast. When he removed the cast two months later he found he had damaged the sciatic nerve by pressure on the wedge. The girl had little power of motion of the flexors and extensors of the foot. Washburne gave up using the wedge, and in his next two cases he found he could easily break the adductors and reduce the dislocation. In his fourth case he had to cut the adductor tendons, but the result, he said, was satisfactory to the patient's parents.

Washburne was made demonstrator in orthopaedics in 1911, and at the same time he opened an office downtown for his private practice. The next year he had the responsibility of teaching a course in orthopaedic surgery.

In 1915 Washburne said that 50 percent of the

deformities seen in the University Hospital were the result of poliomyelitis, with rickets and Pott's disease accounting for the rest. The first recognized epidemic of poliomyelitis had occurred in 1894 in Rutland, Vermont—132 cases with eighteen deaths. Michigan had been comparatively free of the disease, but Washburne estimated there were 1,000 sporadic cases in any one year. There had been small epidemics in Michigan, 20 or 30 cases in 1907 and 1908. In 1910 there were 72 cases in Hillsdale County. Washburne said many had been misdiagnosed by local physicians or by chiropractors and that if they had been recognized no attempt was made to prevent deformities. Washburne condemned the practice of attempting to sterilize the cerebrospinal fluid by giving formalin (Urotropin) or to stimulate the muscles by giving strychnine. Twenty-five percent of the patients recovered without deformity, but a substantial number of the rest came to the University Hospital under the 1913 Afflicted Children's Act, which provided payment for their care. Washburne outlined his surgical treatment.

Arthrodesis is of value in treating joints partially or not at all under the control of normal muscle groups, producing a permanent ankylosis in a useful position. . . . Tendon transference is applicable in properly selected cases as a means of partially restoring function. This operation we have found most useful about the ankle joint, selecting those tendons whose actions most closely correspond to the paralysed muscles they are to replace. . . . Tenotomies are useful in correcting bad contraction deformities at the knee and ankle. This operation has been greatly abused in the past and in the hands of careful workmen is now used only when absolutely necessary. . . . Nerve grafting has marked possibilities, but as yet is too much in the experimental stage to be generally advocated.[28]

When Hugh Cabot came in 1920, Washburne resigned to continue his private practice of orthopaedics.

Finding Nancrede's Successor

Nancrede became one of the elders of surgery. He published numerous case reports and notes on surgical technique, and he frequently gave advice to local medical societies. Near the end of his life he contributed chapters to massive textbooks of surgery. Some chapters were on treatment of gunshot wounds, for Nancrede was very proud of his few

hours under fire at the Battle of Santiago in the Spanish-American War. When he talked on the subject at surgical meetings, surgeons who had been through the Civil War scoffed at Nancrede's experience. He had to reduce his effort in 1914, and Cyrenus Darling was put in charge of the service. Nancrede gave up entirely in 1917.

University authorities did not think Darling had the stature to be permanent head of the department. He was told that he was to serve only until Nancrede's successor was found, and he was made chairman of the committee to find one. Vaughan's telephone call went astray, and Darling did not receive an invitation to the reception for the new head. Darling resentfully refused to attend a dinner in his and Nancrede's honor. Vaughan half apologized and half remonstrated.

Frederick Coller, who knew Darling only after 1920, judged Darling harshly.

He contributed little to medical literature; his main concern was his own practice. As a surgeon he was competent but not brilliant, and his diagnostic abilities, though outstanding, left very little impression on his contemporaries. . . . [H]is strong individualistic ideas kept him from contact with world progress in surgery and made him a strong local rather than a national figure. He was the product of his time—a great individualist with the provincialism of the [Michigan] clinical groups, then overshadowed by the preclinical departments.[29]

Coller had seen nothing of Darling's thirty years of service to the Medical School. At the same time Coller said Nancrede had left little tangible evidence of his great service to humanity. Coller forgot that there had been no department of surgery at Michigan when Nancrede arrived in 1889.

The search for Nancrede's successor was made difficult by the problems of the war, the delay over construction of the new hospital, and the proposed full-time plan. By May 1917 there were seventeen names on a list of prospects. Later Halsted recommended Walter Dandy, and when Evarts Graham applied for the job Victor Vaughan told him he was too young and inexperienced. In July 1919 the job was offered to Dallas Phemister, who declined for the reason he wanted a private practice as well as the professorship. Three months later it was offered to Hugh Cabot, and Cabot accepted.

16
Surgery from 1920:
Hugh Cabot and His Men

Hugh Cabot spent the years 1916–18 at a base hospital of the Royal Army Medical Corps in France. He held the rank of lieutenant colonel in the Medical Corps; he was mentioned in dispatches four times; and he was decorated with the Order of St. Michael and St. George, a reward for those who had served Britain well overseas. When he returned to Boston in 1919 he found his large practice had evaporated,[1] and instead of establishing a new one he came to Ann Arbor.

Cabot found in Michigan's full-time plan the nucleus of the way in which he hoped medical practice would crystallize. Cabot said in 1915 that technological advances and specialization had made obsolete the old-time, individual practitioner of medicine who relied more on judgment and experience than on objective findings. The modern physician, whether he knew it or not, was in fact in group practice, for his patient was examined by an "aurist," an oculist, an orthopaedist, a dentist, a roentgenologist, a chemist, a pathologist, and a serologist. Group practice diminished personal responsibility and increased expense. Competition among groups turned medicine into a business, and medicine was degraded from a profession, whose aims were the advancement of science and the benefit of mankind, into a trade. Cabot told the hearers of his Shattuck Lecture:

> Now if we are to remove from the field of medicine this undesirable kind of competition [for money] then all practitioners of medicine must be paid salaries, and the amounts of these salaries must be determined by persons having no personal interest at stake. This means, reduced to its simplest terms, that we have a choice between the taking over of medical practice by the state or the management of medical practice from institutions or hospitals as a center. In either case, salaries must be paid to all, and the temptation to practice medicine for money must be eliminated as a possibility. . . . I therefore look forward to the development of group medicine with the hospital as its center, such hospitals to be under the management of trustees, who, it is to be hoped, will take their duties much more seriously than do most trustees of today.[2]

This quotation illustrates Cabot's habit of ending an earnest statement with a sting that offends the maximum number of persons.

183

When he came to Ann Arbor Cabot joined a hospital-based group practice in which a lay board of regents had the ultimate responsibility for fixing charges and setting salaries. That is why he came to Michigan. During his ten years at Michigan Cabot faced two problems the full-time plan had not solved: how to provide salaries the staff would consider adequate and how to bring patients of the middle-income class into the scope of hospital-based group practice.

Hugh Cabot's Background

Hugh Cabot graduated from Harvard Medical School in 1898 and served as house officer at the Massachusetts General Hospital. He remained on the hospital's staff until 1919. The seventy or more papers he published before 1920 are the autobiography of a surgeon developing into an authoritative specialist. At first he wrote on the technique of using catgut, on treatment of gastric ulcers, and on fractures,[3] but he soon confined his work to urological surgery. That specialty was well developed at the Massachusetts General Hospital, where Henry J. Bigelow had trained Arthur Tracy Cabot, Hugh's much older cousin, and where Arthur Tracy Cabot trained Hugh Cabot.

Frederick Coller wrote that Hugh Cabot was unusually skilled as a diagnostician,[4] and Cabot displayed his skill in diagnosing stones in the kidneys and bladder. Cabot was candid about others' blunders. He thought errors in diagnosis were grossly underestimated, for mistakes went unreported. Cabot reviewed 153 cases at the Massachusetts General Hospital, where twenty-six unnecessary abdominal operations without relief of symptoms had been performed. Stones in the kidney or ureter had been overlooked. The operations included appendectomy and stripping of the renal capsule for "nephalgia, and as a crowning iniquity, suprapubic cystostomy on a normal bladder for a stone which was situated some two feet away."[5] There were three reasons for failure in diagnosis: reliance on highly misleading localization of pain, the assumption that stone must cause abnormalities in the urine, and the fact that X-ray diagnosis failed 15 percent of the time even in expert hands. On the other hand, no stone had been found in 63 of 300 instances when a provisional diagnosis of stone had been made in the Outpatient Department. Cabot thought that pain, the condition of the urine, and good roentgen plates, in combination, permitted correct diagnosis most of the time.

Cabot wrote frequently on the technique of removing stones from the kidney or ureter.[6] The technique was different for the bladder. From the time of Paré or before,[7] surgeons had invented instruments to remove bladder stones by way of the ureter, but in 1878 Henry J. Bigelow had described how to crush a stone in the bladder and to remove the fragments immediately by irrigation.[8] In one of his first cases Bigelow had crushed and removed a stone weighing 116.8 grams with his lithotrite, and he coined the name for the procedure: litholapaxy. Cabot thought litholapaxy was the operation of choice for stones in the bladder, and he described improved lithotrites and the technique of their use.[9]

Cabot's Practice of Urological Surgery in Boston

By 1909 Cabot was practicing a full range of urological surgery, and he frequently published case reports, descriptions of his technique, and his opinions on controversial subjects. A case report, for example, described treatment of a varix of the papilla of the kidney causing persistent hematuria.[10] He cited examples of misdiagnosis of tumors of the bladder, the result of the surgeon's failure to use a cystoscope correctly.[11] Early diagnosis of hydronephrosis was essential, and that required cystoscopy by an expert plus urethral catheterization. An X-ray examination is valuable but only on the negative side, but pyelography can be done with retrograde injection of silver salts into the pelvis of the kidney.[12] Cabot described management and operative technique in cases of diverticulum of the bladder,[13] and he told how to transplant the ureters to the body wall when total extirpation of the bladder is necessary on account of cancer.[14] Cabot treated urethral stricture by partial or complete resection of the bulbar portion,[15] but at least once he treated "floating kidney," a popular surgical problem, simply by correcting the patient's posture.[16] Cabot said it was his duty to express his opinion about prostatectomy and to give the reasons for the faith that was in him.[17] He thought prostatectomy must be done by some form of intraurethral enucleation. He did not mention Hugh Young's transurethral punch operation.[18] Cabot admitted there is a slightly higher mortality when the suprapubic approach is used, but he thought it far better than the perineal approach. Cabot preferred spinal anesthesia to nitrous oxide and oxygen, and it is clear from his description of the technique that he gave the spinal anesthetic himself.[19]

Phenolsulfonphthalein

In 1911, a year within Rowntree and Geraghty's introduction of the phenolsulfonphthalein test of renal function,[20] Cabot used fifteen pages of detailed tables to report the results of 169 tests in 117 patients.[21] He had followed Rowntree and Geraghty's directions without variation, and he found the test to be more accurate than any other. Cabot thought a Duboscq colorimeter too expensive for most physicians, so he substituted a series of ten standard solutions of the dye. Four years later Cabot measured normal daily variation by repeating the test ten times on one healthy subject, and he determined the effect of anesthesia and operation in 422 cases.[22] Percentage excretion of the dye in the first hour after its initial appearance in the urine averaged 59.3 before ether anesthesia and 46.1 afterward. The decrease was greater the more ether was used and the longer was the operation. Rate of excretion returned to preoperative level in forty-eight hours. Spinal, local, or nitrous oxide anesthesia caused smaller decreases in dye excretion, but there was a profound fall in shock.

Infection

Cabot performed many nephrectomies for tuberculosis of the kidney,[23] but at the Massachusetts General Hospital he made an elaborate study of nontuberculous kidney infections. He had E. G. Crabtree as a resident and then a fellow. In 1916 they published a long and important paper describing bacteriological and autopsy findings in sixty cases.[24] The copy in Michigan's medical library is worn to shreds. They found two types of infection, one by colon bacilli and one by pyogenic cocci. Cabot and Crabtree believed that renal infections by colon bacilli are hematogenous, the bacilli entering the bloodstream from the lower urinary tract, particularly from an infected prostate. Colon bacillus infection often became chronic. It usually did not require surgery, but coccus infection did. Medical treatment using vaccines or a drug breaking down

in the urine to formaldehyde is only moderately satisfactory.

Cabot's Characteristics

In Boston Cabot displayed two characteristics as a surgeon that would be important at Michigan. First, his publications showed that his major interest was high-quality patient care and that he was diligent in telling others of his methods and results. His papers did not describe any new ideas. At Michigan those qualities would be translated into assiduous care of the sick and equally assiduous teaching of medical students and training of surgical residents. Original investigation would be neglected. Second, Cabot had firm ideas, and he spoke his mind freely. Frederick Cheever Shattuck, an equally exalted Bostonian Brahmin, warned Victor Vaughan that Cabot was a strong man who made enemies, and Cabot made them in Ann Arbor.

Cabot's Department at Michigan

Immediately upon arriving in Michigan Cabot began to build a department of surgery consisting of unknown young men who began highly productive careers as surgical specialists. Cabot himself specialized in urological surgery, but he did much general surgery too. His contemporaries thought he was a very competent urological surgeon but only an indifferent general surgeon. For one thing, Cabot sweated profusely, and his sweat fell into the operative wound. This was met by the dictum: "Cabot sweat is sterile." Nevertheless, on at least one occasion a patient had a severe postoperative infection as the result of this break in asepsis. After Cabot had been dismissed at Michigan and had accepted a job at the Mayo Clinic, Edgar Kahn, who had been Cabot's intern, got the courage to buy Cabot a headband, for he knew that Will Mayo would not stand for such behavior.

The young men on Cabot's faculty in the 1920s included LeRoy Abbott, Max Peet, Frederick Coller, Carl Badgley, John Alexander, Carl Eberbach, Reed Nesbit, Edgar Kahn, and Henry K. Ransom. In France Cabot had formed a lasting friendship with Sir Anthony Bowlby, chief surgical consultant to the British Expeditionary Force. In peacetime Sir Anthony was head of surgery at St. Bartholomew's

Hospital, and after the war he sent a succession of young men to work for a while in Ann Arbor with Hugh Cabot. These included Basil Hume, Rupert Corbett, Norman Capener, Herbert Seddon, and Arthur Visick. Most of them had important careers when they returned to Great Britain. By Cabot's last year, 1929–30, there were seven persons of professorial rank, fifteen instructors, and fifteen residents. In addition there were always Chalmers Lyons and a dental intern.

The large staff was required to handle the greatly increased patient load that came when the new hospital was occupied in 1925. Surgical services used eight wards of approximately fifty beds each, and surgeons shared seventy-five private rooms with other services. The surgical wing contained ten full-size operating rooms, two smaller ones, and all rooms required for ancillary services. Only four of the operating rooms had small galleries in which a few spectators could watch the operations. The days of operating in a pit before the whole class were over. Cabot thought students should be discouraged from watching operations; they could satisfy their blood lust in other ways.[25]

Teaching Surgery

During Cabot's time the teaching of surgery assumed very nearly the form it retained until well after World War II, when whole-class lectures to juniors and seniors were eliminated and junior students were sent onto the wards. Early in Cabot's time there were three didactic lectures a week for second-year students on principles of surgery. Cabot did not like lectures that relieved the student of the necessity of reading. He believed clinical presentations were better, and by 1923 the second-year lectures were reduced to Coller's one hour a week on the history of medicine. The medical staff continued to help McCotter teach surgical anatomy to sophomores. In the third year students heard five hours of surgical lectures a week throughout the year, and a little later a quiz hour was added. The lectures were supposed to be clinical presentations rather than didactic. Frederick Coller said that Cabot's own lectures were "excellent. His use of double negatives and of simple, earthy figures of speech and allegories served admirably to emphasize certain points and made his discourses vivid and interesting."[26]

There was work in the outpatient clinic in the third year, and students learned about bandaging. Cabot thought the student the best subject so that he or she could learn the exquisite torture of removing adhesive plaster from unshaven skin, the agony of a too tight splint, and the discomfort of an improperly applied or removed plaster cast.

Senior students were assigned in rotation to a two-week laboratory period in dog surgery where they were taught aseptic principles. Because the dog laboratory was expensive with dogs costing $2.50 each, and because it used a lot of junior staff time, the dog laboratory was reduced to one week in 1925. For a while there were joint clinics with the Department of Internal Medicine, and there were staff seminars to which students were invited but not required to attend. Beginning in 1922 each student was required to submit a thesis of about five thousand words, complete with a bibliography of current literature. The thesis could cover work in the library or the record room, and it was "designed to make the student conversant with the methods that are useful in preparing the subject for publication."[27] For once the faculty did not pretend it was teaching the students to think.

Lectures on the specialties continued, but the bulk of surgical teaching in the fourth year was on the wards. The class was divided into fourths or fifths, and one section was assigned to surgery for nine, later eight, weeks. Each student was assigned to take histories, do physical examinations, and observe X-ray examinations and special procedures such as cystoscopy. Cabot believed there must be an instructor definitely assigned to supervise each student, and the student was expected to follow patients for the duration of the section or until the patients were discharged. The student was to be present at operations upon his or her patients. By 1930 the student was to spend time in the Outpatient Department as well.

Cabot thought the best that could be taught a medical student was the principles and practice of aseptic technique, control of bleeding, avoidance of shock, and the proper application of ligatures and sutures. Actual training in surgery must wait until after graduation.

Cabot did not like the Michigan curriculum in which preclinical subjects were taught in solid blocks in the first two years and the clinical subjects in only slightly less circumscribed blocks in the second two years. He admitted that the block system concentrated the student's mind on the subject at hand, but it made the student think the subject was over when the block was finished. Surgery, he thought, should be taught in conjunction with bacteriology and pathology, but the block system made that impossible. Worse, the preclinical subjects were taught within their blocks as abstract sciences without human association, and the same attitude, when extended to the clinical years, resulted in the German consideration of the hospital as the laboratory for the clinical scientist and the patients as experimental animals. Cabot said that "[n]owhere in this curriculum is there any requirement which would particularly qualify the student or interest him in the mental or psychological behavior of mankind. . . . Hardly anywhere do we even attempt to teach methods of approach and understanding of human beings."[28] Cabot wanted actual contact with patients placed earlier in the curriculum, and he wanted students taught by methods that would lead them to appreciate that patients are human. He was up against Huber, Novy, and Warthin with their monolithic blocks of anatomy, bacteriology, and pathology, and even as dean he could do nothing to modify the block system.

Graduate Training

In Nancrede's time a few medical graduates stayed on as assistants in surgery, but in Cabot's time formal graduate training assumed its modern form. For one thing, "interne" lost the final *e* that had always been part of the title and became "intern." About 1926 an intern began to be called a resident. Some interns and residents were women. Cabot said their number was out of proportion to their number in the medical classes and that they did well. A resident in surgery stayed on for five years, rising in authority and responsibility as experience increased. National boards now set standards, and at the end of training a resident looked forward to a board examination. As Cabot's residents developed a surgical specialty, each of them took further training and qualified for a specialty board as well.

Cabot was particularly interested in training urologists. He said a urologist should not be narrow, confining himself to one organ and one sex. He should have sound medical training including at least a year of medical internship before training in general surgery. Finally, he should become the disciple of a well-trained urologist, and he should spend more than a few months becoming a competent cysto-

scopist. The young urologist will encounter social problems: marriage, divorce, diseases, and disabilities, and he must study social questions.

He will need to bring to these questions the best that his mind affords, for they are intricate, involve time honored if shopworn moral standards, and arouse passionate defense of long standing, if imaginary rights.[29]

Cabot paid particular attention to the graduate training of nurses. He always had his own nurse, who was listed in the faculty roster as assistant to the professor of surgery and who might be promoted to an assistant professorship. At the end of his time in Ann Arbor Cabot cooperated with Mary Giles, an associate professor of nursing at Vanderbilt, to write a textbook of surgical nursing.[30] Cabot and Giles said that previously a doctor had given orders and expected them to be carried out by a nurse as an automaton. Now that a physician depended more on science, the nurse was doing many things previously comprehended under the practice of medicine. In that part of the book dealing with urology Cabot and Giles told the nurse about the anatomy, physiology, and pathology of prostatism and about the principles of its medical and surgical treatment. They explained the preoperative nursing care they expected, and they cautioned the nurse to pay attention to the patient's mental state. Cabot thought hospitals had been designed more for the convenience of the surgeon than for the good of the patient, and he thought too little attention had been given to the psychological damage caused by the hospital experience.[31] Cabot and Giles explained the concentration test, the phenolsulfonphthalein test, and the measurement of blood urea nitrogen, all with emphasis on what the nurse had to do to make the test successful. They concluded with a paragraph on the nurse's part in a cystoscopic examination, and they instructed the nurse how to clean a cystoscope.

Teaching and Practice of Anesthesia

Throughout Cabot's time and until July 1938 Laura Davis Dunstone, R.N., was in charge of anesthesia in the University Hospital. She was an instructor in pharmacology, where lectures on anesthesia were given to second-year medical students. She had directed anesthesia in a hospital in France during World War I, and she had taken courses in anesthesia at the Mayo Clinic, at the Cleveland Clinic, and in New York. Because she did not have the doctor of medicine degree, the faculty considered her incompetent to teach anesthesia to medical students, and she so considered herself.[32] Nevertheless from the early 1920s fourth-year students received practical instruction from her, and they gave from ten to fifteen anesthetics under her direction in various clinics. In 1922 a committee to oversee teaching of anesthesia was appointed with Edmunds as chairman and with Coller as a member. Each year thereafter one of the junior resident surgeons was told to teach anesthesia to the fourth-year students, and this person was always assisted by Dunstone.

Nitrous oxide and oxygen mixtures and ether were the general anesthetics most commonly used. Unconsciousness was often induced quickly by nitrous oxide and then followed by ether. The customary mixture for induction was 98 percent nitrous oxide and 2 percent oxygen, of which the partial pressure of oxygen was no higher than fifteen millimeters of mercury, and consequently unconsciousness was the result of profound hypoxia. Sometimes even 100 percent nitrous oxide was used briefly. The practice might horrify a physiologist, but it was a long time before it was abandoned by surgeons. Later in the operation oxygen was raised to 8 percent, at which hemoglobin saturation is less than 70 percent. Cabot thought the gas should not be used for operations lasting more than thirty minutes. Chloroform, the anesthetic of choice in hospitals near the front during the war, was seldom used.

Ethylene could be given with the nitrous oxide machine, and it was introduced at the University Hospital in September 1924.[33] Three and a half years later it had been used for 11,607 operations.[34] Anesthesia was started with 90 percent ethylene and 10 percent oxygen, and then the mixture was changed to 88 percent ethylene and 12 percent oxygen. Three breaths of 50 percent ethylene and 50 percent oxygen were frequently given, and consequently the patient was not hypoxic. If the patient showed signs of vomiting he or she was flooded with two breaths of 100 percent oxygen. Cabot and Dunstone cautioned against trying to stop vomiting by deepening anesthesia. When the operation was finished, anesthesia was terminated by having the patient breathe pure oxygen. Ethylene alone did not produce adequate relaxation for upper abdominal operations, and in those cases it was supplemented with ether.

When safety was debated Harley Haynes, the director of the hospital, said anesthetic deaths were no more frequent in Ann Arbor than elsewhere. The statistics for early 1930 appear to be typical. In January, 917 general anesthetics were given, and there were two deaths under anesthesia, one during an enterostomy and one as an osteoplastic flap was being made. The next month there were no deaths. Cabot thought that ether was safe enough during operations. He wrote:

It is true that it is remarkably difficult to kill a patient with ether during the operation, a statement eminently justified in view of the many unsuccessful attempts made by utterly ignorant would-be anesthetists in the days before anesthesia had developed to its present high state of excellence.[35]

However, Cabot blamed ether for a large number of postoperative deaths, and he cited the fact that in ninety-three laparotomies performed under ether, there had been fourteen deaths from lung complications. By 1930 he had adopted what he called the most outstanding advance in anesthesia, the practice introduced by Yandell Henderson of Yale of adding 5 percent carbon dioxide to the oxygen used at the end of the operations.[36] He thought that the appropriate use of carbon dioxide diminished the occurrence of atelectasis and was therefore essential in any form of anesthesia, inhalation, regional, or spinal.

There was a problem of safety with ethylene: a mixture of 1 percent with air is explosive. Late in 1927 a patient on the obstetric service was killed by an ethylene explosion, and the use of ethylene was temporarily suspended on Peterson's demand. Cabot told Peterson very firmly that the explosion was the result of gross carelessness: an old machine, not grounded, had been used intermittently in obstetric cases so that a lean, explosive mixture was always present.

Research

Research in surgery came in a poor third to patient care and teaching. Cabot's descriptions of clinical experience might be called research papers, but he wrote few in Ann Arbor. He did controvert the opinion that gastric cancer arises from preexisting gastric ulcer, and in that he agreed with Warthin.[37] Most of his publications were reports of speeches to medical audiences hither and yon in which he warmed over previous concerns: catheter cystitis, nontuberculous infections of the kidney, unnecessary surgery, and the like. His young faculty and residents did not receive enthusiastic encouragement to engage in research. Of them Cabot wrote:

At all times, however, several members of the group are engaged in the study of clinical problems which might be termed "clinical research," and a few members are always engaged in experimental research, generally concerning itself with animal experimentation.[38]

Medicine and Money

Cabot faced problems of medicine and money in three capacities. As chairman of a full-time department he had to find salaries adequate for his junior staff. As dean he dealt with the problem of the private patients of his part-time faculty. As a medical statesman he spoke and wrote on the problem of providing medical care for the middle class between the rich who could afford anything and the poor who received charity care.

Each of Cabot's full-time staff received two salaries, one from the university and one from the hospital. Throughout the 1920s young resident surgeons and faculty members resigned to enter private practice, saying their salaries were insufficient. Carl Badgley, the third orthopaedic surgeon to leave, went to the Henry Ford Hospital in Detroit in 1929. Cabot expressed resentment when he told President Little that Badgley wanted a large income but that he would soon be back after having trouble at Henry Ford Hospital.

Everyone said the full-time plan deprived students of contact with physicians in private practice, and Cabot agreed that U.S. medical schools needed physicians of broad experience and wide knowledge who were prepared to give a large portion of their time to academic work. When he was looking for such an individual for his department he wrote:

[I]t may be pointed out that there comes a time, often not too late in the career of many an active physician, when he comes to believe that his greatest service to the world will not be through his ministrations to individual patients, but through his effect upon students, associates and colleagues; that he may turn, so to speak, from the particular to the general and thus use his accumulated store of wisdom more effectively. I do not at all despair of finding a sufficient supply of such people.[39]

Cabot was describing his own reason for coming to Michigan, but he was never able to bring another senior surgeon into his department.

All other departments except Internal Medicine and Roentgenology were on part time. Each member saw private patients in a downtown office and operated in that office, in patients' homes, or in a community hospital. Occasionally a patient who could not afford his or her doctor's bill was admitted to the University Hospital, but hospital charges were paid from public funds. Some members of the part-time faculty wanted to treat their private patients in the University Hospital. In 1923 Udo Wile, the professor of dermatology, complained that in order to supplement his salary of four thousand dollars he had to spend weekends and evenings seeing his private patients in his office on Maynard Street. He proposed to President Burton that the clinical faculty be allotted beds for their private patients in the University Hospital.

Cabot wanted to modify the full-time plan. As early as 26 December 1919 Cabot proposed that patients capable of paying fees be admitted to the University Hospital and that the fees be collected by the hospital.[40] Cabot believed firmly that the clinical faculty should be salaried, and he proposed that the fees be put in a pool, one of whose uses would be to increase salaries of the clinical staff. The salaries would be limited by the university authorities. Money left over would be used for improvement of hospital equipment or even for the benefit of non-income-producing departments. To physicians in private practice and to county, state, and national medical societies this was fee splitting, and it accounts for the hostility Cabot faced throughout his time in Ann Arbor.

In his inaugural address as dean Cabot said no change was contemplated in the full-time plan voted only two years before,[41] but in 1926 he again proposed in a letter to President Little essentially the same modifications he had outlined in 1919. Nothing was done while Cabot was dean, but immediately after he left the full-time plan was abandoned.

Before Cabot became dean, in an annual discourse to the Massachusetts Medical Society, he expressed general dissatisfaction with private charity as a method of caring for the sick poor.[42] A self-respecting though impecunious citizen, he said, has a right to expect that he can obtain at least average medical care without being driven to bankruptcy. People were now [in 1920] asking if they were not entitled to insurance against illness. During his time at Michigan Cabot made a thorough study of medical economics with an emphasis on the problems of health insurance. He wrote:

The task which I have set myself is to give some account of the background from which the problem of adjusting modern medical practice to the requirements of the community has emerged, to present its economic setting, to set forth the various methods which have been employed in other countries in attacking similar situations, and, if possible, to suggest the principles upon which we must rely in working out for ourselves a proper course to steer in what is, in many respects, an uncharted sea.[43]

Cabot doubted that voluntary health insurance would be satisfactory, but he thought it should be encouraged so that its real limitations might become clear. State insurance of bank deposits had been a failure, and it was likely that health insurance provided by the states would be equally unsuccessful. Cabot did not quite get to the point of proposing compulsory national and universal health insurance, but that was the way his thought was moving. In any event, control by physicians did not seem to him "in the public interest" (276).

The End of Cabot at Michigan

Cabot had been in Michigan only a little over a year. Novy had been an important member of the faculty for more than thirty years, and he was respected. Huber and Warthin had been at Michigan almost as long. Peterson had been at Michigan for twenty years, and he was medical director of the hospital. Each might have expected to be made dean.

Cabot was a strong man, and he accomplished much during his deanship. The new hospital was finished and occupied. The Simpson Memorial Institute was built and staffed. The huge East Medical Building was constructed for the Departments of Anatomy, Bacteriology, and Physiology. The Department of Biological Chemistry was established, and the Department of Physiology was transformed. The Department of Surgery was rescued from collapse and converted into one in which every specialty was in competent hands. Wilson and Newburgh had worked productively in the Department of Internal Medicine, and the organizational problem of that department was solved when Cabot and President

Little made Cyrus Sturgis its head. Throughout the nine years of Cabot's deanship the Departments of Bacteriology, Pharmacology, Dermatology, Neurology, Obstetrics and Gynecology, Ophthalmology, Otolaryngology, Pediatrics, and Psychiatry were stable departments, each under the direction of a man whose abilities ranged from adequate to distinguished. Most departments had productive graduate training programs. If stability meant rigidity in the undergraduate curriculum, the quality of training the undergraduate medical students received was indistinguishable from that of Harvard, Columbia, or Pennsylvania. Cabot did try to lighten the curriculum with preceptorships and tutorials. If not quite so many students received research training as at Johns Hopkins, Michigan students and faculty eventually became officers of their elite specialty societies and editors of their leading journals.

Cabot never was *suaviter in modo,* and he had no velvet glove in the dean's office. His correspondence shows him antagonizing one after another every one of the senior members of the faculty. Cabot knew of their hostility. In 1927 he wrote President Little after a meeting with Huber, Novy, and Gesell that two of the three would rather deal with anyone but himself.

Cabot had enemies outside the school as well. His proposal that physicians be paid from fees collected by the hospital outraged orthodox doctors, and the social Darwinists of the American Medical Association said any form of health insurance is contrary to the principles of democratic government. Cabot effected the demise of the Homeopathic Medical College that the legislature had forced on the university in 1875 by amalgamating it with the "regular" Medical School. Students in the homeopathic school had always taken basic science courses with the other medical students. All Cabot allowed to remain were courses in homeopathic pharmacology and therapeutics, and he made those courses elective. When the remnants of the homeopathic faculty complained that no students elected their courses, Cabot's sympathy was restrained, and he saw to it that the teachers of the empty courses were dismissed. Consequently, Cabot had the enmity of a politically influential sect.

The minutes of the regent's meeting on 7 February 1930 contain this entry and nothing more on the subject.

After a comprehensive oral report by the President and discussion by the Board, the following resolution was adopted:—

Resolved, That in the interests of greater harmony in the Medical School, Dr. Cabot is relieved of the duties of Dean of the School and Director of the Department of Surgery, and the President is advised to appoint an executive committee of five to direct the affairs of the School until such time as some other plan is devised.[44]

Newspaper accounts said that Cabot had been domineering, arrogant, and tyrannical and that there had been long-standing friction in the faculty (fig. 16–1).[45] They also cited disagreement over how the full-time plan should be modified. An account handed down by word of mouth said Cabot had deceived the president as to the faculty's opinion on founding a department of anesthesiology.[46] The real reason, as President Ruthven told Abraham Flexner, was not Cabot's policies but his methods.[47] Letters from Murray Cowie and Frank Wilson to the president tell of a faculty terrorized by Cabot. Cowie said he was the only one who dared speak up in committees against Cabot, and Wilson said Cabot could force the resignation of anyone who disagreed with him as he had forced the resignation of Warfield. A former colleague of Peterson wrote to congratulate the school on having rid itself of a "cross between a rat and a rattlesnake."[48] Peterson, who was himself from Boston, concluded his version of the famous quatrain about the home of the bean and the cod as

Where the Lowells don't speak to the Cabots,
For Hughie's been fired, by God![49]

Whatever precipitated the event, President Ruthven had received a letter in January 1930, signed by all but three of the department heads in the Medical School, requesting the immediate resignation of Dr. Hugh Cabot.[50] President Ruthven would not reveal who signed the letter, and he said the three heads who had not signed did not submit a minority report. Ruthven asked Cabot to save face by resigning, but Cabot refused.

Cabot gave up his chairmanship of the Department of Surgery when Will Mayo offered him a job at the Mayo Clinic. When Cabot died in 1945 Sir Herbert Seddon, who had been one of the young men from St. Bartholomew's Hospital in Great Britain, wrote:

One day, just after lunch, he summoned every member of the department of surgery to his room. He told us quietly and unemotionally how the impasse had arisen; he said that he would not tolerate a state of affairs in which senior men

devoted so much of their time to private work that their hospital duties and their teaching were neglected. For the good of the school the offenders must change their ways. They had refused. . . . "I have failed to get what I believe and know to be right for this medical school. I could capitulate, but I will not. This is an awkward position, one in which I hope none of you will ever be placed. But if you are, however uncomfortable it may be, stick to your principles and don't worry too much about the cost." With these words, Dr. Cabot walked out of the room, and out of the university.[51]

Cabot's Men: Max Peet and Neurosurgery

Max Peet was an assistant professor when Cabot arrived at Michigan, practicing general surgery but edging toward neurosurgery. Peet was a Michigan man who had received his early education in Ypsilanti and who had graduated from Michigan's combined course in medicine in 1910. Peet had a two-year internship at the Rhode Island General Hospital and then spent four years at the University of Pennsylvania as Porter Fellow in Research Medicine.[52] Peet got his name on a hematological paper with E. B. Krumbhaar and John Herr Musser Jr. for having ligated the splenic vein for them. He also cannulated the bile duct for H. B. Lewis.[53] Peet worked with O. H. P. Pepper in showing that there was no difference in fragility of erythrocytes in rabbits made anemic with phenylhydrazine.[54] However, Peet's major work was with the surgeon Charles Frazier.

Frazier was a Pennsylvania graduate who became Penn's professor of clinical surgery after postgraduate work in Berlin. He had been dean of the medical school from 1902 to 1909, and he had established a department of social service in the university hospital.[55] Frazier began as a general surgeon, but by 1904 he had extirpated the gasserian ganglion and operated upon at least six tumors of the cerebellum.[56] After 1918 Frazier limited his practice to neurosurgery, but while Peet was working with him he continued to do general surgery and to confront problems arising from general surgery in the laboratory. Perhaps absorption of toxic substances is responsible for the effects of high intestinal stasis.[57] Frazier and Peet reversed four to five inches of colon above the sigmoid flexure in an attempt to produce colonic stasis, but they found that mere stagnation of colonic contents had no ill effect upon their experimental animals. Peet and Frazier made an Eck fistula

DEAN CABOT OUSTED

EXTRA!   EXTRA!

Regents Demand Resignation of Medical Chief By Noon Saturday

Dean Hugh Cabot, head of the University School of Medicine, must resign before noon Saturday or he will be ousted from the position which he has held for the past nine years. The Tribune has it upon the best of authority that the Board of Regents at its meeting this (Friday) afternoon demanded that Dean Cabot submit his resignation before noon Saturday and that if he did not he would be summarily dismissed.

The exact cause of the demand for the Dean's resignation at this particular time could not be authentically learned, but it is believed to be the culmination of internal dissension that has existed for some time, although it is hinted that when all the facts become known there were other reasons that led to the summary action by the Regents.

Dean Cabot, like Dr. Clarence Cook Little, hails from Boston. He was a great admirer of Dr. Little and was out-spoken in his denunciation of the action of the Board of Regents in accepting the resignation of Dr. Little with such alacrity. And now, scarcely more than a year later, the Dean is himself asked to walk the plank.

As an administrator Dean Cabot has not been overly popular. Those opposed have characterized him as domineering, arrogan and tyrannical. As one doctor recently expressed himself to The Tribune, "the state of Michigan in law and theory may own the University hospital but as a matter of fact Dean Cabot 'owns' it to all intents and purposes."

The medical school was the first professional school organized at the University and has always been very popular. The enrollment has grown year by year in spite of the fact that entrance requirements have been raised from time to time, until they are now among the most rigid in the country. For the past several years the number of applicants for admission has been greater than could be accommodated, which has permitted the medical school to select its students, a plan highly endorsed by Dean Cabot. The University college idea of Dr. Little consequently found a warm supporter in Dean Cabot.

Called here in 1919 as professor of surgery, Dr. Cabot became dean of the medical school in 1921. Up to this time the University had conducted two schools of medicine, allopathic and homeopathic. The year following Dean Cabot's elevation the two were combined on the theory that the teachings of both schools would be open to each student to choose.

Enemies of Dr. Cabot say that the dose which he administered to the homeopathic school through this consolidation was far from a homeopathic one, if one may judge from the bias of its graduates, that homeopaths are almost unknown. Resentment of this school of practitioners toward Dean Cabot is pronounced and deep. They accuse him of deliberately killing homeopathy at Michigan.

Hugh Cabot was born August 11, 1872, at Beverly Farms, Massachusetts, and is one of the family of famous Massachusetts Cabots. He was educated at Harvard University, receiving his A.B. in 1894 and his M.D. in 1898. He received his degree of LL.D. from Queens University, Belfast, Ireland, in 1925.

He began his practice in Boston, in 1900, acting as assistant surgeon and surgeon at the Massachusetts General hospital from 1902 to 1919. From 1900 to 1919 he was

DEPOSED UNIVERSITY OF MICHIGAN OFFICIAL

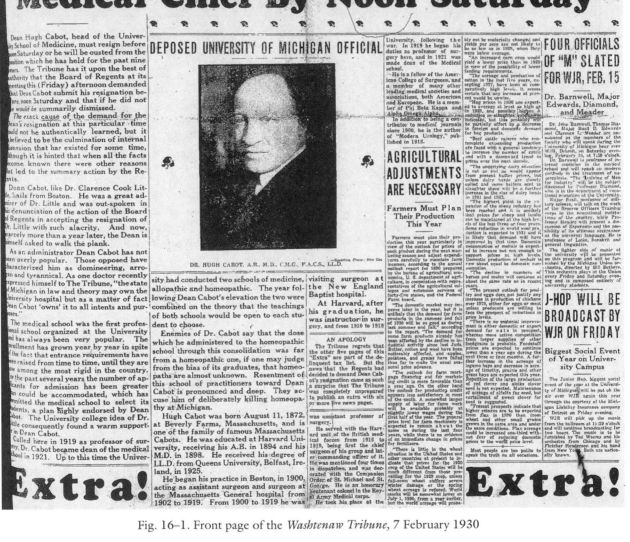

DR. HUGH CABOT, A.B., M.D., C.M.G., F.A.C.S., LL.D.   —Spedding Photo; New Cut

visiting surgeon at the New England Baptist hospital.

At Harvard, after his graduation, he was instructor in surgery, and from 1910 to 1918 was assistant professor of surgery.

He served with the Harvard unit of the British medical forces from 1916 to 1919, being first the chief surgeon of his group and later commanding officer of it. He was mentioned four times in dispatches, and was decorated with the Companion Order of St. Michael and St. George. He is an honorary lieutenant colonel in the Royal Army Medical corps. He took his place at the university, following the war. In 1919 he began his duties as professor of surgery here, and in 1921 was made dean of the Medical school.

He is a fellow of the American College of Surgeons, and a member of many other leading medical societies and associations, both American and European. He is a member of Phi Beta Kappa and Alpha Omega Alpha.

In addition to being a contributor to medical journals since 1900, he is the author of "Modern Urology," published in 1918.

AN APOLOGY

The Tribune regrets that the other five pages of this "Extra" are part of the delinquent tax list. But the news that the Regents had decided to demand Dean Cabot's resignation came as such a surprise that The Tribune was completely occupied and to publish an extra with six or more live news pages.

AGRICULTURAL ADJUSTMENTS ARE NECESSARY

Farmers Must Plan Their Production This Year

Farmers must plan their production this year particularly in view of the outlook for prices of each product during the next marketing season and adjust expenditures carefully to maintain farm incomes, according to the annual outlook report for 1930 prepared by the bureau of agricultural economics, U. S. department of agriculture, in cooperation with representatives of the agricultural colleges and extension services of forty-five states, and the Federal Farm board.

"The domestic market may improve later in the year, but it is unlikely that the demand for farm products in the summer and fall last summer and fall," according to the report. "The demand for some farm products already has been affected by the decline in industrial activity since last June. Butter, cotton and wool have been noticeably affected, and apples, potatoes, and grains have failed thus far to make the usual seasonal price advance.

"The outlook for farm mortgage financing and for marketing credit is more favorable than a year ago. On the other hand the outlook for production credit appears less satisfactory in most of the south. A somewhat larger supply of labor for farm work will be available probably at slightly lower wages during the first half of the year. The general price level for farm machinery is expected to remain about the same as during the last four years, while there is no evidence of an immediate change in prices for fertilizers.

"There is little in the wheat situation in the United States and other countries at present to indicate that prices for the 1930 crop of the United States will be much different from those prevailing for the 1929 crop unless fall-sown wheat suffers severe winter damage or the spring wheat acreage is reduced. World stocks will be somewhat lower on July 1, 1930, from a year earlier, but the world acreage will probably not be materially changed and yields per acre are not likely to be so low as in 1929, when they were below average.

"An increased corn crop would yield a lower price than in 1929 in view of the possibility of lower feeding requirements.

"The acreage and production of cotton in the last five years, excepting 1927, have been at comparatively high levels. It seems certain that any increase at present would be unwise.

"Hog prices in 1930 are expected to average at least as high as in 1929, and possibly higher. A reduction in slaughter supplies is indicated, but this probably will be partially offset by a decrease in foreign and domestic demand for hog products.

"Beef cattle raisers who contemplate expanding production are faced with a general tendency to increase the number of cattle and with a downward trend in prices over the next decade.

"The underlying dairy situation is not as bad as would appear from present butter prices, but unless dairy herds are closely culled and more heifers sent to slaughter there will be a further increase in the size of dairy herds in 1931 and 1932.

"The highest point in the expansion of the sheep industry has been reached and it is unlikely that prices for sheep and lambs can be maintained at the high levels of the last three or four years. Some reduction in world wool production is expected in 1931 and it is likely that demand will have improved by that time. Domestic consumption of mohair is expected to increase but not enough to support prices at high levels. Domestic production of mohair is now about equal to domestic consumption.

"The decline in numbers of horses and mules will continue at about the same rate as in recent years.

"The present outlook for poultry and eggs does not justify any increase in production of chickens unless producers are willing to face the prospect of reductions in price levels.

"There is no material improvement in either domestic or export demand for oats in prospect, whereas more active competition from larger supplies of other feedgrains is probable. Feedstuff prices are expected to continue lower than a year ago during the next three or four months. A further increase in the acreage of legume hays and decrease in acreage of timothy, prairie and other grass hays are expected this year. Repetition of the large production of red clover and alsike clover seed is not expected. Maintenance of acreage of alfalfa for seed, but curtailment of sweet clover for seed is suggested.

"Present prospects indicate that higher returns are to be expected from flax in 1930 than from wheat and other small grains grown in the same area and under the same conditions. Flax acreage could be increased one-third without fear of reducing domestic prices to the world price level.

"Most people are too polite to speak the truth on all occasions.

FOUR OFFICIALS OF "M" SLATED FOR WJR, FEB. 15

Dr. Barnwell, Major Edwards, Diamond, and Meader

Dr. John Barnwell, Thomas Diamond, Major Basil D. Edwards and Clarence L. Meader are announced as the members of the faculty who will speak during the University of Michigan hour over WJR, Detroit, on Saturday evening, February 15, at 7:30 o'clock.

Dr. Barnwell is professor of internal medicine in the medical school and will speak on modern methods in the treatment of tuberculosis. "The Training of Men for Industry" will be the subject discussed by Professor Diamond, who is in the department of vocational education at the University.

Major Basil, professor of military science, will talk on the work of the Reserve Officers Training corps in the educational institutions of the country, while Professor Meader will present a discussion of Esperanto and the possibility of its ultimate acceptance as the universal language. He is professor of Latin, Sanskrit and general linguistics.

The lighter side of music at the university will be presented on this program and will be furnished by the Michigan Union orchestra, directed by Bill Sothern. This orchestra plays at the Union every Friday and Saturday evening and is composed entirely of university students.

J-HOP WILL BE BROADCAST BY WJR ON FRIDAY

Biggest Social Event of Year on University Campus

The Junior Hop, biggest social event of the year at the University of Michigan, will be put on the air over WJR again this year through the courtesy of the Michigan Liability Insurance company of Detroit on Friday evening.

WJR will pick up the music from the ballroom at 11:30 o'clock and will continue broadcasting for two hours. The music is to be furnished by Ted Weems and his orchestra from Chicago and by Fletcher Henderson and his band from New York. Both are nationally known.

Extra!   Extra!

Fig. 16–1. Front page of the *Washtenaw Tribune,* 7 February 1930

so that presumed toxic substances would not be detoxified by the liver, but a dog with both colonic stagnation and an Eck fistula was no different from one with simple reversal of a colonic segment.[58]

Peet had perfected his technique of making an Eck fistula in a cat or dog, and he invented a three-bladed, spring-jawed blood vessel clamp to be used in the operation.[59] Peet found by surveying the literature that formation of an Eck fistula in humans had been attempted twice before, once in France and once in Germany. Peet and Frazier opened the abdomen of a patient with cirrhosis and ascites, but because adhesions were too dense around the hilum of the liver and portal vein they had to abandon their attempt to make an Eck fistula.

Peet's chief experimental work in Philadelphia began as an attempt to produce hydrocephalus in dogs.[60] Frazier and Peet incised the atlantal ligament and lifted the vermes in order to pass a plug of gauze into the lower end of the aqueduct of Sylvius. Their dogs showed no signs of increased cerebrospinal fluid pressure for four to five days, but they became somnolent in two or three weeks, dying with marked dilatation of the ventricles. The plug had been incomplete, for when Frazier and Peet used a mixture of wheat flour and gauze to plug the aqueduct, the dogs died in twenty-four to thirty-six hours.

Frazier and Peet inserted a cannula through the atlanto-occipital ligament and placed the dog on an inclined plane so the cannula was at the lowest point. They connected a graduated glass tube to the cannula in order to measure the rate of formation of cerebrospinal fluid by its rate of progress through the tube. They concluded that secretion of the fluid is an active process, for its rate of flow was unaffected by venous occlusion or by clamping both common carotid arteries. The methylene blue that Frazier and Peet injected into the ventricles slowly appeared in the lymphatic system draining the head, but phenolsulfonphthalein was excreted in the urine in a few minutes. Injection of saline extracts of pancreas, spleen, kidney, liver, ovaries, or testes did not affect the rate of flow, but injection of thyroid extract, fresh or desiccated, inhibited flow for hours independently of any effect upon blood pressure.

This was Peet's last experimental work in neurosurgery. As a general surgeon at Michigan Peet collaborated in an experimental study of the use of a detached omental segment in intestinal surgery as a patch to prevent spread of infection,[61] but he did not use a neurosurgical laboratory. When Peet became a full-time neurosurgeon under Cabot he was faced with the problem of doing preganglionic sympathectomy for the relief of Raynaud's disease of the upper extremities, but the problem of the anatomical arrangement of preganglionic and postganglionic fibers was solved by others.[62] Peet's protégé, Edgar Kahn, "never was particularly interested in doing laboratory research,"[63] and the close association of Elizabeth Crosby with Michigan neurosurgeons did not develop until after 1941.

Peet at Michigan: Specializing in Neurosurgery

When Max Peet returned to Michigan in 1916 he faced the problems of general surgery: finding that a simple enema is better preoperative preparation than a purgative, worrying about how to feed a patient with a high intestinal fistula, and attempting to reduce intrapelvic displacement of the femoral head when the acetabulum is fractured.[64] Ten years later he had confined his practice to neurosurgery.

Nancrede had resected the gasserian ganglion of one patient with trigeminal neuralgia on 6 May 1914,[65] but by that time Frazier at the University of Pennsylvania had done hundreds such operations.[66] Peet did ten the year after he returned to Michigan. He preferred to cut only the sensory root in order to preserve motor function and reduce the possibility of ulceration of the eye. That was possible in only three of his cases in 1917. The alternative treatment was to inject alcohol into the ganglion. Peet said he did not doubt the ability of Carl Camp, Michigan's professor of neurology, to do it, but he thought the procedure unsafe.[67] Thereafter Peet operated upon hundreds of patients with tic douloureux, and occasionally he severed the ninth nerve intracranially to relieve glossopharyngeal neuralgia.[68]

Idiopathic hydrocephalus was then a hopeless condition, but Peet learned to distinguish it from subdural hematoma. If the child with a large head and signs of increased intracranial pressure had a normal face and a dull percussion note over the parietal area, Peet suspected hematoma, and he confirmed the diagnosis by puncturing the fontanel. Peet thought the operation was justified despite the high mortality. Four of nine children operated upon before 1932 survived symptom free.[69]

Max Peet and Edgar Kahn

Edgar Kahn graduated from the University of Michigan Medical School in 1925, and after a brief period in Europe he served a residency under Hugh Cabot. Kahn immediately thereafter became Max Peet's disciple. Except for a short stay with Foster Kennedy in New York in 1928 and five months at Queen Square in the 1930s Kahn was the other half of Michigan's neurosurgical team until Max Peet died in 1949.[70] Kahn as well as Peet sectioned the sensory root of the gasserian ganglion. Peet and then Kahn became experts in performing bilateral chordotomy for relief of intractable pain. The ascending fibers had been identified by Spiller and Frazier at Pennsylvania, and Frazier had performed sixteen chordotomies. In 1926 Peet reported nineteen operations of his own. With the patient under local anesthesia, Peet cut to a depth of three millimeters immediately in front of the dentate ligament and carried the incision directly forward through the exit fibers of the anterior root.[71] Peet and Kahn had done seventy-eight such operations by 1937. At that time Kahn preferred to have the patient under general anesthesia so that the patient did not struggle with pain when Kahn rotated the cord in order to reach its anterior surface. Kahn incised to a depth of five millimeters, and he carried the incision at least two millimeters anteriorly beyond the emergence of the anterior root. He had only one operative death in twelve patients in poor condition.[72]

Peet and Kahn had to deal with tumors, trauma, and infection. Kahn developed a method of dealing with brain abscesses, using increased intracranial pressure to force deep-seated abscesses to the surface. He palpated the abscess with a blunt probe, and he decompressed what he thought was the most superficial part of the brain. Kahn drained the abscess several days later when it appeared at the surface.[73] Later, Kahn used direct transcortical pressure after he uncapped the presenting wall of the abscess and packed the cavity. He instilled six milliliters of colloidal thorium dioxide (Thorotrast), which, when it had been phagocytized by the cellular elements of the capsule, showed the position of the abscess on X-ray examination. Once Kahn fortuitously obtained a film just as the abscess popped through the surface of the brain.[74]

Kahn had failures with abscesses, and Peet and Kahn had other failures as well. When Kahn described a successful excision of an encapsulated tumor of the pineal gland, he said: "In a large series of radical operations on pineal neoplasm and other tumors of the posterior part of the third ventricle, the operative mortality in our cases has been exceedingly high."[75]

The only approach to a systematic account of what happened in the operating room day after day is in Kahn's diary covering the period from 15 February to 7 December 1930.[76] Here are records of two successes.

March 26

I operated on a baby with a lumbar spina bifida. . . . There was no paralysis and the baby was an only child.

When I had dissected down I found a sac which I had to free from the defect and quite easily did. On opening the sac I found a fat pad extending through and tacked onto the lower end of the cord. There was no line of cleavage and I was considerably worried as to causing a subsequent paralysis. The whole thing took two hours and the child stood it very well. It was great to see him kick his legs afterwards.[77]

April 4

Peet operated a boy Robert J. for a suprasellar . . . tumor. He removed the entire tumor as far as we could tell, with almost no loss of blood. He dissected the tumor from the front and back of the chiasm. . . . It was the most beautiful and technically perfect operation I have ever seen. The boy is perfect tonight and one would never know he had been touched.[78]

And a failure.

July 26

R. arrived yesterday. He seemed slightly better so that I decided to put him off until Monday. Started for the farm . . . about 3:30 P.M. Got as far as the Bridge and decided to come back and look at R. He couldn't be aroused. Decided to do him that evening. Turned a left-sided flap and found a large broken down glioma with a hemorrhage into it. Removed as much as I could. Transfused him. The procedure took over three hours and it was terribly hot. . . . [(R.) died several days after the operation.][79]

Surgical Treatment of Hypertension

Because medical treatment of malignant hypertension gave disappointing results, it occurred to Rowntree and Adson at the Mayo Clinic in 1924 "that relative freedom from vascular spasm might be attained through the removal of the vasoconstrictor influence of the sympathetic nerves to the vessels of the leg."[80] The area of diminished resistance could serve as a safety valve for the cerebral and retinal vessels. One of their patients, a young man whose systolic blood pressure ranged from 170 to 200 millimeters of mercury and whose diastolic pressure was 90 to 130, was glad to submit to surgical treatment. In April 1924 Adson removed the second, third, and fourth lumbar segments of both sympathetic chains through a median abdominal incision. There was some postoperative improvement, but six months later the pressure was 220/120 millimeters of mercury.

Peet had done a sympathectomy in 1928 for relief of pain in tabes dorsalis, and in November 1931 he performed his first sympathectomy for hypertension. By 1935 he could report the results of more than one hundred operations.[81] Operative mortality had been 4 percent, and 49 percent of the patients showed "slight" to "marked" improvement. Fifteen percent were tentatively cured.

Peet had amplified the reasons of Rowntree and Adson, and he had extended the operation. In those days it was believed that a patient in shock bleeds to death into the dilated vessels of his or her own splanchnic area. Peet thought lumbar sympathectomy would not only relieve peripheral resistance but would reduce arterial blood pressure by sequestration of blood in the veins. The controversy between Cannon at Harvard and Stewart and Rogoff at Western Reserve over continuous secretion of epinephrine by the adrenal medulla was still raging, and Peet thought that section of nerves to the adrenal glands would eliminate neurogenic secretion, if any, of epinephrine. Others had done partial adrenalectomies for hypertension, attacking the cortex as well as the medulla, but Peet thought that procedure not only futile but dangerous. Long before, A. N. Richards had shown that stimulation of the splanchnic nerves causes contraction of afferent arterioles of the kidney,[82] and more recently Goldblatt had produced persistent hypertension in dogs by renal ischemia.[83] Peet said: "It follows that there must be some cases in which the hypertension is caused by renal artery vasoconstriction which will respond with a rapid improvement in kidney function [to splanchnic section]."[84]

Peet did supradiaphragmatic sympathectomy by means of a subperiosteal resection of a small portion of the eleventh rib near its vertebral articulation. He retracted the pleura and excised seven to eight centimeters of the greater splanchnic nerve, the tenth,

eleventh, and twelfth dorsal ganglia with the lesser and least splanchnic nerves, if present. It took Peet about an hour to do the operation bilaterally, and it was not the total sympathectomy performed later by Reginald Smithwick in Boston.[85]

The preoperative systolic blood pressure in Peet's first patient was 270 millimeters of mercury, and it fell to 140. Peet said this demonstrated that the theory that hypertension is "essential" to provide blood flow to the tissues is wrong; such a plunge in blood pressure would have been fatal if the theory were correct.

Peet's operation for hypertension was done more than eighteen hundred times at Michigan, and through 1947 there were reports of ever increasing numbers of patients treated.[86] For example, of 437 patients followed five to eleven years, 251 were living eleven years after the operation. In 207 of those still living their hypertension had progressed to serious organic disease before operation. Nineteen of 112 patients with the worst form of hypertension, classified as malignant, had lived five to eleven years, and 51 of them had maintained normal blood pressure. Not every operation resulted in a cure. F. Bruce Fralick, the ophthalmologist, found that in eighteen patients where there had been a postoperative fall in blood pressure, there was improvement in the optic fundus in only three.[87] Richard Freyberg measured urea clearance and urine concentrating ability in forty-eight patients.[88] In those whose blood pressure had been substantially lowered, renal function had improved, but in those whose blood pressure had not been changed by the operation, renal function had not improved or had become worse.

Peet gave an example of success.

A 23-year-old woman had presented with occipital headache, retinal changes and arterial blood pressure of 230/145. On April 20, 1938, Peet performed a bilateral supradiaphragmatic splanchnicectomy. Five years after the operation, the woman carried a pregnancy to full-term delivery of a normal infant, and she had no albuminuria while pregnant. Seven years after the operation, her arterial blood pressure was 118/86.[89]

Cabot's Men: John Alexander and Thoracic Surgery

John Alexander won prizes in anatomy, obstetrics, and internal medicine while he was a medical student at the University of Pennsylvania.[90] Soon after graduating in 1916 he served with the U.S. unit attached to the French army, but in 1917 he transferred to the U.S. Medical Corps. At the end of the war Alexander worked briefly in Lyon, learning the technique of paravertebral thoracoplasty as treatment for pulmonary tuberculosis from Leon Bérard. Those thoracoplasties had been successfully developed in Germany, not in France, but in 1919 a U.S. medical officer would not go to Munich to study under Ferdinand Sauerbruch, the most notorious bully in the history of surgery but a superb thoracic surgeon. By 1923 Lyonnais surgeons, Bérard and René Leriche among them, had performed only twenty-seven such operations with eight operative deaths.[91] Bérard had two survivors, perfectly cured after nine and ten years. He described his technique in detail and published a radiograph showing "affaissement énorme de l'hémithorax gauche."[92]

John Alexander returned to the University of Pennsylvania to work under Charles Frazier, but almost immediately Hugh Cabot brought him to Ann Arbor. Many years before, Conrad Georg had performed some experimental pneumonectomies on dogs with few survivors, but in the discussion of Georg's paper Cyrenus Darling had said: "Fortunately we are not called upon very often to operate upon the lung."[93] Alexander started thoracic surgery at Michigan, and he practiced it exclusively after 1928. He began with collapse therapy for tuberculosis, and he invented a knife for stripping the periosteum from a rib as a preliminary to costectomy.[94] His method saved time while avoiding trauma to intercostal nerves and blood vessels. His work was soon interrupted by his own tuberculosis: pleural effusions, renal infection, and Pott's disease. While he was in a body cast at Saranac, Alexander wrote *The Surgery of Pulmonary Tuberculosis*.[95]

Typewriting may be as easily performed in the recumbent position as when sitting. A bedside table that is adjustable as to height and tilt . . . is put across the patient so that its lower edge rests lightly on a small pillow or pad placed on the patient's upper abdomen or on a plaster body-cast as pictured. [The illustration shows the patient, doubtless Alexander himself, typing.] A portable typewriter (the new Corona or the Underwood lend themselves to this use, but not the Remmington, Hammond or old Corona) is then put on the table and caught in a wire rack that is incorporated in the table's edge. With his elbows resting comfortably on the bed, the patient may reach the keyboard with his fingers. Without any especial adjustment of the machine, writing proceeds with the usual speed. Although the keys and writing point are perfectly visible, it is an obvious advantage for the patient to learn the touch system. . . . In fact, teaching oneself the touch system is one of the pleasantest forms of occupational therapy.[96]

An ingenious social worker invented a book holder within reach of Alexander's hand, and the sanatorium librarian brought books and journals. Alexander could type out the manuscript of a book of 356 pages containing five hundred references. The Philadelphia Academy of Surgery awarded him the Samuel D. Gross Prize for his book.

The Collapse Therapy for Pulmonary Tuberculosis

Alexander's book is a review of the literature, not a description of his own experience. It was written to encourage U.S. surgeons to pay attention to European progress in surgical treatment of advanced pulmonary tuberculosis. Alexander collected the results of 1,159 paravertebral thoracoplasties reported between 1918 and 1923, and the literature was almost completely Continental. He estimated there were thirty thousand patients in the United States who would benefit from surgical treatment but would otherwise die of the disease. Only 300 thoracoplasties had been reported by U.S. surgeons; Sauerbruch in Germany had himself done 373. Coller in Ann Arbor had done only 1. Cabot in a brief preface echoed Alexander: surgical attack on tuberculosis had lacked force in the United States.[97]

The object of collapse therapy is to rest the diseased lung. Alexander wrote:

[T]uberculosis . . . heals by fibrous encapsulation. [After resistance of the host,] the next most important factor—the most important one capable of control—is functional rest of the diseased part. . . . It is chiefly because of the interminable persistence of the respiratory movements that pulmonary tuberculosis takes such a fearful toll of death.[98] . . . [When the lung is quiet less toxin-laden lymph flows from it, and danger of spread of disease to other parts of the lung is reduced.] The most striking anatomical result of pulmonary compression is a profuse proliferation of fibrous tissue which encapsulates the tuberculous lesions and closes cavities and renders the disease inactive.[99]

The surgical alternative to artificial pneumothorax is some form of rib resection to collapse the hemithorax and to stabilize the thoracic wall in its new position. Operative mortality and postoperative complications had been high, and in 1925 a U.S. physician had written to Alexander: "My surgical and medical friends here both agree that they have never seen the slightest benefit from the operation of paravertebral thoracoplasty and they do not recommend it in any case."[100] Alexander demonstrated, on the contrary, that the operation as developed by Wilms of Heidelberg and by Sauerbruch had laid the foundation of what Alexander called the revolution in the management of phthisis.[101] By 1937 Alexander himself could publish an enormous book on collapse therapy in which he described his mature operation and nine others, some less radical.[102]

In performing his "modern posterolateral thoracoplasty" Alexander always removed all of the first rib and part of its cartilage, for he demonstrated that adequate collapse could not be obtained if the first rib were allowed to hold up the chest wall. The number of other ribs resected depended upon the size and vertical extent of the lesion. A cavity in the lower lung required resection of all but the twelfth rib. Alexander found that some patients died of cardiovascular collapse or from acute extension of tuberculosis if he resected so much of the ribs that there was excessive paradoxical movement of the operated side, that is, expansion on expiration and contraction on inspiration. He never carried the costal resection sufficiently far as to uncover the anterior surface of the heart, but he did resect ribs sufficiently far as to uncover the left cardiac border when he operated on the left side. Length of resection had to be judged at each operation, but in one patient he removed a total of 197 centimeters of nine ribs. The operation was safer and easier on the patient if it were done in stages, and sometimes Alexander did four or more. A single stage required less than half an hour, but Sauerbruch, in what seemed an act of prestidigitation, had taken from ten to twenty minutes from incision to closure. Sometimes a patient committed suicide on the day before a fifth-stage operation was scheduled.

Operative deaths during thoracoplasty were 52 percent when Alexander returned to Ann Arbor in 1926. Six to eight years later the mortality had fallen to 11 percent, for only 13 of the 119 patients he and Cameron Haight had operated upon between the latter part of 1932 and the end of 1934 had died as the result of their operation or of the disease. Ninety-nine of the patients had closed tuberculous cavities and persistently negative sputum.

Alexander was master of a wide range of other procedures designed to prevent movement of the diseased lung, and he believed that the smallest operation that offered reasonable chance of being effective should be used first. Phrenic paralysis, either temporary or permanent, was one such operation. For temporary paralysis, Alexander exposed the phrenic nerve in the neck, crushed it in a single place, and cut any minor accessory phrenic nerves. Alexander said that in other hands "[t]he vagus, long thoracic, and sympathetic nerves by mistake have been cut, the brachial plexus has been wounded, the thoracic duct torn, the dome of the pleura opened, and the large arteries and veins wounded."[103] For permanent paralysis the exposed nerve was cut and wound on a slowly rotating hemostat. Alexander once evulsed forty-nine centimeters of nerve. In a review of 654 cases Alexander found that in 38 percent of the patients phrenic nerve paralysis had been adequate to close the cavity, and in another 26 percent it had given palliative or partial relief. Unsuccessful temporary paralysis could be renewed or could be followed by a more radical procedure. Temporary paralysis was far better than permanent paralysis. Alexander wrote:

I have seen many tragic instances in which a permanent phrenic paralysis has prevented the performance of a life-saving operation for lesions in the opposite lung which, at the time that the phrenic operation had been performed months or years before, had a relatively innocent appearance.[104]

Another procedure was temporary or permanent multiple intercostal paralysis, and Alexander published superimposed radiographs, one taken at maximal inspiration and the other at maximal expiration, to show that the ribs on the operated side did not move.[105] Only 13 percent of the patients in the Michigan State Sanatorium at Howell had required thoracoplasty if the initial management had been conservative. The choice of operation ultimately depended upon clinical judgment, and Alexander presented eighty-four types of pulmonary or pleural tuberculous lesions with appropriate therapy for each.

Training Thoracic Surgeons

Alexander said in 1928 that there were a shocking number of deaths because "[m]any major thoracic operations are being performed today by surgeons

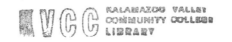

whose only preparation for the work has been the reading of articles and books, and a visit of several days, weeks or months in a thoracic surgery clinic."[106] He began to train thoracic surgeons, and after 1931 Cameron Haight could take over management of the program during Alexander's prolonged winter absences in Arizona.

Alexander could choose graduates of the best medical schools, because there were more applicants than openings. He preferred men who had some special experience in internal medicine, sanatorium practice, anatomy, pathology, physiology, or laboratory methods. They were expected to have had an internship and two years residency in general surgery. A new man immediately became a member of Alexander's team, performing the work of a resident.[107] He participated in frequent conferences with John Barnwell in internal medicine, with roentgenologists and pathologists, and with the staff of the Howell sanatorium. He served nine or ten hours a day, sharing in increasing degree teaching, diagnosis, patient management, and operative work on both ward and private patients. Somehow in the first year he found time to do a complete dissection of the thorax and neighboring parts of the neck and abdomen. The resident began as an assistant in operations, but he soon did simpler operations under direct supervision. In his second year he was able to perform independently virtually every type of major thoracic operation then current. By the end of the year he had done three hundred to five hundred operations and bronchoscopies, and he had acted as first assistant in twice that number.

Alexander said his residents should have intimate contact with as large a number of patients as possible "and that investigative work and study of the basic sciences, important though they are, should be given secondary consideration."[108] The temptation was great to keep a man to share the responsibility of running the clinic, but Alexander sent him away after two years to meet the need for qualified thoracic surgeons outside the University Hospital. Thus, beginning in 1928, Alexander established a program of high-quality patient care and prolific resident training that was to characterize Michigan clinicians for the next thirty years.

Lobectomy

John Alexander had a taste for the history of thoracic surgery. He collected and occasionally published accounts of unsuccessful attempts at lobectomy performed for the treatment of abscess or bronchiectasis.[109] When Alexander was himself making history (fig. 16–2) he wrote: "Until 4 years ago [1931] no patient had ever survived the removal of an entire lung, and until 6 years ago [1929] the danger of the complete removal of a pulmonary lobe was so great as to be prohibitive."[110] Reasons for failure were shock, primary and secondary hemorrhage, pneumonia, overwhelming infection of the pleura and mediastinum, mediastinal emphysema, bacteremia, tension pneumothorax, and mediastinal flutter.

Before Alexander could confidently perform a lobectomy, he treated abscess of the lung by strict bed rest and postural drainage. If an area of the lung were suppurating but not yet abscessed, Alexander established postural drainage, using a bronchoscope to insufflate a solution of 10 percent cocaine and 1:1,000 epinephrine (Adrenalin) to shrink the mucosa. Otherwise he used temporary phrenic paralysis and pneumothorax. If the abscess did not resolve in two months he used more radical treatment such as drainage through the thoracic wall. He said: "The more patients I drain in this stage, the more I am impressed with the futility of delaying drainage for weeks and months in the hope that the cavities will close themselves."[111] Alexander's most radical treatment was patterned after "the staged cautery lobectomy that Evarts Graham has so ably developed."[112] Evarts Graham plunged a large soldering iron heated to red heat into the affected lung. Smoke came out of the patient's nose and mouth like Faffner's while guarding the Rheingold. "Later, as the slough separates and as the open bronchioles begin to discharge pus to the outside, the cough and sputum diminish, the fever disappears, the appetite returns and the patient feels well."[113]

In the early 1930s Alexander developed a two-stage lobectomy as an alternative treatment. By 1935 four clinics had only 10.2 percent mortality in 59 cases, but Alexander said in 1933: "The exceptional difficulty of the technical problems connected with total lobectomy is evidenced by a 53.4 per cent mortality in 127 cases that I have collected from the clinics that have not been importantly connected with the relatively recent advances in technique."[114] Those advanced were largely Alexander's. In the first stage he resected portions of the sixth, seventh, and eighth ribs and separated the diseased lobe from any pleural adhesions. He gently stroked the parietal and visceral

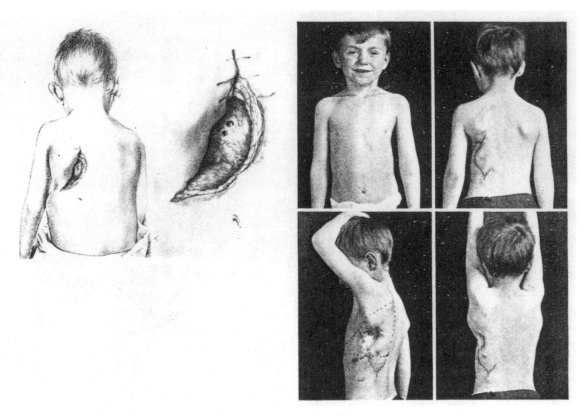

Fig. 16–2. Total basal lobectomy in a five-year-old boy. *Left,* after three weeks; *right,* after solid closure of the wound six months following the lobectomy. (From J. Alexander, "Total Pulmonary Lobectomy: A Simple and Effective Two Stage Technique," *Surg. Gynecol. Obstet.* 56 [1933]: 661.)

pleurae in order to create a protective inflammatory barrier against future infection. The normal lobe became adherent and did not collapse after removal of the diseased one. Nine to twelve days later Alexander freed the diseased lobe from its new adhesions and ligated the hilum as tightly as he could with braided silk.[115] An additional rubber tube ligature around the hilum maintained occlusion of the blood vessels and bronchus as the tissue shrank. If the artery had been successfully occluded, the lobe underwent dry gangrene and became small and shriveled. If the artery had not been entirely occluded, the lobe presented wet gangrene. The wound in the chest wall might be left open or might be temporarily closed. A dry gangrenous lobe fell away spontaneously after a while, or it could be cut off not less than a week to ten days after the second operation. Alexander's most recent patients had been five to thirty-seven years of age, and ten of twelve survived up to the time he reported in 1933.

Pneumonectomy

Given the worldwide progress in the techniques of thoracic surgery occurring in the 1920s, it was inevitable that someone would soon do a complete pneumonectomy and have the patient survive indefinitely. Rudolf Nissen, then a young man in Sauerbruch's Berlin clinic, was the first to do this in 1931.[116] Nissen removed a girl's lung, leaving only a small bronchial fistula. Cameron Haight at Michigan is generally credited with having performed the second successful pneumonectomy and the first in the United States.[117] Haight finished his series of operations on his patient on 14 November 1932, but Eske Windsberg, a surgeon in Providence, Rhode Island, was careful to point out that he himself had completed extirpation of a girl's lung six days earlier, 8 November 1932.[118] When Haight published a very full description of his operation in 1934 he added in press Windsberg's personal communication of his accomplishment. When Windsberg published his case for the second time the next year, he quoted Haight to establish his own priority.[119]

Cameron Haight was not racing for the record book when he assumed charge early in 1932 of a girl who, on 15 January 1932, had aspirated into her left bronchus a piece of the rubber gag used to hold her mouth open during extraction of teeth. When, a month later, A. C. Furstenberg removed the fragment by means of a bronchoscope "an enormous quantity of very foul, thick, yellow pus was liberated."[120] On 29 March Haight temporarily interrupted her left phrenic nerve. Then as a preliminary to thoracoplasty, on 20 July he made a parasternal division of the first to fourth costal cartilage. In a series of four operations separated by about seventeen days Haight removed "moderate lengths" of the first to eleventh ribs. The results of the thoracoplasty, completed on 29 September, were not satisfactory, so Haight did the first stage of a pneumonectomy on 8 November. On 14 November he freed both of the left lobes and developed a satisfactory pedicle for each, which he tied with braided silk and an elastic rubber tube ligature. He did not excise the lobes, but on the sixteenth day he found the upper lobe lying loose in the wound. The lower lobe sloughed off the following day. An abscess in the girl's right lung, found in February 1933, cleared under nonsurgical therapy, and she was discharged on 23 December 1933. She lived to bear a child many years later.

The operation established Haight's reputation as a thoracic surgeon, and it was strengthened when he successfully corrected an instance of congenital atresia of the esophagus with tracheoesophageal fistula in 1941.[121] Haight and Alexander extended their experience with lobectomy and pneumonectomy.[122] Some of Alexander's operations before 1941 were for extrapulmonary neoplasms, and he told other surgeons that immediate removal of a neoplasm, whether it was initially thought to be benign or malignant, would prevent many tragic deaths.[123] Alexander himself died in 1954, and the success of Michigan surgeons trained by him in operating on the heart and aorta came well after the period described in this book.[124]

Cabot's Men: Reed Nesbit and Transurethral Prostatectomy

Reed Nesbit (fig. 16–3), a graduate of Stanford University and of Stanford Medical School, came to

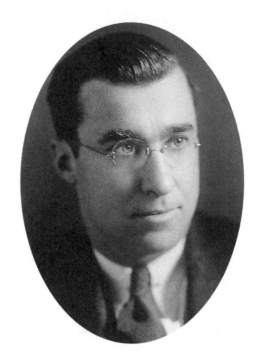

Fig. 16–3. Reed Nesbit

Michigan in 1925 as an assistant resident in surgery to become a urological surgeon under Hugh Cabot's tutelage. He had finished an internship in the Fresno County Hospital, and at first he worked in general surgery at Michigan. Nesbit eventually became Hugh Cabot's disciple, and when Cabot left in 1930 Nesbit was put in charge of the urological service. The service was a busy one, and in 1931 Nesbit reviewed 450 operations for urinary obstruction. Most of them had been suprapubic prostatectomies, and Nesbit found that 17 percent of the patients had epididymitis. After Cabot and Nesbit began to add vasectomy to prostatectomy the incidence of epididymitis dropped to less than 1 percent.[125]

On 10 June 1931 Nesbit attended a symposium in Philadelphia on prostatism arranged by the Section on Urology of the American Medical Association. His imagination was fired, to use his own words, by a paper by Theodore Davis of South Carolina describing the results of 246 operations performed by the transurethral route using a resectoscope that permitted "operation in the minutest detail under direct vision."[126] The patients' hospital stay was a few days rather than several weeks, and there had been no deaths attributable to the operation.

When Nesbit described the history of instrumentation for transurethral prostatectomy,[127] he said that ingenious surgeons from the time of Paré had invented punches and knives to relieve urinary obstruction by transurethral operations, but the revolution announced by Davis was the result of three fundamental discoveries. The first was the invention of an incandescent lamp that could be built into the distal end of the resectoscope. With a good Foroblique optical system designed and built by Reinhold Wappler or his son Frederick there was perfect vision in the surgical field. The second was the Bovie blade using an undamped high frequency current for cutting and a highly damped current for hemostatic coagulation. Surgeons had previously built knives or cautery blades into their resectoscopes, but because they gave unsatisfactory results, the resectoscopes so equipped had fallen into disfavor. The high frequency knife had been invented by William T. Bovie, a 1908 Michigan graduate, but it had first been used by Harvey Cushing. "The cutting is not done by the electrode, which has no sharpened edge, but by the current which forms ahead of the electrode an electrical arc which by volatalizing [*sic*] the tissues separates them as though they were cut."[128] When the current was damped, bleeding was stopped by coagulation. Tissue to be cut was caught in the window and then excised by sliding the Bovie blade through it, the blade being moved by the operator either forward or backward within the sheath. The prostate gland was cut bit by bit, and pieces were washed out with a current of fluid.

Nesbit later discovered that Davis had made extravagant claims, but he set about obtaining a resectoscope and learning to use it. The Liebel-Flarsheim Company of Cincinnati manufactured the apparatus generating the high frequency current, and in October 1931 Mr. G. H. Liebel flew from Cincinnati to Ann Arbor, bringing with him a resectoscope and the electrical apparatus.[129] Nesbit and Liebel spent the night practicing cutting beefsteaks and calves' hearts, and the next morning Nesbit did his first closed transurethral prostatectomy. The patient had complications later, but Nesbit successfully removed his entire prostate gland.

Nesbit himself made a fourth improvement of the resectoscope. He used the McCarthy version in which the fenestra for grasping the tissue was at the end of the sheath. The traveling loop of the knife was moved back and forth by means of a rack and pinion mounted on the sheath. Two hands were needed to control the instrument, one to hold it and the other to move the blade. Another historian of prostatectomy wrote: "Reed M. Nesbit, thinking that no more

than one hand should be used to operate it, placed an internal spring in the handle that would pull the loop into the sheath. The other hand was inserted into the rectum to stabilize the prostate."[130] Nesbit's instrument had a pistol grip on the body that could be grasped with four fingers and a loop on the sliding part that holds the knife. The position of the cutting blade could then be controlled by opening or closing the fist.[131] Contrary to the statement quoted, diagrams prepared by a medical artist under Nesbit's supervision show that the operator's finger, not the hand, was inserted into the patient's rectum. That gave Nesbit a three-dimensional perception of the operative field.

In describing his training of residents Nesbit said:

The operator should spend many hours of practice in cutting pieces of meat under water, for he cannot become a competent resectionist until his reflexes are so well coordinated with the cutting and coagulating functions of the instrument that the mechanical aspects of its use become entirely automatic.[132]

Nesbit thought a resident could learn by working on a relatively small number of patients after mastering use of the resectoscope. The resident, who was present at all operations, began with a few that were completed by the preceptor. The resident was permitted to operate upon progressively larger glands and after doing twenty or thirty resections could remove forty to fifty grams of tissue in sixty minutes. After fifty resections the resident could handle glands of sixty to seventy grams. Because the average gland in a patient with benign hypertrophy weighed less than forty grams, the resident's skill was by then more than sufficiently developed.

Nesbit's Results

Nesbit reviewed his results as he went along. In 1934 he had completed four hundred resections with twenty-five deaths, nineteen of which he thought could have been avoided.[133] This 6.25 percent mortality compared well with the 18 percent mortality that had followed the last four hundred suprapubic prostatectomies performed at the University Hospital. By the end of 1941 Nesbit had perfected his technique and trained fourteen residents. Together they had done more than one thousand transurethral prostatectomies, for Nesbit had used that method to treat 83 percent of his patients with nonmalignant urinary obstruction. Because in transurethral prostatectomy the gland is removed a little at a time, Nesbit used the perineal route for another 10 percent when he thought the gland was too large to be excised within sixty minutes. He used the suprapubic approach for only 7 percent. Nesbit described his technique in detail in *Transurethral Prostatectomy*, published in 1943. His description is clarified by ninety-four drawings by William P. Didusch.

Nesbit had heard Newburgh's message, and he had paid particular attention to the patient's water balance, taking into account water from food and water lost by evaporation. Nesbit found that when he irrigated the site of resection with normal saline solution during resection the patient absorbed so much fluid from the site of operation that his blood was often seriously diluted. He substituted an isotonic solution of glycine, which was not so readily absorbed as the saline. He gave a patient three thousand milliliters of water a day postoperatively.

Nesbit preferred low spinal anesthesia for his elderly and often debilitated patients, and on the patient's account he strictly limited his operation to sixty minutes. He had the anesthetist call out at forty minutes so that he could begin to clean up the operative site, and if he could not finish in another twenty minutes he had the patient brought back for a second operation. At the end of an operation all fluid used for irrigation was diluted to a known volume, mixed, and sampled for measurement of hemoglobin by the acid hematin method.[134] The calculated blood loss was then doubled to take into account postoperative losses. Twenty-two percent of the patients lost 250 milliliters or more, and if the calculated loss was greater than 500 milliliters the patient was transfused. A patient could go home on the sixth to the eighth day if he lived near Ann Arbor; he waited another six days if he lived at a distance.

Nesbit himself had operated upon 645 patients of the last 1,000 operated upon by transurethral prostatectomy in the University Hospital by 1 January 1942, and there had been only eight deaths. His residents had performed the other 365 operations, and there had been thirteen deaths. Nesbit said: "The urologic resident who has just finished his training at the University Hospital [in 1940] performed over a hundred transurethral prostatectomies during his last year without a postoperative death."[135]

Nesbit was not the only one whose imagination

had been fired by Theodore Davis's report. Nesbit said: "Probably every urologist in the North America continent joined the mad rush to obtain the necessary and not inexpensive armamentaria that promised the prostatic millenium."[136] Controversy was the inevitable result. Some tried the operation a few times with disastrous results and thereafter denounced it. After Nesbit had told his story in Boston one surgeon said: "[T]he indications for transurethral removal of the prostate are in direct proportion to the ability of the operator to remove it completely. . . . Dr. Nesbit's contributions to this operation have been considerable."[137] Frederic Foley, whose name has floated to posterity on a balloon, summed it up by saying that the difference in results reflected difference in the resectionist's skill. "Resection is an extremely valuable procedure in some hands where it may be employed in almost all cases and a worthless procedure in other hands where it should be employed rarely if at all."[138] Nesbit and his students continued to use it at Michigan.

The Neurogenic Bladder

Reed Nesbit and other urologists used the word *neurogenic* in the sense of being controlled by nerves rather than in the sense of arising from nerves.[139]

Jack Lapides dedicated his *Fundamentals of Urology* to Reed Nesbit as an "ardent investigator" as well as a "superb surgeon."[140] Lapides's book is the great-grandchild of Nesbit's own little book of the same title, 117 pages lithographed for the benefit of third-year medical students.[141] Nesbit's book covers congenital anomalies, infections and obstructions, neoplasms, and traumatic lesions, but the first edition has not a word on the physiology or pathophysiology of the kidney. Nesbit soon learned of the gap in the students' knowledge, for subsequent editions contained a full account of what students should have learned from Robert Gesell.

Nesbit's book and his lectures to medical students reviewed the extensive experience he simultaneously described in his numerous publications. Beginning as a collaborator with Hugh Cabot, Nesbit wrote on hematogenous coccal infections of the kidney, and he contributed six more cases of bronchial fistula combined with perinephric abscess. He wrote on ketogenic diets for bacilluria, on hypertension associated with unilateral kidney disease, on contrast media, and on many pediatric problems. Nesbit described his corrective operation for hypospadias, his conservative operation for carcinoma of the penis, and his solution of the problem presented by a university student whose penis when erect deviated to the left in the shape of a banana. However, his most substantial publications were on the neurogenic bladder, a series continuing almost until Nesbit retired in 1968. At the end of the 1930s he and members of his staff wrote books and lectures on the neurogenic bladder and its care.[142]

By the time Nesbit became a urologist D. K. Rose of the Barnes Hospital in St. Louis had begun to use cystometric observations to classify disturbances in the nervous control of the bladder.[143] In the 1930s Nesbit displayed his ardor as an investigator by making or supervising more than five hundred such measurements on his patients.

Nesbit used the simplest possible apparatus for cystometry. He catheterized his patient and attached a Y-tube to the catheter. He emptied the bladder and then ran fluid into it from a graduated flask at the rate of 80 drops a minute. He tested temperature sensation by using cold or warm water. Nesbit attached a vertical glass tube to the other arm of the Y, and he measured the height of the fluid, and therefore the pressure in the bladder, by means of a meterstick alongside the glass tube. Later, when someone at the Brady Clinic at Johns Hopkins invented an aneroid ink-writing device to measure pressure, Nesbit bought one, but he still had to calculate intravesicular volume by mean of the graduated flask.[144]

Nesbit found, as everyone else did, that when approximately 50 milliliters have run into the normal human bladder, intravesicular pressure reaches about fifteen centimeters of water and then rises slowly until a volume of about 350 to 400 milliliters is reached. Then, if reflex contraction does not occur, pressure rises steeply. If reflex contraction of the detrusor muscle does occur, pressure rises even more steeply. If the normal bladder is allowed to empty as the result of detrusor contraction, almost no residual volume remains in the bladder. A cystometric curve is difficult to explain on physical and physiological principles.[145] The bladder does not obey the law of Laplace describing the behavior of a hollow vessel with an elastic wall, in part because the wall does not obey Hooke's law, because it becomes thinner as the bladder fills. In addition, there is passive and perhaps reflexly mediated relaxation of the smooth muscle of the bladder as it is distended. Nothing in Nesbit's

publications shows that he worried about these problems; measurement of the pressure-volume relation was sufficient for his purposes. His chief concern was to use cystometry and the neurological examination to determine the level and nature of any neurological disorder responsible for abnormal behavior of the bladder and to provide rational guidance for management of a patient's problems.

Nesbit was sure that the fundamental reflex arc controlling the bladder is confined to the parasympathetic nervous system and reaches the bladder in pelvic nerves, which in turn are controlled by the sacral and caudal regions of the spinal cord.[146] Afferent fibers mediating exteroception, proprioception, and pain travel to the spinal cord along with efferent parasympathetic fibers. Sympathetic innervation is unimportant for bladder function, but Nesbit thought sympathetic impulses might make the internal sphincter contract. He and his student Frederick McClellan found that pain from an intractable bladder infection is caused by spasm of the internal sphincter and that division of the sympathetic nerves to the bladder relieves pain by abolishing spasm.[147]

Nesbit identified three ways the parasympathetic reflex arc can be broken: by destruction of the motor nerves alone as in poliomyelitis, by destruction of the sensory nerves as in tabes dorsalis, or by destruction of the spinal center as by a crushing injury. He described the cystometric findings in each. If the reflex arc is intact but cut off from higher centers, the reflex neurogenic bladder results. Exteroceptive and proprioceptive sensations are absent, and uninhibited contraction occurs before the bladder contains one hundred milliliters. Completely involuntary voiding soon follows. If ascending pathways in the cord are intact but descending inhibitory influences are missing, what Nesbit called the uninhibited neurogenic bladder results. Nesbit and his students identified twenty-five such patients, all having frequency and urgency as well as nocturnal enuresis.[148] In them, exteroceptive and proprioceptive sensations were present. There was no significant infection or irritative lesion in the bladder, but during cystometry the bladder contracted abruptly when the volume reached about one hundred milliliters. In eleven patients the condition appeared to be congenital, and in fourteen it had been acquired. Nesbit deduced that the patients were like infants who had not yet achieved descending inhibitory control of the bladder.

Cabot's Men: Frederick Amasa Coller

Cabot brought Frederick Amasa Coller to Michigan as assistant professor of surgery in 1920.[149] Coller's father, a Michigan graduate of 1880, practiced in Brookings, South Dakota, and young Coller graduated from the state college in his hometown at the age of eighteen. He spent two years studying chemistry before entering Harvard Medical School in the class of 1912. Coller was an intern and a surgical resident at the Massachusetts General Hospital between 1912 and 1915, and therefore he received some of his surgical training under Hugh Cabot.

On 17 March 1915 Coller sailed to Europe with the Harvard unit under the command of Harvey Cushing and containing Elliot Cutler and Marius Smith-Petersen among the resident surgeons. The unit was to serve only three months. Coller remained in France until 1 October 1915, and then he transferred to an English hospital near Devon. After 1 July 1916 Coller returned to the United States to practice in Los Angeles, where his father had moved to escape the rigors of the South Dakota winters. Coller was again caught up in military medicine when the United States entered the war, and he was abroad from 1 July 1918 to 1 June 1919.

When Coller came to Ann Arbor, Cabot had begun to build a large department of surgery with Max Peet in neurosurgery, John Alexander in thoracic surgery, LeRoy Abbott in orthopaedic surgery, and Cabot himself in urological surgery. That left general surgery for Coller. The operating schedule was very full, even in the old hospital, and Coller himself performed twelve hundred thyroidectomies before the department moved into the new hospital in 1925. After 1921 Cabot was busy with the deanship, and Coller in effect gave leadership to the department. He was rewarded with a full professorship in 1929 and chairmanship of the department when Cabot left in 1930.

Thyroid Surgery

Lake Superior water used for drinking in the Upper Peninsula of Michigan contains 0.01×10^6 grams of iodine per kilogram, and deep well water in Mt. Clemens in the Lower Peninsula contains 0.08×10^6. These concentrations can be compared with 2.30×10^6 in Boston.[150] Until iodized salt with 0.2 grams of iodine per kilogram was introduced in 1924,

Michigan was in the heart of the U.S. endemic goiter belt. The incidence of simple goiter in men drafted from Michigan into the army in 1917–18 was 11.43 per 1,000 whereas that from Massachusetts was 0.32. From the beginning Coller had a large thyroid clinic in which he treated patients with simple goiter as well as those with toxic adenomatous goiter or exophthalmic goiter. Coller thought that all adenomatous goiters, whether toxic or not, in patients over twenty-five years of age should be attacked surgically after medication had ceased to be effective.[151] Twenty-six percent of the patients with simple goiter had tracheal compression, and at least a quarter of them, including some with normal basal metabolic rates, had some cardiovascular damage. Six percent showed thyrotoxic psychosis. Only 11 percent of the patients with simple goiter were hyperthyroid in their third decade, but at least a third were so by the age of fifty. Coller thought endemic goiter was a precancerous condition; every instance of thyroid malignancy seen in the University Hospital, 4.03 percent in 1,290 instances, had been found in preexisting simple or adenomatous goiter.[152] Thyroidectomy for simple goiter did not induce hypothyroidism, for Coller found that "almost any amount of adenomatous or colloid gland, no matter how small, if it be enough to protect the parathyroids is enough to carry on normal function."[153]

Coller and his residents, Charles Huggins[154] among them, perfected the technique of thyroidectomy.[155] Between 1 August 1925 and 31 December 1929 Coller operated upon "about 1,200" thyroid glands with satisfactory follow-up in 733 instances.[156] In them there were 184 nontoxic goiters, for the incidence had fallen since 1924. In 95 percent he obtained "good results." Of the 273 treated for adenomatous goiter there were no residual symptoms in 132 and adequate rehabilitation in another 131. Only 10 patients were unrelieved. Among his 267 patients with exophthalmic goiter, 244 were brought to within normal range of basal metabolism though their exophthalmos persisted. Only 22 were unrelieved, and 1 was worse.

Preparation for Thyroidectomy

At Michigan thyroid crisis accounted for more than half the deaths of patients with thyroid disease. From 1925 through 1933, fifty-one deaths from that cause occurred on the medical service before the patients were prepared for operation.[157] Coller emphasized the futility of treatment once thyroid crisis was established, and he tried to prevent it. Coller always encouraged his residents to spend some time in a basic science, and one, Howard B. Barker, earned a master's degree in anatomy as a National Research Fellow under Carl Huber. Barker made a thorough histological study of the effect of injecting absolute alcohol into the thyroid gland of dogs,[158] and then Coller and Barker used the same method on patients for whom all other treatment had failed to make the operative risk good.[159]

By 1926 the use of iodine to prevent the occurrence of goiter was firmly established, and treatment of goiter in adolescent patients was often successful. But Coller said: "It is common to see individuals past thirty with adenomatous goiter who have been carried into a state of marked hyperthyroidism by the use of some form of iodine given with the design of causing disappearance of the tumor."[160] He found administration of a solution of 5 percent iodine in 10 percent potassium iodide (Lugol's solution) most useful in preparing patients with exophthalmic goiter for operation. Coller gave 128 such patients one milliliter of Lugol's solution a day, and he found that in 88 percent of his patients basal metabolism fell slowly to a baseline. Then he operated four to six days after the maximal effect had appeared, for if he did not, basal metabolism rose again. He gave double the dose of Lugol's solution in physiological saline subcutaneously for fifteen days after the operation, but he was not sure the regimen was rational.

Appendicitis and Peritonitis

Coller dealt with two distinct populations of patients with appendicitis. Between 1 September 1925 and 1 March 1930 one population was composed of 128 University of Michigan students referred by physicians of the University Health Service. The average time since the onset of symptoms was thirty hours, and most of that time had elapsed before the student presented him- or herself to the Health Service. Coller wondered why an educated person aware of the dangers of appendicitis would wait a day before seeking help. Nevertheless, Coller could operate before peritonitis had spread, and only two of his student patients died.[161] In a later series of 213 similar patients that he saw within twenty-two and one-half hours the only death was from multiple liver

abscesses resulting from an infected thrombus of the mesoappendix.[162] The other population consisted of 264 patients brought in from the surrounding countryside, and for them the average delay was 9.1 days. Thirteen died of peritonitis.

In the 1920s the death rate following appendectomy had risen to twenty thousand a year, and Coller among others believed that was because surgeons operated upon patients in whom peritonitis had already begun. Consequently, Coller instituted conservative treatment of patients who came to him several days after onset of symptoms. He placed the patient in Fowler's position, recumbent with the head of the bed raised; he applied heat to the abdomen; and he gave a narcotic, usually morphine. The patient was given absolutely nothing by mouth, but saline with glucose was given by vein in amounts up to five liters a day. Formation of a mass around the appendix was recognized seven to twelve days after the beginning of the attack, and it was eventually drained through a lateral incision. The appendix was removed only if it were accessible within the abscess cavity. When the attack had subsided the patient was sent home with instructions to return three months later for an interval appendectomy.[163]

In 1934 Coller told a section of the American Medical Association about his results with deferred treatment of eighty-five patients who had appendicitis on the average 3.3 days before entering the hospital. Seventy-seven had survived. In discussing the paper Alton Ochsner said he was glad Coller knew that Ochsner had proposed exactly the same treatment in 1902.[164]

Immunizing the Peritoneum

Coller said mortality from peritonitis following operations on the colon was as high as 20 percent because the peritoneum was soiled during the operation. Some surgeons tried to protect the peritoneum by rubbing it during the operation in the hope of inducing a protective inflammatory reaction. Bernhard Steinberg of Toledo Hospital and Harry Goldblatt of Western Reserve caused an intense leukocytosis by intraperitoneal infusion of heat-killed *Bacillus coli*. Dogs so treated survived three to eight days after the peritoneum had been soiled by an aqueous extract of dog feces. Four of six treated dogs, but none of the controls, survived when the base of the appendix was ligated and its contents smeared over the peritoneum.[165] Steinberg and Goldblatt reported that they had injected a suspension of heat-killed *B. coli* intraperitoneally into each of one hundred patients twelve to forty-eight hours before an abdominal operation. There had been no peritonitis in patients in whom there had been danger of peritoneal soiling. Steinberg and Goldblatt attributed their success to polymorphonuclear leukocytosis in the abdomen induced by the suspension.

In the 1930s Steinberg, still at the Toledo Hospital, gave Coller his bacterial antigen, a strain of heat-killed *B. coli*, and Coller injected thirty milliliters of a suspension of 200×10^6 organisms per milliliter in 1 percent gum tragacanth in saline intraperitoneally into each of seventy-nine patients scheduled for colon surgery. All had fever and leukocytosis. There was severe pain in twenty and moderate pain in forty-one, and in some the reaction was so severe the operation had to be postponed. Fifty-six of the patients had uncomplicated recovery; twelve had prolonged and complicated recovery; and only one died of peritonitis, that being caused by a large defect in the perineal wound.[166]

In 1939 when Coller reviewed attempts to immunize the peritoneum he thought that if the large bowel had been opened Steinberg's antigen might be used. Otherwise, there was no need for it if the operation were carried out with meticulous technique.[167] Just at that time sulfanilamide became available, and Coller spread crystalline sulfanilamide in the peritoneum of sixty-two patients before 1942. Those were cases in which spreading peritonitis was encountered, those involving resection or anastomosis of the colon, or instances in which the peritoneum had been soiled. Only five patients had evidence of postoperative peritonitis, and the only death from peritonitis occurred in a patient with an open gastric suture line that allowed continuous soiling and chemical necrosis. Two patients with diffuse, purulent peritonitis treated with sulfanilamide died of other causes, and there was no peritonitis or adhesions found at autopsy. However, nine patients treated with sulfanilamide had severe postoperative hepatitis. An experiment with a dog showed that the concentration of sulfanilamide in portal blood rose rapidly after intraperitoneal implantation of the drug and that the drug's concentration in the liver was much higher than in other tissues. Coller advised against implanting more than 5 grams in the peritoneum.[168]

Cabot's Men: LeRoy Charles Abbott and Orthopaedic Surgery

Hugh Cabot completed his recruiting in 1920 by making LeRoy Charles Abbott the surgeon in charge of orthopaedic surgery. Abbott, like Coller, Alexander, and Cabot himself, had been a surgeon in France during the war. Immediately after being discharged from the army Abbott went to Edinburgh, where he studied orthopaedic surgery under Sir Harold Stiles.

At that time a patient with a fractured femur seldom recovered without shortening of the affected leg. During the war a South African surgeon had devised a method of keeping the bone under continuous traction by means of a nonpenetrating caliper engaging the femur just above the condyles. A splint at the knee allowed the leg to be flexed. Abbott introduced the method in Ann Arbor, and he improved it by placing a padded ring firmly against the tuberosity of the ischium that countered the traction applied by the caliper. Eventually Abbott's patients were up and about with a walking splint and legs of equal length.

At a meeting in 1921 Abbott heard Professor Vittorio Putti of Bologna describe his method of lengthening a femur of a patient whose one leg on account of disease or accident was shorter than the other. Putti used an electric saw to make a Z-shaped cut in the bone, and he fixed the limb in traction with a gap between the two ends of the cut. New bone bridged the gap, and Putti achieved lengthening of three to four inches. In Ann Arbor Abbott did almost as well for two patients, obtaining a two-and-one-half-inch lengthening of a united fracture of a boy of twelve and three-inch lengthening of the femur of a poliomyelitis patient of fifteen.

Abbott left in 1923 because Cabot's full-time plan did not provide him a satisfactory income. He went first to St. Louis, where he was consultant to the Shriners Hospital for Crippled Children, and then to San Francisco, where he established a prosperous practice. His relations with Michigan surgeons remained cordial, and when much later he was visiting professor in Ann Arbor he taught them his anterior approach to fusion of the cervical spine.

Carl Badgley

Carl Badgley (fig. 16–4) was born in Cayuga, New York, on 8 October 1893. He entered Michigan's combined course after graduating from a New York

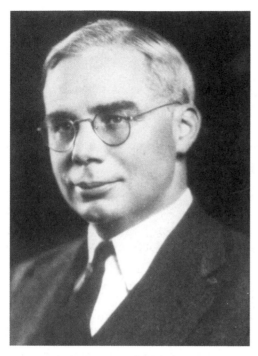

Fig. 16–4. Carl Badgley. (Courtesy of the Department of Surgery, University of Michigan.)

high school, and he received his doctor of medicine degree in 1919. He interned a year in the University Hospital, and then he was trained in orthopaedic surgery by LeRoy Abbott in 1920–22. Badgley tried unsuccessfully to establish a private practice in Detroit, and he returned to the University Hospital when Abbott left in 1923. Badgley went into practice once more, much to Cabot's disgust, at the Henry Ford Hospital, but in 1932 in the depth of the Great Depression when even orthopaedic surgeons could not earn large incomes, Badgley returned to the University Hospital as assistant professor of orthopaedics. His full-time salary was $10,500 made up of $3,300 from the Medical School and $7,200 from the hospital. Eventually, Badgley went on part time at a greatly reduced salary. He and A. C. Furstenberg sometimes debated which of them was paid less by the university and hospital, but they made up any deficiency by seeing private patients in University Hospital and St. Joseph Mercy Hospital.

Badgley participated in the explosive growth of his specialty. As head of a large hospital service he trained 130 orthopaedic surgeons, including some from St. Bartholomew's Hospital under the arrangement made by Hugh Cabot. His students spread throughout the country to meet the urgent demand for qualified men. Badgley's residents were among those Fred Coller sent to teach in Michigan hospitals, and Badgley himself visited clinics for crippled children throughout the state. As a result Badgley could review a large experience, and in 1936 he reported on 113 cases of septic hip joint, in 1937 on 171 cases of nonunion of infected fractures, and in 1942 on 146 cases of tuberculosis of the hip.

Sports injuries were common at Michigan, and Badgley, who was a member of the Board of Control of Intercollegiate Athletics, saw injuries received in swimming, wrestling, hockey, baseball, and tennis as well as football. The type of injury depended upon the sport, and Badgley himself had his shoulder dislocated by the recoil of his gun when he shot a duck rising high and to the right. Badgley found that athletes showed a certain disdain for protective clothing, but time and education increased its use.

Deformities of Childhood

Carl Badgley said that in order to understand acquired as well as congenital deformities of children he had to turn to the basic sciences of embryology and anatomy. Rollo McCotter often helped him, and after 1936 he had Bradley Patten's advice. Badgley displayed a thorough knowledge of the literature, historical as well as contemporary French, German, and Italian literature.

Badgley said that 75 percent of deformities of childhood occur after birth and that many could be prevented. It is a doctor's duty to recognize early changes, for Badgley found that a mother often failed to recognize even a severe deformity until it was pointed out to her. Mothers entertained the idea that a child would outgrow a deformity, a notion Badgley said was based on the fact that a child does outgrow three physiological deformities, bowed legs of a baby, knock-knees of a two year old, and lordosis and pendulous abdomen in a three year old. A child should be seen twice a year in the early years and once a year thereafter that deformities might be detected. Once recognized, a deformity might be corrected. Badgley lamented that even a physician who saw a child regularly failed to examine the bony framework after the child was old enough to dress itself.

Carl Badgley was particularly interested in congenital dislocation of the hip, and after the period covered by this account he made a thorough study of the embryological defect responsible and the surgical means of its correction.

Low Back Pain

Badgley said that the hundreds of patients with low back pain and sciatic radiation he saw in the University Hospital presented a condition known to physicians for centuries that they usually attributed to reflex or referred mechanisms. Badgley said firmly that sciatica is actually not sciatica, for the pain is not distributed along the pathway of the sciatic nerve. It is a condition in which the pain radiates along the pathway supplied by the postaxial and posterior branches of the lumbar plexus. He cited embryological evidence that these branches supply the embryonic limb bud, which in the adult corresponds in its entirety with an area in which the pain of so-called sciatica radiates. Sciatica is a pain referred from the articular facet of the fifth lumbar vertebra.[169]

Badgley read his own X-ray films, and sometimes he saw subtle changes that had been missed on routine viewing, but to gather evidence for his belief he enlisted the cooperation of Ted Hodges, the professor of radiology, who examined the films without knowing the clinical status of Badgley's patients. Hodges saw abnormalities of the lumbosacral and sacroiliac joints in 84 percent of Badgley's 447 patients, and there was narrowing of the intervertebral joint in 220. Hodges used his punch card file to find 185 comparable patients who did not complain of sciatica. In them, only 12 percent showed similar narrowing.

When Badgley and Hodges presented their ideas at a meeting of the American Roentgen Ray Society in 1936, another surgeon said: "I notice that we orthopedists like to ride hobbies, especially in regard to backache and various anomalies of the back. My own hobby is the separate neural arch. We have been very fortunate in hearing Dr. Badgley debunk these hobbies of ours."[170] Then he proceeded to a destructive criticism of Badgley and Hodges's interpretation of their data.

Infection of the Hip

Beginning in 1924 Badgley accumulated experience with twenty-four cases of osteomyelitis of the hip. The patients were seriously ill, and if they survived the acute phase of infection, they had ankylosis or pathological dislocation of the hip. Badgley could find no description of current treatment although he did find that a Lyonnais surgeon had used a radical

one in 1883. Badgley began his own procedure by drainage, and if the patient improved he resected the entire ilium. Mortality was high. Michigan surgeons dealt with many infections of the hip joint, some of them bilateral, and Badgley found that the type of infecting organism largely determined the primary site of infection. Soft tissue changes were more frequent with *Staphylococcus haemolyticus*, and bone lesions were more frequent with *S. aureus*. Patients with osteolytic lesions required radical surgical treatment, whereas those with soft tissue infection could be treated by conservative means. Only 14 of 113 patients treated before 1935 died, but only 7 were discharged with normal hips. The rest had irreparable functional damage.

The Broken Hip

In the nineteenth century European surgeons had attempted to repair a fracture of the neck of the femur by using ivory pegs or screws to unite the fragments, but the pegs or screws displaced too much bone and caused pressure necrosis. Marius Smith-Petersen, working at the Massachusetts General Hospital, had solved the problem in the 1920s by inventing the nail that bears his name. Nails of several lengths were available in the operating room, and an assistant who exerted counterpressure opposed the tendency of the bony fragments to separate as the nail was driven through the lateral surface of the trochanter. The nail provided absolute fixation and did not cause pressure necrosis. Badgley said Smith-Petersen's procedure was "epoch making."

Orthopaedic surgeons, including Carl Badgley, immediately began to modify Smith-Petersen's nail and his methods. The most important modification, devised by an Atlanta surgeon, was a metal plate to be attached to the upper end of the shaft of the femur after the nail was driven home. The plate had a metal ring at its upper end through which the protruding end of the nail could be inserted, and then the shaft of the femur and the fragments of bone were held in rigid alignment. Badgley's own modifications began with a lever he could use in the operating room to adjust the angle that the ring of the bone plate made with the nail. Unlike Smith-Petersen's nail, Badgley's had no head, and after it had been inserted its protruding end could be cut off. An assortment of nails need not be on hand. Soon manufacturers of orthopaedic supplies were advertising the "Badgley Bender" and the "Badgley Nail."

Badgley said that fixation of the fragments of a fractured hip should be accomplished as soon as possible; delay of one week reduces success from 95 percent to 65 percent. Adequate medical care, including X-ray studies and evaluation of the patient's cardiac and renal status, must precede surgery. Success in hip fixation requires adequate reduction of the fragments, which are then secured by internal fixation. If fixation is maintained, the healing power of the bone will prevail. Failure occurs when the screws do not hold or when there is avascular necrosis. Then Badgley had to resort to a prosthesis.

Badgley began to use prosthetic caps to the head of the femur and prosthetic cups in the acetabulum in late 1938, but the story of his struggles with these is beyond the range of this book.

The End

Carl Badgley retired in 1963, and he died on 4 February 1973. Sir Herbert Seddon, who had been one of the young men from St. Bartholomew's Hospital, said that Carl Badgley had "certain attributes of character, the ability to attract the young, to fire their enthusiasm, to make them feel that they count."[171]

17
Frederick Coller's Department of Surgery, 1930–41

Frederick Coller (fig. 17–1) was made chairman of the Department of Surgery as soon as Cabot was dismissed, and he remained chairman until he reluctantly retired in 1957.

Coller's first task was to dispel the hostility of Michigan surgeons caused by Cabot, and he was notably successful. One means was to promote continuing education for physicians, both in Ann Arbor and throughout the state. Coller and G. C. Penberthy of Detroit started their joint summer session for surgeons in 1921, and Coller was always ready to talk to a county medical society. He used his resident training program for the same purpose. He helped surgeons to establish their own training programs by assigning his residents to their hospitals for a while. As a result Coller gained the confidence of the profession, and eventually Michigan physicians were referring their surgical patients to the University Hospital for Coller's attention. They also referred themselves, for many a local surgeon facing a major operation wanted Coller to do it.

Coller's Department: Teaching and Training

Coller complained to Dean Furstenberg that the specialists in his department, Peet, Alexander, Badgley, and Nesbit, would do no clinical work or teaching in anything but their own specialties. That left general surgery and 60 percent of undergraduate teaching and resident training to Coller and his few general surgeons, and Coller frequently asked the dean for more senior staff in general surgery. In 1933 Coller showed the distribution of effort by listing the number of operations done in the previous year.

Neurosurgery	287
Thoracic surgery	629
Genitourinary surgery	379
Bone and joint surgery	1,219
General surgery	3,314

Coller said that in general surgery they treated far more cases of cancer of the rectum than of appendicitis. The combined abdominoperineal resection for cancer of the rectum that

211

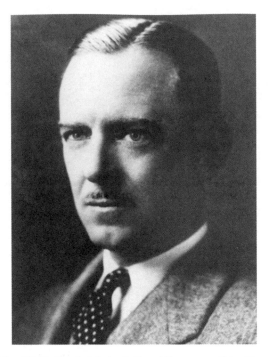

Fig. 17–1. Frederick A. Coller. (Courtesy of the Bentley Historical Library, University of Michigan, Medical School Records, Box 136, "Department of Surgery.")

Coller and Ransom began to use in 1931 took far more time than an appendectomy. Coller divided general surgery into the Red and the Blue Services to divide the burden, and he put Henry K. Ransom in charge of one and Eugene B. Potter in charge of the other. The division of the department into subspecialties was purely informal. Once, when Dean Furstenberg told Coller that the Executive Committee would not approve of the appointment of Carl List for the reason that there would then be too many neurosurgeons, Coller indignantly told the dean that he thought he was chairman of the department with the right to make decisions about distribution of appointments.

Teaching of surgery to undergraduate students was much the same as it had been in Cabot's time. The second-year students heard Coller's lectures on the history of medicine, and third-year students heard relays of specialists three hours a week. One-quarter of the junior class was on the surgical wards at a time. Patients were assigned to students for history taking and physical examination, and students assisted at their patients' operations and with their postoperative care. Each senior student spent six mornings in the dog laboratory where he or she learned some fundamentals of technique.

Coller's residents averaged five years on surgery

after an internship, and each resident spent three years on general surgery before moving to a specialty. The program was designed to produce practicing surgeons for the community rather than professors of surgery. There were, of course, some of the latter: Henry Ransom, who stayed on at Michigan, and those like Walter Maddock and Carl Moyer who became professors in major universities. Forty percent of Coller's two hundred residents eventually practiced in Michigan, consolidating the position of University of Michigan surgery in the state. Because Coller's aim was practical, he insisted on giving the students a grounding in practical sciences. His residents spent a year in pathology, and they learned anatomy by teaching it in the gross anatomy laboratory for one or two semesters. A few of Coller's residents did some research in other sciences, Barker, for example, in histology, and Carl Moyer had worked in physiology before he entered surgery.

Coller's Department: Surgery Described

The nature of surgical activity in Coller's department is illustrated by sixty-six publications in 1935–36, a typical year before the war. Thirteen papers are by John Alexander and Cameron Haight; ten by Max Peet, Edgar Kahn, and Carl List; and seven by Reed Nesbit. The gist of them has already been described. Carl Badgley published two, one on postural deformities and one on results of infection of the hip joint. There were miscellaneous case reports by Henry Ransom and junior members of the staff. Eight of Coller's publications were talks he had given before medical societies, one in Minnesota, one in Nebraska, and one in Wisconsin summarizing work on water requirements of surgical patients to be described later. A major paper by Coller and Luis Yglesias described continuity of fascial planes of the head and neck that permitted spread of infection by direct continuity.[1] The paper is based on numerous dissections, some done by A. C. Furstenberg. The topic was a favorite one of Coller, and it was followed in later years by more papers making the same point. It was also popular with Coller's students, for the copy in the medical library is worn to shreds.

Another long paper, this time by Coller and Ransom, described five-year experience in treating 270 patients with carcinoma of the rectum or the rectosigmoid.[2] Coller and Ransom used the abdominal approach first described by Miles to prevent upward spread of the disease through the lymphatic system.[3] The patients had come late in the course of the disease, and Coller and Ransom attempted curative operations in only 110. When they did the one-stage operation in 27 patients, combining a perineal approach with an abdominal one, there were 7 deaths.

Still another paper by Coller and Ransom described nine years' experience in treating ninety-four cases of external intestinal fistula.[4] Coller joined two pathologists in describing nine cases of Riedel's struma, and he agreed with Warthin that the peculiar features of the iron-hard goiter are largely the result of prolonged iodide ingestion by patients with Graves' constitution.[5] The only papers in the lot describing laboratory work were two by Hermann Pinkus, a German-Jewish refugee given a temporary home in the department as a research fellow while being supported by the Emergency Committee in Aid of Displaced Foreign Physicians and the Ella Sachs Plotz Foundation.[6]

Refugees in Coller's Department

The problem of refugees in Coller's department was typical of that in the rest of the Medical School. Early in 1933 the university began to receive appeals from ad hoc committees and foundations: Did the university have places for German-Jewish refugees? The university's reply was cautious: Michigan could take them only if full support were provided by someone else. Two surgeons, Hermann Pinkus and Carl List, did receive research appointments in the Department of Surgery, the word *research* in their title signifying that they were not paid by the university or hospital. Carl List is the only refugee I have identified who eventually gained a regular appointment in the Medical School.

Hermann Pinkus tried to make his skill in tissue culture useful to Coller during the two years he was at Michigan. Someone had said that passage through tissue culture made homotransplants more acceptable, and Pinkus applied the idea in an attempt to alleviate tetany following parathyroidectomy. In eight of fourteen instances, direct transplantation of the parathyroid gland from one rat into a parathyroidectomized rat prevented tetany in the host, but in only three of thirteen instances in which the parathyroid gland of the donor rat was carried through tissue culture using plasma from the host was tetany pre-

vented. In the face of these unfavorable results, Pinkus carried parathyroid glands from human donors through tissue culture for two weeks before they were implanted into two women with tetany following thyroidectomy. No favorable results were obtained.[7] Coller was not enthusiastic about the work, and Pinkus left Michigan.

Carl List was a neurosurgeon who had worked for a year with Harvey Cushing. List was a research instructor for two years, but in 1936 he was made an instructor and paid from university funds. He held that rank for two years until 1946, when he went to Grand Rapids to practice. His departure coincided with the return of Richard Schneider, later professor of surgery (Section of Neurosurgery), from the army.

List had worked on sweating in Germany, mapping the distribution of sympathetic nerves. He painted the subject's body with 1.5 to 2 percent iodine dissolved in a mixture of castor oil and alcohol, avoiding the eyelids and the external genitals. The subject's skin was greasy yellow until List dusted it with starch powder. List induced thermoregulatory sweating by feeding spicy dishes or emotional sweating "elicited by . . . intellectual strain or painful cutaneous stimulation."[8]

Max Peet had a large collection of patients with well-defined lesions of the sympathetic nervous system, and in a series of five papers List described the sweating in each. The papers are illustrated by numerous lurid photographs of parti-colored patients and by elegant, highly professional diagrams drawn by List himself.[9] Thereafter List published papers characteristic of a versatile and aggressive neurosurgeon.[10]

Anesthesia Again

In 1935 Coller told Dean Furstenberg that Laura Davis Dunstone did not have adequate knowledge or training to teach anesthesia to medical students. She had been teaching them for more than twenty years, and she had taught graduate courses since 1919. Coller said that she gave good inhalation anesthesia but a doctor of medicine trained in anesthesia should be found as soon as possible. In November 1937 the Executive Committee approved the appointment of Fenimore Edison Davis as instructor in charge of anesthesia, and Davis took up his duties in July 1938.

Fenimore Davis had become interested in anesthesia as a junior medical student at Michigan in the class of 1935, and Dunstone gave him special training so that he became proficient in giving ether and nitrous oxide–oxygen anesthesia. Davis interned in surgery at the University of Iowa Hospitals in 1935–36, but as soon as the staff there discovered he could give anesthesia, he was appointed part time as an anesthetist. At the end of his internship Davis took advanced training at the University of Wisconsin, then the country's leading center for research and training in anesthesia. Then he was appointed instructor in surgery at the University of Kansas and director of anesthesia at the Bell Memorial Hospital in Kansas City.

Dunstone's feelings were hurt almost at once. On 27 October 1938 she wrote Dean Furstenberg a long letter complaining that "another person," apparently another nurse-anesthetist, was intriguing against her with Davis. Dunstone said she knew that without a medical degree she had no standing, but she said it was unnecessary to belittle the past in order to demonstrate progressiveness. Dr. Davis had told her that he could order her to do anything he wanted. She said he condescended to ask her opinion on matters of no importance but not on those that made the clinic run smoothly.

Davis left Dunstone in peace when he was called into military service in 1941. Dunstone retired in 1944.

Coller's Department: Part Time

The Medical School began to dismantle the full-time plan as soon as it got rid of Cabot. It voted that beginning 1 July 1931 full time should cease to be mandatory for those now on it. The head of the department and anyone else with the head's approval could go on part time. These physicians would continue to receive a university salary but nothing from the hospital. Their consulting offices would be outside the University Hospital, but a part-time surgeon could admit patients to the fourth and sixth private floors and could use all the hospital's diagnostic and treatment facilities. These physicians could collect fees from private patients for professional services, but all other charges were to be collected by the hospital.[11] In addition, a doctor on part time could practice in a private hospital but was not to have administrative functions there. The regents approved the plan in December 1932.

Coller went on part time in 1935, retaining his university salary of eight thousand dollars. Alexander, Badgley, and Nesbit followed in 1936 with not entirely token university salaries during the Great Depression between three thousand and four thousand dollars. Peet decided to stay on full time for a while.

The Beginning of Coller's Research

There had been very little research in surgery in Cabot's time, but as soon as Coller took charge he wrote to Udo Wile, the member of the Executive Committee responsible for the clinical budget, proposing the establishment of a department of clinical research. In any event, Coller told Wile, he needed a chemical laboratory. No such department was established, and Coller had to make do without qualified professional help until 1935. In the meantime routine work for surgery was done in the hospital's clinical laboratories.[12] Basal metabolism was measured on Coller's thyroid patients with Benedict-Roth machines, some bacteriological work was done for Badgley's osteomyelitis patients, and some chloride measurements were made for Maddock's study of water balance. In 1935 Coller hired Svend Pedersen, a doctoral candidate in biological chemistry, to be his research assistant, and Pedersen did Coller's chemical laboratory work until he went into the army in 1941.

Coller believed research should directly benefit the patient. He admired Harry Newburgh, for Newburgh was a scientist who did fundamental work but also took care of patients. His research results had immediate application in the clinic. Coller's research accomplishment, determination of water and salt metabolism in surgical patients, was directly derived from Newburgh. Coller used Newburgh's methods, and the introductions to Coller's important papers read as though they were written by Newburgh.

Coller told Dean Furstenberg that more than half his day was spent in manual labor in the operating room. The rest went to the multitudinous duties of the head of a department and to the travels of a state and national figure in surgery with a message to impart. Coller himself did none of the actual work of research. As his biographer said,[13] Coller provided the enthusiasm and guidance, and as a reward he frequently put his name first on papers describing work done by others.

Patients were the subjects of Coller's research, but every so often he told one of his young men to do some laboratory work that could not be done on patients. For example, Coller set Franklin L. Troost, who disappeared into general practice the next year, to measuring glucose tolerance in dogs whose livers had been damaged, because Coller had found that patients with liver damage had low fasting blood sugar and abnormal glucose tolerance curves.[14] On another occasion Harry Brinkman, one of Coller's residents, found that abdominal operations on dogs in themselves conferred some degree of immunity against *Bacillus coli* infection of the peritoneum.[15]

Skin Temperature

As a surgeon Coller had to deal with the consequences of inadequate blood flow to the hands and feet. By 1925 he had treated fifty-two patients with peripheral lesions associated with diabetes mellitus. Those were 8 percent of the diabetic patients seen in the University Hospital. Coller found not all lesions were gangrene; twenty-four were infections, and he thought early operation was required.[16] Joslin agreed that one could not operate too soon on a diabetic patient with infected extremities. Patients with Raynaud's disease were coming to the University Hospital, and in the late 1920s Max Peet was doing sympathectomies to alleviate their peripheral vascular spasm. When Walter Maddock finished his residency and began research with Coller in 1929, Coller used measurement of skin temperature to differentiate between local vascular occlusion and vascular spasm caused from excessive sympathetic outflow to the arterioles of the hands and feet.

As the references and discussion of their papers show, Coller and Maddock were well aware that J. J. Morton and Merle Scott of the University of Rochester had already published a series of papers describing the use of skin temperature using normal subjects, patients with occlusive vascular disease, and patients with vasomotor spasm.[17] Morton and Scott had used peripheral nerve block. If, after block, the temperature of the fingers or toes did not rise, occlusion was at fault, but if skin temperature rose to thirty-two degrees centigrade spasm was responsible for low blood flow. An intermediate rise signified a mixed disorder. Therefore, there was nothing new in Coller and Maddock's work, but it did establish a useful technique at Michigan.

Coller and Maddock's partially draped subjects lay recumbent in a room maintained at twenty-five

degrees centigrade, somewhat cooler than the neutral temperature of twenty-eight degrees centigrade. Measurement of skin temperature at thirty-nine points on the body demonstrated the characteristic thermal gradient from forehead at thirty-two degrees centigrade to body, arms, legs, fingers, and toes with the tips of fingers and toes at room temperature. Coller and Maddock then wrapped each subject in a rubber sheet and three woolen blankets, and after an hour they removed the covering only enough to repeat the measurements. Warming obliterated the gradient in thirty normal subjects. Of thirty patients with abnormally cold hands and feet, only one did not dilate blood vessels in the extremities to the extent predicted by the clinical impression when warmed for an hour. That patient did not reach normal vasodilatation, in spite of responses obtained to spinal anesthesia and posterior tibial nerve block, until a hot water bottle was added to the feet. In a patient with Raynaud's disease the hand temperature rose after cervicodorsal ramisectomy and ganglionectomy, and, in a patient with paralysis of the left leg from an old anterior poliomyelitis, the temperature rose in the feet after left lumbar sympathectomy.[18] Other things being equal, skin temperature is symmetrical in a normal person, but Coller and Maddock found that when they induced fever in a patient with generalized arteriosclerosis by injecting typhoid vaccine, the temperature of only one foot rose. Coller and Maddock's conclusions were the same as Morton and Scott's: if temperature does not rise upon heating, sympathectomy is useless. If it rises to normal, sympathectomy is indicated.

Leo Buerger in his comprehensive *Circulatory Disturbances of the Extremities* suggested an etiological connection between smoking and thromboangiitis obliterans.[19] Others had demonstrated by plethysmography that smoking causes vasoconstriction in the hands.[20] Maddock and Coller confirmed the latter result by measuring skin temperature of subjects exposed to room temperature of twenty-five to twenty-eight degrees centigrade. When a normal person smoked a cigarette the temperature of the individual's fingertips fell 3 degrees and that of the toes 1.5 degrees. The response was smaller if the cigarette smoke passed through a filter, and there was none if the subject merely went through the motions of smoking a dummy cigarette. Intravenous injection of one milligram nicotine caused a fall in fingertip temperature.[21]

Buerger in his original description of thrombo-angiitis obliterans had said that "[t]he disease occurs frequently, although not exclusively, among the Polish and Russian Jews."[22] Maddock and Coller repeated their skin temperature measurements, comparing the response of twelve Gentile medical students with that of ten Jewish students. All were male. They also measured the response of a few Gentile girls, but they could apparently find no Jewish girls for comparison. When the Gentiles smoked the temperature of their fingertips fell between 0.4 and 2.1 degrees centigrade. The corresponding data for Jewish males were a range of 0.8 to 5.4 degrees centigrade. Student's *t*-test performed many years later on the data confirmed the statistical if not the medical significance of the difference between Gentiles and Jews. Maddock and Coller thought there were also differences in blood pressure and pulse rate, but the differences were statistically insignificant.[23]

Water Balance

When Coller was a house officer at the Massachusetts General Hospital the standard treatment for severe hemorrhage was to arrest bleeding if possible, keep the patient warm, and perhaps give "1 pint of hot normal salt solution containing 1 dr. [one dram, or four milliliters] of the 1:1000 solution of adrenalin chloride" by hypodermoclysis. Alternatively:

The infusion of 1 pint or more of hot salt solution into a vein is a very valuable remedy; it gives the heart something to contract upon and thus maintains cardiac action. . . . [When the patient has recovered somewhat] fluids and ice are grateful. Frequently sponge the skin with alcohol and water. Milk-punch, koumiss [fermented mare's milk], and beef peptonoids are given at frequent intervals.[24]

The prescription quoted constitutes almost all the material on water and electrolytes amid the 1,697 densely printed pages of the eighth edition of DaCosta's *Modern Surgery* published in 1919.

Coller was sufficiently disturbed by surgical ignorance to ask his former teacher of physiology, Walter B. Cannon, for advice. Cannon said: "Dr. Coller, I admire your interest but you are a surgeon and what do you know about physiology?"[25] This rankled, and Coller repeated his resentment years later. Coller had no opportunity to learn about physiology then, but by 1932 he was a colleague of Harry Newburgh, he was beginning to establish a research laboratory, and

he had help. The result was that over the next few years Coller learned a lot about the physiology of water and salt, and he taught other surgeons to manage them properly.

Newburgh taught Coller that water intake is not simply the sum of water drunk and water included in food and that water output is more than water in urine and feces. Water input also includes the water of oxidation and water released by tissue breakdown. Water output is the sum of all palpable losses and of insensible losses corrected for the patient's daily change in weight.[26] Coller adopted Newburgh's methods of measurement, and he enforced on his service the discipline required. One example of the result is given in figure 17–2.

The patient and the patient's dressings and bed clothing were weighed daily on a balance used for weighing silk, and the patient's weight was found by subtracting the separately weighed clothing and bedding. The patient drank water through a straw from a weighed, corked flask. The patient's meal was weighed before it was served, and the dishes were weighed after he or she had eaten. Stool, vomitus, sputum, the surgical specimen, and fluid drained from the wound were measured. Coller did not use Newburgh's refined calculations based upon respiratory exchanges and tissue breakdown, but they were a second order of importance. At operation the hemoglobin washed with distilled water from instruments and sponges was measured by the acid hematin method and compared with one milliliter of whole blood drawn from the patient.[27] Coller said blood loss is almost invariably greater than believed by the surgeon, and he found losses as great as 1,272 milliliters.

In the discussion following Coller said:

Most surgical patients have been getting along well for many years on the usual regimen, and if one will give a pitcher of water to a patient with a normal gastro-intestinal tract he will automatically maintain his water balance. On the other hand, this information [on water balance] may be of some importance to the very sick patient.[28]

For such a patient who could take little or nothing by mouth or for one of the 20 percent who vomited, Coller laid down rules of management. All losses of fluid must be measured and replaced volume for volume with isotonic sodium chloride solution. Water lost by other routes does not carry sodium chloride with it, and it should not be replaced with sodium

TABLE 1

Table 1. Outline of procedure.*

TABLE 2

DATE 1933	2-14	2-15	2-16	2-17	2-18	2-19	2-20	2-21	2-22
WEIGHT IN GRAMS OF:-			OPERA-TION						
PATIENT	53543	54194	54663	55472	54188	53263	53965	53999	54662
FOOD	1711	1767	0	0	1545	1459	1492	1868	
WATER DRUNK	2943	3009	611	2829	3451	3062	2595	2576	
HYPODERMOCLYSIS			3065						
URINE	1885	2313	712	2587	3896	2064	2101	2768	
SP. GR.	1.013	1.013	1.021	1.007	1.007	1.011	1.011	1.010	
STOOL	281	40	0	0	183	190	124	107	
VOMITUS				85	84				
BLOOD				100					
SPECIMEN				61					
SPUTUM					62				
DRAINAGE SERUM			23						
INSENSIBLE LOSS	1837	1954	1886	1464	1758	1559	1828	1675	
MAX. TEMP °F	98.6	98.8	99.8	101.2	100.8	99.6	99.0	99.0	
TOTAL INTAKE	4654	4776	3676	2829	4996	4521	4087	4444	
TOTAL OUTPUT	4003	4307	2867	4113	5921	3813	4053	4550	

Table 2. Water exchange of a man 51 years of age with an exophthalmic goiter. Basal metabolic rates + 50 per cent, + 27 per cent. Subtotal thyroidectomy under nitrous oxide and oxygen anesthesia on February 16.

*The patient was weighed on a platform scale accurate to 10 grams. other weighings were carried out on a small scale accurate to 1 gram.

Fig. 17–2. Outline of procedure *(top)* and water exchange of a man fifty-one years of age with an exophthalmic goiter *(bottom)*. Basal metabolic rates, plus 50 percent, plus 27 percent. Subtotal thyroidectomy under nitrous oxide and oxygen anesthesia on 16 February. (From F. A. Coller and W. G. Maddock, "Water Balance in Patients with Hyperthyroidism," *West. J. Surg. Obstet. Gynecol.* 41 [1933]: 442.)

chloride solution. Coller calculated that as a general rule a patient loses one liter of water during operation and in the immediate four hours afterward. Thereafter the patient loses another liter through the lungs and skin in the immediate twenty-four hours. Thus, two liters of water must be added to the other water losses. If this water is to be given intravenously, it must be given as a 5 percent dextrose solution that is not made up in saline or Ringer's solution. If water lost without sodium chloride is replaced by saline solution, there is no free water available, and the patient receiving 5 percent dextrose in saline or Ringer's solution retains water and becomes edema-

tous. Dextrose oxidation provides calories and combats ketosis as well. Coller said that the kidneys work on what water is left over, and the amount of free water they need depends upon their ability to concentrate the urine. Coller cited the data of Lashmet and Newburgh: if the maximum specific gravity of the urine is between 1.010 and 1.015 the kidneys need 1,439 milliliters to excrete the daily load of solids. Therefore, the patient's kidney function is adequate if he has a daily urine volume not less than 1,500 milliliters with a specific gravity not greater than 1.015. If the kidneys can concentrate more, less free water is required. Otherwise, blood urea nitrogen will rise.

Dehydration

Coller said a person is dehydrated if the individual does not have enough free water to excrete waste materials in the urine.[29] In one case, Coller and Maddock placed a young man on a diet of constant mineral content to determine the degree of negative water balance required to produce dehydration. They deprived him of water and measured his water exchange. In the preliminary period the subject's weight was 71,500 grams, and it fell to 67,800 grams in three days. By that time the subject showed the clinical signs of dehydration: sunken eyes, hot and dry skin, a dry and leathery tongue, and a slight fever. The specific gravity of his urine had risen from 1.013 to between 1.038 and 1.041, and his blood urea nitrogen had risen from 33.5 to 45.7. He had retained 5.2 grams of nitrogen and 9.9 grams of solids despite his maximally concentrated urine.

This subject's weight loss was 5.7 percent of his initial body weight, and the loss experienced by another subject on the same regimen was 5.8 percent of his initial body weight. Coller and Maddock concluded that in addition to the 1,500 milliliters of free water required by a hydrated person for urine excretion, a seriously dehydrated person requires an additional 6 percent of body weight to replace the water deficit. The usual two to three liters a day given such a patient is entirely inadequate.

Salt Balance

Coller began to think seriously about sodium and chloride in 1936 when he had Svend Pedersen to do the analyses. Someone had said that sodium concentration is reduced in hyperthyroidism, so Pedersen measured sodium in the serum of ten hyperthyroid patients, nine of whom had impaired liver function. He used the laborious uranyl zinc acetate gravimetric method. His values, expressed to a decimal point, were 279.0 to 354.6 milligrams percent, and they were within the normal range accepted at the time.[30] In a large number of instances Pedersen or someone else working for Coller measured serum chloride and expressed the results as milligrams percent sodium chloride.

Rational management of sodium and chloride requires knowledge of the amounts lost, so Coller had one of his young men measure both sodium and chloride in vomitus, hepatic bile, and enterostomy fluid drained from the mid-ileum.[31] In this instance individual values for sodium and chloride were expressed as milligrams percent of sodium or of chloride, but for each pair of values their concentration in milligrams percent sodium chloride was calculated not by adding the two individual values but by assuming all chloride was present as sodium chloride. This particularly misrepresented the data on vomitus, where there might or might not be some approach to stoichiometric equivalence. For example, in one sample sodium ion concentration was 78 and chloride was 88 millinormal; in another sample sodium ion was 3 and chloride was 47 millinormal. Both were presented as so many milligrams percent sodium chloride based upon their chloride concentrations.

Coller told his young men to begin a quantitative study of salt balance in surgical patients. Robert M. Bartlett, a research fellow in surgery; D. L. C. Bingham, fellow of the Royal College of Surgeons, Edinburgh, fellow of the Medical Research Council of Great Britain; and Svend Pedersen did the work, but a preliminary paper describing results obtained on ten patients and the theoretical basis for replacing lost body chloride was signed by Coller and Maddock as well.[32] The definitive paper published in the September and October 1938 issues of *Surgery* was signed by Bartlett, Bingham, and Pedersen alone.[33]

The paper in *Surgery,* "Salt Balance in Surgical Patients," begins with a long discussion of electrolyte balance based on 202 references. "Salt" meant sodium chloride for the reason that all concentrations were based upon determination of plasma chloride, the concentration being expressed as milligrams percent sodium chloride. The reason was simple.

This custom is not scientifically sound, because the sodium content of the plasma is more than equivalent to the chloride content, but it has the great practical advantage of expressing values in terms that are readily understood by the clinician and that can be directly applied in therapy. Thus, most physicians would immediately be confused if it were suggested that a patient be given 400 meq. of chlorine [*sic*], but everyone would immediately understand if the suggestion called for 23.4 grams of sodium chloride.[34]

Measurement of sodium concentration was so time consuming that a clinician could not wait for the result. The amount of "fixed base," chiefly sodium, in the plasma could be estimated by adding the carbon dioxide combining power to the chloride concentration, but the authors did not explain how to add carbon dioxide combining power in volumes percent carbon dioxide to chloride concentration in milligrams percent sodium chloride. Fortunately, they said, correction of chloride deficiency will almost invariably correct sodium deficiency and acid-base balance. The authors said that if chloride is lost in excess of sodium, as from the upper gastrointestinal tract, the result is alkalosis and dehydration. If sodium is lost in excess of chloride, as from the lower gastrointestinal tract, the result is acidosis and dehydration. They did not consider respiratory deviations of acid-base balance, nor did Coller when he wrote textbook chapters on acidosis and alkalosis.[35]

The great bulk of sodium is in the extracellular fluid, and the normal person can regulate its quantity by excreting extra sodium in the urine or by reducing it nearly to zero in times of deficiency. This the young men demonstrated in normal subjects. On the other hand, a seriously ill patient, being unable to regulate sodium excretion, may retain both salt and water and gain weight. Therefore, it is important not to give excess salt to such a patient.

Because Bartlett, Bingham, and Pedersen could not measure extracellular fluid volume or total exchangeable sodium, they relied on measurement of plasma chloride as an index of sodium balance. Plasma chloride concentration might rise in a few patients, but most problems of salt balance occurred in patients who had low plasma chloride and were sodium deficient. Bartlett, Bingham, and Pedersen produced salt depletion in four normal subjects by putting them on a salt deficient diet and then continuously removing their gastric secretion by suction for several days. To this they added data from three patients with continuing upper gastrointestinal fluid loss. In a long, detailed table they reported their subjects' daily body weight, gastrointestinal fluid loss, plasma chloride, and urine volume and composition. After deficiency had been established they gave salt solution and 5 percent glucose solution intravenously and water by mouth. In three equally detailed tables Bartlett, Bingham, and Pedersen demonstrated replacement of salt loss from the upper gastrointestinal tract by twelve patients. With four they replaced lost fluid volume for volume with isotonic salt solution; with four they gave volume for volume of Ringer's solution; and with four they added one thousand milliliters of glucose solution to volume for volume of salt solution. In two more tables they described replacement of salt in seven and eleven patients.

Bartlett, Bingham, and Pedersen said:

All these findings seem to warrant the assumption that the plasma chloride level is a satisfactory index of the chloride concentration throughout the body. . . . On this basis, knowing the normal salt content of the body and the portion of it that has been lost as indicated by the plasma chloride level, one should be able to calculate the number of grams of salt that must be returned to the body to restore the body chlorides to normal.[36]

They took Sherman's figure of 0.15 for the average percentage of chloride in the human body. This is 0.248 percent in terms of sodium chloride. Thus, a seventy-kilogram man contains 173.4 grams of salt. Normal plasma chloride ranges from 560 to 630 milligrams percent, but they chose the lowest value for the reason that many surgical patients are unable to raise their plasma chloride concentration higher. Therefore:

$$\text{Gm. salt needed} = (560 - \text{actual plasma chlorides})/560 \times 0.00248 \times \text{body weight (gm.)}$$

Because clinicians who were confused by milliequivalents were likely to be baffled by such complicated algebra, they restated the rule in italics (621).

For each 100 mg. that the plasma chloride level needs to be raised to reach normal, the patient should be given 0.5 gm. of salt per kilogram of body weight.

Because Coller inspired the work, he took the credit. He told the story to the American Surgical Association in Atlantic City in May 1938. The surgeon who discussed the paper spoke of "Coller's quantitative method." Coller's name was first on a paper in which three figures, four tables, and the conclusion almost word-for-word of the Bartlett-Bingham-Pedersen paper was published in the October 1938 issue of the *Annals of Surgery,*[37] the same month the Bartlett-Bingham-Pedersen paper appeared in *Surgery.* It was published again in the *Transactions of the American Surgical Association.*[38]

The credit Coller received for his career included the presidency of the American Surgical Association and the American College of Surgeons; honorary membership in fourteen surgical associations around the world, including the Royal Colleges of Surgeons of Edinburgh and Great Britain; and five honorary degrees.

1941

The entry of the United States into the war in 1941 put a temporary end to the growth of the Department of Surgery, for most of the staff were called into service. The department had remained remarkably stable since Coller had arrived in Ann Arbor twenty-one years earlier. Max Peet, John Alexander, and Frederick Coller were senior members of the staff, and Carl Badgley, Reed Nesbit, and Edgar Kahn, who had arrived only a little later, were still there. More research had been done than in Cabot's decade, and the research was directed to practical ends. High-quality patient care and prolific training of surgeons for specialty practice were still the aims of Coller and his men as they had been of Cabot and the same men.

18
Obstetrics and Gynecology

Edward S. Dunster, the professor of obstetrics and diseases of women and children since 1874, died on 3 May 1888, and Victor Vaughan had the responsibility of finding his successor.[1] Vaughan chose James N. Martin, Dunster's assistant, instead of going outside. Martin may have recommended himself to Vaughan by publishing on tyrotoxicon, the poison Vaughan had isolated from putrefying milk.[2] The appointment was a temporary expedient, for it was not made permanent until 1891 when Martin was given the title professor of obstetrics and diseases of women. By that time Christopher had brought the care of children under internal medicine. Thereafter George Dock and Murray Cowie were responsible for pediatrics. In parallel with Nancrede, Martin began to establish a university department of gynecological surgery, and although most deliveries occurred in the home he secured a limited number of obstetrical cases for instruction. When he resigned in 1901 after a period of increasing mental instability Martin left gynecological surgery to Reuben Peterson.

Martin's Gynecological Surgery

In Dunster's time no more than seventeen gynecological patients had been seen in the Pavilion Hospital during the six-month academic year. Ovariotomy was the chief operation performed, and sometimes it was done as treatment for epilepsy. Shortly after patients occupied the Catherine Street Hospital in 1892 Nancrede turned over all gynecological surgery to Martin. Nancrede was familiar with surgery on a national scale; Martin, entirely Michigan trained, was not. Thus, Nancrede demonstrated some confidence in Martin's competence. Until his resignation Martin dealt with between six hundred and eight hundred gynecological problems a year in the hospital, and he also operated in patients' homes.[3] Throughout this period Martin had James Lynds, also Michigan trained, as his demonstrator, and Lynds substituted as professor when Martin was on leave on account of blood poisoning contracted while operating. Toward the end of his tenure Martin had two recent graduates as his assistants.

Martin's students had a little gynecological casework on the wards, supplemented by morning sectional clinics (fig. 18–1), but much of the 382 hours devoted to gynecology in the curriculum was spent two afternoons a week from 3 P.M. to 6 or 7 P.M. on the hard benches of

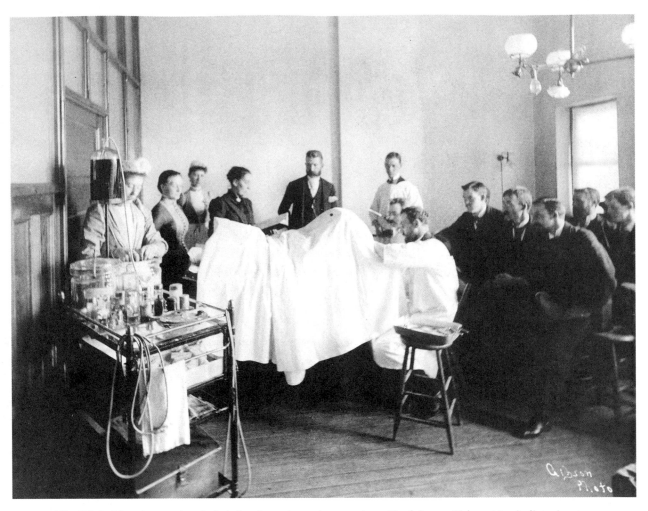

Fig. 18–1. Morning sectional clinic in obstetrics and gynecology. Prof. James Nelson Martin listening to history read by a student. (Courtesy of the Bentley Historical Library, University of Michigan, Medical School Records, Box 136, "Classes by Subject, Surgery and Anatomy Amphitheater Views.")

the operating theater, high above the pit. The students could see nothing and understand little of what was occurring on the operating table. When Peterson succeeded Martin he said that it was not considered good form for a student to sleep elsewhere while he was operating.

Martin early in his career made a thorough study of the anatomy of the female perineum, a subject he thought generally neglected. Carl Huber helped him in his dissections. Martin found how sutures should be placed to repair lacerations and to prevent herniation, and he published his findings with ample illustrations. Martin also tried to teach Michigan physicians. At meetings of the State Medical Society Martin described mistakes he had observed in the diagnosis of ovarian diseases, mistakes made through ignorance or carelessness or both.[5] He told general

practitioners that many of them were too lazy to make a thorough examination.

A little later Martin's colleague James Lynds castigated physicians for the gynecological damage they did by abandoning their patients the minute delivery was complete. In the fifteen hundred to two thousand cases he had seen in eight years in the university clinic three-fourths of the patients suffered from conditions that could have been prevented by proper care. The physician's most important ally was a good nurse, but Lynds would rather have a nurse who had never seen a patient but who would follow directions than an experienced nurse who thought she knew it all and scoffed at antisepsis.[6]

In 1892 Martin reported the results of ten consecutive laparotomies done before the medical class in three months,[7] but Peterson, who was then practic-

Not Just Any Medical School

ing in Grand Rapids, Michigan, capped him with twenty-five.[8] Martin, an invited speaker on a program concerning treatment of pus in the pelvis, advocated section and hysterectomy in most instances.[9] Peterson, who was on the same program, thought hysterectomy justified only in special circumstances.[10] Peterson used a blind method of evacuating pus by the vaginal route, using his finger to break adhesions and to reach the pus pocket.[11]

Reuben Peterson

Reuben Peterson was well known throughout Michigan when he was chosen as Martin's successor in 1901. He was a Bostonian who had graduated from Harvard College in 1885 and from Harvard's three-year medical curriculum in 1888. He received his medical degree from Harvard after completing an internship in three Boston hospitals. One was the Boston City Hospital, where Peterson served on the ward for alcoholics. That experience came in handy later when he was called into consultation about the mysterious illness of a wealthy woman. Peterson immediately recognized delirium tremens.

Peterson began to practice in Grand Rapids, Michigan, and he soon became medical superintendent in St. Mark's Hospital, a hospital about to be desanctified by being renamed Butterworth. He had been favorably impressed by professionally trained nurses in Boston,[12] and he established a hospital nurses' training school. He strongly supported nursing education when he came to Ann Arbor, and he attached a nurses' training school to his private hospital. There were 150 physicians of all schools in Grand Rapids, and in 1895 Peterson persuaded them to organize a medical library.[13] Active membership cost ten dollars a year, and life membership was one hundred dollars. The librarian was paid four dollars a week. The library subscribed to the *Index Medicus* and one hundred journals, very few outside the English language.

Peterson soon began to specialize in obstetrics and gynecology, and his particular interest was gynecological surgery, on which he wrote copiously. In contrast with Martin, whose range was strictly local, Peterson published in national journals, joined a national society—the American Gynecological Society—and frequently attended national meetings. Soon he was making a tour of medical societies, giving advice on the management of pregnancy and on

the indications for operations for pelvic diseases. In 1898 Peterson moved to Chicago, where, in addition to his private practice, he had an appointment in the Chicago Post-Graduate Medical School, an institution giving short courses in the specialties for inadequately trained physicians,[14] and at the Rush Medical College.

Among Peterson's hundred or so publications is the description of his one piece of animal research, done in Chicago just before coming to Ann Arbor.[15] The problem was one that worried Peterson all his professional life: what to do with the ureters in cases of disease of the bladder and urethra. Peterson devised a number of radical operations, creating a vesicovaginal fistula, creating a rectovaginal fistula, and sewing the vagina shut. He transplanted the ureters to the colon, and failures drove him to examining the operation in dogs. He tried bilateral ureterointestinal anastomosis, unilateral ureterointestinal anastomosis, and ureterotrigonointestinal anastomosis. His results were very bad, five survivors out of twenty-one in the last of the three procedures, but he concluded that the trigonal operation was justified in desperate straits.

The Bates Professorship

In 1898 Dr. Elizabeth Bates of Port Chester, New York, left upward of one hundred thousand dollars to the University of Michigan to establish the Bates Professorship of Diseases of Women and Children. She had never visited Ann Arbor, and she knew nothing of the recent developments of the Medical School. Her gift was an expression of appreciation for Michigan's having early, twenty-two years before Johns Hopkins, admitted women to the Medical School on the same terms as men.

The title Dr. Bates specified for the chair gave the university trouble. When the school was founded Abram Sager was professor of diseases of women and children, but by the time the university received the Bates money teaching of diseases of children was firmly in the hands of the internists. The regents solved the problem by the semantic maneuver of naming James N. Martin the first Bates Professor of Diseases of Women and Children and at the same time specifying he was to have the same duties as before. That meant he was to have no responsibility for children. Concurrently the regents said that instruction in diseases of children would continue to be given by George Dock in the Department of Internal Medicine. Peterson succeeded Martin with the same ambiguous title and duties, and until 1923 he was commonly, but improperly, called the Bates Professor of Obstetrics and Diseases of Women.

For many years the Bates endowment was a handicap to Peterson rather than a help. The regents, instead of providing adequately for his department out of general funds and using the endowment as a supplement, charged all obstetrical and gynecological expenses to the income from the Bates endowment. Peterson thought that contravened the intention of Dr. Bates and that the fund should be used to build and equip an adequate maternity hospital or even to support research.

Peterson's Private Practice

Peterson was always in private practice, and he was opposed to full-time clinical appointments. Shortly after Peterson arrived in Ann Arbor in 1901 he rented a house at 1215 South University in which he installed a three-bed ward on the first floor and an operating room and four more beds on the second floor. The next year he leased another house around the corner at 620 Forest Avenue where he had room for nine patients and operating and sterilizing rooms. In 1910 he installed a diet kitchen, and in 1913 he had a laboratory in one of his houses. Over the years he bought or leased more houses on South University and Forest Avenue, and after spending ten thousand dollars for renovation he had forty beds, some of which he leased to Udo Wile and Nellis Foster. Peterson employed fifteen to twenty nurses, and he established a nurses' training school in a house he leased at 614 South Forest (fig. 18–2). After 1920 Peterson confined his work to what he could do in one building, and he discontinued his nursing school.

One evening while Peterson and Lombard were walking home together after a faculty meeting Lombard told Peterson he would have accomplished much more if he had not been in private practice. That night Lombard, overcome by remorse, wrote Peterson a letter apologizing for what he had said and praising Peterson's work. In 1925, when Peterson was growing old, he had come round to Lombard's way of thinking. He then believed the duties of a professor of obstetrics and gynecology could not be combined with a large private practice. The university should have its own clinic in which the professor could work full time, drawing his entire salary from the university or supplementing it to a limited extent by private work done in the clinic. Peterson's attempt to go full time the next year was frustrated by Cabot, who wanted to get rid of him altogether.

Peterson's Staff

Peterson's staff in the University Hospital was always small, young, and inbred. In a typical year he would have one intern, one resident, one or two demonstrators, and one or two instructors. After 1919 he had a succession of assistant professors, each of whom left after a year or two. Only two of the twenty-six men and women who served under Peterson in his first twenty years in Ann Arbor were not Michigan graduates. One had come from Rush with Peterson. All four assistant professors had been his students. In Peterson's thirty years at Michigan no one grew to be a professor with a program of his or her own in Peterson's department as many, including Newburgh and Wilson, had grown in the Department of Internal Medicine or as Cabot's men had in the Department of Surgery. Norman Miller might have been on his way to a professorship, but he left in 1926 for Iowa.

One instructor in 1907–8 deserves to be remembered: Elton P. Billings had a notable talent as a medical illustrator, and many papers by Peterson and others contain highly professional drawings signed with his initials.[16]

Junior members of Peterson's department published frequently, chiefly case reports, reviews of the literature, or descriptions of technique. Peterson's name was never on their papers until 1921, when he signed a paper with J. G. Van Zwaluwenburg on radiological findings in pneumoperitoneum.[17] Peterson was contemptuous of the head of a clinic who kept all the work to himself while his assistants stood around picking up what crumbs they could. The result was that a succession of competent obstetrician-gynecologists left Peterson's department after four years to populate Michigan and the surrounding states.

Peterson as a Gynecological Surgeon

Peterson's standing as a surgeon brought him the presidency of the American Gynecological Society

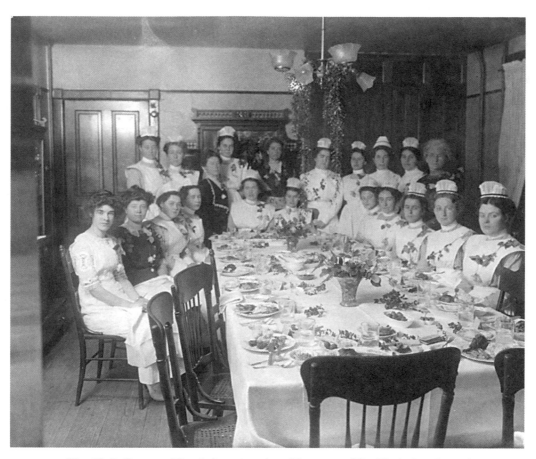

Fig. 18–2. Peterson Hospital nursing class. (Courtesy of Dr. Linda Strodtman.)

and founding membership in the American College of Surgeons. That standing was based on frequent publication of methods and results dealing with the usual range of problems: uterine fibroids, cancer of the cervix, extrauterine pregnancy, and so forth. His first reported series was seventeen operations for suspension of the retrodisplaced uterus using Howard Kelly's newly devised method of suturing the utero-ovarian ligaments to the anterior abdominal wall.[18] In those days the retrodisplaced uterus along with the floating kidney and the dropped stomach gave surgeons a lot of work, for the retrodisplaced uterus was the cause of low back pain, dysmenorrhea, sterility, constipation, hemorrhoids, neuralgia, and insanity. For retrodisplacement, Peterson said that he performed ventrosuspension of the fundus uteri more frequently than any other operation, one that resulted in one or more bands of adhesions two to two and one-half inches long, and that "a number of my patients with suspended uteri have become pregnant and been delivered at full term without

mishap."[19] He sometimes had to deliver a woman by cesarean section on whom he had performed ventrosuspension earlier.[20] Peterson was an expert in performing cesarean section by the vaginal route, and he thought that in cases of eclampsia the uterus should be emptied by that method as soon as possible. Vaginal cesarean section could be performed quickly, and its technique could be acquired by anyone familiar with the rudiments of obstetric surgery.[21] On the basis of 1,066 laparotomies for pelvic disease Peterson said that in addition to inspecting the appendix the surgeon should palpate the gall bladder, looking for stones. Therefore, the incision should be large enough to permit thorough exploration of the abdominal contents.[22] George Dock tried once when Peterson was operating, but he failed. It seemed to him as if the incision was about two feet from the liver.[23] On several occasions Peterson substituted the anal for the vesical sphincter in cases of inoperable vesicovaginal fistulas.[24]

Peterson kept careful records of his results, and his

file in the Bentley Historical Library contains hundreds of mimeographed questionnaires returned by former patients. There are also many copies of letters sent to physicians in attempts to locate missing patients. Those documents show the public and private distribution of Peterson's work. For example, of the sixty-six women with prolapse of the uterus that Peterson saw in 1906, forty-five were treated in the University Hospital and twenty-one in his private clinic.

Peterson was candid about his problems, for he said: "If a man operate[s] long enough and often enough he can illustrate in his own practice almost every surgical complication."[25] That remark was made in a paper describing tetanus in a nineteen-year-old university student for whom Peterson had done a hysterorrhaphy. He had recently switched from commercial catgut to catgut prepared by his own technician, and he thought sterilization had been inadequate. The young woman recovered.

Peterson's cases in the University Hospital were used for teaching. Each case was assigned to two students for workup and diagnosis. Their written report was read before a small section of students in the operating room, and immediately afterward their diagnosis was tested by surgery.

Obstetrics to 1931: Buildings

Sager, Dunster, and Martin had been professors of obstetrics, but there were essentially no clinical obstetrics at the time, and it was possible for a medical student to graduate and to go into practice without having seen a delivery. Sager had lectured on segmentation of frogs' eggs and performed one cesarean section. Dunster had been called the most eloquent lecturer in the history of the school. Most women were delivered at home and with good reason: mortality from puerperal fever could be 25 percent in a hospital. Medical students could be excluded from deliveries for reasons of propriety, and obstetric manipulations were done beneath a sheet. After 1889, what practical training students had was with a mannequin, but if a student were lucky he or she might see one of the ten or twelve obstetrical patients cared for during the school year.

Beginning in 1901 Reuben Peterson had the task of obtaining a satisfactory obstetric ward and finding the women to fill it. He complained that the Catherine Street Hospital was poorly designed, poorly

maintained, and septic. Patients with contagious diseases could not be isolated, and if scarlet fever, diphtheria, or smallpox appeared the entire hospital would be quarantined for weeks. A few contagious patients could be admitted to a makeshift pesthouse. The problem was solved in 1914 when the people of Ann Arbor voted a bond issue of twenty-five thousand dollars to build an isolation hospital to be managed by the university. Peterson as medical director of University Hospital traveled east to inspect similar buildings, and he supervised planning and drew up regulations for a twenty-four-bed contagious disease hospital perched on a ridge in back of the Catherine Street Hospital overlooking the Huron River. The hospital served the University Health Service as well as the city, and in its first year it housed patients with chicken pox, whooping cough, diphtheria, Vincent's angina (necrotizing ulcerative gingivitis), tuberculosis, and pneumonia.

The Catherine Street Hospital's small obstetrical wards could hold no more than five patients, and because it was customary for a woman to be hospitalized for weeks before and after delivery the number of patients seen during the year was small. When the Palmer Ward was opened in 1903 Peterson, through the courtesy of George Dock, who was in charge of the ward as a children's hospital, used a part of it as an obstetrical ward. In 1905 and again in 1908 wooden buildings, formerly dwellings, were moved to a site just west of the West Ward (Medical Ward), and one of those served as a maternity cottage for eighteen to twenty waiting patients and the other as a hospital for women in labor. When the university built a spur from the Michigan Central Railroad to carry coal to its heating plant on Huron Street, Mortimer Cooley, the engineer and an important figure in the university administration, ran the track between the two buildings. Peterson was furious. When one of his patients was hurried from the "waiting building" to the delivery building she broke a leg tripping over a rail.

Peterson's obstetrical buildings were used as "Exhibit A" to demonstrate how horrible things were when a legislative committee visited the Medical School. The governor told President Burton that something must be done, and the regents appropriated fifteen thousand dollars to repair the obstetrical buildings. In 1925, when everyone else moved into the new hospital, the hospital director allowed the old Eye, Ear, Nose, and Throat Ward, a building constructed in 1910, to be converted into an eighty-two-bed obstetrical hospital for Peterson's "much despised obstetrical patients." Peterson said the hospital director, Harley Haynes, was the only true angel that he had found since he had come to Michigan.

Obstetrics to 1931: Patients

Peterson's obstetrical patients in the University Hospital were charity patients. In 1889 and again in 1915 the legislature provided that "obstetrical cases as a public charge" should be cared for in the University Hospital, but the legislature also provided that the charges be paid by the respective counties, not the state. Consequently, the law was totally ineffective in getting such patients to Ann Arbor. County officials could not refuse to send their gynecological patients to the University Hospital, but they could save money by sending their pregnant, unmarried girls to their own county poor farm.

Peterson's battle for more patients was with the university itself. He resented that those responsible for training medical students failed to provide adequately for essential teaching. When Peterson went to James Henry Wade, the secretary of the university and the professional watchdog of the university treasury, with the plea that obstetrical patients be admitted free of charge, the secretary was amazed and said such a request was ridiculous. It was sufficient that every medical student witness one delivery in the hospital theater. Victor Vaughan had similar trouble with the same man and called him "a village tradesman, selected by the regents to manage the finances of the university and incidentally to dictate to professors."[26] Both Peterson and Vaughan must have been amused when, during an audit of the university accounts, the secretary found it convenient to visit relatives in Chicago and to resign quietly.[27]

Pressure intensified in the 1920s when Fred C. Zappfe, the executive secretary of the Association of American Medical Colleges, made his accreditation visit. Zappfe told President Little that Michigan was meeting its accreditation requirements only by what amounted to perjury. Both Zappfe and Cabot told President Little that the situation could only be remedied by adjunct facilities in Detroit. In reply President Little said that hospital cases involving the birth of children to unmarried mothers are not good teaching material. Peterson was astounded.

Obstetrics to 1931: Peterson's Teaching

When Peterson had his maternity hospital more or less in working order third-year students were able to observe labor. They had three hours of lecture a week throughout the year, and in keeping with Michigan tradition Peterson provided the students with a short crammer: *A Manual for a Demonstration Course in Obstetrics,* a lithoprinted typescript.[28] In outline form it told the student the minimum he or she needed to know about normal and problem deliveries. Peterson's gigantic textbook, *The Practice of Obstetrics,* was also available.[29] Peterson had edited that 1,087-page book but had written none of it.

Senior students in groups of two were assigned a pregnant patient whom they followed to delivery and during three or four weeks of hospitalization thereafter. In the outpatient clinic they were taught the management of delivery in the home, and after delivery they made postpartum calls.

In 1912 the students could have seen 109 obstetrical patients of whom 104 delivered.[30] There were three maternal deaths, one of a patient who arrived moribund. One other died of pulmonary embolus and the third of peritonitis following cesarean section. Four premature infants died, and there were five stillbirths. The major complications were gonorrhea in thirteen patients and syphilis in nine. Some of the syphilis had been detected in unsuspecting patients by the Wassermann test, for Peterson was a firm believer in its routine use, as were most of his contemporaries practicing obstetrics and gynecology.

Most of the patients delivering at the University Hospital were unmarried, and their babies were kept in the hospital for weeks before being put out for adoption or assigned to a home. In that time medical students studying obstetrics were taught the principles of infant feeding in a manner somewhat simpler than that used by Murray Cowie in teaching infant feeding to students in pediatrics.[31]

Belief in the thymicolymphatic constitution prevailed in the Department of Obstetrics as well as in Pathology. In 1924 Peterson reported that in 120 consecutive births, 20 of 54 female infants and 32 of 66 male infants had abnormally enlarged thymus glands. Such prevalence might have encouraged Peterson to revise his definition of normality. Every infant so diagnosed was immediately treated with X rays to prevent stridor, cyanosis, and convulsions, for Peterson believed it to be absolutely essential that every baby with lymphatic symptoms be so treated.[32]

Abortion and Sterilization

Peterson had to deal with abortion and sterilization. He said that we may not destroy one life to make another life easier. Only in advanced cases of tuberculosis in the mother should a fetus be aborted. He had to answer the question, Under what circumstances is craniotomy on the living child justifiable?[33] In answer Peterson said the medical profession likes dogmatic statements. One such is that it is never justifiable to perforate a living fetus. But the profession is also good at finding exceptions to general rules, and "the terrible butchery of the unborn went on until the various operations having to do with the delivery of the child had been so perfected as to give the mother a fair chance when they were resorted to."[34] Yet much craniotomy continued to damage the mother as well as the child. Peterson laid down his own rules.

The conditions under which craniotomy on the living child may not only be justifiable but clearly indicated can be stated as follows:

1. When the mother is septic.
2. When the child is feeble and not likely to live under any conditions.
3. When the fetus is a monster or so badly defective as to make its future existence problematic.
4. When from the necessities of the case the choice must be made between craniotomy and the major obstetric operations in unskilled hands.[35]

As for sterilization, Peterson said that in twenty-five thousand cases in his clinic to 1926 he had performed "primary sterilization" only eight times. Four were for imbecility, two with and two without court order. The other four were to prevent attacks of eclampsia or to prevent pregnancy in cases where there was serious kidney or heart disease or marked debility. He thought sterilization during the course of other operations another matter, and he had done it 105 times. Sixty-five of those were for instances of marked uterine prolapse, and the reasons for the other 40 ranged from debility following multiple pregnancies (13) to feeblemindedness (2). Peterson said: "In every instance the reasons for sterilization should be stated in writing and the request for sterilization made in writing by both patient and husband with the distinct understanding that after the operation, pregnancy cannot take place."[36]

The Detroit Affiliation

In Peterson's last year at Michigan the final blow came from someone he had always thought a friend: Udo Wile, as a member of the Executive Committee replacing Cabot, had persuaded President Ruthven to force Peterson to make an alliance with the Woman's Hospital in Detroit. Four seniors were to be sent to Detroit each week, where they would receive obstetric instruction under a man who had been trained by Peterson. The fourteen women and four African Americans in the class were to be excluded from the rotation. Peterson said it was horrible to talk to the students who had returned from Detroit. They did not get any obstetrical experience to speak of but were instead talked to by men who were not trained in obstetrics and who were opposed to Peterson's teachings. They saw the wrong things in the delivery room, and Peterson cited an example of inappropriate use of forceps that had resulted in the death of the baby.

Peterson's Retirement

Peterson resigned in May 1922, effective at the end of the academic year. He gave no reason, but his hatred of Dean Cabot was reason enough. Peterson rescinded his resignation, but the conflict with Cabot continued. In 1926 Cabot wrote a long letter to President Little, denying Peterson's request for a two-thousand-dollar raise that would allow Peterson to go on full time. He said Peterson was now sixty-four years old and surgeons of that age were placed on the retired list in many hospitals. Later Cabot wrote Peterson that he had read in the newspaper that Peterson had been out of town during term time. Cabot sharply reminded Peterson that he should have asked leave. Teaching suffered when the professor was away, and interns must not be expected to do it. Furthermore, Peterson had been late in turning in examination grades.

Peterson remained until age forced him to retire in 1931. He did not want to be made professor emeritus, and he asked to be made consultant obstetrician. The university would not allow that. Peterson had no pension, but Novy, who was now chairman of the Executive Committee, allowed Peterson to continue on a salary of two thousand dollars to be paid from the administrative account. Peterson moved to Duxbury, Massachusetts, where he amused himself with the occupation characteristic of a superannuated professor: writing a history of the University Hospital. Dean Furstenberg carried on a lively correspondence with him, sending Peterson news, copies of documents, and volumes of *Regents' Proceedings.* Peterson repeatedly asked the university for secretarial help, but when the subject of support was brought to President Ruthven, the president's response was a groan. The finished manuscript was rejected for publication by the university; it was too chatty, it contained personal items that might well have been omitted, and it did not include an account of research accomplishments.[37]

Peterson's Successor

Norman Fritz Miller had been promoted rapidly, for he was an assistant professor five years after graduating from medical school in 1920. He was promoted equally rapidly in Iowa, for he was a full professor there before being brought back to Ann Arbor in 1931 to be Peterson's successor.

When Miller left for Iowa Dean Cabot asked him what might be done to strengthen the department at Michigan. Miller replied that he had some very definite ideas, but out of loyalty to Peterson he would keep them to himself.

Miller inherited what had been almost a one-man department managed by a man heavily committed to practice gynecological surgery in his own forty-bed hospital. Miller himself moved to part time in 1935, but his private practice was in the University Hospital. Peterson had deplored the separation of obstetrics from the more glamorous subject of gynecological surgery that had occurred, for example, at Johns Hopkins, but he had not been notably successful at promoting obstetrics at Michigan. Miller was primarily a surgeon, but he did better by obstetrics. He quickly developed a better-balanced university department. Unlike Peterson, Miller raised many younger men to professorial rank, but, like Peterson's, Miller's department was inbred. Twenty-two of the twenty-four physicians who served him as instructors or assistant professors before 1942 were Michigan graduates. The other two were from Harvard.

Posture and Dysmenorrhea

Miller thought gynecologists had addressed themselves to unusual problems; common disturbances

had been neglected. Many women were constipated, but few physicians were willing to take the time to do more than to tell the patient to take mineral oil or to eat more roughage.[38] Forty-five percent of menstruating women had some discomfort during their periods, and 15 to 20 percent were seriously inconvenienced or incapacitated.[39] Endocrinologists had contributed something to understanding dysmenorrhea, but gynecologists had neglected mechanical factors, of which posture was the most obvious.

When Miller went to Iowa he constructed a frame in which he could photograph the anterior-posterior and lateral silhouettes of women of the entering class of the university and of the nurses' training school.[40] Miller measured twenty-eight dimensions of the anterior-posterior silhouettes and eighteen of the lateral ones, and he classified posture as "excellent," "good," "fair," or "poor." When at first he correlated posture with menstrual history he found that women with poor posture were more likely to have dysmenorrhea and that correcting posture reduced discomfort during menstruation. Miller found that 33 percent of the women with fair or poor postures in 1927 had better grades of posture in 1929. All those had dysmenorrhea in 1927; none had it in 1929.

Miller attributed dysmenorrhea to congestion resulting from the upright position. In a biped most of the blood volume is below the heart level. The pelvic organs have thin-walled veins, and the veins empty into others that have no valves. Therefore, he argued, the generative organs are particularly susceptible to conditions causing congestion, and the physiological congestion occurring during the menstrual period superimposed upon continuing congestion causes the dull pain of dysmenorrhea. Poor muscle tone and bad posture exacerbate uterine congestion.

Some years later Miller worked up his complete data on 302 young women, and he could not substantiate his earlier conclusions.[41] He could find no cause-and-effect relation between posture and dysmenorrhea. All Miller could say was that taller women are less likely than shorter ones to have dysmenorrhea. Now Miller thought malposition of the uterus may cause dysmenorrhea, but more often it does not. He published an elaborate analysis of the factors producing retroversion of the uterus, illustrated with twenty-nine diagrams. The factors included a full bladder, a full rectum, loss of pelvic support, trauma, faulty posture, changes in intraabdominal pressure, and gravity.[42] Miller wrote: "Yet the thousands of symptomless retroversions indicate that such cause and effect relationship [between retroversion and symptoms] is not the rule. . . . Obviously surgery directed primarily toward correction of the retrodisplacement is never indicated until a symptom cause and effect relationship is proved. In most cases [correction] may be accomplished by manual replacement of the uterus and use of an appropriate, properly fitting pessary to keep the replaced organ in position."[43]

On another occasion he told the Canadian Medical Association that surgical intervention for dysmenorrhea should be "thoroughly premeditated."[44] Peterson's days of enthusiastic hysterorrhaphy were over.

Miller's Gynecological Surgery to 1941

Miller entered the surgical literature when he was still a resident by describing the case of a fourteen-year-old girl with pain in the left lower quadrant who had been ineffectively operated upon elsewhere for appendicitis. The correct diagnosis of congenital double uterus was not established until operation at the University Hospital, and by the time her several anomalies, including a rudimentary left kidney, had been sorted out her pelvic organs had been so damaged that all had to be removed.[45] A little later Miller told how he had used the fistulous tract to construct an anal outlet for a girl, age fifteen, with atresia ani vaginalis. He thought the procedure was simple and practical, and in this instance it gave the patient normal anal sphincter control.[46] By the time Miller moved to Iowa he had developed a fascia-pleating procedure for correction of cystocele, and he reported results obtained in one hundred cases. He said the size of the cystocele had ranged from " 'enormous,' the size of an average orange," to " 'small,' the size of a bantam's egg or plum," for food rather than a centimeter ruler was apparently available in the operating room. He had obtained complete cure in seventy-two instances and improvement in twenty-two. Miller recommended his procedure as a simple one; other operations were too complicated except for highly trained gynecologists.[47]

In 1935, after he had returned to Michigan, Miller demonstrated his interest in the history of his subject by beginning his description of his method for correcting a vesicovaginal fistula with a long, amply illustrated account of methods and results obtained since 1854. Sims, reporting in 1860, had obtained cures in 216 of 261 cases, and others had been successful between 64 and 95 percent of the time. Miller's own method, inversion of the bladder mucous membrane and eversion of the vaginal mucous membrane after extensive mobilization of both, had been successful in all fifteen of his cases.[48]

Miller deplored the long waste of time between the first appearance of symptoms and the diagnosis and definitive treatment of uterine cancer.[49] Adenocarcinoma and uterine fibroids coexist sufficiently often to be clinically important. Age, pelvic findings, and type of bleeding are not sufficient to permit diagnosis of adenocarcinoma associated with uterine fibroids, and consequently, Miller said, diagnostic curettage should always precede treatment of fibroids. Between 1931 and 1935 he had made the diagnosis of uterine fibroids in 244 patients. Of these, 102 had been admitted to the University Hospital for treatment, and in 12 of them coexisting carcinomas had been found. Miller said that if curettage reveals cancer, preoperative irradiation should be followed in five or six weeks by total hysterectomy and salpingo-oophorectomy.[50] Sometimes fracture of the neck of the femur followed irradiation for gynecological malignancies.[51] By 1940 Miller could report statistics in 183 cases of carcinoma of the body of the uterus. Of 156 patients he had treated by total hysterectomy, 68 had survived five years.[52]

Miller accumulated large experience.[53] Between 1934 and 1938 he dealt with 899 instances of extensive benign lesions of the cervix in older women. His method was to excise a cone of glandular tissue from the cervix with an electrical Bovie knife. Healthy tissue returned to the cervix in five to six weeks.[54] He saw approximately one hundred new cases of carcinoma of the cervix every year, and of the 676 cases seen between 1931 and 1938 he obtained five-year cures in 24 percent by radium irradiation.[55] Miller reported his surgical technique for correction of inversion of the uterus and of the vagina.[56] After another long historical introduction Miller described surgical treatment of 182 patients with complete perineal tears.[57] The average duration of the tear had been nine years, and many of the patients had been unsuccessfully operated upon by other surgeons. Miller insisted upon exact definition of results rather than the vague statement the patient had been "cured." He said function was "improved" when the patient had control over normal stools but no control over liquid stools or gas. Function was "restored" if she had complete control of feces but not entirely satisfactory control over gas. Using these criteria, Miller restored function in 87 percent of 38 patients in his latest series, improved function in 8 percent, and failed in 5 percent. He hoped that others would give equally thorough and candid descriptions of their methods and results.

Like other Michigan professors Miller traveled frequently in the 1930s to lecture to medical societies on his methods and results.[58] He followed Cabot's example by collaborating with a nurse in writing a thoroughly practical textbook, *Gynecology and Gynecologic Nursing,* that told the second scrub nurse exactly where to stand and how to hand the surgeon the instruments.[59]

Birth Control

In 1932 Miller told Harley Haynes, the director of the hospital, that he was teaching birth control, and he asked to be allowed to set up a birth control clinic for patients. Haynes did not want such a clinic; he was afraid of the criticism it would arouse.

Miller was chairman of the Section on Gynecology and Obstetrics of the Michigan State Medical Society that year, and in September of the next year he told members of the section assembled in Kalamazoo that it should undertake three projects. First, there were ninety thousand births in Michigan each year, but birth certificates were seriously defective. Physicians should work to have the certificates provide more information about pregnant and puerperal states and about complications of delivery. Second, the section should undertake controlled clinical trials of controversial procedures. Third, the section should give consideration to birth control. Miller was not arguing for or against it, he said, but it should be made a topic for discussion at the next annual meeting. Miller appointed a committee to report then.[60]

The secretary of the five-man committee was Norman Kretzschmar, Miller's assistant professor, and other members represented Catholic and Protestant opinion. Physicians in Michigan returned 1,846 questionnaires, and the replies were worked up by the university statistician. There were no differences in their attitudes according to specialty; 83.3 percent of physicians were in favor of birth control. There was likewise no difference when results were tabulated by county; rural and urban physicians thought alike. Of those objecting to birth control, 45 did so

on religious grounds, 14 thought birth control unnatural, and 11 said it promoted race suicide. Fifty-four percent (988) of the responding physicians prescribed birth control in their practice, and 659 said they gave information without specific reasons of health. One thousand twenty-three physicians thought there was a need to establish contraception clinics in their communities, and this opinion was stronger in the cities than in the country. Of the 532 who answered no to that question, 74 thought local physicians should be used, and 43 said clinics were already present in their communities. Sixty percent of the physicians teaching contraception recommended methods considered standard, and 39 percent prescribed diaphragms with spermicidal jelly.[61]

The committee also questioned heads of departments of obstetrics and gynecology throughout the country. Twenty-seven said they taught contraception, six said they did not, and five said they taught only general principles, whatever they are.

Kretzschmar, who wrote the report, said in conclusion that the report suggested a more general use of contraception might aid in decreasing the incidence of abortion with its attendant fetal and maternal morbidity and mortality. He appended the opinion of the Catholic member of the committee that the Catholic Church was unalterably opposed to any form of contraception but that Protestant churches were edging toward "natural" methods. Kretzschmar ended by thanking the anonymous physician for his generous offer of funds to cover the cost of the survey. Was Miller that anonymous physician?

Problems with Obstetrics: Patients and Money

Norman Miller inherited Reuben Peterson's problems with obstetrics, and in October 1934 he prepared "A Statement Concerning the Needs of the Obstetrics Division of the University of Michigan Medical School."[62] He said the teaching of theory and fundamentals had never been difficult. If anything, it had been overdone as a defensive reaction to the lack of clinical material. He documented that lack by comparing the number of students with the number of deliveries in the University Hospital year by year from 1902. In 1902 there had been 84 students and 38 deliveries; in 1933–34 there were 100 students and 257 deliveries. Approximately 25 percent of the current seniors never conducted a single delivery; 40 percent conducted 1 delivery; and 20 percent conducted 2. The remaining 15 percent managed to get 3 to 4 deliveries, usually by remaining on call during vacations or by special arrangements with other hospitals. The Detroit affiliation permitted students to see good as well as bad obstetrics, but it did not help much. In 1933–34, 32 students had rotated through the Woman's Hospital in Detroit and had seen 85 deliveries. Michigan was not meeting the State Board of Registration requirement of 6 deliveries a student.

Miller said the situation was appalling and an outrage against humanity. It was a crime against womanhood to expose a woman to such untrained physicians as graduated from Michigan. A recent graduate was not expected to be able to perform surgery but was expected to be fully qualified as an obstetrician. In the first place, Michigan needed an up-to-date maternity hospital. The present hospital, converted from the old Eye, Ear, Nose, and Throat Ward, was so much better than the previous one that its problems tended to be overlooked (fig. 18–3). In the second place, there should be provision for twelve hundred deliveries a year in the University Hospital.

A large number of expectant mothers applied to the University Hospital, but there was no money to pay their bills. At Miller's urgent solicitation the Rackham Fund gave fifteen thousand dollars in 1934, and in 1934–35 that money subsidized 472 obstetric cases in the University Hospital. That increased the number of deliveries 62 percent. After the Rackham money was exhausted Harley Haynes said that it had recently cost the hospital twelve thousand dollars for 250 deliveries. On 27 December 1937 Haynes ruled that as of 31 December 1937 free service was to stop. In 1941 Haynes raised the rates for paying obstetric patients without telling either Miller or Dean Furstenberg, and the dean said that that would cut the number of deliveries in half.

Obstetrical Teaching to 1941

Norman Miller used Reuben Peterson's *Manual* in teaching obstetrics to medical students. In 1937 Peterson published another edition, but by then he had moved away from Ann Arbor. In its preface he thanked Miller and his staff. The book differs from the earlier edition by recommending transfusion of blood in case of hemorrhage or 4 to 6 percent gum acacia followed by 6 percent glucose if blood were not available. Miller's name was added to a third edition published in 1943 but copyrighted in 1940, and Miller must have been responsible for its preparation. That edition has more frequent admonitions to transfuse blood. Blood was available in the University Hospital, for Fred Coller had established a blood bank in 1939. The book also contains six pages of outline on analgesia and anesthesia though both Peterson and Miller disapproved of what Miller called the fad and fancy of twilight sleep.[63]

Another fad Miller cautioned against was "the experiment with so-called prophylactic, academic, or outlet forceps. . . . Prophylactic outlet forceps, like its principal instigator, obstetric analgesia, is on probation awaiting the verdict of accumulated experience and time."[64] Joseph DeLee described the procedure in 1920: "When the head has passed the cervix and rests between the pillars of the levator ani and has begun, just begun, to part them and to stretch the fascia between them . . . the patient is put to sleep with ether, and a typical perineotomy . . . is performed. Under the minutest possible control of the fetal heart tones . . . the forceps are applied and delivery accomplished."[65] DeLee, who himself deplored the rapid spread of the craze for twilight sleep, cautioned against general adoption of his procedure on the grounds that conscienceless accoucheurs would hastily terminate labor "for their own selfish ends."[66] In 1938 Miller said the operation was unquestionably abused but that it did have a place provided it could be done with *safety* and *benefit*.

When Miller surveyed errors in gynecology and obstetrics in 1941, after castigating belief in the "excessive evil attributed to retrodisplacements of the uterus" and the "generous sacrifice of the uterus, tubes and ovaries, especially in middle-aged women," he said that error in obstetrics arose from perpetuation of obsolete standards. Good obstetrics was not cheap, but insurance companies allowed a doctor only twenty-five dollars for a delivery. Another error was home confinement. "Four walls and a light" did not make a delivery room. A student trained in home delivery and certified by a passing grade and graduation from a medical school contributed abundantly to the disrespect commonly displayed for obstetrics.[67]

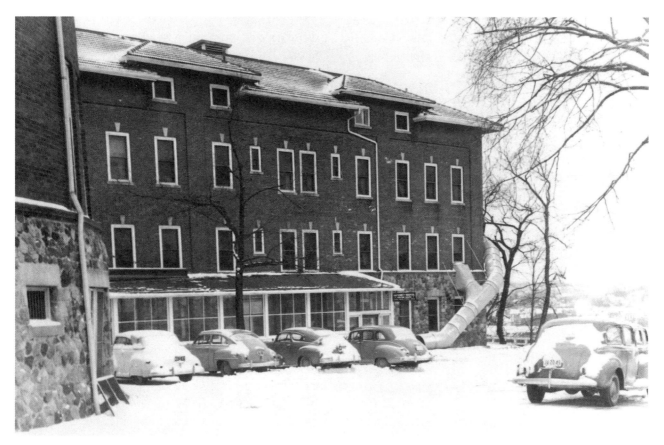

Fig. 18–3. Maternity Ward (Old Mat). (Courtesy of the Bentley Historical Library, University of Michigan, Medical School Records, Box 136, "Medical School Photographs, Buildings, Including Hospitals.")

Research

In contrast with the Department of Internal Medicine, where Newburgh and Wilson did their own research, Miller hired a man not qualified in medicine to do the research in the Department of Obstetrics and Gynecology. James T. Bradbury had received his doctor of science degree from Michigan in 1932 for work in the Department of Zoology on factors affecting lactation in mice.[68] He was to study endocrinology, called by Miller "the beautiful romantic young maiden of modern medicine, who keeps us dizzy with her therapeutically provocative gyrations."[69] The work was supported by grants from the Faculty Research Fund and a few thousand dollars from here and there.

Miller said that laboratory and clinical research are important, but he thought it not always fair to judge an individual's worth or the sum total of that person's ability by research productivity. It is a mistake to force a young physician to write papers in order to achieve recognition. Miller's strictures did not mean that his young faculty did not publish. Between 1931 and 1941 seventeen of them produced twenty-two papers on such topics as dermoid cyst of the ovary, so-called essential uterine bleeding, and the influence of iron and diet on the blood in pregnancy.

Bradbury helped the clinicians. For Udo Wile he measured androgens by the capon comb method and estrogens by the rat vaginal smear method in the urine of normal persons and of men and women with acne.[70] Wile and Bradbury thought there was an increase in androgen excretion in patients with acne and a decrease in estrogen excretion. In the custom of the times Wile and Bradbury made no statistical analysis of their data, and in fact the differences have no significance. Bradbury in conjunction with Sprague Gardiner measured uterine contractions of women six to nine days postpartum who were given posterior pituitary extract (Parke, Davis and Company).[71] Bradbury studied the masculinizing effect of crude gonadotropic extracts upon rats.[72] Willis Brown, a young gynecologist, wanted to see what the extracts did in human subjects, and he and Bradbury needed patients with well-known menstrual histories who could be studied over a long time. They used women in the Ypsilanti State Hospital who were "fairly stationary in regard to their psychoses." In those days the investigators did not need to obtain permission from an institutional review board, but they did seek permission from the hospital superintendent. Seven of the twelve women given daily injections of anterior pituitary-like extracts of pregnancy urine (Antuitrin-S) for four to six weeks showed no alteration in menstrual rhythm, and five had amenorrhea lasting one to five months.[73]

19
Pediatrics

Pediatrics at Michigan was under the administration of internal medicine by the time George Dock arrived in Ann Arbor in 1891. The American Pediatric Society had been founded in 1888 with Abraham Jacobi as its first president and William Osler as a member. Pediatricians were practicing and teaching in the large cities of the United States. Walter Christopher, a Cincinnati pediatrician, had been professor of medicine at Michigan for a year, and when he went to Chicago in 1891 he became a leader of a group of fellow pediatricians. Dock as a student of Osler did not neglect children, and the practice of pediatrics was not separate from the practice of internal medicine at Michigan until well after 1900. Love M. Palmer, Alonzo B. Palmer's widow, gave the university twenty thousand dollars in 1901 to build a children's ward on Catherine Street, and the regents added five thousand dollars. The Palmer Ward was ready in 1903, but for a while its upper floor was a nurses' home, and the roentgenology laboratory was housed in the basement along with David Murray Cowie's laboratory for milk analysis. In the press for space, the ward's seventy-five beds were shared with orthopaedic surgery, oral surgery, dermatology, and gynecology patients so that in 1916 only twenty beds were available for general pediatric patients.[1] At times beds for children were placed in the glass-enclosed corridor connecting the East and West Wards of the University Hospital, and Cowie thought the need for children's beds was a major factor in persuading the legislature to appropriate money for the new hospital.

From 1913 to 1933 children's beds were kept full by the legislative provision that children were to be treated at the University Hospital at public expense (fig. 19–1). In addition to the funds for erection of the Palmer Ward, Mrs. Palmer had given an endowment of $15,000, and its $750 a year income helped to pay for children's care. Additional support came from several charities. By 1933 another act of the state legislature provided that care could be given in other hospitals at public expense, and the number of children coming to the University Hospital was reduced. Cowie thought the act had dealt a serious blow to his effort to develop a children's clinic adequate for teaching.

Cowie's assumption of responsibility for the subspecialty pediatrics was recognized in 1905, when he was given the title instructor in pediatrics (fig. 19–2). "Diseases of Children" had been listed as a division of the Department of Internal Medicine in the Medical School

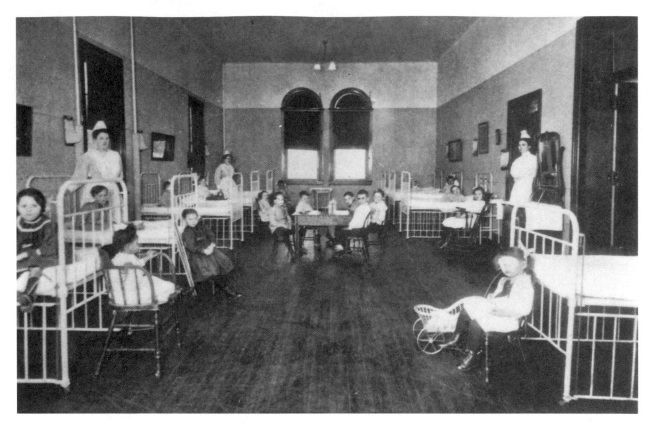

Fig. 19–1. Pediatric patients in the Palmer Ward, Catherine Street Hospital. (Courtesy of the Bentley Historical Library, University of Michigan, Biomedical Communications Records, Box 5, "Misc. Wards.")

Annual Announcement since 1901.[2] Cowie held various titles within Internal Medicine until 1921, when he was made head of an independent department with the rank of professor. At that time the parent department had been without a permanent head for three years. Cowie remained in charge of pediatrics, with a brief leave in 1908 to work with Ludolf Krehl in Heidelberg, until he died of myocardial infarction shortly after midnight on 27 January 1940 at the age of sixty-eight.

Cowie was in general private practice from his graduation from medical school in 1896. He died in his own twelve-bed "Cowie Hospital" at 320 South Division Street, a hospital he had opened in 1912. The hospital included chemical and bacteriological laboratories, and papers published by Cowie and the assistants he employed were footnoted "From D. M. Cowie's private laboratory."[3]

Michigan's Pediatrician

David Murray Cowie had been born into a medical family in Moncton, New Brunswick, in 1872. He came early to Michigan for college education in Battle Creek and medical education in Ann Arbor, but he expressed his interest in his homeland late in life by making a substantial collection of books on the history of Acadia. His wife gave the collection on her husband's death to the University of Michigan Clements Library.[4]

As a medical student Cowie took care of animals for Arthur Cushny in pharmacology, and he worked in George Dock's clinical laboratory. For about ten years Cowie worked on problems of infection and gastroenterology,[5] and he dealt with general medical problems. Once, for example, a very debilitated woman was admitted to the University Hospital with the hopeless diagnosis of an enormous abdominal

Not Just Any Medical School

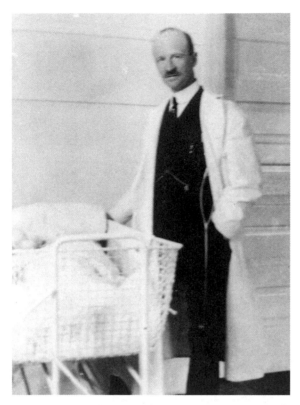

Fig. 19–2. David Murray Cowie, 1910. (Courtesy of the Bentley Historical Library, University of Michigan, Medical School Records, Box 136, "Photographs, General, Faculty, Individuals.")

tumor. Cowie waited impatiently for a photographer to take a picture of the patient's distended abdomen, and then he cured her of her tumor by catheterizing her bladder and withdrawing two quarts and half a pint of urine.[6]

Cowie's Staff and Courses

Cowie usually had an assistant, one or two interns, and an instructor to help him after he became head of the pediatric section in 1905. A social worker joined his staff in 1914. After he became head of an independent department in 1921 he had two or three interns and three or four instructors. In 1925 the new University Hospital and the Contagious Hospital provided 110 beds for children, and there were 90 more beds for pediatric surgery patients. Consequently, Cowie's staff grew to two assistant professors, three or four instructors, two or more interns, a dietician, a chemist, and a technician.

The Medical School *Annual Announcement* described the steady increase in courses in pediatrics:

from lectures and demonstration clinics twice a week in 1905–6 to lectures, laboratories, and ward work occupying 140 to 150 hours in both the junior and senior years in the 1930s. The babies from the obstetrical ward who had been born to unmarried mothers were artificially fed, and each medical student was expected to become familiar with the practice of bottle-feeding. What Cowie taught about that will be described in the section "Teaching Infant Feeding." Students were assigned cases to be presented before the class, and while doing ward work they learned how to perform sensitization tests for tuberculosis and diphtheria, how to give serum by intraspinal injection, and how to transfuse by way of sinus puncture. The pediatric program looked good on paper, but student perception was different. The student committee report of 1934 said that the majority of students thought pediatric training was inadequate and that except for instruction in contagious diseases the work was haphazardly organized. The Executive Committee reached an even harsher conclusion just before Cowie's death.

Adult Gastric Secretion and Emptying

Perhaps Cowie's problem with his own peptic ulcer, a problem causing him to be bedridden for eight months in 1910 while his wife took care of his private practice, encouraged him to conduct a study of gastric secretion. He thought diseases of the stomach are more often than not the result of neuroses, and he took up the problem of the nervous control of gastric secretion in adults. Cowie knew of von Noorden's work on the occurrence of hyperacidity in melancholia,[7] and he may have known that Carl Anton Ewald, a leading German gastroenterologist, thought "hyperacidity and hypersecretion of the gastric juice [are] sensory neuroses of the secretory function."[8] Accordingly, Cowie went to the Michigan Asylum for the Insane in Kalamazoo where he might find hypersecretion in neurotic patients. He performed gastric analyses on twenty-eight female patients, thirteen with melancholia, ten with dementia, three with mania, one with hysteroepilepsy, and one with hypochondria.[9]

Cowie gave the asylum patients a test meal composed of sixty to eighty grams of white bread without crust and three hundred milliliters of water. Cowie knew that Walter B. Cannon had shown that salivary digestion of carbohydrate continues in the stomach, and he examined gastric contents recovered by stomach tube for all carbohydrate digestion products down to dextrose and maltose. Cowie removed small samples of gastric contents every five or ten minutes for an hour in order to estimate gastric secretion. He titrated each sample to the end point of Töpfer's reagent, about pH 3.5, to determine free acid and then to the end point of phenolphthalein to determine total acidity. Cowie stated that the normal acidity of a sample obtained at the end of an hour was between fifty and sixty, but he did not state his units. They were the "clinical units" defined by Ewald, and they also happen to be millinormality.[10] Cowie also examined gastric contents for fermentation products: acetic, lactic, and butyric acids. He determined the peptic power of gastric contents by Mett's method in which a length of a column of coagulated egg white in a small glass tube is measured before and after immersion in gastric juice for twenty-four hours.

Cowie had no means of measuring the volume of gastric contents or their rate of emptying, and he had trouble defining hypersecretion on the basis of acid concentration alone. Ewald had said that the normal concentration of acid one hour after a breakfast test meal like Cowie's is between forty and sixty-five clinical units and that hyperacidity begins when the amount of acid is between sixty and seventy.[11] Using Ewald's criterion, Cowie found hypersecretion in seventeen of his twenty-eight asylum subjects. In two, total acidity was over one hundred clinical units. Hypersecretion could be the result of functional neurosis.[12]

During his work at the Kalamazoo Asylum for the Insane Cowie repeated his gastric secretion measurements many times on adult patients in the University Hospital.[13] At the University Hospital, the test breakfast was thirty-five grams of granose (whole wheat processed into crisp flakes, John Harvey Kellogg, Battle Creek, Michigan) and three hundred milliliters of water. Granose could not be swallowed without being thoroughly mixed with saliva. He found in "stomach cases" admitted to Dock's clinic that secretory response to a protein meal is greater than that to a carbohydrate meal. However, "[m]ilk, a nitrogenous food, has little stimulating effect; it binds quite large amounts of acid and will often take the place of antacids for the relief of pain."[14] Otherwise Cowie recommended a diet rich in carbohydrate as treatment for hyperacidity.

Cowie learned from reading Ivan Petrovich Pavlov that fat inhibits gastric secretion in experimental animals,[15] and he undertook a long series of experiments on the effect of olive oil on gastric secretion in humans.[16] In this series, he gave each of thirty-two University Hospital patients thirty grams of shredded-wheat biscuit followed by three hundred milliliters of water, and he recovered samples at five-, ten-, or fifteen-minute intervals. At the end of an hour he washed out the stomach with a known volume of water in order to recover residual contents. After performing control experiments as many as fifteen times on one patient he gave one or two ounces of olive oil before, with, or after a meal. He determined the effect of olive oil in one patient sixteen times. Secretion and gastric emptying were reduced when olive oil was given before or with a meal, but olive oil given after a meal for some strange reason had no effect upon previously occurring secretion or emptying. The effect of oil was temporary, for it had no effect upon a subsequent meal unaccompanied by oil.

Gastric Secretion and Emptying in the Newborn

Cowie made 107 observations on fourteen breast-fed infants and twenty-eight bottle-fed infants from one day to two months old in order to determine the stimulating effect of food in normal infants and how secretion and emptying are altered by addition of alkali to the feeding formula. He did not have to obtain prior approval from an institutional review board, for there was none. The formula was introduced by stomach tube, and samples were removed for analysis at fifteen- or twenty-minute intervals for as long as ninety minutes. Most samples contained only a trace of free acid and from three to sixty-five millinormal combined acid. Rennet was active from the first day of life, for curds were found in all samples. Pepsinogen was invariably present, but in most instances there was not enough free acid to permit peptic digestion of casein. Sodium citrate or lime-water, a solution of calcium hydroxide, was added to the formula to control the acidity of the milk that had been standing without adequate refrigeration. Cowie found that, when the formula was made alkaline to phenolphthalein, casein did not coagulate in the baby's stomach and that gastric acidity did not rise to control values.[17]

Cowie knew about Cannon's theory of acid control of the pyloric sphincter: that acid in the antrum causes the sphincter to open and that acid in the duodenum causes it to close. He attempted to identify acid control of gastric emptying in his infant patients. Because Cowie had no way of knowing the acidity of duodenal contents, he could not distinguish between the effect of acid in the gastric antrum and acid in the duodenum. All he could do was to see whether neutralization or acidification of a meal slows or hastens emptying. He found that when the formula was neutralized with sodium citrate, emptying was delayed. On ten occasions in one baby he gave seventy-five milliliters of fluid by stomach tube and recovered its gastric contents forty-five minutes later. When he gave seventy-five milliliters of water none remained, but when he gave seventy-five milliliters of twenty-five millinormal hydrochloric acid he recovered forty-five milliliters. As a control, he twice gave a nearly neutral formula, recovering zero or three milliliters. When Cowie titrated the formula to thirty millinormal combined acidity but zero free acidity before giving it, the stomach emptied completely in forty-five minutes, but when he made the formula sixty millinormal in combined acidity and ten millinormal in free acidity he recovered forty-five milliliters.

Cowie attempted to distinguish anatomical and reflex pyloric stenosis in infants by adding 2.5 grams of sodium bicarbonate to a meal fed to each of six patients with grossly delayed gastric emptying, and he compulsively repeated his observations thirty-three times on one patient.[18] In all six infants there was little gastric emptying in an hour when the meal was given without alkali, but there was complete emptying when bicarbonate was added to the formula. Cowie concluded the duodenal closing reflex had predominated, causing what he called pseudopyloric stenosis.

The Intestinal Gradient

Cowie was impressed by Walter Alvarez's idea that an intestinal gradient of activity controls movement of gastrointestinal contents,[19] and he himself did some experiments confirming Alvarez's observations that the frequency of intestinal contraction decreases from duodenum to ileum.[20] He also demonstrated a metabolic gradient by measuring the time it took for an isolated segment to turn Locke's solution acid to phenol red. Cowie applied the gradient idea in treating some infants who vomited their liquid formula. He thought pinching the gut reverses the intestinal

gradient and causes reverse peristalsis, hence vomiting. The liquid formula was too bland to stimulate the intestine. Thick cereal heightens the gradient, starts orthograde peristalsis, and therefore should stop vomiting. Cowie's treatment worked, for babies fed thick cereal no longer vomited.[21]

Infant Feeding: Milk

Cowie had to deal with problems of milk supply, the composition of cow's milk as compared with mother's milk, the constitution of formulas, and the amounts fed.

Milk was delivered to Ann Arbor from as far as fifty miles away, but Cowie thought milk was delivered more quickly than to cities.[22] Cream was seldom more than twenty-four hours old in Ann Arbor, whereas it might be three days old in Detroit. The local health officer and staff were responsible for seeing that milk was clean, and the health officer had the authority to revoke the license of a dairy that did not, after a warning, reach acceptable standards. Herds were tested for tuberculosis, but Cowie preferred pasteurized or sterilized milk to certified milk. He said pasteurization or sterilization could be done at home.[23] He had seen cases of abdominal tuberculosis caused by unpasteurized milk certified to be tuberculosis free. The authorities also enforced the regulation that milk delivered to Ann Arbor must have the legal minimum of 3.5 percent fat and total acidity not over twenty-five.[24] As usual, the units of acidity were not specified. The acidity, as Cowie expressed it, is the titratable acidity to the phenolphthalein end point given as the number of grams of lactic acid per hundred milliliters of sample multiplied by one hundred. The titratable acidity is not entirely lactic acid, for proteins neutralize a small amount of alkali used for titration. That could be accounted for by subtracting ten from the final figure. Milk does not taste sour until the acidity is over thirty.

Cowie published analyses in the 1900s of the fat content of milk from fifty-two local dairies. Fat was 4 percent or more in twenty-five samples, between 3.5 percent and 4 percent in seven samples, and below 3.5 percent in eight. One sample had 10 percent fat, but the inspector detected fraud. Low fat was usually the result of poor feeding of the cows, but sometimes it was the result of dilution by skim milk. In the 1900s milk could not be refrigerated adequately on the farm or during delivery, and iceboxes in the home did not cool the milk well. As milk remained near room temperature bacteria multiplied, and titratable acidity rose. Cowie's assistant in his private laboratory found that the bacterial count increased in geometrical progression but that there was no constant relation between bacterial count and titratable acidity.[25] Local dairies usually bottled milk soon after milking and then put the remaining milk in tanks. Inspectors found more contamination in milk transported in tanks, for the tanks were not thoroughly cleaned between uses.

Cow's milk contains approximately three times as much protein as mother's milk, and cow's milk was diluted before being fed. Dilution reduced the fat and sugar content, and pediatricians such as L. Emmett Holt published tables showing the proportions of cow's milk, cream, and sugar to be mixed to obtain a satisfactory formula.[26] Cowie said that many doctors carried cards in their pockets bearing tables from which they read the formula they thought appropriate for a given child. Cowie himself used gravity cream, that is, cream that rose to the top of the bottle, rather than centrifugal cream. Many physicians used lactose rather than cane sugar, but Cowie thought cane sugar satisfactory except in rare instances of intolerance. Cow's milk has a higher total salt content and even when diluted has more calcium than mother's milk. Calcium was often increased by the practice of adding limewater to the formula to neutralize its acid. Cow's milk is very low in iron, but Cowie made no special provision for increasing it. After about 1915 he was aware of the need for accessory food factors, but he thought milk contains enough fat-soluble vitamins. However, if milk had been pasteurized or boiled its vitamin C content was low. Cowie recommended boiling, for in addition to making milk safer, boiling made the curds smaller and more easily digestible.[27] Therefore, Cowie regularly supplemented the formula with a daily teaspoon of orange or tomato juice.

Teaching Infant Feeding

Cowie described his method of infant feeding in 1912.[28] At that time he was using Holt's percentage method, and he gave each student a table showing the percentage of fat, sugar, and protein in twenty-four mixtures together with the caloric value of each component and mixture. For example, a mixture of 2.5 percent fat, 5 percent sugar, and 1 percent pro-

tein contains 6.97, 6.15, and 1.23 calories, respectively, from each for a total of 14.35 calories per ounce. An infant should receive 45 calories per pound for the first six months, declining to 40 or 36 in the latter months of the first year. Cowie thought the student must be impressed with the need to meet the basic protein requirement, and he supplied another table showing that a child two weeks old requires 0.68 grams of protein per pound of body weight and that a child two to twelve months old requires 1.10 to 1.5 grams of protein per pound.

For a class exercise Cowie gave each student a blank chart and another table showing the weight in pounds and ounces of a particular child for fifty-six days from birth. He told the students to calculate the energy required each day. When plotted on the chart, the data gave the "energy line." Then, using the composition and number of ounces for the formula fed, the students calculated and plotted the calories the child had been given. The child began to lose weight in the sixth week, and Cowie required the students to discuss in writing the probable reasons, for example, simple dyspepsia as the result of overfeeding according to the energy line.

The exercise involved one and a half hours, and in the next class Cowie gave the students a more complicated example of a child who lost 1.5 pounds beginning in the third week of life. Thereafter Cowie took up the problem of sugar tolerance, illustrating it with data of one child who tolerated large amounts of lactose and of one who did not. He took a case of salt excess from the literature: the problem of a child fed milk from which the protein had been removed (Eiweissmilch). The problem was further illustrated by an instance in which a child had been given fifty grams of 1 percent sodium chloride solution and one hundred grams of 4 percent sodium chloride solution by gavage on two successive days. The child's temperature had risen following the four grams of sodium chloride. In contrast, another child given four grams of sodium bicarbonate had no reaction. Therefore it is the chloride and not the sodium that causes "salt fever."

After the students had completed these exercises and some more homework they were ready to go on the wards and to follow their cases. Cowie said: "Since developing this chart method an interest in even the usually uninteresting cases has been awakened. The student feels that he is really doing something and although his visits night and morning to the ward are kept track of, the tendency to bolt has practically disappeared."[29]

By 1923 Cowie taught a simplified method of feeding he had used for the last seven or eight years. He still calculated the energy line at 45 calories per pound, and he said that after it had been reached 30 calories should be added for optimum growth. All upward additions should be gradual. Now Cowie used whole milk as delivered from the dairy, for it contained 4 percent fat and 21 calories an ounce. An infant weighing ten pounds would require 450 calories a day, and if 1 ounce of sugar containing 120 calories were added to the formula, 15.5 ounces of milk would supply the remaining 330 calories. The rest of the formula was to be made up with water. The amount of the formula to be diluted was based on the rule that an infant's stomach will hold 1 ounce more than it is months old, up to 8 ounces, 8 ounces being the maximum size feeding for the first year. The formula should be pasteurized or boiled, and Cowie preferred boiling. Orange juice or tomato juice should be given to ward off scurvy. Vegetables and cereal should be added after the eighth month.

Managing the Contagious Hospital

The new Contagious Hospital for which the city of Ann Arbor had provided twenty-five thousand dollars was occupied on 9 August 1914 (fig. 19–3). It had been planned to house patients with all varieties of contagious diseases. Reuben Peterson and David Murray Cowie had visited Providence, Rhode Island, where the practice of the aseptic method in the contagious pavilion of the City Hospital demonstrated that cross infection could be avoided. First, each of the twelve rooms on the main floor of the hospital opened onto a wide porch through a door wide enough to admit a hospital bed. An infectious patient could be brought in through the door without coming into contact with other patients or could be given the benefit of fresh air during clement weather. Each person, nurse, staff, and students, entering a patient's room put on a gown and on leaving thoroughly washed his or her hands and arms. The patient's dishes were sterilized after he or she had eaten, and nightclothes and bedding were also put in a bag that was sterilized.[30]

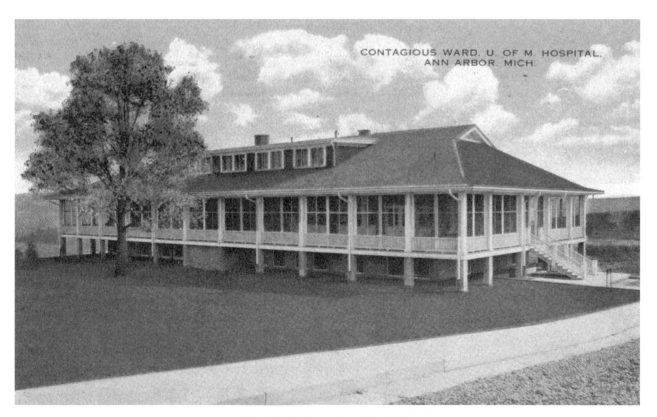

Fig. 19–3. Contagious Hospital

In the first eleven months the hospital housed 223 patients, referred chiefly from the city, the University Health Service, and the Palmer Ward. There were 29 cases each of chicken pox and mumps, 26 of scarlet fever, 27 of acute tonsillitis, and 49 of diphtheria. Thirty-five nurses served an average of forty-six days each on the ward, and twenty-two doctors, in addition to Cowie's staff of three, visited patients more or less regularly. In addition, eighty students made over eight hundred visits to the bedside. Cowie's intern contracted scarlet fever, but no others, including the janitor who handled the infected linen and the maids who handled the dirty dishes, were infected. Five cases of cross infection occurred among the patients, and Cowie carefully traced the cause of each. Cross infection could not be traced to students, but nurses and interns were most likely responsible. One nurse with faulty technique "terminated her services in the hospital." As a rule, if a nurse broke technique she was reassigned to another service.[31]

The aseptic ritual continued through the 1930s, but it was not well observed when a transporter took an infectious child in a closed cart to the main hospital for X-ray or other examination. Students leaving the Contagious Hospital through the ground floor walked over cocoa mats saturated with mercuric chloride to prevent carrying the infection with them on their shoes, but despite such precautions an occasional epidemic of chicken pox or measles swept from one end of the pediatric ward in the University Hospital to the other.

Dealing with Epidemics

Between 23 September and 11 November 1918, 131 patients with influenza were admitted to Cowie's service in the University Hospital. The first patient, a soldier visiting from Massachusetts, came in nine days before the epidemic became general. Local patients were mostly students in the Army Training Corps and in the nurses' training school. There were three deaths among patients with already established pneumonia, and there were eight deaths among those who developed pneumonia in the hospital. Cowie concluded that all deaths from influenza resulted from bronchopneumonia.[32]

Cowie was impressed by symptoms resembling adrenal insufficiency in his patients: asthenia, prostration, and lowered blood pressure. Others had seen hemorrhages in the adrenal glands of persons dying of influenza, and in six of Cowie's patients coming to autopsy there was adrenal hypoplasia but no hemorrhages. In 1918 there was still no generally recognized clear distinction between the roles of the adrenal medulla and adrenal cortex, and despite his large caseload Cowie found time to test the effect of epinephrine upon blood pressure and blood sugar in some of his patients. He concluded that administration of epinephrine was not therapeutically useful.[33]

During the 1931 Michigan poliomyelitis epidemic Cowie took care of 125 patients in the University Hospital. Eighty-one were admitted in the preparalytic stage of the disease and 44 in the paralytic stage. All patients in the preparalytic stage were given intravenous infusions of serum or whole blood from convalescent poliomyelitis patients, whole blood from adults who had not had the disease, or a combination of all three. The dose was 50 to 200 milliliters, but one patient received 325 milliliters of whole blood. One of the 81 patients was not under Cowie's care, but of the ones whose course he observed, 77 did not develop paralysis. Of the 3 who did become paralyzed, involvement was slight, and none was paralyzed when Cowie reported the cases in 1934.[34]

Rabies vaccine was regularly prepared in the Bacteriology Department's Pasteur Institute by H. W. Emerson, and Emerson made a similar poliomyelitis vaccine for Cowie, a 5 percent emulsion of cord tissue preserved in 0.7 percent phenol. Cowie vaccinated three monkeys with daily increasing doses over twenty-eight or twenty-nine days, and when he injected a paralytic dose of poliomyelitis virus provided by Simon Flexner into the frontal lobes of the monkeys, two of the three survived. The two surviving monkeys were not protected against a second inoculation of the virus. One of four unvaccinated monkeys inoculated with the virus survived, but Cowie thought it had been improperly inoculated.[35]

Therapeutic Adventures

Cowie had used nonspecific protein therapy in treating patients with arthritis, and he used it for his patients with influenzal pneumonia. One patient, Dr. H., had developed pneumonia after being admitted on 5 November 1918. Following an intravenous injection of 500 million dead typhoid bacilli Dr. H. had a chill followed by a fever of 106 degrees Fahrenheit. He recovered, as did three others similarly treated. Five died.[36]

Cowie reported his early experience with arthritis in a paper containing thirty-two pages of detailed tables and eleven figures, all to describe ten patients.[37] Some had been given as many as ten successive intravenous injections of typhoid vaccine, and all patients had reacted violently with paroxysms similar to those of malaria. Leukopenia was followed by leukocytosis, and Cowie thought the leukopenia was the result of migration of leukocytes into the tissues. Some patients had improved, and some had not.[38]

Cowie frequently used similar nonspecific protein therapy in treating infections.[39] He injected horse serum into seven children with pyuria, obtaining cure in one and improvement in the others.[40] Later in the 1920s when bacteriophage therapy was being used by many others, Cowie was more successful in treating urinary infections. He isolated bacteriophage from stools of patients with pyelitis, chicken pox, measles, and typhoid fever, but his attempt to cure a child with pyelitis with the lytic principle was unsuccessful.[41] Cowie improved his technique by adapting the bacteriophage to the patient's particular strain of infecting bacterium. He isolated bacteriophage from sewage, and then he repeatedly fed it with nine-hour cultures of *Bacillus coli* or *B. typhosus* found in the patient's urine. After the bacteriophage had been built up by feeding and had been tested on agar plates or in broth, Cowie injected one, two, or three milliliters of filtrate subcutaneously into the patient's arm, repeating the injection daily three to eight times. In eighteen instances the primary infection was promptly terminated, and it did not return. Chronic infections were more resistant, but eleven were cured or improved, so Cowie said.[42]

The Beginning of Goiter Prophylaxis in Michigan

In 1924 R. M. Olin, the Michigan commissioner of health, wrote: "That the state of Michigan has an abnormally high percentage of persons affected with goiter has been a matter of common knowledge for years, but of no great concern either to the public or to the medical profession."[43] If the public were indifferent, by 1924 health authorities and alert members of the medical profession were aware of the magnitude of endemic goiter in the state and of the recently demonstrated means by which it could be prevented.

The State Department of Health had begun to collect data on the incidence of simple goiter in 1919, and in 1924 a systematic survey of children in four Michigan counties had been completed. The counties formed a diagonal band from Houghton County in the far northwest of the Upper Peninsula through Wexford and Midland Counties to Macomb County in the southeast corner. Houghton County is almost completely surrounded by the iodine-free waters of Lake Superior, and water in Wexford County also contains no iodine. There was some but not much iodine in water used in Midland and Macomb Counties. Incidence of goiter was 64.4 percent in Houghton County, 55.6 percent in Wexford, 32.7 percent in Midland, and 26.0 percent in Macomb. By this time, largely as the result of the work of David Marine, then a pathologist at Western Reserve in Cleveland, Ohio, iodine deficiency had been accepted as the cause of simple goiter.[44] Marine had deduced that iodine deficiency causes goiter in fish and mammals, and he had proved that administration of small amounts of iodine prevents the occurrence of goiter in many species and the involution of goiters in animals having them.[45] The last glaciation had scoured iodine-containing soil from the rocks underlying Michigan, and all analyses of Michigan water supported the correlation of the incidence of goiter with iodine deficiency.[46]

At 11:30 A.M. on 7 December 1922 Marine told the Second Annual Conference of Health Officers and Public Health Nurses in Lansing, Michigan, how to prevent goiter by giving schoolchildren one hundred to two hundred milligrams of iodine in any form twice a year. He had used the method since 1917, and the results had shown what Marine often said: endemic goiter is the easiest known disease to prevent.[47] At the next year's conference O. P. Kimball described the experiment that Marine, with Kimball's help and with the full cooperation of the school board and with the approval of the county medical society, had conducted in Akron, Ohio.[48] Girls in grades 5 through 12, with written permission of their parents, had filled sanitary drinking cups with water to each of which the teacher had added a teaspoon of sodium iodide solution. The teacher was careful to see that the girls actually drank the mixture. Of 2,190 girls taking two grams of iodide twice a year, in ten divided doses over two weeks, five had developed goiters. In the 1,182 whose thyroid was enlarged at the beginning, the gland had decreased in size in 773. There had not been a single incidence of hyperthyroidism among the girls, and the bugaboo of jodbasedow raised by Kocher[49] had been laid to rest, at least for the girls with early goiter. Among the 2,305 girls not taking iodide, the thyroid gland enlarged in 495, and of the 1,049 among them with initially enlarged thyroids the gland shrank in only 145.[50] Kimball told his Michigan audience that similar means of preventing endemic goiter among schoolchildren were already being used in Switzerland, Italy, and New Zealand and that like measures were being adopted in New York, West Virginia, Ohio, Indiana, Wisconsin, Minnesota, Utah, Oregon, and Washington.

Kimball had told the same story to the Michigan State Medical Society on 8 June 1922, when the society held its annual meeting in Flint, and he emphasized the fact that he was talking about simple goiter, not hyperthyroidism, not Graves' disease, and not Basedow's disease. He spoke in a symposium together with surgeons and internists, and the immense discussion following the talk demonstrated that his hearers were more interested in the conflict between surgeons and internists over treatment of goiter than in its prevention.[51]

The Pediatric Section of the society had been organized the same day, and F. B. Miner, its chairman, appreciated how Kimball "and Dr. Marine had worked out a definite method of prevention of simple goiter, through prophylactic treatment of children."[52] Miner proposed an advisory committee of the Pediatric Section, and in his enthusiasm he assigned the committee the duties of setting standards for artificial feeding of infants, of proposing improved care of undernourished and pretuberculous children, of examining the care of nervous and mentally deficient children, and of devising a method of procedure and treatment in the prevention of simple goiter in children. Ex officio members of the committee were Thomas B. Cooley, the incoming chairman of the section, and Lafon Jones of Flint. Others were Miner himself, Guy L. Bliss of Kalamazoo, F. J. Larnard of Grand Rapids, and D. J. Levy of Detroit. David Murray Cowie was chairman of the committee.[53]

Putting Iodine in Table Salt

Cowie did not assemble his committee until after he had been gently chided by Lafon Jones in December for his long delay.[54] When the committee met on the afternoon of 24 January 1923 in the Michigan Union its members decided to concentrate their efforts on the prevention of simple goiter, and they set themselves the task of deciding the best means of assuring an adequate intake of iodine.

By this time there had been many programs in which schoolchildren had been given periodic doses of sodium iodide in chocolate. Kimball preferred that as being more acceptable to children. Because only a tiny fraction of water supplied to a city is drunk or used in cooking, iodination of the general water supply would be too expensive and wasteful.[55] Marine had told the Michigan Public Health Conference: "Perhaps ultimately the household use of iodized or sea salt will become the preferred plan."[56] One Swiss canton had begun to use table salt containing ten milligrams of iodide per kilogram, and eighteen cantons used it in the next year with the result that 55 percent of the Swiss population received iodine in table salt. In fact, two cantons allowed sale of iodine-free salt only by prescription.[57] Consequently, Cowie was following the current trend when he talked to his committee about the possibility of adding a small amount of iodide to table salt.

After dinner Cowie introduced William J. Hale to the committee, and Hale spoke on the same subject. Hale was a Harvard doctor of philosophy in chemistry who, after the customary German training, had risen from instructor to professor of chemistry at the University of Michigan. In 1917 he had married one of Herbert Dow's daughters, and he had become director of organic research at the Dow Chemical Company in Midland, Michigan. The foundation of the company had been laid on the separation of halides, and Hale was in the position to speak authoritatively on the iodination of salt. As a result, the committee's work was concentrated on iodination of table salt to reach the general population. The committee became known as the Committee on Iodized Salt.

Cowie waited more than eight months to call the next meeting on 5 September 1923. In the meantime one member had worked up data from the Michigan Agricultural College on iodine in Michigan water, soil, and food. Another member passed on the word that the data on iodine collected by McClendon in Minnesota were the most comprehensive.[58] Cowie himself had been busy estimating the average salt consumption of a Michigan family, his own, finding it to be about four to five pounds a year. He concluded that two milligrams a week intake of sodium iodide would be both adequate and safe.

Cowie rashly planned to have a bill introduced into the state legislature requiring that all salt used for food in Michigan contain a prescribed percentage of iodine. Fortunately, he brought Clyde J. Holmes to the meeting. Holmes was an attorney for the Consumers Power Company and an expert lobbyist. He persuaded Cowie and the committee that any attempt to mandate the use of iodine in salt would arouse formidable opposition and would certainly be defeated. He advised an educational campaign through the press and an agreement with the manufacturers of table salt. Means of educating the public, not only through the press, were at hand in the Extension Division of the university, which in concert with the State Department of Health had provided 196 lectures on public health problems to audiences totaling twenty-six thousand persons in 1922. W. D. Henderson, the division's director, was in chronic need of more physicians to lecture on health matters, particularly on goiter. Cowie's committee helped to fill the need by preparing an outline and by shipping sets of lantern slides to speakers in all parts of the state. Some 170 doctors told luncheon clubs, women's clubs, parent-teacher associations, and schools about the efficacy of small amounts of iodine, and as a result Michigan citizens, for the most part, were ready to accept iodized salt when it appeared.

In the next two months Cowie introduced himself to the "salt men," representatives of companies refining and distributing salt in Michigan. He and his committee met several times with the Salt Producers Association in Detroit. William Hale helped by explaining how iodine could be added to mass-produced salt without detriment. At that time salt was usually treated with 1 percent magnesia so that it would run freely in any weather, and sodium iodide could be added at the same time as magnesia. No one knew exactly how much iodine to use, and Hale suggested that at first sodium iodide be added in a minimum of 0.01 percent and a maximum of 0.02 percent. The salt producers, with the exception of the Morton Salt Company, became anxious to put iodized salt on the market. They planned to begin a campaign on Sunday, 16 March 1924. They wanted to say in the newspapers that the amount of iodine contained in the package was that recommended by the State Medical Society, but they planned to go ahead whether or not they had the endorsement. Cowie drafted a referendum to be presented to the society's executive council on 12 March 1924, and passage of the referendum by the council would have

the effect of endorsing iodized salt on behalf of the State Medical Society. On 15 March F. C. Warnhuis, the society's secretary, telephoned Cowie that nine members of the council had voted for the referendum and three against. Two members had not been heard from. Iodized salt went on sale in Michigan on 1 May 1924 with the label:

This salt contains 0.01% [or 0.02%] sodium iodide, the amount approved by the Council and advocated by the Pediatric Section of the Michigan State Medical Society as a preventative of goiter. *Individuals using this salt must not take any other preparation of iodine without the advice of their physician.* TO BE EFFECTIVE, THIS SALT MUST BE USED FOR COOKING AS WELL AS FOR TABLE USE.

The Morton Salt Company joined the others in September (fig. 19–4).

Iodized Salt in Michigan; The Result

In 1930 the largest distributor had shipped 58,643 cases of iodized salt and only 7,057 cases of plain table salt. Other distributors said they shipped eight cases of iodized salt for every one of the other kind.[59]

Cowie reported the results of six surveys of the iodine content of salt bought over the counter throughout Michigan.[60] In sixty-three samples obtained in the first survey in 1926 the content found in the laboratory of the Michigan Department of Health ranged from 0.006 to 0.03 percent, and in almost all instances the content was lower than that claimed on the label. By the time of the last survey in 1938–39 the content was much more uniform, but it still tended to be low. In thirty-five of forty-four instances the state analyst found a substantial fraction, sometimes more than half, of the iodine claimed on the label to be in the pasteboard of the carton.[61] Cowie said the amount of iodine actually present in the salt was seldom below the level his committee had estimated to be sufficient to prevent goiter in children. The problem of the loss of iodine from salt was solved in 1940 by chemists at the University of Wisconsin who added reducing agents.

In October and November 1935 physicians working for Cowie's committee and the State Board of Health and with the assistance of O. P. Kimball examined schoolchildren in the same four Michigan counties surveyed in 1924. Those making the new survey attempted to discover whether each child used

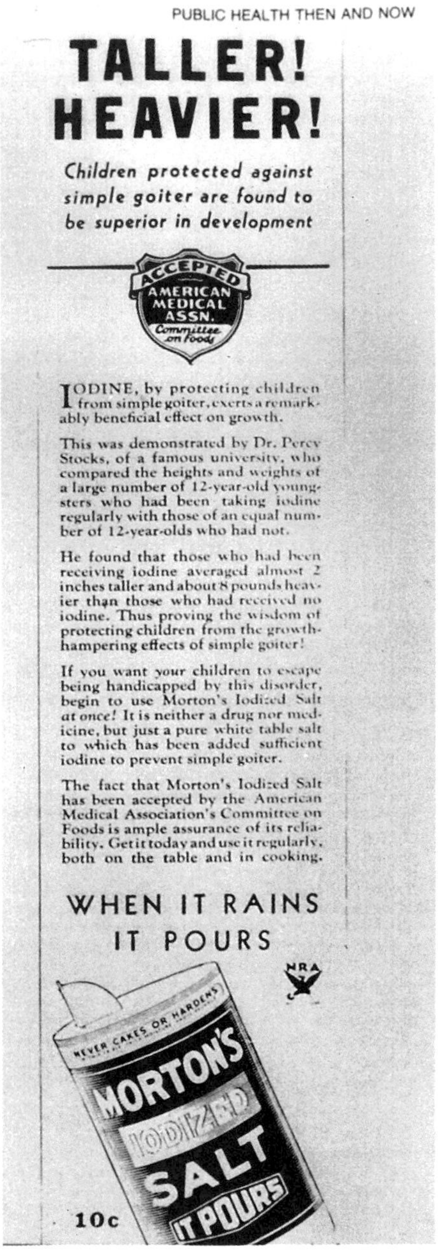

TALLER! HEAVIER!

Children protected against simple goiter are found to be superior in development

ACCEPTED
AMERICAN
MEDICAL
ASSN.
Committee
on Foods

IODINE, by protecting children from simple goiter, exerts a remarkably beneficial effect on growth.

This was demonstrated by Dr. Percy Stocks, of a famous university, who compared the heights and weights of a large number of 12-year-old youngsters who had been taking iodine regularly with those of an equal number of 12-year-olds who had not.

He found that those who had been receiving iodine averaged almost 2 inches taller and about 8 pounds heavier than those who had received no iodine. Thus proving the wisdom of protecting children from the growth-hampering effects of simple goiter!

If you want your children to escape being handicapped by this disorder, begin to use Morton's Iodized Salt at once! It is neither a drug nor medicine, but just a pure white table salt to which has been added sufficient iodine to prevent simple goiter.

The fact that Morton's Iodized Salt has been accepted by the American Medical Association's Committee on Foods is ample assurance of its reliability. Get it today and use it regularly, both on the table and in cooking.

WHEN IT RAINS IT POURS

NRA

MORTON'S IODIZED SALT IT POURS

NEVER CAKES OR HARDENS

10c

Fig. 19–4. Morton Salt ad, 1934. (From H. Markel, " 'When It Rains It Pours': Endemic Goiter, Iodized Salt, and David Murray Cowie, MD," *Am. J. Public Health* 77 [1987]: 225. Copyright 1987, American Public Health Association.)

iodized salt at the time, had once used it, or had never used it. Cards containing the reports on each child were sent to Ann Arbor, where Cowie and Harry Towsley sorted them on the Ping-Pong table in Towsley's basement and tabulated the information.

In the two northern counties, Houghton and Wexford, goiter had decreased by 74 and 78 percent.

Expressing the results as percentages concealed the fact that there was still an incidence of 15.8% in Houghton County and 12.2% in Wexford County. The Great Depression had hit the Upper Peninsula hard; many of its citizens were not buying iodized salt in the grocery stores but were using uniodized salt provided in barrels. In the two southern counties, Midland and Macomb, incidence of goiter had fallen from 32.7 and 26.0 percent to 5.2 and 3.6 percent, respectively. The greatest reduction was in children of families who, according to the children's reports, were using iodized salt at the time of the survey, but there was also a marked decrease in goiter incidence in children who reported they had never used iodized salt. To explain this, Cowie suggested it was "not improbable that these children were unconsciously using iodized salt at least part of the time. When one asks for salt at the grocers in Michigan he is perhaps more likely to be given iodized salt. Whosesalers and our educational propaganda have encouraged them to do so."[62] At the same time an experienced thyroid surgeon in Detroit said: "Without the presence of endemic goiter nodular and toxic diffuse goiter operations have been reduced 50 per cent."[63]

Cowie's Reputation

"With the iodinization of table salt, the prevention of simple goiter was established on a firm basis." So said Arthur F. Abt in the *Abt-Garrison History of Pediatrics*.[64] Cowie got none of the credit. His name appears only on another page, where he shares a single sentence with three other pediatricians and where he is said to have studied serum disease and the intradermal reaction to diphtheria antitoxin.[65] Otherwise Cowie lives in medical history as a local figure who made no permanent contribution to pediatrics. When the American Pediatric Society planned a book to memorialize "men who had exerted a *national* influence" upon the specialty, Cowie was omitted.[66] His name occurs in the volume only twice, once as the man preferred by the University of Michigan as its professor to the eccentric Thomas B. Cooley and once as a man who could always be depended upon to present a paper at the society's annual meeting, a paper described as being on work done by some assistant whose import Cowie occasionally failed to grasp.[67] This sour comment may have been provoked by Cowie's 1930 paper in which he reported measurement of nitrogen balance over 105 days in a six-year-old boy with glomerulonephritis. Urine and stool nitrogen were determined daily, and serum nonprotein nitrogen, albumin, globulin, chloride, calcium, phosphorus, carbon dioxide combining power, sugar, cholesterol, and creatinine were measured at intervals while the child was carried through four periods in which he was fed 2.6, 1.5, 1.0, and 3.8 grams of protein per kilogram of body weight. Edema and ascites were induced when the protein intake was low, but Cowie said: "The edema in this patient cannot be ascribed to a lowered osmotic pressure of the blood. The chlorides were almost invariably above normal; there was no consistent increase in the ascitic chlorides, and the organic crystalloids were normal. The salt and crystalloid content of the blood more than offset the loss of colloid."[68]

Dr. Cowie, may I introduce Professor Starling? He will explain that edema occurs when the hydrostatic pressures of blood in the capillaries and water in the interstitial fluid are normal but the *difference* between the colloid osmotic pressures of plasma and interstitial fluid is reduced. When your patient was on a low protein diet the concentration of albumin in his plasma, which is responsible for almost all of the plasma's colloid osmotic pressure, and therefore the *difference* between colloid osmotic pressure of plasma and interstitial fluid, was reduced. An increase in salt and crystalloid content of the blood could not offset a reduction in the *colloid* osmotic pressure of the plasma.[69]

The End

Throughout the 1920s Cowie was in conflict with Dean Cabot over the pediatric budget, and later there was a long and complicated struggle with Dean Furstenberg over hiring a dietician. The dean wanted the pediatric diets to be prepared by the hospital's dietician, but Cowie wanted his own dietician. There were other troubles, some recorded in the dean's office files. On 4 June 1936 the Medical School Executive Committee, with Dean Furstenberg and Doctors Bruce, Coller, Edmunds, and Weller attending, made this entry in its minutes.

Following considerable discussion the Executive Committee approved *unanimously* the following resolution: "that the Department of Pediatrics is inadequate in its teaching and also in its care of patients; that further, a radical reorganization of the Department is necessary.[70]

Anyone who has served on the Executive Committee knows that such an uncharacteristically intemperate resolution inserted in the minutes followed an even more intemperate discussion.

The problem of the Department of Pediatrics disturbed the central administration of the university as well, for on 30 March 1939 Dean Clarence Yoakum of the Graduate School wrote to Cowie suggesting that it would be highly desirable for Cowie to spend more time on his research and that Cowie would find the time by handing over to someone else the distractions of administration and the current problems of the clinic. A few days later Dean Furstenberg attempted to get Cowie out of the way by making the same suggestion. Cowie replied he would give up neither administration or his clinical work.

When Cowie's conflict with the administration was resolved by Cowie's death in 1940, Dean Furstenberg appointed a committee consisting of Coller, Wile, and Edmunds to recommend a successor. After compiling the usual long list of names the committee reported on 28 February 1941 that Charles F. McKhann, then a Harvard associate professor at the Children's Hospital in Boston, was by long odds the outstanding candidate. McKhann was said to be anxious for the Michigan job, and he accepted the appointment. The Kellogg Foundation promised the university one hundred thousand dollars to be spent over ten years to rehabilitate the Department of Pediatrics. Pediatrics at Michigan was off to a false new start, for McKhann soon resigned.[71]

20
Ophthalmology, Dermatology, and Neurology

There were no specialists on the faculty when the Medical School opened in 1850; three clinical professors taught medicine, surgery, and diseases of women and children. They dealt as well as they could with all the problems that would be attacked by specialists. Fifty-five years later ophthalmology, otolaryngology, dermatology, neurology, and psychiatry were in the hands of men with professorial appointments. Roentgenology was practiced by a technician under the professor of surgery, but it, too, soon became an independent specialty.

The Beginning of Ophthalmology at Michigan

Ophthalmology was the first specialty to differentiate at Michigan. George E. Frothingham was a Bostonian educated at Phillips Academy, Andover. He was apprenticed to William Warren Greene, a surgeon who had graduated from the University of Michigan Medical School in 1855.[1] Perhaps Greene, as a Michigan graduate, suggested that Frothingham study medicine at Michigan, and Frothingham graduated from Michigan in 1864.[2] When Greene was called to Ann Arbor as professor of surgery in 1867 he brought Frothingham back from Boston with him. At Michigan Frothingham taught gross anatomy as well as surgery. He quickly acquired skill as an ophthalmologist, and in 1870 he was appointed lecturer on ophthalmology. "Aural surgery" was added to his title when he was promoted to a professorship in 1872. Thereafter, whatever his title, he was responsible for everything included in otorhinolaryngology.

In the 1870s Frothingham had a general private practice as well, and in 1878 he was Victor Vaughan's "beloved preceptor." Soon he confined his practice to his specialty, leaving his general practice to Vaughan. Frothingham operated in the Eye and Ear Clinic attached to the Pavilion Hospital during the six months of the year it was open, and he operated in his office throughout the year. Ophthalmological surgery literally overshadowed general surgery in the hospital, not only in the frequency of operations but in physical fact because the clinic cut off light for the hospital's operating room. In 1879–80 Frothingham treated 433 cases of eye and ear disease in the hospital and performed 173 operations. Thirty-six operations were cataract extractions. Nevertheless, practice in Ann Arbor was too limited to suit Frothingham or Donald Maclean, the surgeon who succeeded Greene. In 1889 both were dismissed by the regents for their intemperate campaign to prevent a new University Hospital being built in Ann Arbor. Frothingham moved to Detroit, where he taught and practiced until his death in 1900. He was succeeded as professor of ophthalmology by Flemming Carrow.

Flemming Carrow

Flemming Carrow had been born in Still Pond, Maryland, and he attended Columbian University, later George Washington University, in Washington, D.C. He graduated bachelor of arts in 1870 and doctor of medicine in 1874. Then he studied ophthalmology in New York, London, Berlin, and Vienna. In about 1875, the year of his marriage, he went to Canton, China, where he succeeded a medical missionary who had founded a busy ophthalmological hospital there.[3] Carrow said that in his seven years in China he served as physician for the Chinese Army, for the Chinese Custom Service, for the British Consulate in Canton, and for British gunboats in the harbor. At Michigan he frequently decorated his lectures with "many tales of his service in China, in all of which he occupied the character of the hidden hero."[4] Carrow returned to the United States in 1882, on account of his wife's declining health.

Carrow at Michigan

Carrow was in private practice in Bay City, Michigan, when he was called to the university in 1889. His appointment was strongly supported by the regents and professionals in his locality and in Detroit. Vaughan, however, mentioned Carrow only twice in his autobiography: once to note his appointment and once to note his resignation.[5] Carrow appeared to meet Vaughan's first criterion of faculty selection in that he was a "gentleman."

Carrow established a private practice in Ann Arbor. He operated on private patients in his office and on charity patients in the University Hospital. When Carrow performed a cataract extraction he merely washed out the patient's eye with boric acid solution although he knew it had little antiseptic power. He began with puncture and counterpuncture exactly in the sclerocorneal line and finished in the clear cornea with an upward incision. He made a small iridectomy and a thorough rent in the capsule. He removed the speculum prior to delivery of the lens so that, should the vitreous prolapse following delivery of the lens, the lids might be quickly closed to prevent the loss of a large quantity of vitreous humor. Carrow thought that loss of a small amount of the vitreous humor was not important. Even in unilateral operations he bandaged both eyes firmly shut, and the patient was discharged after twelve days in the hospital. The patient was fitted for glasses two weeks later. In eighty-one cases done in one year there were two failures: one as the result of suppuration of the corneal wound and one in which the lens was displaced into the vitreous during the operation by a sudden movement of the patient. Of eighty-one patients, sixty-eight had "good results," defined as 20/40 vision with glasses.[6]

Parke, Davis and Company gave Carrow a preparation of epinephrine (Adrenalin), whose use they were promoting in 1902. He responded by declaring that epinephrine is a valuable aid in surgical work on mucous surfaces; he used it routinely in eye work and in operations within the nasal cavity.[7] Otherwise Carrow's publications were case reports in local medical journals: laryngectomy and partial removal of the upper jaw for pharyngeal growth,[8] foreign bodies in the eyeball,[9] and venereal affections of the eye.[10]

Carrow examined 681 students at the Michigan State Normal School in Ypsilanti in response to an invitation from its faculty.[11] He found 379 to be hypermetropic, 79 myopic, 47 astigmatic, and 2 color blind. Carrow believed the myopia resulted from bad lighting and ventilation in the school buildings and that schoolwork made students progressively myopic. His Ypsilanti results confirmed his belief. Someone had found 19.5 percent of Philadelphia schoolchildren to be myopic. Carrow attributed his figure of only 11.6 percent to the fact that Ypsilanti students, destined to be teachers, had only a limited education and were therefore less exposed to conditions causing myopia than Philadelphia students.

Carrow's Teaching

Students attending Carrow's clinics had an even worse time than with Nancrede's or Peterson's. They could see nothing of the operation from the benches; only Carrow's assistants could profit from his instruction. For lectures, Carrow appeared in "clothes of the most recent cut, with piqué facing to his vest and a perfect color combination of sox and neck-ties."[12] Before starting, he stood in silence, withdrew a silk handkerchief from his coat pocket and cleaned the lenses of his pince-nez. His lectures were fully written and typed double spaced, ready to be read. Every so often Carrow inserted a note to himself: "(relate case)" or "(explain)." The lectures covered all topics of ophthalmology, otology, and laryngology in detail; that on diseases of the cornea occupied thirty-four typewritten pages, and there were five complete lectures on the ear. They demonstrate that the clinical faculty's compulsion to read the textbook to students still stood. Carrow recognized that most students would not specialize in his field, and he insisted only that they know the difference between iritis, glaucoma, and cataract.

One former student described Carrow's methods of teaching as "not orthodox" but considered him "one of the best of that day [because] he had a way of impressing students with facts that made them remember them always."[13] By 1895 the junior class was divided into sections, and for five weeks each section was drilled in the use of the ophthalmoscope and laryngoscope, using models, mannequins, healthy subjects, and patients (fig. 20–1).

Carrow and Money

Carrow's practice of admitting private patients to the University Hospital got him into trouble. When he described his results on cataract extraction to the Michigan State Medical Society one physician said: "I am glad to have the opportunity of pitching into him for operating before his class on a patient worth $80,000; this practice is entirely wrong."[14] Carrow

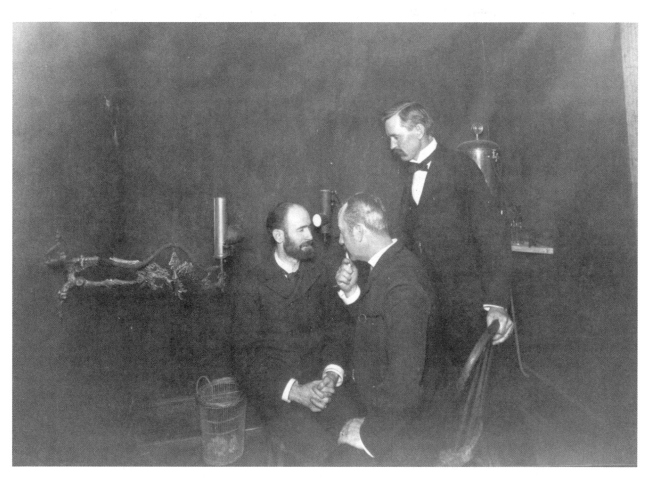

Fig. 20–1. Flemming Carrow using a reflecting ophthalmoscope in the darkroom at the Catherine Street Hospital. (Courtesy of the Bentley Historical Library, University of Michigan, Medical School Records, Box 136, "Gibson #3.")

thought otherwise. On 27 May 1904 the regents received a letter from Carrow asking them to resolve that and related problems. What should be done with patients needing immediate attention when the hospital beds were full? Could they be sent for private care? If a patient appeared on what was not a clinic day, should he or she be sent to a private office? If a patient in easy circumstances applied for clinic care, not knowing of a private office, should the patient be sent to one if willing to go? "Some of us have felt that we could take patients who were abundantly able to pay to our private offices."[15] The Board of Regents replied at once, firmly and at length, saying in part: "In no case shall any patient coming to the University Hospitals for treatment be subjected either directly or indirectly to any influence, pressure or inducement . . . to leave the hospital, and go to the private office, or private hospital, of any of the Hospital Physicians."[16] Furthermore, the superintendent of the hospital was the only one to provide glasses to hospital patients, and that was to be done at hospital expense. Carrow immediately resigned and went into private practice in Detroit.[17]

Carrow's Successor: Walter Robert Parker

The regents divided Carrow's chair; in September 1904 they appointed Walter R. Parker as clinical professor of diseases of the eye and Roy Bishop Canfield as clinical professor of the diseases of the ear, nose, and throat. Parker was made clinical professor because he wanted to keep his large private practice in Detroit, where he lived. In May 1905 his title was changed to professor of ophthalmology "upon the condition that he shall become a resident of Ann Arbor by the 1st of October next."[18] In May the next year, "On the motion of Regent Dean, it was voted to call the attention of Dr. W. R. Parker to the condition upon which he was appointed Professor of Ophthalmology, viz.: that he should become a resident of Ann Arbor."[19] Nevertheless, Parker continued to live in Detroit for the next forty-nine years and to maintain a private practice there. He commuted to Ann Arbor two days a week to operate in the University Hospital, to teach medical students, to train residents, and to engage in the private practice of ophthalmology in a downtown office with George Slocum. He retired in

1932 and died in his house in Grosse Pointe on 1 April 1955.

Vaughan chose Parker out of a hundred persons applying for Carrow's job. Parker graduated from Michigan's Department of Engineering in 1888, and he received his medical training at the University of Pennsylvania. He was trained in ophthalmology at the Wills Eye Hospital, Philadelphia. He began to practice his specialty in Detroit in 1894; he studied briefly in Vienna in 1896; and he was appointed clinical professor in the Detroit College of Medicine in 1899. When Parker was appointed at Michigan he was well established with privileges at two Detroit hospitals, and he was well known for frequent papers given before the Michigan State Medical Society. He published in local journals, and he was abstract editor for the *Physician and Surgeon*.

Parker's Staff and Teaching

George Slocum, Parker's associate in his Ann Arbor private practice, was the mainstay of Parker's staff in the University Hospital. Slocum was responsible for most of the formal instruction of resident graduates and about half of the instruction given to medical students. As acting assistant professor he managed the department while Parker was in the military service in World War I.

Parker thought that undergraduate teaching in the specialties should be limited to that necessary for a thorough general education. A professor such as himself, one with broad clinical experience, was best fitted for that kind of teaching. Technical aspects could be taught by assistants, and development of specialists should be left to postgraduate work.[20] In Parker's first years at Michigan teaching of ophthalmology was still combined with teaching of otolaryngology, and the two occupied 195 hours in the junior and senior years. They were separated in 1913 when ophthalmology was given 108 hours. By 1919 there was an eight-week course in the junior year in which students in sections learned to use trial cases of lenses, the retinoscope, the ophthalmoscope, and the perimeter. Students heard whole-class lectures in the senior year, and again in sections they saw patients and studied refraction and external diseases of the eye. This occupied about 100 hours. During a spasm of curriculum reform in 1930 Parker agreed to cut the required work in half and to make the rest optional.

Parker began graduate instruction in ophthalmology limited to three graduates at a time, each serving three years after one year as intern in a general hospital. A graduate in training rose to become an assistant and then an instructor. F. Bruce Fralick finished the program and Carl Badgley was interested for a while, but A. C. Kerlikowske was encouraged to leave it for less demanding work as a hospital administrator. The training was mostly practical, but there were systematic lectures in embryology, anatomy, pathology, and physiological optics. In the second decade of the century Parker opposed efforts to establish a school of optometry in the university, and by 1918 he had a man doing refraction and teaching it to postgraduate students. Trainees who held a college degree were eligible to earn a master's degree, and all were expected to meet the qualifications of the American Board of Ophthalmology, the first medical specialty board, of which Parker was a founder and long a member.

Parker's Ophthalmology

Most of Parker's seventy or so publications are reports of cases seen in the University Hospital, and they show the range of problems encountered and the methods of treatment. There were infections of the eye, including tuberculosis and manifestations of syphilis treated with arsphenamine (Salvarsan).[21] Parker used the Krönlein operation, entering the orbit through the lateral wall, to remove a dermoid cyst,[22] and he occasionally reconstructed the face and lids with skin grafts.[23] There were many reports of one or two cases of this and that.[24]

Parker found epinephrine useless in treating glaucoma, but when he reported his results in seventy-three cases treated by operation he said he was surprised at the high percentage of good results. They were good in thirty-one for whom he had done scleral trephination, usually with a 1.5-millimeter opening. He had six poor results and twenty-six failures.[25] Parker also used scleral trephination combined with incision of the choroid or retina to treat detached retina, and of eleven patients vision was improved in four, unimproved in five, and worse in two.[26] Someone measured visual fields in fifty patients diagnosed as having hysteria. When Parker read his paper describing the results at a meeting a physician asked if the fields had been correctly determined, for there was much possibility of error with such patients. Parker replied: "The few I saw were

taken carefully, and I believe all of them were."[27] Parker reported dyschromatopsia in thirty-six patients.

Cataract

Parker repeatedly published the story of his experience with cataract: 300 cases in 1911, 1,320 in 1920, and 1,421 in 1921.[28] The last series contained 156 simple extractions and 1,123 combined extractions. Simple extractions were done without iridectomy, and combined operations were done with it. For those extractions, Parker used much the same technique as Carrow, but by 1911 he was using aseptic methods combined with careful preliminary antisepsis. In his series of 1,421 operations there were only seven infections. He made a large corneal incision including a large conjunctival flap, for he thought that making too small an incision was a common error. He cut the capsule or tore it with forceps and then removed the cortical parts of the lens after the nucleus had been extracted. When Parker reviewed his data he found that in many instances results were "not recorded," and he thought that unfortunate for the reason that patients with the most successful results left the hospital early and did not return for study. Those with complications remained. Failure, defined as vision less than 6/60, occurred 111 times in patients with the combined operation. There were 88 accidents, including 11 as the result of injury by the patient him- or herself. One accident was the result of postcataract delirium in which a woman tore the bandages from her eyes and rushed from the hospital.[29] Other failures were the result of corneal or vitreous opacities.

Among Parker's 1,421 cases were 91 "Indian operations." This was not the traditional Indian procedure of "couching for cataract" in which the suspensory ligament was torn from behind and the lens abruptly pushed into the vitreous, where it remained.[30] Western ophthalmologists estimated that the operation was no more than 10 percent successful. Parker's Indian operation was the one described by Major Henry Smith of the Indian Medical Service.[31] There was characteristic controversy over the merits of the operation, and it was condemned chiefly on account of danger of loss of the vitreous. In 1906 Parker said: "I determined to give it a trial and here report my first case." His patient was a fifty-eight-year-old farmer. "A high corneal incision (midway between upper pupillary border and limbus) was made. With a large squint hook, pressure was made on the cornea below, counterpressure above with spatula. The iris seemed rigid, or I was too timid and failed to deliver the lens. An iridectomy was made, after which pressure was applied as before. The lens immediately took a position with its long axis vertical, the upper edge presenting in the wound, but not until the pressure had been exerted for several seconds did the attachments give way, after which the lens in its capsule was delivered without loss of vitreous. . . . The result in this case certainly confirms all claims made by Major Smith."[32] This may have been the first Indian operation in the United States.

Choked Disk

Parker received the Knapp Medal from the Section on Ophthalmology of the American Medical Association for his paper on the relation of intraocular pressure to the choked disk.[33] This was the only experimental work he published. Parker had seen that choked disk in six patients was greater in the eye with less tension. Parker used twenty dogs to measure intraocular pressure in each eye and then to do a scleral trephination in one eye to reduce its tension. Intracranial pressure was most successfully raised in those dogs in which he inserted a sponge between the dura and the skull. In them the disk became choked in the eye with lesser tension. He repeated the experiments with twelve monkeys, obtaining the same results, and he concluded that choking is simply the result of a pressure difference.

When Stewart Duke-Elder reviewed the many competing theories in his chapter on diseases of the optic nerve he said: "In a general sense it may be said that papilloedema results when the normal pressure relationship of the circulation on either side of the lamina cribrosa is disturbed." After citing Parker's results among many others, Duke-Elder concluded that "the mechanism of the formation of papilloedema has excited an immense amount of research and controversy, but to-day [1941] the question is still unsettled."[34]

Parker's Reputation

Parker was prominent internationally through his work in professional organizations, civilian and military. He was the first person from the state of Michigan to be elected a member and president of the American Ophthalmological Society. He was chairman of the Section on Ophthalmology of the American Medical Association and president of the American Academy of Ophthalmology and Otolaryngology. In World War I, Colonel Parker was chief of the Division of Surgery of the Head. Parker's place among contemporary ophthalmologists is described in the 109-page chapter, "Operations," in the ninth edition of his friend and colleague de Schweinitz's textbook, where, amid copious citations of others, Parker is mentioned twice, once for suggesting that greasing the skin with sterilized petroleum jelly (Vaseline) facilitates cutting a graft and once for observing that iritis is less likely to develop if iridectomy is done during sclerocorneal trephining.[35] In another contemporary textbook with an ample bibliography Parker's name appears once alone and once "among others."[36] However, upon review of his career, two universities bestowed on him the degree of doctor of science.

Parker's Benefactions

Parker's wife died long before he did, and in her will she left $30,000 to the university for research and scholarships in ophthalmology. In addition, she donated her art collection, with Dr. Parker retaining control over the objects during his lifetime. (The Parkers had previously given the university money to support Walter Koelz, which brought a spectacular collection of Tibetan Buddhist paintings [*tankas*] to the university that are now in the Museum of Anthropology.) The Margaret Watson Parker bequest was transferred to the University of Michigan Museum of Art in four groups. The first, in 1937, was her collection of Pewabic pottery, made by the leading producer of art pottery in Detroit. In 1947, 84 Japanese Ukiyo-e prints were donated. The third group, in 1953–54, consisted of 158 prints plus paintings and drawings by James McNeill Whistler, other paintings and prints by Western artists, Asian ceramics, sculpture, and lacquer, and her personal library of 170 volumes. The final group of objects came to the museum at Dr. Parker's death in 1955. He left $25,000 to be added to the ophthalmology fund established by his wife, but he also left cash and securities worth $136,968 to the museum to establish the Margaret Watson Parker Art Fund, which the museum has used to purchase Asian art, with the result that his connection with the university is commemorated in galleries in the Museum of Art named for him and his wife as well as in the Department of Ophthalmology.

George Slocum

George Slocum was promoted to a professorship and made head of the Department of Ophthalmology when Parker retired in 1932. Slocum was sixty-seven years old, and he had twenty-eight years of faithful service in the department and twenty-five years of private practice with Parker to recommend him. He died of a heart attack on 24 March of the next year.

Slocum had deep Quaker conscientiousness, and he was shy.[37] Perhaps these qualities kept him from pushing himself forward by frequent publication. Aside from a few highly detailed case reports,[38] Slocum published only two major papers. When Parker learned that Hewlett was doing a systematic study of nephritis he assigned Slocum the task of making ophthalmoscopic observations on Hewlett's patients. Fully aware "that the conditions studied have already been described in the minutest detail," Slocum published his own minutely detailed findings.[39]

On 16 September 1921 Slocum had performed a cataract extraction on a badly frightened, uncontrollable patient, and more by accident than design he made a conjunctival bridge. Bridges, as Slocum well knew, had often been described, but Slocum thought his particular modification worth reporting. He had first deliberately used it in June 1925, but he delayed publication until he had a sufficient number of cases to furnish a background of comparison with the procedures of others. Slocum began with the customary puncture and counterpuncture one millimeter above the horizontal median, and he carried his incision upward as though he were making a broad corneal flap. When the incision was two-thirds completed he began to make a bridge. He carried an incision six to eight millimeters above the limbus on the temporal side and another incision four to five millimeters on the mesial side. Then he made a horizontal cut from the upper edge of the lateral incision to a point four millimeters above the upper end of the mesial cut. The flap could then be reflected mesially and downward, giving sufficient exposure to permit easy expulsion of the lens. Slocum's description of successful results in 568 instances turned out to be a posthumous publication.[40]

F. Bruce Fralick and the Department to 1941

Bruce Fralick was called back from the University of Chicago when George Slocum died. Fralick had gone to Chicago in 1931 to be an instructor in ophthalmology, and when he returned to Ann Arbor he was made an associate professor and acting chairman of the department. The university left the professorship vacant until 1938, when it was given to Fralick as chairman.

Fralick progressed rapidly through Parker's training program after he had graduated from medical school in 1927, and he was made an instructor in 1929. While holding the John E. Weeks Scholarship for Research in Ophthalmology, Fralick applied Reuben Kahn's new test for syphilis to aqueous humor drawn from the anterior chamber with a twenty-seven-gauge needle. He found the Kahn reaction to be positive when there was syphilitic involvement of the eye, although blood and spinal fluid reactions might be negative.[41] Immediately upon returning to Ann Arbor Fralick had opened an office downtown for the private practice of ophthalmology, and most of his publications before 1941 were reports of cases seen in his office or in the University Hospital. One described a unique case of luxation of the lens into the subretinal space through a retinal tear.[42] Another written with Russell DeJong described a single case of neuromyelitis optica.[43] By the end of the decade Fralick was giving advice to medical societies on the posterior approach for removal of magnetically susceptible intraocular foreign bodies,[44] the management of glaucoma,[45] and the management of strabismus.[46]

Fralick continued Parker's training program until the war, although he had a very small department, and it supplied him with a few instructors. He did not need much staff for teaching, because he had only seventy-seven hours in the curriculum in which to give the usual didactic lectures and to instruct in the use of ophthalmological instruments. Senior students spent only nine hours on the ophthalmological wards, one hour a day for nine days.

William F. Breakey and the Beginning of Dermatology

In 1909 the university celebrated with considerable pomp the fiftieth anniversary of William F. Breakey's doctorship, for Breakey had been a beloved teacher since 1868, beginning as prosector of surgery and demonstrator of anatomy. He had graduated from the Medical School in 1859, when the curriculum was chiefly a series of lectures on major medical subjects. His graduation thesis, "Irrational Medicine," was a florid denunciation of quackery, but he agreed that the so-called regular profession was also full of folly. His early practice in a nearby village was interrupted by the Civil War, and Breakey was badly wounded at Gettysburg. After the war he practiced in Ann Arbor, and for many years he was chairman of the town's Board of Health. When Breakey was made lecturer on dermatology and syphilology in 1890 with thirty-two hours of lecture and sixty-four hours of clinic, the subject was established as an independent medical specialty at Michigan.

Breakey was self-taught in his specialty. He could have learned little about it in medical school, and he did not study for any appreciable time in Boston, New York, or Philadelphia, where European-trained dermatologists were teaching. When he went to Europe in his old age it was as a medical tourist. Nevertheless, Breakey was well informed and progressive. He cited publications of Unna and Duhring, and he used microscopic and culture techniques to confirm his diagnoses.[47] He used Finsen's light method to treat tuberculous lupus,[48] and he studied conditions that influence treatment of epithelioma by X rays. Most of his papers were purely descriptive, saying there is no effective treatment and prognosis is guarded. A member of his staff did, however, remove a disfiguring nevus from the nose of a young girl by application of carbon dioxide snow.[49]

Breakey's Syphilology

Breakey began to practice and teach syphilology at the time Palmer thought syphilis was rare in Michigan. Treatment was with mercury in many forms. An example of the state of the subject is given by one of Breakey's contemporaries, who reported in a local medical journal that he had fruitlessly treated a young woman for intractable headache. Only when she mentioned that she had once had a sore throat did the diagnosis of syphilis immediately become clear. Her headaches disappeared when she was given a few injections of mercury bichloride (corrosive sublimate).

The Wassermann reaction entered clinical practice in 1906, and arsphenamine (Salvarsan, "compound 606") was introduced in 1910. Both were at the end of Breakey's career. In 1910 Mark Marshall, who was teaching practical therapeutics as well as internal medicine, treated seven patients with ten doses of "606" given him by Simon Flexner of the Rockefeller Institute for experimental purposes.[50] At the same time a member of Breakey's staff at the University of Michigan treated two cases, obtaining no cure in one and improvement in the other.[51] Breakey opposed the common practice of cauterizing the initial syphilitic lesion. Antiseptic dressings were enough, and mercury given in the early stages was not only futile but dangerous.[52] Treatment was expectant, and the physician should wait until secondary lesions appeared before beginning specific treatment. "A free and pronounced eruption occurring at about the average period is regarded as a favorable symptom."[53] Occurrence of a rash was necessary to establish the diagnosis, for many primary lesions that appear to be syphilitic are not. Syphilis is curable, but many cases are never cured. Breakey thought it safe to assume that syphilis is caused by a virus, and he hoped that discovery of the syphilitic factor and an antitoxin would sweep away the disease as well as speculations about it.

Public Health

Breakey, the local authority on contagious and communicable diseases, had to deal with the smallpox epidemic of 1888–89. He deplored the citizens' panic and extreme actions, and he thought isolation of the sick and disinfection of their bedding would control spread of the disease. Like George Dock, Breakey favored partially compulsory vaccination. His colleague William J. Herdman, as professor of neurology and diseases of the mind, had to treat tabes and general paresis, and Herdman agreed with Breakey that the medical profession has the obligation to mount a persistent campaign of education in hygiene and public health.[54] Each medical society should have a standing committee to disseminate information, and the committee should include lawyers and clergy as well as physicians. A woman physician of the right sort is particularly useful. True to his profession, Breakey inspected the kitchens and the food lockers of the ship on which he went to Europe. The kitchens were clean, but food was kept too long in the lockers. Breakey got ptomaine poisoning on shipboard after eating some elderly fish. He was horrified to see a child with whooping cough playing with other children on the foredeck.

Breakey's Successor: Udo Julius Wile

When Breakey retired in 1912 Rufus Cole recommended the thirty-year-old Udo Julius Wile as Breakey's successor, and the faculty agreed that Wile was the most promising candidate (fig. 20–2). Wile, a member of a New York mercantile family, had been an undergraduate at Columbia and had studied medicine at Johns Hopkins, where Cole knew him and where W. H. Welch suggested that he specialize in dermatology. After graduating from Johns Hopkins in 1907 Wile studied dermatology in Europe, first at the Charité Hospital in Berlin and then in Bern and Paris. For several months he lived in the Hamburg home of P. G. Unna while he worked in Unna's private clinic and hospital. Wile went to London carrying a letter from his former teacher, William Osler. He showed his silver-stained tissues to Jonathan Hutchinson and gave the first dark-field demonstration in the British Isles.[55] When he returned to New York Wile began to practice with Sigmund Pollitzer, who, like most leading dermatologists, had also studied under Unna.[56]

Wile asked permission to open an office in Detroit for private practice of dermatology when he was appointed at Michigan. Vaughan was in favor, but Peterson opposed. During a long debate in the faculty meeting of 3 July 1912, it was moved that Wile be allowed to open a free dermatology clinic in Detroit for the exclusive purpose of developing an adjunct to the University Hospital. Canfield objected on the ground that it would imply that Ann Arbor facilities were inadequate. Lombard's motion to table the proposal was carried. Upon arriving in Ann Arbor Wile immediately opened an office on the corner of Liberty and Maynard Streets, and he continued in private practice until he retired thirty-five years later.

Wile's Teaching

Dermatology and syphilology as a specialty occupied only a minor place in the undergraduate curriculum but a major place in patient care and graduate train-

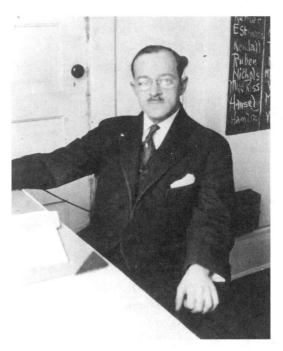

Fig. 20–2. Udo Julius Wile. (Courtesy of the Bentley Historical Library, University of Michigan, Medical School Records, Box 136, "Photographs, General, Faculty, Individuals.")

ing. There were the usual didactic lectures to the third-year class and a histopathology laboratory that was made elective in 1929. Wile's junior staff, instructors, residents, and interns made his department larger than those of other specialties. Until 1921 Wile himself was the only one holding professorial rank, but after that there were always assistant and then associate professors as well. From the beginning interns moved through the ranks, often spending a year as research assistant, until they became instructors. As instructors they engaged in clinical research, and a substantial fraction of Wile's publications in which he was always senior author described the clinical experience of residents or instructors. Instructors moved to responsible positions elsewhere after serving under Wile for several years. Through 1937 a total of twenty-seven men were trained by Wile. The first of these, John H. Stokes, graduated from Michigan the year Wile arrived, and after his graduate training he established the Section of Dermatology at the Mayo Clinic and then became Duhring Professor of Dermatology at the University of Pennsylvania. Others held professorships at Illinois, Temple, and Oregon, and some gave their names to diseases of the skin.[57]

Wile said that dermatology had abruptly established itself in Vienna when dermatoses were classified on the basis of their morphological characteristics. "Dermatologists became expert diagnosticians of disease entities for which an awkward name existed, and for which, for the most part, they had no adequate explanation."[58] The names persisted, but within Wile's lifetime ideas changed radically. Dermatological diseases were recognized as manifestations of systemic disease. Skin diseases themselves had been narrowed to local infections and malignant growths.[59] Consequently, medical and graduate students must approach dermatology from the standpoint of general medicine. Next to the basic sciences a reading knowledge of French and German is of paramount importance, and Wile thought that the liberalization of the premedical curriculum, particularly the substitution of humanities for foreign languages, would handicap all medical students. Wile said this just at the time Dean Cabot was proposing elimination of French and German in favor of humanities.[60]

Wile's Publications

Wile published 150 papers before 1941. At least 49 of them were case reports. He began in 1907 by describing the autopsy findings at Bellevue Hospital in a woman with previous ventral suspension of the uterus for "falling of the womb" who died of a posterior rupture of the uterus during labor.[61] He continued with 11 more papers, each reviewing the literature and reporting a single case. Wile then published similar reviews and reports of 2 cases,[62] 3 cases,[63] 5 cases,[64] 6 cases,[65] and so on, until he reached 88 cases of Charcot's arthropathy in 1930[66] and 425 cases of cancer of the lip in 1937.[67] Most of the papers were on syphilis.

Wile's Syphilology

Wile said that every dermatologist was necessarily a syphilologist, and a syphilologist's first problem is identifying syphilitic patients. Wile began just at the time the Wassermann test was introduced, and he said it was his good fortune to be one of the first U.S. students of the complement fixation test and to have learned the test under one of Germany's foremost serologists.[68] That was in 1907–8 in the Berlin Dermatology Clinic, where Wile in the study of 100 cases found the test to give positive results for both

serum and urine in 50 instances.[69] In his paper Wile thanked Dr. Franz Blumenthal, under whose direction the work was done. Twenty-eight years later Franz Blumenthal as a refugee was research professor of dermatology in Wile's department at Michigan supported by three thousand dollars a year from the Rockefeller Foundation.[70] Blumenthal eventually became head of the Dermatology Clinic at the Wayne County General Hospital. As the Wassermann test was made more sensitive, Wile became skeptical of "serological cure" of syphilis. In the latter part of the second decade of the century he found that of 459 patients with syphilis in all stages, 50 would have been considered negative by earlier tests.[71]

In the early 1920s, when Reuben Kahn was still employed in the State Laboratories in Lansing, Wile and a resident compared the Kahn test with the Wassermann. In 154 control patients the Kahn test gave three false positives, and both tests gave positive results in 193 cases of syphilis. Wile thought the Kahn test was simple and rapid and less susceptible to errors. It might replace the Wassermann test.[72]

Wile believed all patients should be compelled to submit to a serological test before admission to the hospital, not only for identification of latent syphilis but for protection of the staff. Dentists, physicians, and surgeons had been accidentally infected by patients in the septic stage of their syphilitic infection, and if a patient were infectious, an operation should be postponed.[73]

Beginning in 1920 Wile wrote a series of articles for the *Archives of Dermatology and Syphilology* that almost constitutes a textbook of visceral syphilis. He began by demonstrating that syphilis of the liver is more common than generally supposed. He reviewed the literature and then gave the incidence, symptoms, differential diagnosis, prognosis, and treatment.[74] He continued with similar articles on syphilis of the kidney, ureter, suprarenal glands, stomach, pancreas, spleen, intestines, and lung. Then Wile described occult cardiovascular syphilis.[75] A large number of syphilitic patients came to his clinic entirely unaware of heart trouble. In the seven-year period 1930 to 1936, he saw 210 cases of cardiovascular syphilis, one-third symptomatically occult.

Spirochetes in the Brain

For years psychiatrists had debated whether general paresis is caused by syphilis. One said: "Without syphilis, no paresis," and another said: "I desire to make it clear that progressive paralysis is not a specific syphilitic disease of the brain."[76]

In 1913 J. W. Moore of the Central Islip State Hospital in New York prepared sections of seventy paretic brains preserved in formalin, and he stained them by the Levaditi reduced-silver method, the procedure Warthin found unsatisfactory.[77] He sent duplicates to Hideyo Noguchi at the Rockefeller Institute for Medical Research, and Noguchi identified *Treponema pallidum* in twelve sections.[78] A little later Noguchi found spirochetes in forty-eight of two hundred brains of patients dying with paresis and in twelve spinal cords of patients with tabes.[79] In the same year Noguchi, using six brains in a fresh state, found spirochetes by dark-field examination in one, and he inoculated testicles of thirty-six rabbits with the infected tissue. The Wassermann reaction became strongly positive in one rabbit, and there were spirochetes in the testicular lesions.[80] Others working at the Army Medical School in Washington, D.C., also succeeded in transmitting syphilis to rabbits from brains of patients dying with syphilis.[81]

About the same time Forster and Tomaszewski, working in the psychiatric and dermatology clinics of the Berlin Charité Hospital, demonstrated that spirochetes could be found in the brains of living paretics.[82] They casually referred to their method as the "Neisser-Pollaksche Hirnpunktion" as though it were a well-known procedure. Udo Wile was present at two of their operations, and he was more explicit when he described the work in the *Journal of the American Medical Association.*

The patient's head is first shaved and the anterior portion of the skull thoroughly painted with tincture of iodin [*sic*]. The point of operation selected is over the frontal convolution from about ½ to 1 inch from the midline and well forward of the middle meningeal artery. The region is frozen with ethyl chlorid and a revolving dental drill is thrust quickly through the skin and deeper tissues. A few rapid revolutions of the drill in the hands of an assistant suffice to pierce the skull. The borer, or drill, is then removed and a long, thin trocar needle is inserted in the hole through the skin and bone; this is pushed firmly and deeply into the cortex. The wire obturator of the trocar is withdrawn and a syringe barrel is attached to the end of the needle. By suction, a small cylinder of brain substance containing both gray and white matter is drawn into the syringe, together with more or less fluid from the ventricle. This material, transferred to a sterile Petri dish, is examined at once with

a dark field illumination. Thus far the organisms have been found in gray matter only.[83]

Wile repeated Forster and Tomaszewski's work in 1915, using six paretics in the Pontiac State Asylum. He found spirochetes by dark-field illumination in fresh tissue, and he gave samples to Paul de Kruif, then a graduate student of bacteriology at Michigan, who had been assigned to help Wile. De Kruif injected the tissue into a testicle of a large rabbit on 11 June 1915. A month later Wile and de Kruif found many spirochetes in fluid aspirated from the testicle, and the next month they succeeded in cultivating spirochetes from the testicle on ascitic-agar plates.[84]

As soon as Wile's papers describing this work were published there was a national spasm of moral indignation led by antivivisectionists and continued by newspaper editors. Wile was denounced for using human subjects in experiments that were not intended to benefit those patients, for using human subjects without their consent, and for infecting rabbits with syphilis, driving them crazy with a "loathsome disease." Wile said he was indifferent to public opinion.

Walter B. Cannon and W. W. Keen were particularly disturbed by Wile's work. Cannon was chairman of the Committee for the Protection of Medical Research of the American Medical Association, and Keen had spent almost thirty years defending animal experimentation from the antivivisectionists. Both thought Wile's experiments undermined their work by providing an example open to legitimate criticism. Cannon read Wile a sermon in the form of a long letter with a copy to Dean Vaughan, rebuking Wile for saying he was indifferent to public opinion. Wile had not only violated the principle that an individual has the exclusive right to determine the use of his body but he had greatly endangered the freedom of research. Keen wrote a series of less restrained and more indignant letters to Vaughan, who replied uneasily that he thought Wile's work was justified. Vaughan said it proved that general paresis is a syphilitic infection.

In an editorial in the *Journal of the American Medical Association* Cannon, without naming Wile, singled out each action for which Wile could be criticized.

Occasionally, however, reports appear which indicate that investigators have made tests on human subjects which possibly may not have been intended directly for the benefit of the person concerned. In some instances it has not been clear that the consent of the subject was obtained. In other instances, in which dependents have been subjects, the superintendent of the hospital or asylum has been responsible for his charges, and it has not been clear whether he has given his consent or secured the sanction of relatives. . . . The medical profession is certainly not called on, in any sense, to support the physician who transgresses the elementary principles of ethics.[85]

Keen in a letter in the same issue of the journal was more forthright.

These investigations, however, in my opinion, were wholly unjustifiable. . . . Hence I wish to register here my condemnation of Dr. Wile's experiments and a protest against any similar experiments in the future.[86]

Keen, however, diluted his criticism with a detailed attack on an antivivisectionist for lying.

In 1917 Wile described finding spirochetes in the spinal fluid of patients with tabes dorsalis, general paresis, and cerebrospinal syphilis.[87] He had not seen spirochetes in spinal fluid itself, but he found them in rabbits inoculated with the fluid. In 1923 he treated spinal fluid samples with 95 percent alcohol and examined the resulting clot. He found spirochetes in 9 of 115 samples.[88] No one commented on the moral difference between searching for spirochetes in spinal fluid and looking for them in the brain.

Wile's Treatment of Syphilis

Udo Wile established his syphilis clinic in 1913, and he thought his patients were treated under ideal conditions in the University Hospital. They were not "treated in the ambulatory fashion" but remained in the hospital, chiefly in bed, for eighteen days.[89] Breakey had thought treatment should not begin until secondary manifestations appear, but Wile believed treatment should start at once and be vigorously prosecuted. He said the appearance of late sequelae is an indictment of inefficient early treatment.[90] Beginning in 1916 Wile repeatedly demonstrated that the nervous system is frequently involved in early syphilis before there is any other evidence of hematogenous spread. "The fate of every syphilitic with regard to the incidences of cerebrospinal lues . . . is determined in the first months of the infection."[91] If the central nervous system is not involved

early, it is seldom involved later. Wile also found that bones and joints were affected in 60 of 165 cases of early syphilis.[92]

Arsphenamine (Salvarsan) began to replace mercurial ointments from which volatile mercury compounds were inhaled and mercuric chloride, salicylate, or tannate given by injection at the beginning of Wile's career.[93] A little later Wile found neoarsphenamine (Neosalvarsan) easier to administer and less toxic than arsphenamine.[94] He soon learned to give intradural injections of neoarsphenamine, and by 1914 he had experience with fifteen cases of tabes dorsalis, general paresis, cerebrospinal syphilis, and taboparesis.[95] Unfortunately, patients were likely to experience severe pain immediately after injection and to die in a day or two.

Wile said he had no routine treatment for syphilis; every case must be considered individually. He made this clear when he outlined the principles of treatment of cardiovascular syphilis.[96] The best treatment is prophylaxis, twenty or thirty injections of an arsenical with interim bismuth in the early stages. He said there is a small group of patients who have arrhythmias during treatment, and he thought invasion by spirochetes of tissue previously damaged by some other event is responsible. Such patients should have bed rest and standard antisyphilitic treatment. There are patients, chiefly middle-aged men, who might have four-plus Wassermanns but who are otherwise in perfect health. Treatment to reverse their positive blood test did more harm than good. A patient with syphilitic heart failure should receive the same treatment as that for failure from any other cause, but his syphilis should be treated cautiously. Vigorous treatment might produce a therapeutic paradox, making the patient worse instead of better, for the syphilitic heart seems to do better when the process of repair is slow.[97]

The Cooperative Clinical Group

In the 1930s Wile joined the Cooperative Clinical Group, whose purpose was to discover the optimal treatment for syphilis and to determine what treatment accomplishes. Wile's student John H. Stokes of Pennsylvania was chairman, and other members included H. N. Cole of Western Reserve, P. A. O'Leary of the Mayo Clinic, and Joseph E. Moore of Johns Hopkins. The group was assisted by members of the U.S. Public Health Service, including Thomas Parran Jr. and R. A. Vonderlehr, and it was supported by an anonymous donor and the Milbank Memorial Fund. The group drew 5,293 patients whose spinal fluid had been examined twice from a pool of 75,000 syphilitics.

The group said optimal treatment must begin with arsphenamine; no other drug would do. Treatment must be continuous and last at least eighteen months with not less than twenty and preferably thirty-two injections of 0.3 to 0.6 gram of arsphenamine. In a total of 105,942 injections the group found mild reactions to arsphenamine in 14.7 percent and severe reactions in 2.2 percent. Treatment with a heavy metal is required as an adjuvant, and bismuth is better than mercury. If bismuth is used, injections of arsphenamine should be interrupted five times so that a total of forty-two injections of a water- or oil-soluble bismuth preparation could be given in a dose of 0.1 to 0.2 gram twice weekly. Bismuth medication should be accompanied by 2 to 3 grams of potassium iodide three times a day. In the meantime, the patient is advised to practice continence, but because the advice is seldom followed absolute mechanical protection during intercourse is required.[98]

Wile and other members of the group understood the relative benignity of untreated syphilis, but they could not determine correctly the efficacy of treatment unless they could compare their treated patients with an untreated group. Only a retrospective study was available in 1934.[99] The physician in charge of the syphilis clinic in Oslo's Royal Hospital between 1891 and 1916 believed that syphilitics did as well untreated as with the mercurial treatment then in vogue. As a consequence 2,181 patients infected in that period had gone untreated. In 1925–27 another Norwegian physician identified 473 of the original patients. There were no signs of syphilis in 27 percent of the 309 then living, and only 37 percent of the 164 who had died had lesions of late syphilis. To provide a comparable prospective study, the U.S. Public Health Service, with the advice and participation of the Cooperative Clinical Group, began a long-term study of untreated syphilis in African American males in Macon County, Alabama. The progress of the study was published in the open literature for thirty years, and tragically no one raised an objection until 1972, when the public was informed of the Tuskegee Study by Jean Heller of the Associated Press.[100]

Malaria Therapy

Wile began to treat syphilis with malaria in the University Hospital in 1925, and by 1941 he had treated over one thousand patients. Twenty-nine had died as the result of treatment, twelve with circulatory collapse and five each of pneumonia or hyperpyrexia. Two patients had committed suicide.[101] Wile induced malaria by patient-to-patient transfusion, and he usually allowed ten to twelve paroxysms before he aborted the malaria. Occasionally he allowed as many as fifteen and once seventeen.

Wile first used malaria therapy for dementia paralytica. He found early results disappointing, but he thought that was because he picked the worst cases for treatment. His eventual conclusion was that the treatment prolonged life but had little effect on the dementia. He observed good results with tabes, obtaining improvement in sixty-three of eighty-seven patients, and he extended the treatment to other forms of neurosyphilis.

Will Herdman and His Three Specialties

William James Herdman was responsible for three specialties long before Udo Wile came to Ann Arbor: neurology, psychiatry, and electrotherapeutics.

Herdman had graduated from the University of Michigan Medical School in 1875, when the two-year curriculum was still in effect, and he immediately went into private practice in Ann Arbor. He soon began to specialize in neurology, but he continued to have a large miscellaneous private practice until his death. He was also surgeon to the Ann Arbor Railroad, a position providing passes on trains, and he taught the university's law students about railway injuries and expert testimony.[102] Within four years of graduation Herdman began to help Corydon Ford teach anatomy in the dissecting room. He published a tiny *Guide to the Dissection of the Human Body* that in thirty small pages attempted to answer the students' questions: "Where shall we begin? What ought we to look for? What should we do next?"[103] A little later he began to teach pathological anatomy as well, but when he followed the course of a patient with a cyst of parasitic origin at the base of the brain, the autopsy was done by Gibbes.[104]

From 1888 Herdman was professor of neurology with a part-time appointment, and after the four-year curriculum was adopted he lectured and taught neurology in a clinic on Wednesday afternoon. He was assisted by Jeanne Cady Solis, who was appointed immediately after graduation in 1892. George Dock's clinical notes show that patients were referred between his clinic and Herdman's. In 1890 diseases of the mind were added to Herdman's responsibilities, and because he was an enthusiastic practitioner of electrotherapeutics he was made professor of the subject. Herdman began to practice and to teach roentgenology in 1896 because he had the electrical equipment available. That will be described in chapter 21.

In a campaign beginning in 1901 Herdman and the regents persuaded the legislature to appropriate fifty thousand dollars to build a psychopathic hospital next to the East Ward of the University Hospital on Catherine Street. It would be the central laboratory of the state system of asylums, and it was to be supported by the state through the Joint Board of the Asylums for the Insane. However, it was to be staffed and managed by the university. At that time there were four asylums in Michigan, and the state was spending a million dollars a year to maintain them. The hospital in Ann Arbor was to be a modern mental health research institute where the physicians and surgeons of the Michigan faculty could obtain more accurate knowledge of "the nature and causes of insanity" by systematic observation, investigation, and treatment.[105] This would save the state money in the long run. Because it was one of the state hospitals, patients could be brought to it from other hospitals, and incurable patients could be transferred out to make room for more useful subjects of investigation. Family physicians were to be helped, and the public was to be educated. Construction started in 1902, and the hospital was opened in February 1906. Fifty-five patients were brought to it from asylums in Pontiac and Kalamazoo. George Dock sent his fourth-year students to perform physical examinations on the patients. Ten days later the students had not done them. The patients were "excited a little"; the house physician would take the cases. Dock sent them back to the Psychopathic Hospital to try again.

In 1906 Herdman was given a full-time salary and leave of absence to study psychiatry in Europe. He started out, but on his way he developed intestinal obstruction and died after an operation in Baltimore at the age of fifty-eight without seeing the results of his progressive idea. Albert Moore Barrett, a neuropathologist from Massachusetts, was put in charge of the Psychopathic Hospital, and what he did will be described in chapter 22.

Herdman as a Neurologist and Psychiatrist

Herdman's obituary notice in the *Journal of the American Medical Association* says he was one of the most prominent U.S. neurologists,[106] but it is hard to account for that opinion. He was successful enough as a medical politician to be elected chairman of the American Medical Association's Section on Neurology and Medical Jurisprudence and eminent enough to be invited to lecture on topics of general medical interest, but his published work on neurology is trivial. He described simple neuritis for the benefit of Michigan general practitioners[107] and primary lateral sclerosis for which treatment was the usual course of potassium iodide.[108] He thought exophthalmic goiter is a neurological disease resulting from congestion of a center in the spinal cord or in sympathetic ganglia that might be treated with galvanism in addition to digitalis, iron, bromides, and nerve tonics such as arsenic, phosphorus, and zinc.[109] When he described in great detail at a meeting of the Michigan State Medical Society what he thought was a case of trophoneurosis he was challenged by a discussant who suggested the patient really had a vascular disease.[110] Herdman had no satisfactory reply.

The neurology Herdman taught can be judged from some of the examination questions he posed at the end of the first semester of 1899–1900.

1. Give the etiology, pathology, symptoms and treatment of amyotrophic lateral sclerosis.
2. Give the differential diagnosis of ataxic paraplegia, posterior spinal sclerosis, and Friedreich's ataxia.[111]

The remaining three questions were more of the same, and so were the first four of the five questions set at the end of the second semester. Herdman's teaching of neurology paralleled McMurrich's course on neuroanatomy, and the Michigan tradition of neurology firmly based on neuroanatomy was established.

In 1899–1900 diseases of the mind were covered by the fifth question

5. What are the characteristics of delusional insanity (Paranoia)? What medico-legal significance does it possess?

Do the statutory enactments of our states deal justly with this class of defectives?[112]

In 1895–96 the corresponding question had been

5. What are the characteristics of simple mania and melancholia and how should cases of each be treated?[113]

Until 1906 Michigan medical students had little opportunity to study psychiatric patients for themselves. Beginning about 1894 Herdman took the medical class to visit "two insane asylums, where the most interesting cases of mental disease are selected and used for clinical instruction."[114] Later, superintendents of Michigan asylums lectured to the senior class each year. The regents allowed them traveling expenses but no honorarium.

Henry Mills Hurd, the Michigan medical graduate of 1866 who was the superintendent of the Eastern Michigan Insane Asylum in Pontiac, told his Ann Arbor audience how to recognize simple mania and how to begin its treatment. First, turn out all injudicious relatives and curious neighbors. "Don't bleed the patient, don't shave the head and apply a blister, don't blister the back of the neck, don't fancy you have cerebro-spinal meningitis and apply croton oil along the whole length of the spine, don't give large doses of opium."[115]

For Herdman in 1904, Emil Kraepelin of Heidelberg was the "commander-in-chief in the present campaign against insanity," and his work was a model of what should be done at Michigan.[116] Kraepelin thought mental manifestations are nothing else than functions of the brain: "Mental disorders are diffuse illnesses of the cerebral cortex."[117] Kraepelin rejected psychoanalytical implications. Herdman's attitude was equally materialistic. Fatigue, for example, in neurasthenia is literally the result of fatigue of nerve cells exhibiting chromatolysis. The normal condition of fatigued cells is usually resumed in a few hours, but if the cells are forced to continue to function, more intense chromatolysis and neurasthenia result. The sympathetic nervous system becomes unstable, and in a vicious cycle metabolic disturbances affect already devitalized nerve cells. Higher centers are permanently affected, making neurasthenia a psychic disorder.[118] On the other hand, simple mania is not associated with demonstrable organic brain disease; cortical hyperemia accounts for the excessive ideation. Simple melancholia is a form of moral insanity in which

the surplus stock of animal spirits and *vis nervosa* is soon exhausted.[119]

Neurasthenia can be treated by S. Weir Mitchell's method.[120] The physician must take over and dominate the patient, who is to be given "a combination of entire rest and of excessive feeding, made possible by passive exercise obtained through the steady use of massage"[121] and systematic stimulation of unused muscles by induced currents. Patients with simple mania should be taken to the open country or go on long sea voyages between attacks. Hot baths and cold compresses to the head are useful, but hypnotics should be avoided. Attacks of mania are likely to recur, ending in dementia. Melancholy turns into catatonia. Treatment is usually ineffective in the long run, and patients end in an asylum.

As for etiology, diseases of the mind follow pneumonia or typhoid fever, and they may be caused by gout or phthisis. Alcohol and drugs are important causes. Syphilis is responsible for some but by no means all cases of paretic dementia, "for paretic dementia is . . . the result of a chronic inflammatory process of an angio-paralytic nature, whose essential element, the vaso-motor weakening, is due to overstrain of the encephalic vaso-motor centre."[122] Psychic events, emotional problems, harsh treatment, failures in business cause insanity, but above all they must act on hereditary disposition. Some persons remain normal in the face of the same provocations, because they do not have the hereditary trait of insanity. Everyone agreed that "heredity plays a most important part in the production of mental disease. The vast majority of insane persons inherit a susceptibility to insanity from some ancestor."[123] Therefore, marriage of such persons should be prohibited.

Electrotherapeutics

The Psychopathic Hospital carried Herdman's influence upon medicine at Michigan into the indefinite future, but his favorite specialty, electrotherapeutics, died with him.

Electrotherapeutics flourished in the second half of the nineteenth century. There were journals of electrotherapeutics, schools of electrotherapeutics in many cities and towns, and a national society of electrotherapeutics of which Herdman was once president. Electricity was used in three forms: galvanic, static, and faradic.

Galvanic current was at first produced by an array

of batteries, but when Edison wired cities with direct current it was drawn from the mains. Current flowed through the patient between an indifferent electrode and one designed for application to a particular surface or for insertion into an orifice. Direction of flow was important: current from the negative pole is electrolytic, and current from the positive pole coagulates. Galvanic current was used to treat every recognized disease: exophthalmic goiter, cerebral syphilis, parasitic infestations of the skin, and so on, through the list. According to textbooks of electrotherapeutics, treatment was successful.[124] Georges Apostoli, a Parisian gynecologist, had demonstrated that uterine fibroids could be dissolved by galvanic current from an intrauterine negative electrode,[125] and he soon extended galvanism to treatment of dysmenorrhea. His practice was enthusiastically followed in Ann Arbor by Herdman and his disciple Jeanne Cady Solis.[126] Solis also found that faradic current stimulation of the uterus was nutritive and sedative. Galvanic current delivered by a rectal electrode dissolved rectal strictures, and current delivered by a urethral electrode treated strictures in the male.

For treatment with static electricity the patient was placed on an insulated platform and touched with an electrode connected to a large electrostatic generator. For an "electric bath" a large ring-shaped electrode was held above the patient's head, causing an "electric breeze" that made his or her hair stand on end (fig. 20–3). Solis thought this particularly useful in treatment of neurasthenia, and she recommended that it be applied ten minutes twice a day. "A discharge of sparks from between the shoulders over the organic spinal centers finishes the treatment."[127]

Faradic current produced by a variety of induction coils and interrupters ranged upward to the very high voltage and frequency of a Tesla coil. It was applied by stigmatic electrodes for the identification of motor points and defectively innervated muscles. Faradic current was also applied through urethral electrodes to treat strictures in the male or incontinence in the female. It could be applied by a "brush" electrode, and for treatment of impotence "the dry faradic brush to penis, scrotum, and inner sides of the thighs is also at times an efficient method of producing erections."[128]

Herdman and his associates taught all this to Michigan medical students. He gave an optional course in electrotherapeutics in 1889 when the three-year curriculum was in effect, but it was required when the four-year one was introduced. There was a

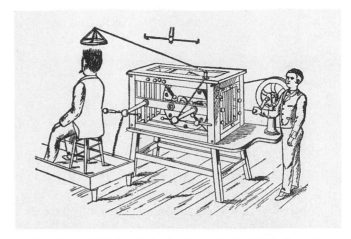

Fig. 20–3. The electric bath. (From G. A. Liebig Jr. and G. H. Rohé, *Practical Electricity in Medicine and Surgery* [Philadelphia: F. A. Davis, 1890], 269.)

laboratory course, every day for six weeks, and it cost a student a dollar. The nature of the course can be seen in the inevitable locally published *Laboratory Manual of Electrotherapeutics* by Herdman and his assistant, F. W. Nagler.[129] Students were taught the principles of direct current: Ohm's law, parallel and series circuits, and so forth. They learned how to construct a Daniell cell, a Bunsen cell, and a bichromate cell, how to make a cautery knife, and, quite practically, how to solder. For faradic currents the students were taught the principles of magnetism and induction and the use of the "physician's induction coil." For static electricity they were introduced to the Wimshurst machine and taught how to apply sparks to the patient. By 1898 the course included instruction in how to generate and detect roentgen rays. There was little on application in the laboratory course; that came later in Herdman's demonstrations and lectures, one afternoon a week. Herdman had no doubts whatever about the efficacy of electrotherapeutics or the importance of his subject. He even gave a correspondence course in electrotherapeutics.[130]

The elevation of electrotherapeutics to a required course could not have occurred without Victor Vaughan's approval. Vaughan's scientific and clinical judgment was not sufficiently penetrating to make him critical of the claims of electrotherapeutics, and at the same time he was touting his nucleinic acid as a treatment for tuberculosis. Nevertheless, when Herdman died electrotherapeutics was immediately made optional and dropped two years later.

Not Just Any Medical School

21
Roentgenology

When roentgenology became a medical specialty early in 1896 there were no roentgenologists.[1] In many cities physicians practicing other branches of medicine trained themselves to deal with X rays. In Detroit, for example, Preston M. Hickey learned to use X-ray tubes and soon became a member of the new band of specialists. That did not happen in Ann Arbor, for until Herdman's death roentgenology in the University Hospital was in the hands of a technician with the rank of instructor under the supervision first of the neurologists and then of the surgeons and internists. Finally in 1913 the Department of Roentgenology was created, with J. G. Van Zwaluwenburg as head. When Van Zwaluwenburg died in 1922 Preston M. Hickey was brought to Ann Arbor to take charge of roentgenology and to plan the facilities in the new hospital. In turn, Fred Jenner Hodges succeeded Hickey.

The Beginning of Roentgenology at Michigan

In 1896 electrotherapeutics was a respectable discipline at Michigan although it was beginning to be considered quackery elsewhere. Soon after Roentgen told the world in December 1895 that the apparatus Herdman had in his private office and in the Electrotherapeutics Laboratory was capable of generating X rays, Herdman became a roentgenologist.

The Crookes tube was a simple device: a partially evacuated glass bulb containing two electrodes. When a large potential difference was established between the electrodes, positive ions in the gas remaining in the tube hit the cathode and stimulated emission of electrons that streamed toward the anode. When the electrons hit the anode, X rays were generated. There was a Crookes tube in every physical laboratory at the time, for the study of electrical discharges in gases occupied many physicists. The physicists did not know their tubes were emitting X rays until Roentgen told them so. Likewise, every physicist had a means of generating the high potential difference, an induction coil producing alternating current or an electrostatic generator producing direct current. Consequently, when the news of Roentgen's discovery that the Crookes tube, or Hittorf tube as it was called in Germany, emits a ray that penetrates flesh and casts the shadow of a bone on a photographic plate became known, hundreds of persons in Europe and the United States made X-ray photographs.[2] Sometime in February 1896

Michael Pupin had photographed a New York lawyer's hand containing buckshot, and shortly thereafter someone brought a patient with a bullet in his foot to Ann Arbor. Professor Henry S. Carhart of the Physics Laboratory and Herdman rigged up a Crookes tube and photographed the foot. Nancrede removed the bullet. The next year roentgenograms of a bullet in the hand, of one in the collar bone, of a needle in the foot, and of a diseased knee were published in the *Michigan Alumnus* (fig. 21–1).[3]

In 1902 the regents appropriated one thousand dollars to purchase X-ray equipment that was to be in the charge of Mr. Vernon J. Willey, instructor in electrotherapeutics, and they provided three hundred dollars to be used to fit up a room in the basement of the Palmer Ward to hold the equipment. The regents allowed a salary not to exceed four hundred dollars for an assistant who was to attend to photography and to do routine work. That item was carried in the surgery budget. The regents also tackled the perennial problem of jurisdiction over roentgen rays by ruling that Willey alone was to operate the equipment.

By 1903 Nancrede and his staff used X rays for treatment as well as diagnosis.[4] Nancrede gave thirty-four exposures to an ulcer on a patient's upper lip, and he unsuccessfully treated a woman with a massive genitourinary growth referred to him by Peterson. Nancrede, with his customary conservatism, tried to avoid superficial burns, and he said burns could be avoided by a short exposure of fifteen minutes. He warned against trying to make a diagnosis by X rays alone.[5] He had found a large stone in the bladder although the X-ray plate had shown nothing. The stone, consisting of uric acid, was radiolucent. At the same time George Dock began to show students in his diagnostic clinic skiagrams of the chests of patients with tuberculosis, and he described treatment of the enlarged spleen of a leukemic patient and of an exophthalmic goiter with X rays. X rays were apparently used routinely for diagnosis and treatment in the University Hospital in the early 1900s.

Vernon J. Willey's Roentgenology

Willey described his methods in detail.[6] When he used the electrostatic machine to generate the potential difference he achieved a dry atmosphere in which the machine worked best by putting a lighted kerosene lamp in its cabinet. He preferred the slightly more reliable high voltage delivered by a large induction coil. Current flowing through the primary coil had to rise and fall in order to induce current in the secondary coil. In the early days only direct current was available, either from a set of chromate batteries or from the Edison Company's lines, but it could be interrupted by a mechanical vibrator acting on the principle of a doorbell. Willey thought the Wehnelt electrolytic interrupter more satisfactory. A platinum electrode protruded into a 20 percent solution of sulfuric acid through a ceramic tube, and the other electrode in the solution was a sheet of lead. When the platinum rod was the anode current, flow was interrupted by alternating formation and collapse of an insulating coat of bubbles about its exposed tip.

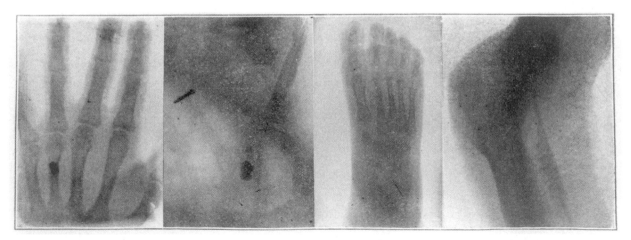

Fig. 21–1. Skiagraphs (radiographs) of cases in the surgical clinic of the University Hospital, 1899. (Courtesy of Dr. William Martel.)

Not Just Any Medical School

Amperage could be controlled by varying the exposure of the tip, but there was no means of controlling or even measuring the frequency. By 1908 the city of Ann Arbor delivered three-phase alternating current at 220 volts to the University Hospital, and Willey built an autotransformer with ten taps to provide more stable and predictable alternating current to his induction coil.

The induction coil could be constructed to supply any desired voltage, but the fact that the current alternated in direction posed a serious problem. X rays are generated when electrons hit the anode. In all tubes the cathode was constructed to focus the electrons on the anode where the X rays were generated, and the anode was constructed to dissipate heat. If electrons flowed in the opposite direction the cathode would be damaged, and that occurred when the alternating current reversed. That was called the inverse current, and the electromotive force responsible could be suppressed by putting a rectifier in the secondary circuit. Willey occasionally used a Lodge valve, whose operation as a rectifier depended upon the geometry and composition of its electrodes. One electrode was a large coil of aluminum that occupied the body of a gas-filled glass tube. The other electrode was a small steel disk well back in a narrow arm of the tube. When the aluminum coil was the cathode it was bombarded by positive ions of the gas and emitted a copious stream of electrons carrying a large current. When the steel disk was the cathode it emitted few electrons that carried only a little current. Consequently, current in effect flowed in only one direction through the tube. Willey also used an electrolytic rectifier that consisted of two electrodes immersed in an alkaline solution. One electrode was aluminum and the other steel, lead, or carbon. If alternating current was passed through the solution for a few minutes, the aluminum electrode became polarized by a coat of aluminum salts. Thereafter resistance to flow of current in one direction was higher than resistance to flow in the other direction. Alternatively, Willey used a spark gap, one pole being pointed and the other flat. Because a spark leaps more easily from a point than a plate, the spark gap rectified the current.

Willey, like other roentgenologists, measured the potential difference by means of a spark gap. The rule was that the voltage supplied equaled ten thousand volts plus another ten thousand volts multiplied by the length of the spark in inches. Willey thought that an induction coil should deliver at least a nine-inch spark, but he preferred one at least fourteen inches long.

Rays emitted by Willey's tubes were either hard or soft, hard being the most penetrating and soft the least. Penetration was measured by a set of platinum windows of graded thickness, but Willey made his own penetrometer by gluing aluminum disks and lead and brass strips to a sheet of cardboard. He could judge the hardness of the rays by examining the penetrometer fluoroscopically, but he was careful to shield his hand with lead while doing so. The hardness of the rays generated by a particular tube depended upon the vacuum, and the vacuum changed as it was used. Gases adsorbed on the glass were released. Willey went to a good deal of trouble to measure the characteristics of his tubes in order to correlate hardness with such quantities as the age of the tube and applied wattage, and he had at least five different tubes, each for a specific purpose. A new tube gave soft rays, and an exposure of twenty or more minutes was required for photography. An aged tube emitted homogeneous hard rays giving a satisfactory exposure time in 0.5 to 10 seconds. Length of exposure was important, for a patient could not be immobilized long.

Willey told his readers that they should develop their own plates and not rely upon portrait or landscape photographers, whose aims in producing a negative are different. He described solutions and procedures needed to obtain the sharpest contrast with the shortest exposure. Michael Pupin had used a fluorescent screen to intensify a photographic image in 1896, but Willey did not anticipate the 1912 commercial availability of intensifiers by making his own.

Secondary rays blurred the image. Some came from the tube itself, and some came from the cones used in an attempt to collimate the rays. Willey recommended a diaphragm to cut off the secondary rays from the tube. The most troublesome rays were generated within the subject him- or herself, and they constituted as much as 80 percent of the radiation reaching the photographic plate. The problem was solved by inserting a grid between the subject and the plate and then making the grid move during exposure of the plate. That occurred shortly after Willey left Michigan.[7]

Willey went to medical school while he was working as a roentgenologist, and he graduated from Michigan in 1909. He became head of the Section on Roentgenology at the Mayo Clinic in July 1909, but he left the clinic in 1911 and died of heart failure in Kalamazoo in 1912.

Roentgenology, 1909–12

Nancrede was nominally responsible for the X-ray service, but the actual activities of the service were in the hands of James Gerrit Van Zwaluwenburg, a young instructor in the Department of Internal Medicine. Van Zwaluwenburg had the practical skill required in dealing with the technical aspects of roentgenology.

Van Zwaluwenburg prepared at Hope College and earned a bachelor's degree from Michigan in 1898, studying chemistry under Moses Gomberg. Van Zwaluwenburg wanted to study medicine, for he was inspired by his much older brother Cornelius, a surgeon. Because he was too poor to go to medical school, he worked five years as a chemist and metallurgist in Canada, Missouri, and New Jersey. When he did enter medical school in 1903 he laid the foundations of his profound knowledge of human anatomy by assisting in the dissection room.[8] After graduating in 1907 he served a year under George Dock, and when Dock left in 1908 he served under Walter Hewlett. Van Zwaluwenburg's contributions to Hewlett's work with occlusion plethysmography have already been described.

Sometime around 1910 Van Zwaluwenburg and Luther F. Warren, another instructor in internal medicine, undertook a study of the dimensions of the heart using orthodiagramography, a method for outlining any object seen by X rays without distortion. Orthodiagramography had been described in 1900 by Prof. Dr. Moritz of Munich.[9] The method had been improved by others, chiefly Franz Groedel, and an enormous German literature on the subject had sprung up.[10] A Crookes tube was mounted on a movable frame below the table on which the subject lay, and an arm having an aperture with a small lead spot in its center was fixed to the same frame above the subject but below a fluorescent screen. The small lead spot was directly above the anode of the Crookes tube, and it maintained its position relative to the anode as the frame was moved in either horizontal direction. The observer guided the frame so that the small lead spot followed the shadow on the fluorescent screen to be outlined, and a pen or pencil attached to the frame traced the path of the spot on paper. The University Hospital had such a device in 1910, and its use demonstrates Van Zwaluwenburg's familiarity with roentgenology before he left the Department of Internal Medicine.

Van Zwaluwenburg and Warren used the method to outline the heart shadows in 187 subjects, 9 of them long-distance runners on the track team.[11] Other subjects were patients with mitral stenosis or regurgitation, aortic regurgitation, myocardial insufficiency, and so on. They made an elaborate geometrical analysis of their figures. The area of the heart measured with a planimeter borrowed from the Engineering Department was not useful, for there were no distinctive differences among the patients with different heart diseases. In addition, the heart might be greatly enlarged in other directions although its horizontal dimensions are normal. Instead, they chose linear dimensions they thought represented chiefly the size of the auricles or of the ventricles, and they found that they could distinguish among normal subjects, the athletes with slightly enlarged ventricles, and patients with mitral stenosis and aortic regurgitation. Van Zwaluwenburg and Warren reported their results to the referring physicians to be compared with results determined by percussion, but they did not relate any comments made by the physicians. Van Zwaluwenburg remained an enthusiast for orthodiagramography for the next ten years.[12]

In May 1913 Nancrede asked to be relieved of the responsibility for roentgenology at the end of the academic year, and Van Zwaluwenburg, out of a sense of duty, agreed to take full charge. He was appointed clinical professor of roentgenology with a salary of two thousand dollars, the title and the salary indicating that he was expected to earn the rest of his living by private practice. There was only one X-ray tube in the hospital, and the regents agreed to provide some new equipment. They gave Van Zwaluwenburg four hundred dollars for an assistant. Otherwise, the department was expected to be self-supporting. Van Zwaluwenburg spent the summer of 1913 traveling to Boston, New York, and Philadelphia to learn more about roentgenology. At the beginning of the school year Van Zwaluwenburg, like every other person who has assumed direction of a department of radiology, complained bitterly about the state of the equipment he had inherited. He said forward progress had stopped in 1906, the date of Herdman's death, and thereafter there had been only retrogression, both in the physical condition of the equipment and in the character of the work. Repairs had been woefully neglected, and some valuable apparatus had fallen into disuse. Van Zwaluwenburg with his practical experience and his ability to build equipment was a good man for the job. He was also able to pick and train good technical assistants. He could find any plate that he had ever made in a few minutes or tell where it had gone if it had been borrowed. Dean Cabot praised Van Zwaluwenburg's capacity for organization and his knowledge of business methods. He was the first man in the University Hospital to use a Dictaphone, and his typed reports reached the referring departments quickly.

Roentgenology, 1913–22

Before Van Zwaluwenburg's time the X-ray laboratory was a purely service enterprise. Because there was no formal teaching of roentgenology, George Dock had to explain to his students that a skiagraph represents the subject as seen in a mirror and that the plate is a negative with the densities reversed. Van Zwaluwenburg immediately instituted a course of lectures once a week on diagnosis and therapy for senior medical students, but his major effort was providing service for the clinical departments. Providing good service was a way of teaching the staff. He said that a surgeon could learn continuously by relating roentgenological findings to operative findings, and in 1917 Van Zwaluwenburg described fifty-six such instances.[13] His diagnoses before operation were made blind, for he insisted that clinical findings and laboratory results not be sent to him along with the patient. Knowing the findings might prejudice the roentgenologist, who might tend to confirm the diagnosis or lean over backward to disprove it. There had been perfect agreement in twenty-six of the cases, and Van Zwaluwenburg was particularly pleased with his success in diagnosing gallbladder disease. In another twelve his diagnosis had been incomplete, but operation was justified. He said three cases had no redeeming features; the correct diagnosis had been missed by both the roentgenologist and the surgeon. Even a correct diagnosis might be medically wrong. He cited the example of a nurse with abdominal discomfort and morbid fear of gastric carcinoma. He found nothing wrong with her stomach, but he saw an enlarged gallbladder containing seven stones. A surgeon (and—Van Zwaluwenburg carefully pointed out—not one working in the University Hospital) had removed her gallbladder and

confirmed Van Zwaluwenburg's count. Because the stones had doubtless been present for years without causing symptoms and because the operation did not relieve the patient's discomfort, Van Zwaluwenburg thought both he and the surgeon had made a mistake.

Almost every month Van Zwaluwenburg showed lantern slides derived from his previous month's work to the Clinical Society of the University of Michigan. In one month in 1916, for example, he described twenty-six cases: bone disease and fractures, an unerupted tooth, a brain tumor, a bullet in the tip of the frontal lobe that Nancrede removed, a safety pin in the esophagus, and carcinoma of the stomach.

Van Zwaluwenburg regularly reported to Dean Vaughan as well, and the summary of his first three yearly reports shows the growth of his service. In the two calendar years before he took over, 609 and 830 plates had been exposed, and billings had been $1,064.27 and $1,369.00. In the next three academic years with Van Zwaluwenburg in charge 1,271, 1,457, and 2,217 plates were made, and billings had risen from $3,895.35 in the first of the three years to $8,546.85 in the third. Receipts did not quite keep up with billings, for only $7,363.87 had been collected in the last year. That was not enough to keep the department going, and Van Zwaluwenburg told the dean he absolutely had to have another $2,000 in his current account to get through the rest of the year and $500 for repair of a machine.

Van Zwaluwenburg could not do all that work as a clinical professor, and in 1915 he was back on full time as an associate professor. He was promoted to full professorship in 1919. In the same period Van Zwaluwenburg had only technical assistants: two, three, or four men without degrees. Finally in 1919–20 he had one man with a medical degree to help him, and the next year he had two physician instructors: one senior intern and one junior intern. When Van Zwaluwenburg died suddenly of pneumonia in the early morning of 5 January 1922, leaving his family destitute, two instructors carried on for the rest of the academic year and saw Van Zwaluwenburg's last publication through the press.[14]

Van Zwaluwenburg's Roentgenology

Van Zwaluwenburg preferred to use a fluoroscope when examining a patient thought to have a peptic ulcer. If he took a film he could examine only two or three patients a day. Because the viscera move, he had to make frequent exposures, and that ran up the cost. With a fluoroscope he could examine twenty to twenty-five patients a day. In 1915 he used bismuth as the contrast medium, but he switched to barium in 1917. Bismuth subnitrate or barium sulfate was suspended in fermented milk, a mixture he thought more acceptable than a suspension in water. The acid in the milk delayed gastric emptying by exciting the pyloric reflex. Van Zwaluwenburg found that "the great diagnostic wastebasket labeled 'Gastric Neurosis' show[ed] gradual and consistent shrinkage of its contents" as he became more expert.[15]

Stereographic roentgenograms had been made since 1896, but Van Zwaluwenburg with his mechanical ability devised his own method of displaying pairs so they could be viewed sitting down.[16] He used the stereographic method to improve localization of foreign bodies in the eye,[17] and "after struggling some time with the methods available in the face of an unsympathetic surgeon" Van Zwaluwenburg succeeded in differentiating "the confusing shadows of the structures of the base of the skull" and cervical spine when he took stereographic views of the skull for the purpose of diagnosing accessory sinusitis.[18] Van Zwaluwenburg also used stereographic technique when he devised pelycography for Reuben Peterson.[19] A local anesthetic was infiltrated into a woman's skin one inch below the umbilicus, and a needle connected to an anesthesia bag full of carbon dioxide was plunged through the skin. One and a half liters of gas was insufflated, or two liters if the patient did not complain too seriously, and then the patient assumed the knee-chest position with a plate changer beneath her. Van Zwaluwenburg took stereographic pairs by shifting the tube on the long axis of the body. He used carbon dioxide because a patient filled with oxygen was uncomfortable for twenty-four to forty-eight hours. The procedure meant that he had to make his plates in the gynecological examining room with portable apparatus, because the carbon dioxide disappeared by absorption by the time the patient reached the X-ray laboratory. It is not quite clear why Peterson could not have done the insufflation in the latter place. By 1920 Van Zwaluwenburg had examined more than forty patients by this method.

Van Zwaluwenburg examined a large number of patients with pulmonary tuberculosis, and he was surprised to see that a lung collapsed by spontaneous or therapeutic pneumothorax is less X-ray dense than a normally expanded lung. That made him think that most of the shadow is contributed by blood in the lung. After going to a great deal of trouble to get exactly comparable films, he demonstrated that the lung shadow is darker during forced inspiration on a closed glottis when the lung capillaries are relatively full than during a forced expiration on a closed glottis when the lung capillaries are relatively empty.[20]

Van Zwaluwenburg examined stereopairs of chest X rays, and he found "a clear line usually seen along the inner surface of the second rib and separated from its shadow by a clear space of perhaps 3 or 4 mm. wide. It may also be seen at times beneath the first rib and sometimes it extends downward further into the axilla or becomes continuous with the shadow of the thickened pleura left by a preceding pleural effusion."[21] Van Zwaluwenburg saw this "pleural cap" in 10 percent of all chest X rays in the University Hospital, but he saw the cap in 93 percent of patients showing tuberculous deposits in the faucial tonsils. When Van Zwaluwenburg reviewed a large number of films of tuberculous and nontuberculous patients he thought that the route of infection is from the tonsils through the cervical lymph glands to the pleura and finally to the apex of the lungs.[22] In the last year of his life Van Zwaluwenburg made stereograms of the entire first- and second-year medical classes, and he obtained 258 satisfactory pairs of films. Ninety-six pairs showed the pleural line, and 16 gave evidence of tuberculosis. Those sixteen students were independently examined by internists.[23] Eight were found entirely free of tuberculosis. Seven had healed and inactive tuberculosis, and one had suspicious findings. Van Zwaluwenburg thought it would be particularly interesting to follow the students with apical caps, but he did not live to do so.

Preston Manasseh Hickey

Within three weeks of Van Zwaluwenburg's death the regents chose Preston M. Hickey to be professor of roentgenology, and Hickey took up his appointment in the autumn of 1922 after a trip to Europe. Hickey gave up a large private practice in Detroit to accept a full-time appointment at Michigan carrying a salary of twelve thousand dollars.

When Hickey graduated from the university's Literary Department in 1888 he had accumulated ninety-two hours' credit in Greek, Latin, Sanskrit, French, German, and Italian, and reading Greek remained a lifelong recreation. About the time he graduated he formed a friendship with Aldred Warthin, who had just arrived in Ann Arbor to begin his medical studies. Hickey earned his doctor of medicine degree from the Detroit College of Medicine in 1892, and at first he practiced pathology. Later his interest in pathology and his friendship with Warthin resulted in a jointly conducted interdepartmental conference on Friday afternoons.[24] Early in Hickey's Detroit career he switched from pathology to otolaryngology, and he practiced that specialty with E. L. Shurly, whose views on tuberculosis were closer to Gibbes's than to Warthin's. Shurly bought one of the first pieces of commercial X-ray apparatus to be used in Michigan, and that together with Hickey's hobbies of photomicrography and landscape photography turned Hickey toward roentgenology about 1900. When Hickey trained himself as a roentgenologist he was already a competent clinician, and all his life he insisted that a roentgenologist must be a broadly based clinical consultant rather than a mere technician.

Hickey quickly established himself as an expert roentgenologist and as an elder statesman of the new specialty. In 1906 he was founding editor of the *American Quarterly Journal of Roentgenology,* and he remained editor for ten years. He was elected president of the American Roentgen Ray Society in 1906, and for the rest of his life he was active in the society's affairs. He was particularly interested in setting professional standards. Hickey was a part-time professor of roentgenology at the Detroit College of Medicine, and he conducted his private practice in his own suite of rooms at the Harper Hospital. When he was designing that space he said: "No waiting room is provided, the hall serving for outpatients."[25] Older persons will remember a similar uncomfortable arrangement in the 1925 University Hospital's Department of Roentgenology planned by Hickey where inpatients waited on gurneys in the hall for hours. Hickey went to France with the Harper Hospital unit in World War I, but he was soon detailed to serve as consultant to all U.S. forces in France.[26]

In contrast with other pioneer radiologists who died lingering deaths as the result of burns, Hickey was never injured by X rays. That may be because he avoided doing fluoroscopy before the days of lead-impregnated gloves.

Hickey's Department at Michigan

Hickey protested that hospital superintendents put the Roentgenology Department in the basement near to the coal cellar and that architects gave it inadequate wiring. He found the Michigan department in the basement of the Palmer Ward, and he shared his main transformer with another heavy and unpredictable load.[27] The regents gave him ten thousand dollars for some new equipment, but his chief concern was that he could plan the space for his new department in the hospital under construction. He was proud of the department he occupied in August 1925.[28]

Hickey's new department occupied twelve thousand square feet on one floor of the Surgical Wing, and it was entered at its center through a corridor from the main building. A corridor at a right angle to the east led to rooms for patient examination and treatment, and a corridor at a right angle to the west led to rooms for the staff.

Hickey did get his own transformer delivering current at 220 volts through large enough wires, and he saw to it that all electrical arrangements were safe. In addition, he had base plugs installed throughout the rest of the hospital capable of carrying thirty amperes for a portable machine.

The examining rooms were grouped around the photographic rooms. Hickey carefully specified the characteristics of the light traps for exchanging cassettes, the temperature control of the developing tanks, and the arrangement for turning on and off the lights in the film-changing room to minimize damage to expensive intensifying screens. He even provided for recovery of silver from the developing solutions. Hickey thought most delay occurred in waiting for patients to change clothes, so he built a row of dressing rooms that patients could enter from the waiting area in the hall and leave into the examining rooms. In one examining room there was a ten-kilowatt tube over a horizontal table fitted with a Potter-Bucky diaphragm, and there was another tube under the table for fluoroscopy. Because the room was used for barium enemas, there was a toilet nearby. A separate, similar room served for the Graham test, for gallbladder visualization was in heavy demand. The room containing the vertical fluoroscope with its orthodiagraphic frame was indirectly lighted at floor level so that patients could find their way and examiners not lose dark adaptation. There was also a fluoroscopy room on the surgical floor fitted with a clock adding seconds and minutes of radiation exposure of the patient. There were smaller rooms for head and dental work. The treatment room, separated from the examining rooms, contained a 250,000-volt tube for deep therapy, and its floor was battleship linoleum over a thick layer of barium plaster. Hickey found there was no stray radiation in the room below. The department also had one hundred milligrams of radium and apparatus to collect radium emanation, all bought in 1928 with thirty-five thousand dollars voted by the regents. Finally, there was a shop for instruments used in measurement of radiation.[29]

Hickey was particularly concerned to have adequate ventilation, and he insisted that there be large windows, even in the darkrooms, fitted with lightproof wooden shutters. He did not trust the hospital ventilation system, and he wanted to have plenty of blowers on hand.

At the staff end of the hall there was an office for Hickey and his secretary, and offices were found for others as the staff grew. Because Hickey preferred teaching in small groups, there was a classroom for section teaching as well as rooms for film viewing where Van Zwaluwenburg's stereoscopic device was still in use. Current films were filed and kept in the department for two or three years and then transferred to a fireproof vault for a year. After that they were permanently filed in another vault with a smokeproof door.

Hickey as a Roentgenologist

His friend Warthin said of Hickey: "His mind was not primarily scientific; he was not preëminently an investigator."[30] Hickey regarded himself first of all "as a clinician, and one of his residents said that under him we students had not that lack of confidence in his clinical knowledge which is so evident in the case of certain men who have spent all of their lives in academic work."[31] When Hickey wrote a long account, "The First Decade of American Roentgenology," he described the accomplishments of numerous clinical practitioners, but he did not mention Walter B. Cannon.[32] Otherwise, as a roentgenologist Hickey was, in a nonpejorative sense, a highly accomplished technician.

Twenty-two of Hickey's publications before he came to Michigan are editorials, addresses, and discussions of papers given by others. Nineteen are case

reports, treatment of diphtheria carriers by means of roentgen rays,[33] the intralaryngeal application of radium for chronic papillomata,[34] and X-ray evidence of ulcers.[35] Thirty-five papers are one-, two-, and three-page notes without references describing how to take stereoroentgenograms, detection of a scarf pin in the right lung, the advantages of a lateral view of the hip or spine, the roentgen demonstration of a pulmonary abscess, a simple method of immobilization, and teleoroentgenography of the head.[36] The last note he published from Detroit told how to start colonic peristalsis during a barium enema by allowing the fluid to drain into a bucket.[37] After Hickey had settled in his new quarters his less frequent papers ranged from a description of how to measure the lumen of the esophagus to how to make roentgenographic demonstrations of the trachea and bronchi. For the first Hickey made bougies of various size by punching out barium-impregnated gelatin with cork borers. He began by having the patient swallow the smaller ones, and he worked up to a size that would not pass the obstruction. The observer could stop a bougie at any point if he or she passed a stout thread through it by means of a darning needle.[38] The second was described in a much longer paper written with A. C. Furstenberg.[39] It began by saying that the average roentgenologist—not, it implied, Preston M. Hickey, who had been a laryngologist—does not have the skill to introduce iodinated oil into the trachea without laryngeal irritation. Hickey and Furstenberg preferred supraglottal introduction of the oil by indirect laryngoscopy. The laryngologist, after first anesthetizing the soft palate, the base of the tongue, the epiglottis, and the larynx with a swab of 10 percent cocaine, injected ten to twenty milliliters of oil into the trachea. Alternatively, the oil could be introduced into the trachea of a reclining patient by means of a Jackson bronchoscope. Almost immediately thereafter the roentgenologist began the examination before the oil became emulsified and its shadow blurred. They had only one accident: interstitial emphysema in the neck and shoulders of a child that soon cleared.

Hickey as a Teacher of Roentgenology

Hickey revised teaching of roentgenology at Michigan from the ground up. He persuaded George A. Lindsay of the Physics Department to add a twelve-week section on the physics of X rays to his course on physics for premedical students. Laboratory experiments included measurement of high voltages, the characteristics of gas-filled and Coolidge tubes, X-ray absorption coefficients, measurement of the spectrum and wave length, and determination of dose.[40] Because many Michigan medical students were graduates of the university, they came to Hickey with some knowledge of his subject. Hickey required his residents in training to take the course, and Lindsay taught them informally when he helped Hickey and his staff measure the output of their tubes.

Hickey thought the introduction of large basic science courses had deprived students of the early stimulation they received when medical education was largely by apprenticeship. He tried to remedy this by introducing roentgenology into the first two years,[41] not for its own sake but to "inject something of the practical side of medicine so as to stimulate the enthusiasm of the students."[42] With Huber's consent roentgenologists gave lectures on anatomical topics such as development of the skeleton, and Huber installed viewing boxes in the dissection rooms so that students could see pyelograms and films of injected arterial and venous vessels, of injected bronchi, and of the paranasal sinuses. Hickey praised Walter Meek's use of X rays in measuring cardiac output, for he must have heard Meek lecture on the subject when Meek was in Ann Arbor as a candidate for the chair of physiology. Otherwise, Hickey, who must never have heard of Walter B. Cannon, said physiologists had been backward in the use of X rays, and he hoped they would begin to do so. In this and other connections Hickey said nothing about restricting the use of X rays to trained roentgenologists.

Hickey disliked large class lectures in which students slept in the dark while roentgenologists showed slide after slide, but he moved the lectures on roentgenology from the senior to the junior year so that students could know something about the subject when they were on the wards in the fourth year. He gave no quizzes throughout the year, but he provided students with one hundred study questions upon which the final examination would be based.

Senior students in small groups rotated through the department, and Hickey offered short elective courses on film reading, X-ray technique, and radiotherapy. He was pleased to see how many students took the electives. Senior students were expected to be present when gastric or pulmonary patients were fluoroscoped, and all students could see their patients' films.

Residents intending to become roentgenologists spent two years with Hickey after completing a rotating internship. They began moving through a graded curriculum by making roentgenograms of autopsy and operating room specimens. Because Hickey thought a roentgenologist should be a clinician first and a roentgenologist second, he had his residents take histories and do physical examinations before beginning fluoroscopy on patients. Hickey insisted that a resident achieve technical mastery of the subject, and he had only two technicians, one for the photographic darkroom and one for dental work. Otherwise, residents were to master the techniques of exposure and film development. One resident remembered "many weary months" with portable apparatus.[43] Residents had to know how to measure dosage, and two of them together had to verify and sign for filters in deep therapy. Hickey called a resident on the carpet for sloppy work, but he was lavish in praise of good work. He introduced his residents to the economics of roentgenology, and he gave them training in public speaking.[44]

Hickey taught his students how to write roentgen-ray reports, for he found that in general reports submitted by a roentgenologist were far inferior to those of a pathologist and were haphazard and without respect for scientific accuracy.[45] A report might consist of two words only, or it might be a long disquisition on the nature of the disease and end with impertinent suggestions to the referring physician for therapy. He said: "A simple statement that there is a fracture of the lower end of the radius is usually confirmatory evidence of what the patient has known since the accident,"[46] and he gave examples of the outline of a report on a fracture that would exactly describe what was seen on the roentgenogram. He said candidates for membership in the American Roentgen Ray Society should be required to submit one hundred reports written in conformity with standards set by the society.

Because courts had decided a physician was guilty of negligence in treating a fracture if the physician failed to obtain an X-ray examination of it, Hickey gave a short, intensive course for the general practitioner located in a small town who wished to use X rays in his or her practice. In addition, he gave another short and intensive course in pulmonary diseases, urology, and so on. At another level he gave courses in the technique of dosimetry for technicians.

As Hickey became more and more disabled he could not travel from his home on Cambridge

Avenue to the hospital. He moved into the hospital to be near his beloved department, and he died there on 30 October 1930. A few years earlier a Philadelphia roentgenologist had summed it up: "At Dr. Hickey's school there is no complaint, but I doubt whether there is another medical school in the country where roentgenology receives anything like the same recognition as at his school."[47]

Intermezzo: Physical Therapy

Electrotherapeutics contributed to the origin of roentgenology and then disappeared from respectable medical schools, but it lingered into the 1920s as an exuberant quackery, often called physical therapy. Morris Fishbein, the editor of the *Journal of the American Medical Association,* wrote a series of lively articles in 1925 and 1926 denouncing physical therapy as it was practiced then and calling for reform.[48] In May 1925 the American Medical Association established the Council on Physical Therapy in imitation of its Council on Pharmacy and Chemistry, which had combated quackery in the form of patent medicines. The council was chaired by a surgeon, and its members included an internist, a dermatologist, a roentgenologist, and two pathologists. Other members were Walter B. Cannon, W. T. Bovie, and Arthur H. Compton. The new council began its work by describing the current state of physical therapy. It said physical therapy had found a legitimate place in medicine during World War I and that in 1925–26 it was in a state of transition. Its province was the therapeutic use of heat, light, electricity, massage, baths, and exercise. Physicians should be trained in the subject, courses should be taught in medical schools, and there should be a careful study of its efficacy by clinical trials.[49] The council issued rules for acceptance of therapeutic devices, and it outlined the nature of training required.

Aldred S. Warthin was one of the pathologists on the council, and in 1927 in an editorial in the *Annals of Clinical Medicine,* a short-lived journal he edited, Warthin said that medical schools were "slumbering in the period of *Drug Therapy* [whereas] the actual practice of medicine has slipped past [them] into a new era of *Physical Therapy.*"[50] Warthin cited the progressive action of Michigan, where a faculty advisory committee had devised a three-year curriculum to train medical students in physical therapy, and he sounded a note loudly repeated in all discussions of the subject: technicians should help but in no way usurp the perquisites and privileges of the physician therapists!

Hickey was sympathetic with the aims of the Council on Physical Therapy, and the Michigan program was begun under the direction of Hickey, the orthopaedic surgeon Carl Badgley, and Ernst A. Pohle, who had some experience in heliotherapy.

Pohle, a German-trained roentgenologist who had come to Michigan in 1925, was particularly interested in calibrating roentgen radiation by means of the electroscope, and Hickey said Pohle was available to calibrate X-ray apparatus throughout the state.[51] At the same time Pohle worked with members of the Physics Department to define the characteristics of ultraviolet lamps and to calibrate their output.[52] At Michigan he treated some seven hundred patients with ultraviolet light, and he found in agreement with others that it is useful in treatment of rickets and is especially efficacious if the patients are sensitized by being fed 0.1 gram of eosin. Ultraviolet radiation seemed to be useless in treatment of tuberculosis.[53]

Pohle left Ann Arbor in 1928, and the next year he was replaced by Willis S. Peck, who had graduated from the Syracuse Medical School and had spent three years in the private practice of physical therapy. Hickey was made head of a new department of physical therapy with the responsibility for supervising Peck, and Huber and Warthin were Hickey's advisers. When Fred J. Hodges replaced Hickey in 1931 he recommended that the department and the hospital's physiotherapy unit be combined in a subdepartment of the Department of Roentgenology. Hodges also recommended promotion of Peck to an assistant professorship, and he gave Peck full authority for developing a program of physical therapy. In the mid-1930s physical therapy was given a home of its own on the ground floor of the southeast wing of the hospital, where an exercise pool was installed with Rackham money.

Peck gave a brief course of lectures and demonstrations to second-year medical students and an elective course in the clinical use of physical therapy in the junior year. He taught students the principles of measuring X radiation, how to test muscles with electric currents, and how to treat paralyzed extremities. He had an assistant who taught a few young women to be physical therapy technicians. Peck gave talks to associations of technicians, telling them the kinds of jobs they might find and warning them that although they might disagree with a physician prescribing physical therapy, they should defer to the physician.[54] Peck also published a few papers on the use of fever in treatment of intractable asthma and on the use of ultraviolet radiation in preparing wounds of an extensive burn for skin grafting.[55]

The physical therapy content of the courses was gradually submerged in roentgenology, and the 263-page syllabus prepared in 1939 by Peck and Hodges for an introductory course contains not a word on physical therapy.[56] "Physical therapy" as a separate entity was totally submerged in 1939 when it was transferred to the Department of Surgery. Peck left for private practice, and physical therapy did not arise from its submersion again until after World War II.

Hickey's Successor: Fred Jenner Hodges

A search committee compiled a list of every senior academic roentgenologist in the country, but on 9 January 1931 Udo Wile reported on behalf of the committee recommending Fred Jenner Hodges, a relatively junior roentgenologist. Wile said that Hodges's experience was shorter than desirable, and the appointment, if offered, should be for three years. If Hodges proved inadequate, the appointment could be terminated. On 15 January Hodges telegraphed he would be happy to accept the three-year appointment beginning 1 April.

Fred Hodges, always called "Ted" Hodges to the confusion of strangers, had earned his medical degree at Washington University in St. Louis, and he had served as an assistant resident in pathology at the Barnes Hospital for a year. He rose from instructor to professor of roentgenology at Wisconsin while working as roentgenologist for St. Mary's Hospital in Madison between 1925 and 1931.

J. A. E. Eyster and Ted Hodges's elder brother, Paul, had gone to a great deal of trouble to measure the size of the normal heart by X rays,[57] and Ted Hodges continued the work after his brother left Madison. In 1926 Ted Hodges and Eyster published what they intended to be a definitive estimation of the transverse diameter of the heart in adult men.[58] They used teleoroentgenography and orthodiagramography, and they concluded from the study of eighty normal male subjects that the normal transverse diameter in millimeters is (0.1094)(age in years) $- (0.1941)$(height in centimeters) $+ (0.8179)$(weight in kilograms) $+ 95.8625$. If the heart were "5 mm. wider in its greatest transverse diameter . . . the chances are three to one that the widening is pathologic."[59]

For years Hodges told medical audiences about the clinical value of roentgen measurements of the heart size,[60] but in 1939, after Hodges had given a masterly description of fifteen years' work, one cardiologist in discussing Hodges's paper said determination of heart size was becoming unimportant. On the same occasion Samuel Levine, the famous cardiologist at the Brigham, said: "But it is not very often that those of us interested in clinical heart disease have to lean heavily on the roentgenologist."[61]

Rehabilitating the Department at Michigan

Ten years after he came to Michigan Hodges wrote about "the splendid plant conceived and developed under [Hickey's] direction,"[62] but it did not appear splendid when he arrived. In April and June 1931 Hodges wrote long letters to the Executive Committee outlining his plans and stating the needs of the department. He said the department should render clinical services as complete, as excellent, and as modern as any department in the school, that it should be "second to none" in undergraduate and postgraduate teaching, and that it should make creditable contributions to knowledge. The department had a generous amount of floor space; the salary budget seemed adequate; equality with other departments had been established; and the hospital administration was cooperative. There was an esprit de corps among the professional staff. "World-wide good-will" had been accumulated by Hickey.

But the floor space was badly used; the department was congested; and it was impossible to handle the patient load. The darkroom facilities were inexcusably bad and in need of a thorough renovation. The dressing rooms were poor. Equipment was antiquated; methods of technical procedure were poorly coordinated; and routine badly needed reorganization. Reports lacked uniformity and were not rendered with dispatch. The staff was not given proper status as consultants, "and the pernicious practice of weighing other diagnostic data of a case *before* rather than *after* unbiased film study by the department staff appears to be the rule." The professorial staff should be expanded from two to four. Finally, students in training were allowed to use patients to gain technical experience; employment of a few technicians would better serve the patients' welfare. The goodwill left over from Hickey could not be expected to endure, and "unsatisfactory conditions overshadowed by his reputation must be rather quickly remedied."[63]

Hodges's Statistics

Shortly after Hodges came to Ann Arbor the hospital staff organized a clinical investigation of cancer in which neoplasms encountered on all services were discussed at a weekly tumor conference. At approximately the same time the hospital records were centralized, and H. M. Pollard was made the first medical statistician. Patient records were coded on Hollerith punch cards, the precursors of the IBM punch cards that were for a time ubiquitous. Hodges was put in charge of the actual operation of the punching, sorting, tabulating, and printing machines, and the dean's files for the next few years contain many letters from Hodges about trouble with the machines.

Hodges was also in charge of records accumulated in the investigation of cancer, and he was the senior author of successive annual reports.[64] Hodges had each patient's record transferred to punch cards in duplicate so they could simultaneously be sorted by patient registration number and tumor type, thus saving sorting time. When the cards were fed into the listing machine, the printout gave each case history. Hodges could describe, for example, the 1,341 tumors encountered in the 1939 calendar year among hospital registration of 27,808 patients. His published tables gave the distribution of tumors by reporting service and by county of patient residence, anatomical location of the tumor, pathological diagnosis, nature of treatment, and cause of death.

Hodges said that record keeping in a department of roentgenology was a major problem and that files were useless unless they were kept in an orderly manner.[65] Furthermore, cross-indexing of roentgenological impressions was required for all departments that aspired to qualify as approved teaching institutions. He developed a system of cross-indexing that began with "Category I, Major Divisions of the Diagnostic Code Used at Michigan," and ended with "Category X, Female Genital Organs." Case numbers were indexed versus findings and entered in loose-leaf notebooks containing green pages for normal findings and red pages for abnormal findings. Among examples Hodges gave was

Case 1004

IMPRESSION: 1.   Sinus tract (visualized by lipiodol injection) extending from the region of the left popliteal fossa to the upper part of the thigh.
V-28*

V meant "lower extremity"; *28* meant "sinus tract injection"; and * meant "special interest."[66]

With his sorting system Hodges could easily work up statistical studies of the success of roentgenological diagnosis. In an early paper from Michigan Hodges answered the question: "In how many cases [of brain tumor] was it possible on the basis of neurological examination alone to predict the location of the tumor correctly?"[67] The answer was that in 98 of 190 cases the neurological examination was sufficient. Sixty-eight times the neurologist and the roentgenologist together had not been correct, and nine times the two together localized the tumor. Fifty-nine times the tumor had defeated all preoperative effort. Hodges concluded that tumor localization is a group effort requiring the neurologist, the roentgenologist, the neurological surgeon, and the pathologist.

Before 1941 Hodges published similar papers describing the results of 2,380 examinations of the colon in twenty-seven months,[68] the findings in 2,781 oral cholecystograms in two years,[69] and the diagnoses in 1,000 consecutive patients subjected to complete gastrointestinal examination.[70]

Hodges and the Physics Department: Treatment of Cancer

In 1935 Michigan's Physics Department dismantled its Van de Graaff generator and began to build a cyclotron. One of the Rackham funds administered by the Graduate School gave the department $25,000 that year, $20,350 for construction and $4,650 for salaries. In later years less was earmarked for equipment and more for salaries. Through 1941, when the project was suspended on account of the war, a total of $110,000 was appropriated from Rackham money. Some physicists believed the money would not have been given so generously had it not been for the medical implications of the project.[71]

Hodges wanted to use the cyclotron to treat cancer, and he was involved in planning the project from the beginning.[72] On his own he investigated sources and cost of high voltage equipment to be used with the cyclotron, and he even offered advice on likely sources of iron for the magnet. Hodges told Harrison Randall, the head of the Physics Department and director of the cyclotron project, that cancer patients were sent to the University Hospital at the rate of fourteen hundred a year. Those with skin cancer were treated in Hodges's department with X rays generated with a maximum of 90,000 volts, and deep therapy was given with one of two 200,000-volt tubes. Michigan lacked extremely high voltage equipment. Hodges had visited high voltage installations throughout the country, and he was not impressed with the advantages claimed for even the 1,000-kilovolt machine at the California Institute of Technology. In May 1935 Hodges proposed a joint clinical research program to Randall. He hoped the cyclotron would generate radiation having wavelengths approaching those of gamma rays from radium. Hodges was familiar with Ernest O. Lawrence's neutron therapy project in the Crocker Laboratory at Berkeley,[73] and he thought neutrons might be superior to X rays. Perhaps radioactive material produced by the cyclotron could be used for cancer therapy. In the meantime Hodges sent Isadore Lampe, whom he considered the most outstanding young man ever to come under his observation, to the Physics Department for graduate training, and he arranged for Lampe to spend the summer of 1936 at Berkeley.

Hodges was more sensitive to the possible harmful effects of radiation than were the physicists, and he arranged with Cyrus Sturgis for blood tests on those working with the cyclotron. Isaacs, to whom Sturgis assigned the job, reported to Randall on 22 March 1937 that he had detected very slight changes that might be seasonal. It was, however, a change in the direction to be expected with X rays, and it occurred in quite a number of persons at the same time.

In 1936 some of the Rackham money was used to clean out and fit up a room in the basement of the West Medical Building for Lampe. The room was conveniently close to the cyclotron in the building next door. In 1938 Lampe earned a doctor of philosophy for work done "to determine whether or not neutrons and roentgen rays differ in their compara-

tive action upon different tissues *in the same individual organism,* or *in the same species of organism.*"[74] The emphasis was Lampe's.

Lampe determined the lethal dose of neutrons for mice, but because the mouse is large in relation to the beam of neutrons within the target chamber, the distribution of neutrons within the mouse's body was not uniform. Someone carefully measured the distribution of ionization within the target chamber, and Lampe was able to determine the effect of the neutron beam on *Drosophila* eggs and wheat seedlings. He collected eggs on disks of fermented banana agar containing enough lampblack to provide a convenient background for counting the eggs. Normally 97 percent of the eggs hatched, and Lampe's criterion of effectiveness of radiation was the percentage decrease in hatching. Lampe found a big fall in sensitivity to X rays or neutrons as the eggs aged from 1.5 hours to 6 hours, but the ratio of X irradiation to neutron irradiation required to kill an egg was 2.0 to 2.8 over that period. Lampe grew wheat seedlings on water-saturated paper, and he irradiated groups of thirty when the primary roots were two to four millimeters long. The dose of X rays required to reduce growth to 70 percent of the control rate measured forty-eight hours after irradiation averaged 6.2 to 11.8 times the dose of neutrons required to produce the same inhibition of growth. Lampe attributed the greater effectiveness of neutrons to the close spacing of ion tracks of secondary particles released in the tissue by neutrons, and he speculated that, from a clinical standpoint, neutrons might have a selective action different from that of X rays.

Despite the structural limitations of the Michigan cyclotron Lampe and Hodges followed up Lampe's suggestion by comparing the X-ray and neutron doses required to cause complete aspermatogenesis in rabbits.[75] Michigan physicists inserted a beryllium probe through the tank wall into the deuterium beam within the D electrodes to get an intense neutron beam. The collimator had to be outside the evacuated chamber. Lampe and Hodges placed an anesthetized rabbit in a fixed position so that the animal's genitals were adjacent to the collimator orifice. A dose in the range of 356 to 800 n (units of fast neutron radiation) was given at a time, and that required the cyclotron to run continuously for two to four hours. Four months after irradiation the animal was killed, and slides of the testes were prepared and read by Carl V. Weller.

Others had found that the dose of roentgen radiation required to produce complete aspermatogenesis in a rabbit also caused severe and lasting damage to the scrotal skin. Lampe and Hodges confirmed this when they irradiated the testes with their 200,000-volt X-ray tube. The scrotal skin of six rabbits with aspermatogenesis had not healed in four months. On the other hand, the scrotal skin of six rabbits in which neutron radiation had caused aspermatogenesis had healed by the time the rabbits were killed. Therefore, neutrons appear to have some selectivity.

While this work was going on Hodges became impatient with the Physics Department. On 27 February 1939 he wrote Randall a stiff letter saying that he and Dean Furstenberg had decided his work was so important that he should receive preferential use of the cyclotron. Randall replied mildly that, in fact, the expenditures in both time and money during the preceding year had been exclusively for Hodges's benefit.

Hodges had planned to spend his sabbatical leave in Europe, but he was prevented by the war. Instead, he spent the fall term of 1940 at Berkeley, where he could use the neutron beam of the Crocker cyclotron to finish his work with rabbits. Because money to build the cyclotron had been raised on consideration of the cyclotron's potential medical use, Hodges was able to preempt cyclotron time to the detriment of the physics program. Michigan and Berkeley physicists had cross calibrated the beams, and Hodges could report to Dean Furstenberg that his experiments were going well. Hodges also had the pleasure of seeing the Michigan football team defeat California forty-one to nothing on 28 September.

Hodges on Part Time

Before Hodges left for California he planned to change from a full-time appointment to a part-time appointment when he returned. He wrote Dean Furstenberg a long letter on 20 June 1940 outlining his plans and asking them to be approved so that he could assume his new status on 1 April 1941, the tenth anniversary of his beginning at Michigan.

Hodges preferred to carry on his private practice in the University Hospital rather than in an office downtown, and he asked for the use of approximately 750 square feet for office and laboratory near the X-ray department. He would pay for alterations and for installing complete diagnostic, therapeutic, and film processing equipment. He would pay for all supplies used, and he would rent radium from the hospital at the going rate. He would pay for patient registration, for technical services, and for part of the departmental secretary's time. Hodges would impose, collect, and keep all private patient fees, and he would be paid a part-time salary of seventy-five hundred dollars by the Medical School and hospital.

When Hodges went on part time in 1941 the "full-time plan" of 1919 was dead.

22
Neurology Again and Psychiatry

Soon after Will Herdman died in December 1906 Victor Vaughan brought Carl Dudley Camp, a twenty-seven-year-old instructor in neuropathology at the University of Pennsylvania, to Ann Arbor to be Michigan's professor of diseases of the nervous system with responsibility for both neurology and psychiatry. Eventually Albert Moore Barrett made psychiatry an independent discipline, and Camp's title was changed to professor of neurology. He continued in that rank until he retired in 1950. His appointment was always part time, and in 1928 he told Dean Cabot that he spent his mornings in the University Hospital and his afternoons in his private office at 304 South State Street.

Carl D. Camp's Background

Camp had graduated in medicine from the University of Pennsylvania in 1902, and after a year's internship he began to work with Charles W. Burr, Pennsylvania's professor of diseases of the mind, and with William G. Spiller, the neurologist.[1] Camp published frequently with both men, and he often exhibited patients before the Philadelphia Neurological Society with them or by himself. Most of the twenty-five or so papers Camp published between 1904 and 1907 dealt with the usual range of neurological problems: two cases of multiple sclerosis with autopsy findings, peripheral obliterating arteritis as a cause of triplegia, a case of cerebellar tumor with autopsy findings, the difficulty of distinguishing between cerebrospinal syphilis and disseminated sclerosis, and so on.[2] After he came to Michigan, Camp continued for a while to publish on material accumulated at Pennsylvania. Spiller was interested in tracts in the spinal cord and in sensory deficits resulting from central lesions. In a similar fashion Camp described his deductions about paths of fibers mediating pain, sensations of heat and cold, tactile sensations, and the sense of position derived from a study of four patients, one of whom went to autopsy.[3]

Camp's major publication at the end of his Philadelphia period was a long paper, eighteen tall columns of small type in the *Journal of the American Medical Association*, describing the pathology of paralysis agitans.[4] Camp reviewed the literature, citing 104 references, but his own contribution was based on original investigation of fourteen cases, all with partial or thorough necropsies. He said fourteen was a large number, for an 1899 review had turned up only twenty-four that had been examined histologically.

After a long analysis of theories of the disease, Camp concluded that paralysis agitans is not a neurosis nor the result of senility. Camp's most constant finding was fibrosis of the capillary blood vessels of the spinal cord, but he concluded that changes he and others saw in the nervous system are simply the normal ones of advancing age. Camp's most significant findings were in one muscle biopsy and in samples of muscles obtained in nine necropsies. Muscle fibers were swollen; there were changes in the number of nuclei; and there was overgrowth of connective tissue. Muscle spindles were hard to find, and their muscle fibers showed the same changes as the surrounding muscles. Camp said that resistance of muscles was the same whether the limbs were moved quickly or slowly and that moving a patient's limb was like bending a lead pipe. Therefore, the rigidity is very different from spasticity; it is not reflex in origin but arises from changes in the muscles themselves. Tremor is a disturbance of muscle tonus caused by affection of the muscle spindles.

Camp concluded that paralysis agitans is probably a general toxemia. He was impressed by the correspondence between the symptoms he saw and the results obtained by his friend W. S. Carter with parathyroidectomized dogs. Camp examined the parathyroid glands in two of his cases; both were distinctly pathological. He deduced that paralysis agitans is the result of alteration of secretion of the parathyroid glands.

Camp was sufficiently proud of his paper to publish it twice in German,[5] but by 1934 Camp had decided that paralysis agitans results from degeneration in the lenticular nuclei and that changes in the muscles are secondary.

Camp's Department and Teaching

If we discount the staff of the Psychopathic Hospital that was nominally associated with neurology until 1920, Camp always had a small department with a light teaching load. When Camp succeeded Herdman, Jeanne Cady Solis withdrew to private practice, and Vernon J. Willey stopped being an instructor in electrotherapeutics. Theophile Klingman remained Camp's demonstrator for thirteen years. At first Camp had one intern on his service and a senior

medical student who lived in the hospital and acted as a junior intern. In 1920 Camp began a formal training program in neurology. A physician in the program served one year as a rotating intern and then a year each as assistant resident, junior instructor, and a senior instructor. After the new hospital was occupied in 1925 Camp had a staff of four instructors, each of whom served for two years. Raymond Waggoner and Russell DeJong, both Michigan graduates, were eventually promoted to assistant professor.

From 1907 Camp gave a series of didactic lectures in the second semester of the junior year, and similar lectures were continued for senior students. Those students also attended a Wednesday afternoon clinic and had some ward work as well. By 1910 seniors spent two hours a week on the wards for seven or eight weeks, and some ward work in the afternoons brought their total experience in neurology to fifty hours. When Raymond Waggoner became an assistant professor elective courses in lumbar puncture technique and neuropathology were offered.

In 1934 Leonard E. Himler, Camp's current instructor, published a 250-page lithoprinted transcript of Camp's lecture notes, and consequently it is possible to reconstruct Camp's lectures in detail.[6] The first 235 pages take the student through methods of examining the patient, diseases of the spinal cord, diseases of peripheral nerves, and diseases of the brain. The copy surviving in the Taubman Medical Library is liberally marked up by a student, and the following excerpt with the student's underlining and marginal marks demonstrates that Camp satisfied the Michigan medical student's need to know exactly what he or she was expected to reproduce on the examination.

NEURITIS

Neuritis by definition means inflammation of nerves but the term is commonly used for all pathological conditions of the peripheral nerves
✓ and includes cutting and parenchymatous degeneration even where there is no inflammation. Severing a nerve fiber interrupts its conductivity. Partial interruption slows up the impulses which it conveys.
✓ The idea that irritation of a nerve increases its conductivity is not true. Disease always results in impairment or loss of function, never an increased function. Some physical agents such as warmth which do not cause destruction, may increase conductivity, but this is slight. Physical, toxic or traumatic agents generally decrease or destroy it. Therefore

*   in any <u>neuritis</u> the <u>reflexes are diminished</u> or <u>lost</u>, never <u>increased</u>.[7]

Trigeminal Neuralgia

When Camp came to Michigan he knew that Frazier at Pennsylvania had frequently cut the sensory root of the gasserian ganglion to alleviate the pain of trigeminal neuralgia, and he soon learned that Nancrede did the same operation. Camp also knew that some neurologists injected osmic acid into the nerve after it had been exposed and that others injected the nerve with alcohol where it exits from the skull.[8] Camp read about injecting alcohol into the ganglion itself, and "after some practice in the anatomical laboratory, injected [his] first case, April 19, 1912."[9] By 1914 Camp had seen forty cases of trigeminal neuralgia at Michigan, and he had injected three. He described his technique, using drawings and photographs to show how he got the point of his needle into the ganglion. Nancrede was alarmed; the anatomy of the region is variable, and there are major blood vessels in the area. He said that "I do not say Dr. Camp's operation is impossible, for he has succeeded, and I recently referred a private case to him for this operation, but I do say that I am perfectly sure if injection operations be tried often enough, serious accidents will occur."[10]

Camp and the Psychoneuroses

Camp, like Weir Mitchell and many other neurologists of the day, earned most of his living practicing some form of psychiatry. He treated a large number of patients in his private office, never in the University Hospital.[11] He also saw students suffering from "nervous breakdown."[12] Camp said 40 percent of them had "bad heredity" or "congenital defectiveness." For some, the cause of the breakdown is abnormal strain or nervous irritation, ranging from pediculosis capitis to badly fitting shoes. For others, the cause is worry, chagrin, or depression.

The year after Camp came to Michigan he told Michigan physicians that every doctor should be able to diagnose functional nervous diseases and to use psychotherapy "so successfully that it can never more be said that a quack or a charm can cure a case of disease in which a physician has tried and failed."[13] There is no routine method of treatment, for each disease and each patient is distinct.[14] In treating simple anxiety "[t]he physician should be firm and insist that the patient realize the truth."[15] Suggestion therapy is a time-honored method exemplified by a shrine or a prayer, and it is not the same as persuasion, command, or punishment. Camp said psychoanalysis is a rational method of treatment, but it is primarily a method of diagnosis. It is applicable only to selected cases and is difficult in older patients. The general practitioner should not try to use it.[16]

When Camp reached his mature view of the etiology of the psychoneuroses he thought that Gestalt psychology fitted his ideas completely. Quoting Janet, professor of psychology at the Sorbonne, he said: " 'When an organism perceives the necessity of adapting itself to its environment and at the same time perceives its inability to adapt itself—then there results a series of phenomena that collectively we speak of as an emotion.' . . . Note that the individual must perceive the necessity for adapting himself to the environment. . . . He must also see his inability. No matter whether his perceptions are true or false, the results are the same for him."[17] The conflict over adaptation is repressed to the unconscious. As Freud had demonstrated, the patient suffers because he continues to have the unconscious conflict, and this is the psychopathology of the psychoneuroses. As an example, Camp cited the case of a woman with emotional glycosuria simulating true diabetes mellitus that was traced to her unconscious wish to displace her mother in her father's affections, an Oedipus complex as described by Freud.

Camp used psychoanalysis to uncover the conflict: "By a psychoanalysis I mean taking a very careful and complete life history of the patient with particular reference to their education and social contacts. . . . Although such a history often furnishes many clews to the trouble it does not reveal the repressed idea and the real psychoanalysis is then carried on by association reactions, reaction time tests, dream analysis and other methods of that sort. The actual uncovering of the original mental conflict is usually attended with an increase in the emotional phenomena and this reaction may sometimes be severe; in fact it is one of the dangers in psychoanalysis but its occurrence is perhaps the best evidence that the analysis is needed and may benefit."[18] The galvanic skin response to certain words or Jung's method of reaction time might be revealing. Camp instanced a girl with hysterical blindness in the left eye whose lengthened reaction time to the words *fire* and *brother* led to the discovery that her brother had once thrust a hot poker toward her eye.[19]

When the cause of the conflict is uncovered the patient at first denies it, but he admits it "after the facts are pointed out to [him]."[20] A cure that is usually only temporary is achieved when the therapist makes a statement of fact that the patient must accept.

Camp's Later Days

Camp's rate of publication on miscellaneous neurological topics, including syphilis, did not fall off until about 1920, but in the years 1926 to 1941 he published only eight papers. One was an obituary notice of Albert Barrett, and three were addresses to medical societies. At the same time his interest in his professorship declined, for he would appear in the hospital between 10:00 and 10:30 A.M., dictate the findings of his cursory examinations of patients to his secretary as he walked down the ward, and disappear about noon.

Two of Camp's later papers described his continuing interest in the problem of sleep. When Camp was in Philadelphia he had a patient who fell asleep for a few minutes many times an hour, and he could not stay awake long enough for Camp to hypnotize him. At first Camp tried to explain sleep and its pathology with ideas based on Sherrington's *Integrative Action of the Nervous System*. One reflex may be totally inhibited by another of greater importance in preserving the individual. To Camp sleep is a reflex inhibition of the brain. Later he decided the waking state is a conditioned reflex and that sleep is a form of areflexia that may result from lack of appropriate stimuli or from a break in the reflex arc.[21]

In the 1930s most publications from the department were by Camp's students Raymond Waggoner and Russell DeJong. DeJong was a Michigan graduate of 1936 who succeeded Camp as department chairman in 1945. He wrote on medical history[22] as well as on central nervous complications of subacute bacterial endocarditis, delayed traumatic intracerebral hemorrhage, Horner's syndrome, and electroencephalography.[23] Internists at the time were treating diseases with megadoses of vitamins, and DeJong did the same. He gave patients with amyotrophic lateral sclerosis as much as 240 milligrams of α-tocopherol a day. None improved, nor did those with the Guillain-Barré syndrome to whom he gave large doses of thiamin.[24]

The Psychopathic Hospital

Albert Moore Barrett came to Ann Arbor in 1906 with the titles of associate professor of neural pathology, pathologist to the state asylums, and director of the Psychopathic Ward. Both Adolf Meyer and August Hoch had been approached by Herdman and his advisers, but they were unavailable. Both had just settled as directors of New York State hospitals and as teachers at Cornell Medical School. When Herdman died in December Barrett was promoted to a professorship and given the additional responsibility of managing the business of the Psychopathic Hospital. He was forced to become a full-fledged psychiatrist as well as a neuropathologist.[25]

The Psychopathic Hospital had been created as a part of Michigan's asylum system largely through Herdman's efforts, and, as Herdman said, its purpose was to obtain knowledge of the nature and causes of insanity, to clear the way to removal of some of the causes, and to effect cures in some cases then practically incurable and thus to relieve the state of the burden of their care. The Psychopathic Hospital was expected to stimulate research in other Michigan asylums and to educate the public in prevention and treatment of insanity.[26]

Barrett described how the hospital worked after he had been running it for more than a decade (fig. 22–1).[27] The hospital was controlled by four from among the trustees of the state hospitals and four from among the regents of the University of Michigan. They provided intimate connection between the rest of the state hospital system and the resources of the university. Barrett thought an important aspect of the hospital was its flexibility, enabling it to take up special problems as they arose, and a major advantage was that patients with mental diseases directly related to physical disease could be treated by the medical and surgical staff of the University Hospital. The hospital was the right size with its sixty-two beds, not too large and not too small. The staff saw about 325 inpatients a year. Fifty-three percent of the admissions were voluntary, and 43 percent were at public expense. Although psychiatric treatment was prolonged, 69 percent of those discharged had been in the hospital less than three months, and 84 percent recovered within that time. Less than one-quarter of the patients ended in district hospitals for custodial care.

As Barrett's diagram shows, he emphasized the hospital's community functions. It served as the cen-

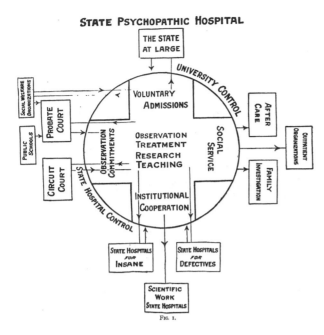

Fig. 22–1. Functions of the State Psychopathic Hospital at the University of Michigan. (From A. M. Barrett, "The State Psychopathic Hospital," *Am. J. Insan.* 77 [1920–21]: 312–13.)

tral pathological laboratory, doing diagnostic work impossible in the district hospitals. Six hundred outpatients were seen each year, and another twelve hundred were seen in a satellite clinic in Detroit. Theophile Raphael, one of Barrett's staff, worked in the Student Health Service. Both inpatients and outpatients required the services of psychiatric social workers who were trained in the hospital. Barrett and his staff worked with the probate and circuit courts in accepting commitments and in giving advice, but by 1920 Barrett was beginning to be disillusioned about the ability to make Michigan judges and lawyers see mental illness from a psychiatrist's point of view.

Barrett's Background

Albert Barrett grew up in Iowa City, where his father, a Presbyterian clergyman learned in the New England tradition, was a pastor. Barrett attended the University of Iowa for his academic and medical degrees, graduating in 1895. This was long before the school was reformed on Flexnerian lines. Students were admitted to the three-year course directly from high school. In the medical school

Barrett developed skill in histology and pathology, and upon graduation he became pathologist at an Iowa hospital for the mentally ill. In order to improve his technique Barrett spent a year at the Kankakee State Hospital in Illinois, where Adolf Meyer had recently assumed the responsibility of reorganizing that institution hitherto afflicted by political corruption. Meyer moved to a similar position at the Worcester Lunatic Hospital in 1896, and Barrett after a year back at Iowa once more went to work under Meyer. Meyer found his pupil to be a "well balanced and well focused inquirer, . . . thoroughly sophisticated and unbiased, sensibly and practically interested in doing justice to the task and opportunity of studying the brain."[28] However, Meyer complained that he would have preferred to have Barrett wholeheartedly devote himself to obtaining a telling history of the newly admitted patients, some of whom might come to autopsy and provide material for a neuropathologist.

In 1900 Barrett went to Germany, where he made the rounds of the neuropathological institutes: Nissl's, Weigert's, and Alzheimer's. He was particularly impressed by Kraepelin, under whom he did some bedside work, and for the rest of his life Barrett liberally cited Kraepelin's publications. Upon returning to the United States Barrett became neuropathologist to the Danvers State Hospital in Massachusetts and an assistant in neuropathology at Harvard.

The Somatic Basis of Mental Disease

Adolf Meyer said that when he first knew Barrett the young man's intention was only to acquire the techniques of neuropathology and that Barrett had "nothing of an ulterior yearning or an immediate desire to determine 'the' pathologic basis of insanity."[29] Most of Barrett's early publications and those for some time after he came to Michigan were straightforward reports of autopsy material: disseminated syphilitic encephalitis, spinal cord degeneration in acromegaly, diffuse glioma of the pia mater, and so on through some twenty papers.[30] Nevertheless, while he was still at Danvers, Barrett attempted to correlate gradual changes in behavior with the development of arteriosclerosis.[31] As Adolf Meyer said, Barrett's clinical responsibilities and his obligation to teach psychiatry drew him into the domain of personality functions.

Barrett was well aware of Freudian psychoanalysis as it was understood in the United States about 1910. In that year Louville E. Emerson, formerly an instructor in philosophy in the university, began to treat patients in the Psychopathic Hospital by a version of psychoanalysis that involved a great deal of word association and reaction times.[32] Emerson knew what was going on in Vienna, for he complained that the psychoanalytical literature was piling up so fast that he could not keep up with it. A little later in discussing anxiety neurosis Barrett said: "The theories of Freud and others have at least developed a line of thought which has ultimately made amenable to treatment a large group of hitherto obscure neurasthenic cases."[33] Nevertheless, Barrett's brand of psychiatry remained rooted in somatic considerations.

The somatic basis was easy enough to find in some instances. The spirochete is ultimately responsible for general paresis, but Barrett wondered why some paretics are depressed while others have exalted moods. After Barrett came to Ann Arbor he described the clinical courses of eight patients whose symptoms differed from the presbyphrenic form of senile insanity and from the arteriosclerotic form. At autopsy Barrett found scattered and circumscribed alterations in cerebral arteries that had been encapsulated by neuroglial fibers, and he thought many symptoms could be referred to specific organic changes in the brains.[34] But in many instances he could find nothing in the brain responsible for the symptoms, and one of his biographers said that at the end of his life Barrett was disappointed in being unable to see anything in his slides that might account for schizophrenia.

Sometimes Barrett could find medical reasons, hypo- or hyperthyroidism, for example. In 1920 he published two case histories relating toxic mental disorders to the occurrence of tetany.[35] The patients were depressed and confused over many weeks, but nothing in the histories gave any clue to the cause of the tetany or its relation to the patients' confusion. Often Barrett was reduced to blaming constitutional and hereditary factors. In 1922–23 he published a long paper describing three patients with differing types of psychopathic personality: an excitable young man "with a chip on his shoulder" who had frequent outbursts of passion and who acted without thought or reason, a pathological liar with a marked degree of mental deficiency who actually believed his own stories, and a man with weakness of character who, lack-

ing in will, was unconcerned about his frequent delinquencies. Barrett thought these and others, the spendthrift, the dipsomaniac, and the destructive and querulous person involved in endless litigation, were suffering not from a disease engrafted upon a healthy personality but from malformation of character. Because Barrett could say nothing about etiology, he could only prescribe treatment to protect society by banishing the man with outbursts of passion to a farm and by confining the delinquent to prison for long periods.[36]

Barrett thought that constitutional defects are inherited, and he wrote at least four papers on hereditary and familial factors in the development of psychoses.[37] His data were drawn largely from the massive German literature of Kretschmer, Kraepelin, and the like, in which family histories of nonpsychotic and psychotic patients were compared. In one population of 1,193 nonpsychotic persons, for example, 67 percent were found to have some hereditary taint—psychoses, nervous diseases, alcoholism, epilepsy, senile dementia, or suicide—among their parents, grandparents, great-grandparents, siblings, or collateral relatives. In comparison, in a population of 650 manic-depressives, 84.13 percent had similar tainting that appeared to be hereditary as a simple, dominant Mendelian factor. Barrett himself collected family trees to determine inheritance of mental illness. In one instance the propositus, a "deteriorating schizophrenic," had two sisters and a brother with "schizoid personalities" and one with "abnormal character." The mother was a manic-depressive and came from a family with many instances of similar psychoses. Although the father never developed overt psychosis, he was moody and excitable. Barrett did not speculate on what living in such a family was like.

Barrett's Staff and Teaching

Barrett always had a comparatively large staff to meet the demands of the Psychopathic Hospital. At first he and most of his staff were paid by the state, but they had obligations of teaching in the university beyond the Medical School. Barrett's staff gave a course in psychiatry for nursing students and another for students of sociology. Barrett himself cooperated with Walter Pillsbury, professor of psychology in the Literary Department, in teaching abnormal and experimental psychology. Barrett's university functions were recognized in 1920 when the Department of

Diseases of the Mind and Nervous System was divided into a new Department of Psychiatry with Barrett as chairman and a Department of Neurology under Camp. State support decreased during the Great Depression, but in 1934 the Rockefeller Foundation, in an effort to improve teaching of psychiatry, gave the university fifteen thousand dollars that Barrett used to support members of his staff. The grant was renewed for several years.

Barrett usually had one, two, or three instructors or assistant professors and two or more resident physicians. In the early days a pathologist, sometimes a woman trained by Warthin, ran the neuropathology laboratory with the help of technicians. After 1930 Konstantin Löwenberg, a German neuropathologist, reorganized the neuropathology laboratory, and neuropathology remained in the Psychopathic Hospital and in the Department of Psychiatry rather than in the Department of Pathology until long after 1941. Until the central hospital laboratory was established under Reuben Kahn there was a serologist with an assistant in the Psychopathic Hospital. The director of Social Services and an occupational therapist served patients and trained apprentices.

Second- and third-year medical students heard Barrett lecture on psychiatry, and fourth-year students spent thirty-six hours in the Psychopathic Hospital over eight weeks. In the 1930s Barrett himself or Löwenberg offered an elective course in neuropathology. Students reporting to the dean on the curriculum in 1934 said they wanted more psychiatry.

Barrett's Successor: Raymond W. Waggoner

Barrett died suddenly in the early hours of 2 April 1936 at the age of sixty-five, and Dean Furstenberg immediately began to search for his successor. The Rockefeller Foundation gave the university $250 for travel expenses, and Furstenberg went east and H. M. Pollard went west to interview candidates. By autumn they had accumulated a list naming every senior academic psychiatrist in the country and some promising juniors as well. F. G. Ebaugh of Colorado declined an offer, and others may have done so. Nevertheless, Furstenberg thought the field was barren. His opinion of the ability of psychiatrists to minister to the general run of medical and surgical patients was never high, and it occurred to him that a good neurologist could do the job. To the astonishment of many, Furstenberg offered the job to Raymond W. Waggoner, then an associate professor of neurology under Camp. In a letter to President Ruthven, Furstenberg listed thirty psychiatrists and justified his choice of Waggoner by saying that Waggoner's "qualifications appear to be as satisfactory as those of any of the above candidates who are available for the post at Michigan. We know him well, he is reliable and dependable, and a man who is animated by an enthusiasm for teaching, investigation, and clinical practice. He is capable of independent thinking, has demonstrated courage and self-reliance, and presents credentials which are at least equal to those who might be attracted to this Chairmanship."[38]

When Dean Furstenberg's cable reached him with the offer, Waggoner was in London on sabbatical leave, working at the Queen Square and Maudsley Hospitals. He intended to return in February 1937. The dean said there was a revolt in the Department of Psychiatry over Waggoner's choice, and he said Waggoner should return a month early to settle it. The dean also agreed with Waggoner's plan to turn his attention to the review of psychiatry.

Waggoner accepted by cable; and he took over leadership of the department in January. The regents made the appointment effective 1 March 1937. Harley Haynes, the director of the University Hospital, assumed management of the business of the Psychopathic Hospital, relieving Waggoner of that task.

Raymond Waggoner's Background

Raymond Waggoner earned his medical degree at Michigan in 1924, and after an internship at the Harper Hospital in Detroit he served as resident at the Orthopedic Hospital and Infirmary for Nervous Diseases in Philadelphia under T. H. Weisenburg, who offered Waggoner a three-year Commonwealth Fellowship. Waggoner also worked at the Philadelphia General Hospital while earning a degree of doctor of science from the University of Pennsylvania's Graduate School of Medicine. He returned to Ann Arbor in the 1930s as assistant professor of neurology.

In Philadelphia Waggoner presented patients before the Philadelphia Neurological Society, and he published clinical and pathological studies of a case of thrombosis of the superior cerebral vein and of extraneural anomalies in Friedreich's ataxia.[39] In the latter paper he described a family with four frank cases and two in the abortive form in one generation, all having associated spina bifida occulta and degenerative changes in almost every organ system. However, Waggoner's most elaborate studies in Philadelphia were on the development of the plantar reflex in normal children and in children with chorea.

In describing work on the plantar reflex Waggoner said: "This research began as a study of general reflexes, but we [Waggoner and his collaborator, W. G. Ferguson] soon found that the scope of such a problem was altogether too large and were forced to limit ourselves to the examination of the plantar reflex. We believe that we have shown three things: that the condition of the patient, particularly whether asleep or awake, is of considerable importance in the type of reaction obtained; that the type of stimulus and its strength are important, and that the reaction type varies considerably at various stages in the age development of the child."[40] Waggoner and Ferguson had borrowed a device from the neurophysiologist Grayson McCouch with which they could stroke the plantar surface with a predetermined pressure.[41]

Encephalography

Walter Dandy had performed encephalography by exchanging air for cerebrospinal fluid by way of lumbar puncture,[42] but because neurologists at the University of Pennsylvania in Waggoner's time thought the procedure dangerous they did ventriculography by injecting air into the ventricles by way of a small trephine hole.[43] Waggoner, encouraged by his chief at the Infirmary for Nervous Diseases, revived the method of lumbar puncture, and he found it was not so dangerous as others thought.[44] Waggoner used a lumbar puncture needle connected with a manometer. One arm of a three-way stopcock placed in the needle's hub was connected with a ten-milliliter syringe, and the other was connected with a closed graduated cylinder containing air. Waggoner withdrew three to five milliliters of fluid at a time, and, while keeping the pressure as constant as possible, he replaced the fluid with the same or a slightly smaller quantity of air. He performed the exchange with the patient lying on his or her side, and then he moved the patient to the upright position for the X-ray exposure. Because handling the patient that way was awkward, Waggoner devised a chair "so constructed that the patient can be placed in either an upright or a prone position which can be varied at will while he remains in the chair. It also has an adjustable head rest which will hold the head firmly during the injection of air and may be adjusted to any position during the procedure. . . . The chair is placed on a platform sufficiently large to counterbalance any change in weight caused by shifting the position of the patient. The platform is in turn mounted on large casters which simplify the movement of the patient from the operating room to the x-ray room" (fig. 22–2).[45] When Waggoner returned to Ann Arbor the roentgenologists provided a special mounting for the X-ray tube and a cassette holder with a Bucky diaphragm.[46] The paper describing Waggoner's technique in detail has Camp's name ahead of Waggoner's for the reason that Camp was head of the department. By 1936 Waggoner and Russell DeJong had performed more than 150 encephalographies in the University Hospital.[47]

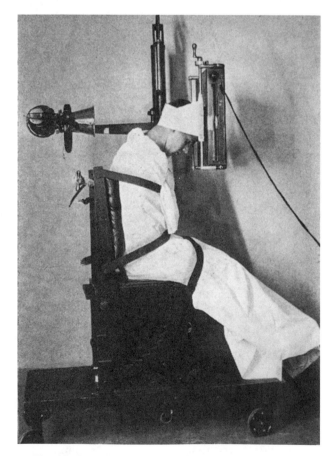

Fig. 22–2. Waggoner and Hickey's encephalography. (From R. W. Waggoner and D. M. Clark, "A New Position Used in Encephalography," *Am. J. Roentgenol.* 25 [1931]: 533.)

The Neuropsychiatric Institute

The old Psychopathic Hospital was in bad condition when Waggoner took over psychiatry, and he complained that it had only one shower and no elevator. The legislature had designated $300,000 for its replacement in 1929, but the money was not forthcoming. Waggoner told the State Board of Asylums that in the year 1936–37, 3,777 outpatients had been seen and that there had been 5,874 interviews. In the first six months of 1937, 171 patients had been admitted. Within four days of his confirmation by the regents Waggoner told his plans to Dean Furstenberg. Waggoner's relations with the powers in the state capital were always good, and nineteen days later bill 197 was introduced in the state senate proposing to transfer the Psychopathic Hospital to the university and appropriating $400,000 for establishment of a Neuropsychiatric Institute.

The five-story building housing the Neuropsychiatric Institute cost $456,000, the extra money coming from the hospital depreciation fund. It was attached to the north of the University Hospital, and it contained offices, treatment and recreation rooms, laboratories, and eighty-five beds (fig. 22–3). According to Waggoner, the institute was to be a center for clinical and laboratory research in psychiatry, for the study and interpretation of mental disease with a view to prevention, for the study of methods of treatment, for service to mentally ill children, and for the training of physicians.

From Neuropathology to Neuropsychiatry

In Waggoner's first years as a psychiatrist he continued to be a neurologist and neuropathologist, and he and Löwenberg published eight papers together. They also traveled to scattered state asylums to give clinical and neuropathological demonstrations, and they drew material for their papers from those hospitals. Four of their papers are simple case reports, and others describe familial incidence of neurological diseases: two members of a Traverse City family with Friedreich's ataxia; a father, three daughters, and a son with Alzheimer's disease; a kinship with agenesis of the white matter and idiocy in six siblings; and still another family group displaying hereditary cerebellar ataxia.[48]

Löwenberg and Waggoner described the neuropathological findings in three patients who died in

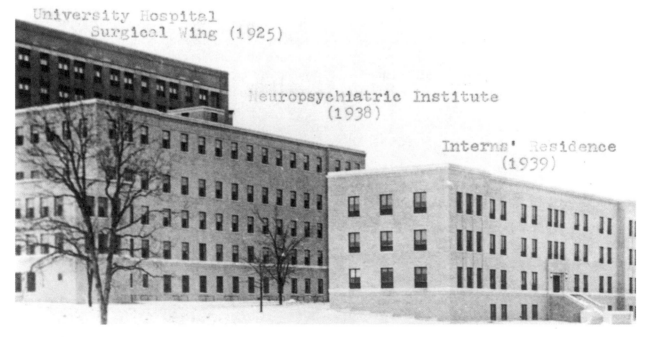

Fig. 22–3. Neuropsychiatric Institute. (Courtesy of the Bentley Historical Library, University of Michigan, Medical School Records, Box 136, "Medical School Photographs, Buildings, Including Hospitals.")

Neurology Again and Psychiatry

287

the University Hospital during nitrous oxide anesthesia.[49] Löwenberg and Waggoner did not state in their case histories the percentage of oxygen used, but the anesthesiologist they cited recommended rapid induction with pure nitrous oxide and then a mixture containing 5 or 6 percent oxygen until the patient "leveled off." After that "a secondary saturation" with 100 percent nitrous oxide may be necessary "to secure the desired relaxation."[50] The anesthesiologist did not think the patient's cyanosis is a reliable indicator of oxygenation, and giving the moribund Michigan patients 100 percent oxygen did not cause them to recover. This convinced Löwenberg and Waggoner that the brain damage they found was caused by a specific toxic action of nitrous oxide, rather than by profound and prolonged hypoxia.

The reason for the astonishment at Waggoner's appointment as professor of psychiatry was that his Michigan colleagues thought of him only as a neuropathologist; they did not remember that his University of Pennsylvania doctor of science thesis had been a study of the personality of children with chorea minor, also called Sydenham's chorea or St. Vitus' dance.[51] Waggoner said that the disease usually occurs in children between the ages of five and ten years and that it frequently presents mental symptoms: emotional instability, fretfulness, peevishness, and unreasonableness. The patient is tearful, cries at the slightest provocation, and is difficult to manage. Sleep is frequently disturbed by horrifying dreams whose content is not remembered. Loss of memory may be marked and associated with deafness and confusion.

Waggoner attempted to understand the family background and in particular the parents' attitude to the child's disorder. He found some parents overprotective and indulgent with the result that the child traded on the disability. Other parents failed to realize the nature of the affliction and scolded or punished the child for awkwardness. The attitude of schoolmates affected the child. One who was apt to be the butt of jokes developed a recessive attitude and became sensitive and timid. Waggoner's probing of the state of mind of the parents and child was not so deep as one would expect from a practicing psychiatrist, and he tended to take statements about whether the child had been wanted or not, the extent of its knowledge of sex, and the like, at face value. Nevertheless, the thesis demonstrated Waggoner's early orientation toward psychiatric problems.

In 1941 Waggoner demonstrated a deeper understanding when he described twenty-five cases of juvenile aberrant sexual behavior.[52] He divided his patients into three groups: those whose families were overprotective and who were emotionally infantile and without personal independence; those rejected by their parents whose leading feelings were insecurity, inferiority, and inadequacy, and those with defects in personality whose powerful instinctive drives were not controlled by weak or missing inhibitory mechanisms. Waggoner, who cited no literature, appeared to take a position midway between those who thought the cause of aberrant sexual behavior is a constitutional disturbance and those who thought it shaped by unspecified psychological and emotional influences. He said that adult sexual perversion does not spring de novo but that the pattern and necessity for perverted expression are determined to a great extent by early emotional and environmental influences.

23
Otolaryngology

When Flemming Carrow resigned as professor of ophthalmology and aural surgery in 1904 the regents divided the chair, appointing Walter R. Parker in ophthalmology and Roy Bishop Canfield in otolaryngology. Canfield, unlike Parker, lived in Ann Arbor, but like Parker he always maintained a private practice with an office on South State Street. His range of practice included Detroit, and stories about the whopping bill, twenty-five thousand dollars, he submitted to Henry Ford for the care of Edsel still circulate in Ann Arbor.[1]

Roy Bishop Canfield, always called Bishop Canfield, had grown up in Ann Arbor. He attended the Ann Arbor High School, and he took the combined course in the Literary and Medical Departments of the university. When Canfield graduated from the Medical School in 1899 he worked under Flemming Carrow for a couple of months, but he soon left for training at the Massachusetts Eye and Ear Infirmary in Boston. He spent one and a half years in Germany, where he rose to be chief of Albert Jansen's clinic in Berlin, and upon returning to the United States Canfield went into practice in New York City, where he was appointed assistant surgeon at the Manhattan Eye, Ear, and Throat Hospital. He was thirty years old when he was called to Michigan.

Canfield's Early Experience

Canfield submitted his candidate's thesis to the American Laryngological, Rhinological and Otological Society at the time he returned to Ann Arbor, and he was duly elected a member. Canfield described in his thesis his "observations upon some two hundred cases of chronic disease of the different nasal accessory sinuses, treated radically, and upon one hundred and ten cases treated conservatively."[2] He thought conservative treatment was successful nine cases out of ten in uncomplicated conditions and that it should be tried first. Radical treatment consisted of surgical drainage of a pus-filled sinus, followed by irrigation. Canfield drained frontal sinuses by the Killian operation, opening the anterior wall of the sinus and making a permanent opening from the sinus into the nose. He was careful to leave a bridge of bone over the orbit. At that time rhinologists often drained the maxillary antrum by drilling a hole through the socket of an extracted tooth, preferably the first molar. After the sinus had been irrigated, the hole was plugged with iodoform gauze. Later, in order to prevent closure of the hole, a dentist fitted it with a rubber plug or cannula. Alternatively, the antrum was approached by the Caldwell-Luc route: an incision in the gingivolabial recess. An opening over the canine fossa was made with a chisel and mallet and enlarged with bone-cutting forceps. A counteropening was made in the antronasal wall large enough to allow drainage during the process of healing of the anterior opening. At first Canfield thought the Caldwell-Luc operation was to be used, but he soon discarded it in favor of his own approach through the inferior nasal meatus.

Canfield at Michigan

Canfield did not operate before the class as Nancrede and Peterson did, but he established an operating room under the stairs leading to the surgery theater. It was just large enough for Canfield, the patient, and the anesthetist, and Canfield's nurse stood in the hall, passing instruments through the door. In 1910 Canfield and Parker moved into the new Eye, Ear, Nose, and Throat Hospital that had been built at the cost of twenty-five thousand dollars (fig. 23–1). Its operating room was large enough for a small group of students to see what Canfield was doing. His new equipment, costing an additional ninety-six hundred dollars, included a bronchoscope, a gastroscope, and additional drills. The building contained offices, cubicles for examining outpatients, fifty-three beds for inpatients, and quarters for interns. By that time Canfield had a corps of graduate assistants, and there were two or three senior medical students earning room and board by helping care for patients. Those students were expected to be present at all operations. Fifteen years later Canfield had still better facilities as he and Parker moved into the new University Hospital, leaving the old one for Peterson's "despised obstetrical patients."

About 1907 Canfield perfected his submucosal resection of the lateral nasal wall for treatment of intractable chronic suppurative disease of the antrum, ethmoid, and sphenoid.[3] He infiltrated the lateral and anterior walls and floor of the nose with 0.25 percent cocaine and 1:10,000 epinephrine (Adrenalin) and then began with an incision through the soft parts of the nostril from the middle of the lateral wall to the pyriform opening. He extended the incision to

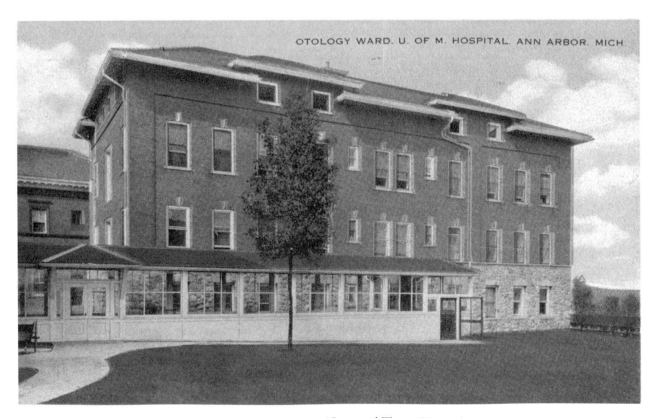

Fig. 23–1. The Eye, Ear, Nose, and Throat Hospital

the floor of the nose. Canfield elevated the mucous membrane and periosteum of the lateral and anterior antral walls and then removed the inferior half of the lateral wall of the pyriform opening and of the lateral wall of the nose. He enucleated much of the bone of the inferior turbinate and removed enough of the anterior and median walls of the antrum to allow a view into the antrum so that he could perform any necessary curettage. That part of the operation permitted continuous drainage of the deepest parts of the antrum and prevented formation of granulation tissue. Then if an operation on the ethmoid and sphenoid was indicated, Canfield entered the ethmoid after enucleating the bone of the middle turbinate and removed the anterior wall of the sphenoid. He completed the operation by forming a flap of mucous membrane of the median wall of the antrum and carefully approximated it to the floor of the antrum. The patient was left with cavities of the sinuses in free communication with the nasal passage.

Canfield wrote that for the surgeon "[t]he difficulties of the operation are mainly those encountered in the sub-mucous resection of the nasal septum, increased somewhat by the fact that the lateral wall of the nose is sharply concave and that the bone of the lateral wall of the pyriform opening is very dense and requires the energetic use of the mallet and chisel or a strong rongeur."[4] For the patient the difficulty was living with the result of the operation, and every so often Canfield and A. C. Furstenberg, his successor and disciple, had to listen to denunciations of their "butchery."[5]

Canfield thought that simple opening and draining of the mastoid process is not sufficient in treating acute mastoiditis. All infected structures should be removed and free communication with the inner ear established.[6] In treating chronic suppurative otitis media, Canfield converted the mastoid, antrum, middle ear, and external auditory canal into one cavity with smooth walls, and after he sealed the tympanic orifice of the eustachian tube, he covered the entire cavity with Thiersch skin grafts from the patient's thigh.[7] Invasion of the labyrinth could occur without symptoms, and although Canfield might suspect suppuration of the labyrinth, he usually made the diagnosis at the time of a radical mastoid operation. Then he performed complete exenteration of the labyrinth.[8]

Because tumors or infections of the sinuses or of the ear readily enter the cranium, Canfield perforce became a brain surgeon. When Canfield operated

upon one girl of fourteen years for suppurative middle ear disease he found the bony wall of the cerebellum was destroyed and the cerebellum exposed. Despite Canfield's efforts to wash away the pus, the child died. Canfield thought his mistake was not to have operated earlier.[9] He was more successful with a child of four years whose frontal lobe abscesses followed frontal sinus infection. Canfield drained the abscesses in four operations, and the child recovered.[10]

Canfield believed that the theory of focal infection was well established and that the nose and throat, and in particular the lymphoid ring of adenoids and tonsils, are the most important sites of focal infection.[11] Bacteria lodged there may give no sign of their presence, but they elaborate toxins that produce symptoms of disease in distant organs. Focal infection in an adult may cause loss of energy without demonstrable disease. If adenoids and tonsils are the site of focal infection, they must be removed. However, the surgeon must wait until the child is about six years old, for in earlier years the adenoids and tonsils as well as the thymus gland have a repressive action on endocrine glands. If they are removed, hyperthyroidism becomes evident as shown by increased susceptibility to infection. Another function of adenoids and tonsils is to regulate body size and weight. If they are removed early, children grow taller than their parents. These functions are less important as the child grows older.

A. C. Furstenberg

David Murray Cowie wrote: "Returning from a consultation trip, driving at high rate of speed as was his custom, passing a truck with a trailer a few miles east of Ann Arbor at a little after 1 A.M., May 12th [1932], [Canfield's] car for some unknown reason left the road, striking a tree. Death was instantaneous."[12] Canfield's widow endowed a fellowship in his memory, and a committee consisting of Udo Wile, Cyrus Sturgis, Norman Miller, and Carl Weller recommended that A. C. Furstenberg be appointed Canfield's successor (fig. 23–2).

Furstenberg had earned his doctor of medicine degree at Michigan in 1915, and he immediately began training under Canfield. When Canfield left to serve in various base hospitals in 1917, Furstenberg was made acting assistant professor in charge of the Department of Otolaryngology, and when Canfield

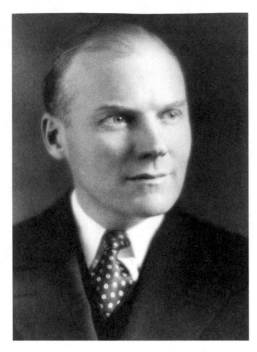

Fig. 23–2. Albert C. Furstenberg. (Courtesy of the Bentley Historical Library, University of Michigan, University of Michigan Faculty and Staff Portrait Collection, Box 2, "Furstenberg.")

returned in 1919 the "acting" was removed from the title.

Canfield's publications dropped off to a few trivial case reports after his practice was well established, but Furstenberg's increased steadily in frequency and importance. By the end of the 1930s Furstenberg had become one of the elder statesmen of his specialty, and his publications gave the benefit of his broad experience to his contemporaries.[13]

Laryngectomy

Canfield attempted laryngectomy around 1911, because cancer of the larynx had 100 percent mortality. The results were so disappointing that the operation was abandoned until 1923, when Michigan surgeons adopted the technique of John E. McKenty.[14] Consequently, by 1931 Furstenberg could report on a series of 135 patients with cancer of the larynx he had treated. Of those, 36 were living with "wonderful morale" after total extirpation of the larynx.[15] Furstenberg found that cancer of the larynx occurred seven times as frequently among men as among women and that 75 percent of his patients were public speakers, auctioneers, singers, preachers, and

teachers who habitually overused their voices. He thought that the best treatment for a precancerous condition signaled by persisting hoarseness is complete silence, not even a whisper, for weeks or months. Unfortunately, patients delayed seeking relief, and 70 percent of the ones he saw had symptoms of purulent and blood-stained sputum and were beyond reach of surgical intervention. Not one of the patients had consulted a laryngologist within two months of the onset of symptoms. When operation was possible, Furstenberg preferred complete laryngectomy to any attempt at submucous resection, and he trained nurses in postoperative care to guard by use of suction against allowing any discharge to enter the lower air passages. Later, many survivors developed a distinctly audible whisper.

The Spread of Infection

Furstenberg was a master of radical operations, but his attitude was conservative. He thought that conservative measures would suffice in the majority of cases of acute infection of the nasal sinuses. He put the patient to bed for a week and gave the patient morphine if necessary to control the pain. When Furstenberg reported the results of 300 cases from the University Health Service and the University Hospital he found 296 asymptomatic on return visits. The four who developed chronic maxillary sinusitis were among the twelve who had been treated surgically elsewhere.[16]

One reason for conservatism was that Furstenberg found, in eighty-four cases of diffuse osteomyelitis of the cranial bones, fifty-two had followed bone work during acute infection of the accessory nasal sinuses.[17] Infection spread by continuity of tissue and by retrograde thrombosis of veins and resulted in early injury to the inner table of the skull. Brain abscesses then followed from extradural spread of infection and eventual penetration of the dura.[18] Treatment then must be radical: removal of full thickness of bone and maintenance of massive drainage of the exposed dura. Furstenberg said there is no need for apprehension in removing large portions of the cranial vault, for he often found that regeneration of bone obliterated the defect.[19]

Furstenberg said that the most charitable treatment of infection of the parotid gland is a wide incision that secures massive drainage. Otherwise infection of the neck is distributed through the pharyngomaxillary fossa.[20] Furstenberg and a young surgeon named Luis Yglesias demonstrated the route of spread of infection to the mediastinum by making gross dissections of the cervical region and thorax, carefully reflecting the planes of the body commencing with the skin and following in an orderly sequence. "Thus, as one would read and turn the leaves of a book, from the first to the last page, the true story of an anatomic dissection is revealed and the relative importance of its component parts determined through a careful and orderly study of the adjacent structures of the body. In this way one may obtain, as by no other means, an explanation for the clinical behavior of many of the deep-seated suppurations of the neck and mediastinum."[21] By study of longitudinal and cross sections of adult cadavers (fig. 23–3), by injection of iodized oil followed by roentgenography, and by examination of embryological specimens, Furstenberg and Yglesias showed how the mediastinum is exposed from all sides to suppuration secondary to retropharyngeal abscesses. Furstenberg described his success in one case and failure in another when he applied his knowledge to drainage of the mediastinum.[22]

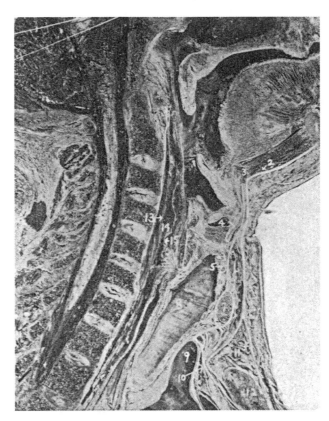

Fig. 23–3. Sagittal section of the neck and upper mediastinum showing the deep cervical fascia. (From A. C. Furstenberg, "Acute Mediastinal Suppuration," *Trans. Am. Laryngol. Rhinol. Otol. Soc.* 35 [1929]: 218.)

The Nervous System

In addition to the neurological work with Elizabeth Crosby summarized in chapter 10, Furstenberg described lesions producing laryngeal paralysis based on a study of a large series of neurological patients and of pathological material obtained at autopsy.[23] He outlined the corticobulbar fibers carrying motor impulses to the lower motor neurons supplying the larynx, and he summarized the facts necessary for localizing central lesions causing laryngeal paralysis. In particular Furstenberg differentiated the causes of the spastic form from the flaccid types of paralysis.

Furstenberg worked with Max Peet in studying patients Peet treated for hypertension by splanchnicectomy, because patients with hypertension often consulted an otolaryngologist first on account of headache. Thirty percent of such patients had vertigo that could be differentiated from Ménière's disease. When Furstenberg made audiograms on patients before and after Peet's operation he found that a decrease in blood pressure was associated with an improvement in hearing.[24]

Furstenberg found that nearly all the hypertensive patients he saw were emotionally disturbed. They

were despondent, irritable, anxious, and apprehensive. In fact, he said that an otolaryngologist sees a great many patients who are suffering from illness of psychological origin, and he gave many examples. He wrote: "The otolaryngologist may be a poor psychotherapist but experience soon teaches him the fundamentals of psychopathology so that he is not lacking in his judgment of anxiety states, depressions, phobias and obsessions, so commonly observed in the patients who consult him."[25]

Furstenberg had no faith in the ministrations of the psychiatrists.

Medical Treatment of Ménière's Symptom Complex

When Furstenberg considered Ménière's symptom complex—a violent attack of vertigo with deafness, nausea, spontaneous nystagmus, and persistent tinnitus together with total disability during attacks and terror of impending ones—he found that the sum total of proposed treatments had been of little use to the patient. Once Samuel Kopetsky, a professor of otology at the New York Graduate School of Medicine, asked Furstenberg a series of questions.

What class of individuals have vertigo? Why are dizzy attacks frequently seen in patients with cardio-vascular-renal disease? The answer . . . lies in some disturbance in the metabolism of water which gives rise, perhaps, to a water-logged condition of the static labyrinth. Why don't you study water balance in these patients?[26]

When Furstenberg searched the literature he found only one paper on the subject, that by Dida Dederding of the Copenhagen City Hospital.[27] Dederding had dealt with 135 patients with morbus ménièri, chiefly studying factors affecting bone conduction. Dederding concluded that the disease is "not only a matter of local but also of universal disease" associated with abnormal accumulation of water.[28] Treatment consisted of restricting water intake and promoting loss by gymnastics, fresh air, Finsen light, baths, and sweating induced by injections of pilocarpine. Hearing, at least, was improved and attacks decreased.

Furstenberg thought that Dederding's conception of water balance was as confused as the treatment. He was not a colleague of Harry Newburgh for nothing, and he knew that it is not water alone that is retained in extracellular fluid but water plus sodium salts. He had Floyd Lashmet, one of Newburgh's young men, to help him and Frank Lathrop, a medical student working his way through school, to prepare the salt-deficient diets.

As was the case with Coller's papers, Newburgh might well have written Furstenberg's description of the principles and methods of measuring water balance. Furstenberg described in detail the clinical course of one man who had two or three attacks a week for two years and a seizure daily for the past six months. Furstenberg, Lashmet, and Lathrop put the patient on a constant diet containing only 87 milliequivalents of sodium a day, and they measured his water balance every twelve hours. Attacks disappeared, but when they gave the patient 348 milliequivalents of sodium he retained water and had a very severe attack. In order to separate the effects of water retention from those of sodium they dehydrated the patient, and while he remained dehydrated they gave him 261 milliequivalents of sodium, precipitating another attack.

By 1934 Furstenberg had followed fourteen such patients, all hospitalized for thirty days or more while their water balance was studied. "In not one instance did we fail to produce an attack by the administration of sodium, and not once were we disappointed in obtaining complete relief by the medical therapy above described." Furstenberg prescribed a regimen of a low sodium diet supplemented by three grams of ammonium chloride with each meal to promote sodium loss.[29]

Others found Furstenberg's treatment useful,[30] and by 1941 he could report "uniformly satisfactory" results with "more than 150 patients."[31] Thirty-five patients made return visits, and among them were six failures as the result of dropping off the diet for one or another reason. Furstenberg reached an additional sixty patients by questionnaire, and 52 percent of them reported that they were entirely free of attacks. In the case of complete failure Furstenberg sectioned the vestibular portion of the eighth cranial nerve.

Teaching Otolaryngology

Canfield in his inaugural address at Michigan described his relation as a specialist to the general practitioner. His concept of that relation governed his undergraduate teaching and that of Furstenberg after him.[32] Lectures and section work were designed to teach medical students to examine the ear and to recognize its diseases. Canfield said that many signs and symptoms of disease pass unnoticed by the general practitioner, but proper treatment will prevent 50 percent of the deafness of "middle life." In cases of measles, scarlet fever, and diphtheria it is the duty of the student once he is in general practice to look at the ear each day. Most of the disease of the middle ear originates in disease of the nose and throat, and the physician should look for hypertrophic adenoids. Purulent disease of the brain can arise from a single infection of the ear, and a general practitioner must be able to distinguish between acute ear inflammation and cerebrospinal meningitis in a child. Having made the diagnosis, the general practitioner should refer his patient to a specialist and not try to do the surgery. In turn, the specialist must be careful to return the patient with a courteous explanation of his treatment. Furstenberg's letters were always distinguished by their elaborate courtesy.

Canfield's major teaching effort was to train specialists in his own image, and the result was, as

Furstenberg said, "that every man now living who has finished such a training at the University of Michigan is one of the outstanding otolaryngologists in his community and a much respected member of the profession."[33]

Furstenberg thought that the days were over when a physician could make himself a specialist in otolaryngology by independent thinking, courage, and self-reliance.[34] In Canfield's time the program of graduate training began for an intern fresh out of medical school and continued with two years of increasing experience and responsibility. At first there were only three interns at a time, but when Canfield's department moved into the new hospital in 1925 the program expanded to as many as four interns at once, all rising to instructorships in two or three years. When Furstenberg succeeded Canfield he required his postdoctoral students to complete a rotating medical or surgical internship first. A student coming on to Furstenberg's service as an assistant resident was assigned to the wards to do physical examinations. The student, after learning to use the examining instruments and a head mirror, was allowed to assist in minor surgical procedures such as tonsillectomies. The next year as a resident the student worked in the Outpatient Department and was permitted to perform operations of a more technical nature, a submucous resection, for example. The resident, having been promoted to junior instructor in the third year and put in complete charge of the Outpatient Department, had practical experience in major operations and taught otolaryngological anatomy to junior medical students. A senior instructor in the fourth year of training had major surgical responsibility, supervised junior residents, and taught clinical otolaryngology to senior medical students. Furstenberg said: "The residents on our service spend two years in studying and teaching anatomy, in association with clinical otolaryngology before they are permitted to perform a radical operation upon the nasal accessory sinuses. Even then they are carefully supervised and directed during the performance of at least fifteen such surgical procedures before they are permitted to assume full responsibility for the results of their efforts and the life of the patient."[35]

Furstenberg deplored the rigid separation of preclinical and clinical subjects in the curriculum, and as dean he could do nothing to change the practice, but in his graduate training program he tried to extend the study of anatomy, physiology, and pathology throughout the four years.

Dean Furstenberg

When Frederick Novy retired in 1935 President Ruthven made Albert Carl Furstenberg dean of the Medical School without consulting anyone on the faculty. Fifty years earlier, when Victor Vaughan became dean, the school had an inadequate basic science building, the Anatomical Laboratory, the Chemical Laboratory, a part of the Physics-Hygiene Building, and the Pavilion Hospital with sixty beds, one operating room for general surgery, and one for ophthalmology. There were nineteen members of the faculty with the rank of instructor, assistant professor, or professor, and there were eleven assistants. In the early years of Furstenberg's deanship there were two large basic science buildings and several hospital buildings with 1,330 beds. Sixteen thousand patients were seen each month in two outpatient clinics, and twenty-seven thousand were admitted to the hospital each year, where one thousand operations were performed every month. There were more than two hundred physicians on the hospital staff and one hundred men and women on the faculties of the basic science departments.

Dean Furstenberg was a busy man until his retirement in 1959. As an otolaryngologist in private practice he had an office on South Main Street; he had an office and he operated in the St. Joseph Mercy Hospital; and he had an office and operated in the University Hospital. His dean's office was in the West Medical Building, where Vera Cummings and H. M. Pollard as recorder and secretary of the faculty, respectively, did much more than routine work. Because Dean Furstenberg had trouble meeting appointments in all those places, he was known as "the late Dr. Furstenberg."

Dean Furstenberg was the ideal representative of the Michigan faculty as it had become by 1941. Of all the senior members of the clinical faculty, only L. H. Newburgh and Frank Wilson were not on part time and enjoying an eminently lucrative private practice. Each department chairman or section head ruled his department or section with a firm hand, and his juniors were absolutely dependent upon him for professional and financial advancement. There were inbreeding and provincialism. By the end of the 1930s every member of the Departments of Physiology and Surgery was trained at Michigan, and some other departments were not much different. Because the dominant members of the faculty thought alike, they determined the tone and policies of the school. Acting as a sort of Polish parliament[36] with the dean presiding, they respected each other's prerogatives, and nothing could be done over the veto of one of them.

Dean Furstenberg was "by choice and training a practical man in medicine . . . [whose] chief concern is with cause, effect, and the cure of disease."[37] He had only a cursory interest in "inquiries into the 'whys and wherefores' of phenomena," and that was the attitude of many of his clinical colleagues. Consequently, basic research was neglected in many of the clinical departments, but when it was done it could be very good indeed. Harry Newburgh was among the half-dozen U.S. leaders in the study of metabolism, and Frank Wilson's work in electrocardiography had worldwide influence. Fred Coller with all his private practice and other commitments led a team that made the understanding of a patient's water and electrolyte balance an obligation for every progressive surgeon. Reed Nesbit used apparatus costing only a few dollars to define the characteristics of the neurogenic bladder.

Dean Furstenberg's set of mind made him a poor judge of what was going on in the preclinical departments. He knew that Robert Gesell was a poor teacher and H. B. Lewis a good one, because the students told him so. He could not make an independent judgment of the quality of research in the preclinical departments, and he had to rely on hearsay or on the assumption that if an individual, Robert Gesell, for example, were on the Michigan faculty he must be a good scientist.

Dean Vaughan and those who cooperated with him made Michigan what a well-informed historian of U.S. medicine called "not just any school," and that school lasted until the bad days of World War I. Dean Furstenberg and his colleagues made an entirely different kind of school that lasted long after World War II.

Epilogue: Building the Modern Medical Center, 1941 to Present

Janet Tarolli

In the brief span of an epilogue, I can offer only an outline of the remarkable expansion of the University of Michigan Medical Center from 1941 to the present and mention a few of the leaders of this growth.

The Medical School in the Early 1940s

In 1940 the U.S. government was deferring all medical students from military service for the duration of medical school and a one-year internship. The army, navy, and public health service needed ten thousand doctors to serve an army of 1.4 million. Since U.S. medical schools only graduated five thousand annually, medical schools were considering whether to add to enrollments, shorten the preprofessional curriculum, reduce the required hours of medical training, or accelerate the program by continuous study through the summer months. Enrollment at the U-M Medical School was 472, with 131 in the first-year class.

The census at University Hospital remained depressed, owing to the decreased state appropriation for the care of crippled and afflicted children. The average census for 1940–41 was 843, compared with 739 in 1939–40. In July 1941, when a new photofluorographic unit was placed into operation, a new program was begun to check all who registered at the hospital for unsuspected chest conditions, particularly tuberculosis. With the advent of the hospital service plan in Michigan and its coverage of improved services, many new demands were being made on the hospital. More semi-private rooms were added, and cubicles with privacy curtains were installed on each ward, a process that had been started in the 1936–37 academic year. There were needs for a modern maternity hospital, a modern fireproof building for patients afflicted with contagious disease, and a special hospital unit for carrying on research in the treatment of rheumatism.

In 1941–42 it became apparent that every physically qualified male medical student was destined for the armed forces. The army expected to recruit fifty-five thousand doctors by October 1942. There were approximately sixty thousand able-bodied physicians under the draft age of forty-five. During 1942 sixty-six of seventy-eight medical schools in the United States and Canada, including ours, instituted an accelerated program to graduate medical students in three years instead of four. The teaching staff suffered a reduction of 40 percent. Subjects of military importance were being stressed: preventive medicine, tropical diseases, aviation medicine, sexually transmitted diseases, fractures, industrial medicine, and psychiatry.

On 12 March 1942 the 500,000th patient registered at University Hospital. There continued to be an acute shortage of personnel in all classifications because many had joined the armed forces. Hospital volunteers and extra service by regular personnel helped with the work. The average daily census was 843. Just over 51 percent of patient-days represented days of care to indigent patients who were hospitalized under various public statutes (sent to University Hospital by county governments), down from 80 percent in the 1937–38 academic year. There was an increase in patients referred to the hospital by private physicians (clinic patients), and an increase in private patients. A block method of instruction for senior medical students was adopted by many of the departments. Small groups of students did full-time work on inpatient and outpatient units, and there was a decrease in didactic instruction. This caring for patients by students helped offset the loss of junior medical staff. A group of medical and nursing staff had departed Ann Arbor by train in June 1942 to staff the 298th General Hospital, which served in England, France, and Belgium.

Dean Furstenberg said in his 1943–44 annual report, "We view with anxiety the effect of the accelerated program upon medical education."[1] The effects of rapid schedules invite "decadent trends." He believed there was no need for alarm about a peacetime shortage of doctors. Before the war, there was 1 doctor for 700 people. It was estimated that in 1949 there would be 1 doctor for 733 people. "The great need now," he said, "is the establishment of well-equipped hospital centers in various parts of the country which will attract groups of well-trained specialists and thus distribute adequate service to all our population, economic as well as geographic."[2]

Almost 50 percent of patients were paying the hospital directly for care, and the percentage of patients whose hospitalization was paid for by the state steadily decreased. A new program called the Emergency Maternity and Infant Care Program reimbursed hospitals for the cost of care given to the wives and infant children of men in the four lowest classifications of the armed forces.

In one of the old Catherine Street Hospital buildings, 125 beds were made available for the U.S. Public Health Service to establish a Rapid Treatment Center for patients with sexually transmitted diseases. Another of this group was made over into a dormitory for student nurses, who were badly needed. The only new building in the 1940s was the Veterans Readjustment Center, a fifty-bed psychiatric facility that was built and equipped entirely from funds from the state legislature. It opened in October 1947 and was a source of pride because it was the only one of its type operated by a teaching institution in the United States. The next new building was the long-awaited Maternity Hospital (Women's Hospital), which was occupied in February 1950.

The 1950 Medical School Centennial

The one hundredth anniversary of the opening of the University of Michigan Medical School was celebrated during three days in September 1950 and written up in the *University of Michigan Medical Bulletin*. The medical faculty, supported by the regents, had decided that the Medical School "should be quartered in a modern Medical Center providing facilities for all of its activities: undergraduate and postgraduate teaching, the care of clinic and hospital patients, and continuous medical research."[3] The 1925 University Hospital, with its various additions, was the nucleus for this project. Proposed plans for a complete medical center included a pediatric hospital, an outpatient clinic, clinical research facilities, and a new medical science building for preclinical teaching and research, including the medical library and offices for medical school administration. Through the generosity of the S. S. Kresge Foundation, the Institute for Clinical Medical Research was planned and was soon under construction. The state legislature provided funds for the planning of a seven-story outpatient clinic east of the Neuropsychiatric Institute and connected for several floors with the surgical wing of University Hospital. The pediatric hospital

Not Just Any Medical School

and new medical science building remained unfunded, and it was expected that the medical center, as envisioned, might not be completed until 1960.

In 1951, the Medical School was expanding its enrollment by admitting a class of two hundred, but it would have to make do with some overcrowded conditions temporarily. In addition to the building program, the curriculum committee sought to bring about "complete modernization of the plan of medical instruction at Michigan,"[4] so that basic sciences could be taught in close association with clinical studies and faculty members could mingle. By the fall of 1954, after three years of admitting approximately two hundred students, Medical School enrollment was 775, the largest in the United States and Canada. The following June, 176 medical students were graduated, the largest group from any single medical school in North America. The large class sizes continued through the 1970s.

The new Outpatient Clinic Building was ready for occupancy in January 1953. Twenty thousand outpatients were seen there monthly in its twenty-four departmental clinics, compared with 16,022 visits per month in 1947 and a *yearly* total of 11,500 outpatient registrations in 1925. Construction of a new five-hundred-bed general hospital for the Veterans Administration was well along less than a mile away. This hospital, along with the eight-hundred-bed University Hospital and Outpatient Clinic, promised to be very important to the Medical School for its clinical facilities. Both hospitals would be needed to accommodate the inordinately large number of medical students. The Veterans Administration Hospital was dedicated in September 1953. At the same time "a program of rehabilitation" was launched by Director Albert C. Kerlikowske to modernize University Hospital completely, at a cost of $6 million. There was a backlog of requests for private and semiprivate rooms.

The Kresge Medical Research Building was dedicated in May 1954, providing offices for 128 laboratory units and such features as walk-in incubator rooms and air-conditioned animal quarters. One wing was designated as the Kresge Medical Library. Two years later a pleased Dean Furstenberg estimated there were three hundred research projects in operation concerned with nearly every aspect of the basic sciences and clinical medicine. When a portion of the first unit of the Medical Science Building was completed in April 1958, the Department of Pathol-

ogy moved into its new quarters, and the Departments of Pharmacology and Biological Chemistry and Medical Administration soon followed. Other preclinical departments remained in the East Medical Building on main campus, awaiting the construction of the second unit. With generous amounts of state money available for mental health, a seventy-five bed hospital for children with emotional disorders was built in 1955, but a general pediatric facility, C. S. Mott Children's Hospital, was not completed until 1969. The Mental Health Research Institute, established in 1955, moved into a building of its own in 1960.

In 1959 Albert C. Furstenberg retired after twenty-four years as dean, the last of the deans to combine chairmanship of a department, private practice, and medical administration. President Harlan Hatcher recommended the appointment of William N. Hubbard Jr., who had spent most of his time as an internist and medical administrator at New York University. In his first annual report Dean Hubbard said: "In the next decade, this faculty will face an unprecedented demand for its services to both patients and the community: it must confront the need of the community for an extraordinary increase in the number of physicians and must undertake research which will lead to new concepts and techniques in preventing and treating malignant and degenerative diseases."[5]

The Medical Center in the 1960s

By 1961, the Polio Respirator Center had grown into a children's rehabilitation center, serving children with cerebral palsy, cystic fibrosis, and other conditions. The first grumblings about the aging University Hospital were voiced. Dr. Kerlikowske wrote in his 1960–61 annual report: "Facilities for children are crude and antiquated. The ancient, eighteen-bed adult wards, with the inadequate work areas adjacent, were never designed for the number of medical and nursing students and faculty now frequenting them."[6] In August 1962 the Veterans Readjustment Center terminated its patient services following loss of state funding. In a few months it reopened as the North Outpatient Building, to serve as an extension of the main Outpatient Building.

In his annual report of 1962–63, Dean Hubbard acknowledged the election of James V. Neel, professor of human genetics and of internal medicine, to membership in the National Academy of Sciences. He said, "It is becoming increasingly evident that, in the next decade, there will be many advances in the field of genetics. The research program which Dr. Neel directs provides The University of Michigan with the foundation for studies commensurate with the promise of this important new discipline."[7] New facilities for basic research on hearing and human genetics were completed in 1963 and 1964, respectively.

Quantitative demands for health services were increasing at a rapid rate. In the annual report for 1964–65, Dean Hubbard identified the following reasons: increasing numbers of people, an increasing percentage of people between the age groups over sixty-five and under ten, increasing expectations of health care for all people, and increasing ability to pay for services. One million patients had been treated at the University Hospital in the forty years between 1925 and 1965, and a new children's hospital remained a critical need. By 1968 there was an increasing national focus on the "health manpower problem," especially the shortage of physicians, and the "mal-distribution of health workers, the inadequate organization of the health care delivery system, and the escalating cost of medical care."[8] The first three human heart transplants in Michigan were performed at University Hospital that year, with much media fanfare.

The centennial of University Hospital was celebrated with more than forty programs, special events, and conferences during 1969. About five thousand medical and hospital specialists were expected to attend one or more of the events, many of which were held in the newly opened Towsley Center for Continuing Education. Themes of the major programs included biomedical instrumentation, the education of hospitalized children, infection control, practice and research in nursing, the service unit and new patterns of hospital care, and trends for the hospital of the future. In its centennial year, the eight-hundred-bed University Hospital continued to be the major clinical resource for 800 medical students, 750 nursing students, and 400 interns and residents in twenty-two medical specialties.

In July, Dean Hubbard assumed additional duties as director of the University of Michigan Medical Center. In the medical center, it was felt that teaching, patient care, and research were inseparable. Dr. Hubbard kept the position less than a year, leaving to accept a position as a vice president of the Upjohn Company in April 1970. Dr. John A. Gronvall, who had come to the university in August 1968 as associate professor of pathology and associate dean, was acting dean and director from April to January.

The Medical Center in the 1970s

In January 1971, President Robben Fleming announced the appointment and approval by the regents of Dr. Gronvall as dean and director of the medical center. Dr. Fleming said, "Solutions to the complex problems of health care in our state and in our nation require the vigor, the skill and the scholarship of young leaders as Dr. Gronvall."[9] Dr. Gronvall was thirty-nine, the same age as two previous U-M medical deans when they were appointed, Dr. Hubbard and the late Victor C. Vaughan.

In his first annual report as hospital director (1969–70), Mr. Edward J. Connors listed some of the events of public interest: U-M surgeons successfully reattached a severed arm of a man involved in an accident; the first press briefing on the transplant program was held; Dr. J. G. Turcotte, head of the kidney transplant team, delivered the Henry Russel Award Lecture; the Upjohn Clinical Center for Pharmacology was dedicated; Philip T. Barnum, Michigan's first and the world's fiftieth heart transplant recipient, died; U-M's first lung transplant was attempted; thirty-five kidney transplants were performed this academic year; and *Time* magazine reported U-M's treatment of urinary tract infection.

In the fall of 1971, 225 first-year students entered the Medical School, one of the largest first-year groups in the United States. Applicants were accepted on the basis of their intelligence, aptitude for science, and evidence of concern for society. Doctor of medicine degrees were awarded to 203 graduates in 1973. One featured speaker at the ceremony was the actor Robert Young, who, Dr. Gronvall said, "through an authentic and sensitive portrayal of 'Dr. Marcus Welby' on television has greatly enriched the rapport between the American people and their physicians."[10] That issue of the *University of Michigan Medical Center Journal* (April–June 1973) also reported that record-size classes were expected to continue, since "the Medical School [was] now enrolling almost 250 in its freshman classes toward a goal of 300 students entering by 1980."[11]

In 1972, fifty exceptional students were admitted to the Medical School directly from high school as part of the Inteflex program (Integrated Flexible Premedical/Medical School Curriculum). This program, which is still in existence, was designed to graduate well-rounded, highly trained physicians in six years.

In his 1973–74 annual report, Dean Gronvall said the Medical School was faced with declining federal support and increasing federal and state control and program expectations. There were 237 entering freshmen in the regular M.D. program, and total of 947 students. More than 50 percent of the clinical education of medical students occurred at hospitals other than University Hospital. Affiliates included Henry Ford Hospital (new that year), St. Joseph Mercy Hospital in Ann Arbor, Veterans Administration Hospital in Ann Arbor, and Wayne County General Hospital. After geometric increases in federal support for medical research, a plateau in funding had been reached. The research laboratories were having trouble keeping pace with the effects of inflation. (Inflation had been so severe in 1971 that President Nixon had issued an executive order to freeze all prices and wages under the Economic Stabilization Act.) In addition, there was a significant redirection of federal support toward targeted research. In November 1973 a new Medical Service Plan was endorsed by the regents. The plan represented a fundamental revision in the management of professional fee income and established a clinical faculty salary system with incentive elements.

During the next academic year (1974–75), a decision was made to defer plans for further student enrollment increases and continue at the same level (237), owing to constraints on federal and state funding for medical education. By the 1975–76 academic year, the school would have moved to enrolling 280 "first-year" students, with 237 students in the regular program and 40 to 50 students in the fourth year of the Inteflex program. Now, however, the sum of the regular students and fourth-year Inteflex students would equal 237 for that academic year.

In 1974–75, plans were developed for the establishment of a new family practice residency, and a decision was made to mount a major research effort on development and application of recombinant DNA methodology. The Department of Human Genetics initiated negotiations with the U.S. Energy Research and Development Administration toward the establishment of designated laboratory status for the conduct of large scale assessment of the effect of environmental pollutants on the genetic composition of humans. Of particular interest was the genetic effect of the atomic bombs dropped on Japan during World War II.

The new federal government position in 1975–76 was that the nation did not need more physicians, but it must pay attention to their geographic distribution. In the fall of 1975, the percentage of women matriculants was 28 percent, up slightly from 25 percent the previous year. The actual numbers and percentage of minority applicants was decreasing, prompting the Medical School to obtain a federal grant to support an outreach recruitment program. An unprecedented debate on the risks and benefits of recombinant DNA research occurred nationally and locally. Jeptha Dalston was appointed the new hospital director in August 1975. Premium costs for malpractice insurance escalated rapidly. More progress was made toward the establishment of the Department of Family Practice, and formal action was to occur in the next year. The Health Professions Education Act of 1976 authorized almost $3 million for health manpower training.

The Replacement Hospital Project

In December 1971 an independent engineering firm released a state-funded report on building conditions, which served as a baseline study for future planning in the entire medical center. Certain buildings were slated for "eventual demolition": the Neuropsychiatric Institute; the Interns' Residence (now the Clinical Faculty Office Building); North Outpatient Building; Victor Vaughan House; Simpson Memorial Institute; and the Kresge Medical Library wing. Women's Hospital, the Outpatient Clinic, and Children's Psychiatric Hospital were deemed structurally adequate. University Hospital was judged to be in marginal condition for its present use as an acute inpatient care facility and it was recognized that there was a need for a new hospital.

Patient acceptance of the hospital was declining. Patients expected semiprivate or private rooms, not open wards containing four to eighteen beds. They expected private bathrooms and telephones by the bed, and adequate heating and air conditioning. University Hospital could not provide these basic amenities.

Structurally, the loading capacity of the floors was less than half of current hospital design load requirements. Some new equipment was too heavy to place anywhere but in the subbasement. Floor-to-floor height limited the capacity for installing new electrical, plumbing, and ventilating systems. Space was limited and running out. Hallways were being used as storage areas, waiting rooms, and classrooms. It was increasingly difficult to attract and retain high-quality professional staff.

Old Main had to go. The replacement hospital and the A. Alfred Taubman Health Care Center were completed and occupied in February 1986. Former hospital director Jeptha W. Dalston, in his 1986 draft report on the history of the Replacement Hospital Project, said: "The University Hospital takes care of sick people on two levels. It serves as a community hospital for those who live nearby and who go there to have their babies delivered and their gall bladders removed. But it is also a center for the most advanced and sophisticated diagnosis and treatment. As such, it serves the entire State. If that logger on the distant Upper Peninsula has a severe medical problem that his local doctors can't solve, they may very well refer him to Ann Arbor for definitive care.

"There's a circle here. As the newly trained doctors fan out over the State to practice, the level of care in the community hospitals rises, and they're able to treat locally many patients who once would have had to be sent to Ann Arbor. At the same time research advances are bringing new methods of diagnosis and treatment to University Hospital so that they are now able to help patients who might not have been sent there a few years ago because so little could have been done for them.

"Medical educators are fond of referring to a place like University Hospital as a stool. It stands solidly on three legs—patient care, education, and research—but will collapse if any one of them is taken away."[12]

The Medical School in the 1980s

There was a significant decrease in the number of applicants to medical schools nationwide in 1979 and 1980. Nationally, 24.4 percent of medical students were women, but 30 percent of students at U-M Medical School were women in 1980. In a special report on the views of medical students about the critical medical issues today (May 1980 issue of *Michigan Medicine*) a University of Michigan medical student listed the development of family practice as a specialty, national health insurance (he was against

it), the rising cost of medical education, and the importance of patient education. In 1981 the Taubman Medical Library moved to new facilities constructed on Catherine Street.

At the University of Michigan the combined dean of the Medical School/director of the medical center had long been abandoned. In 1983, the position of vice provost for medical affairs was created to directly oversee the dean of the Medical School and the director of the hospital. This position was filled by Dr. George D. Zuidema in 1984, and he remained in that capacity until 1994, when the office was disbanded. Soon after he arrived, M-CARE was developed as a preferred provider organization, and plans were made to develop a health maintenance organization. Zuidema oversaw the completion of the Replacement Hospital Project and activation of the Taubman Center. In addition he developed a strategic plan, a mission statement, and goals for the medical center to follow into the 1990s. In the medical center's strategic plan relating to the Medical School, priority scientific areas were identified as bioengineering and biotechnology, oncology, molecular genetics, the neurosciences, and aging.

John Gronvall left the university in 1983 to become deputy chief medical director of the Veterans Administration Hospital System, and Peter Ward served as interim dean until 1985. By 1983–84 the entering class had been reduced by thirty over the previous two years, which had helped the school implement recommendations of the Neidhardt Report (Report of the Joint LS&A/Medical School Task Force on Medical Education), adjust to the loss of the Westland Medical Center (formerly, Wayne County General Hospital) as a site for clinical placements, and "adapt to changes in the nature and quantity of the patient base available for teaching."[13] A further reduction from 207 to 177 was being contemplated sometime after 1986–87.

The Medical School initiated a two-semester curriculum (AIMED Program) in 1984–85 to improve the qualifications of educationally disadvantaged students. Efforts to maintain the diversity of the classes were successful. The class entering in the fall of 1986 had 167 students, including 50 women and 29 members of under-represented minority groups. Forty Inteflex students entering the first year of medical school at that time included 18 women and 1 minority. Eighty-five percent of the class of 1987 received one of their top three choices of training site for a residency. Placements included Brigham and

Women's Hospital, Rush Presbyterian, Johns Hopkins, Massachusetts General Hospital, University of California at San Diego, Strong Memorial Hospital, and Washington University, St. Louis.

Joseph E. Johnson III served as dean from 1985 to 1990, a period of continued growth in external research funding and turbulence in medical education. Under Dean Johnson plans were made for a major curriculum revision to include, for example, improved teaching in the ambulatory care setting and more emphasis on preventive care. Medical Science Research Buildings I and II were activated in 1986 and 1989. The Howard Hughes Medical Institute, established in 1984, grew to a complement of ten investigators, greatly enhancing the university's strength in molecular genetics. The clinical departments participated in developing "Centers of Excellence" for cancer (Max Wicha), geriatrics (Jeffrey Halter), multi-organ transplantation (Jeremiah Turcotte), and substance abuse (Department of Psychiatry).

Giles G. Bole, dean from 1991 to 1996, oversaw the construction of Medical Science Research Building III and the renovation and remodeling of Medical Science Buildings I and II. The new medical student curriculum was implemented, and the school received a Robert Wood Johnson Scholars Program grant. After Dr. Bole's retirement, Dr. A. Lorris Betz, the Crosby-Kahn Research Professor in Neurosurgery, served as interim dean until 1998, establishing funds for translational research, technology development, and educational innovations. John Forsyth became executive director of the hospital in 1985. When he resigned in 1996, one of his assistants, Larry Warren, was appointed as interim executive director and then, in 1998, as executive director. In his list of seven priorities, number one was "putting patients and families first."

The University of Michigan Health System

The University of Michigan Health System (UMHS) consists of the Medical School with its faculty group practice; the hospitals and a network of ambulatory care services; Michigan Health Corporation, which facilitates joint ventures and networking; and M-CARE, which offers health maintenance organization, point of service, Medicaid, and Medicare plans. In a position that was created in November 1996,

Gilbert S. Omenn, M.D., Ph.D., is executive vice president for medical affairs, chief executive officer of the health system, and professor of internal medicine and human genetics. The Medical School dean and the executive director of the health system/hospitals report to Dr. Omenn, who reports to the president of the university.

Dr. Omenn has been clear about the goals of the UMHS. "Along with a caring and viable operation and a strong commitment to the academic mission, we explicitly state our goal to create healthy communities in our region."[14] The first letters of the values of the health system spell "partners," acknowledging that clinicians and health care organizations can improve the health of communities through community-based partnerships. For example, the health system has joined with St. Joseph Mercy Health System and the local health department to focus on issues such as infant health, abuse and neglect, violence, and access to care. Ford Motor Company and UMHS have crafted a health plan called Partnership Health. In addition, medical students, faculty, and staff participate in a host of "healthy lifestyle" programs at the hospitals and health centers and in community organizations.

The Medical School

The Medical School, based administratively at Medical Science Building I, has academic departments in fifteen clinical areas, six basic sciences, and two units. Over sixteen hundred faculty at the school work in instruction, primary research, or the clinical departments and participate in the education of medical students, graduate students, residents, post-doctoral fellows and U-M undergraduate students. Faculty in clinical departments provide care to patients at the University Hospitals and U-M Health Centers, which record more than 1 million visits per year.

The most recent additions to U-M clinical facilities are located at the East Medical Campus, a setting for community-based care, and the Comprehensive Cancer and Geriatrics Centers. These centers were designated "Centers of Excellence" by the regents for their multidisciplinary, patient-focused care. The three Medical Science Research Buildings provide state-of-the-art biomedical research facilities in a triangular configuration, designed to provide direct access to core facilities and ample window space in all laboratories.

The A. Alfred Taubman Medical Library, connected to Medical Science Building II, owns one of the largest medical collections in the nation. It primarily serves the faculty, staff, and students of the Medical School, the School of Nursing, the College of Pharmacy, and the hospitals and institutes of the medical center, but it is also a campus and community-wide resource. The library has over 400,000 volumes and current subscriptions to over three thousand medical, nursing, pharmacy, and science journals. It is also an excellent source for medical historical information. The Learning Resource Center, in the lower level of the library, provides computers and multimedia instructional programs.

In 1997, 660 medical students were enrolled in the M.D. program. As a result of the 1992 curriculum revision (MD21), medical students are exposed to small-group instruction, student-centered exercises, multidisciplinary conferences, early introduction to patients, and increased experiences in ambulatory and primary care. One early experience includes work with a preceptor in community care. The University Hospitals serve as the core facilities for clinical teaching. Underrepresented minorities comprise 15 percent of the medical student enrollment, and women comprise 41 percent. In the graduate programs, these figures are 10 percent and 41 percent, respectively.

Through the Horace H. Rackham School of Graduate Studies, the Medical School offers Ph.D. and master's degree programs in the basic sciences. Currently 266 students are enrolled in the basic sciences programs. In the Medical Scientist Training Program, one of thirty-three NIH-funded programs in the United States, students with significant research experience and potential may earn both a doctor of medicine degree and doctor of philosophy degree. Currently fifty-nine students are enrolled in this program.

Residency and fellowship programs are offered in all fifteen clinical departments as well as several subspecialty areas in internal medicine, surgery, and pediatrics and communicable diseases. Currently there are 834 interns and residents at the University Hospitals, Veterans Affairs Medical Center, and other affiliated hospitals and clinics.

The Medical School administration consists of Dean Allen S. Lichter, M.D., thirteen associate and assistant deans, and six directors. The department chairs are as follows:

Anatomy & Cell Biology, Bruce Carlson, M.D., Ph.D.
Anesthesiology, Kevin Tremper, M.D., Ph.D.
Biological Chemistry, Jack Dixon, Ph.D.
Dermatology, John Voorhees, M.D.
Family Medicine, Thomas Schwenk, M.D.
Human Genetics, Thomas Gelehrter, M.D.
Internal Medicine, H. David Humes, M.D.
Medical Education, Roland Hiss, M.D.
Microbiology & Immunology, Michael Savageau, Ph.D.
Neurology, Sid Gilman, M.D.
Obstetrics/Gynecology, Timothy Johnson, M.D.
Ophthalmology, Paul Lichter, M.D.
Otolaryngology, Gregory Wolf, M.D.
Pathology, Peter Ward, M.D.
Pediatrics & Communicable Diseases, Jean Robillard, M.D.
Pharmacology, Paul Hollenberg, Ph.D.
Physical Medicine & Rehabilitation, James Leonard, M.D.
Physiology, John Williams, M.D., Ph.D.
Psychiatry, John Greden, M.D.
Radiation Oncology, Theodore Lawrence, M.D. (interim)
Radiology, N. Reed Dunnick, M.D.
Surgery, Lazar Greenfield, M.D.
Unit for Laboratory Animal Medicine, Daniel Ringler, D.V.M.

The Hospitals and Ambulatory Care Facilities

Inpatient care facilities include 872 licensed beds in University Hospital (the main adult hospital) and in the Maternal and Child Health Center, comprising C. S. Mott Children's Hospital, Women's Hospital, the Child and Adolescent Psychiatric Hospital, and the James and Lynelle Holden Perinatal Hospital (fig. E-1). In 1998, about thirty-six thousand people received inpatient care. Ambulatory care services are provided through the A. Alfred Taubman Health Care Center; U-M Comprehensive Cancer Center; U-M Geriatrics Center; W. K. Kellogg Eye Center; Turner Geriatrics Center; MedRehab (rehabilitation services); MedSport (cardiac and sports medicine); Briarwood Radiology; U-M Center for Occupational Rehabilitation & Health; Chelsea Arbor (substance abuse treatment); and U-M Primary Care Network, a network of thirty community-based health centers in Washtenaw, Livingston, Oakland, Wayne, Monroe, and Jackson Counties. This health care network handled 1.2 million outpatient visits in 1998. Air transport services include two Survival Flight twin-engine helicopters and a fixed wing aircraft that services

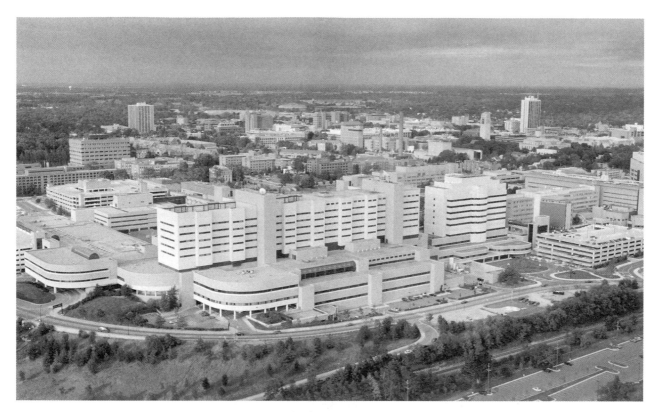

E–1. The University of Michigan Medical Center, 1998. The view of the medical center from the northeast encompasses the A. Alfred Taubman Health Care Center *(left)*, the Towsley Center for Continuing Medical Education and the Maternal and Child Health Center *(behind Taubman Center)*, University Hospital *(center, with twin towers)*, the Comprehensive Cancer Center and Geriatrics Center building *(adjacent to the right)*, Medical Science Buildings I and II *(forming a T shape)*, a corner of Medical Science Research Building III *(triangular, beyond Medical Science II)*, and patient and visitor parking structures *(lower right foreground and far left)*. To the southwest other research and patient care facilities, student dormitories, and campus buildings form the background. Consideration was given to blending the hospital design into the environment. University Hospital faces the Huron River and Huron River Valley. The windows in patient rooms were designed to allow a patient lying in bed to see outside, and large curved windows were placed in the cafeteria. The emergency entrance and parking area is to the right of the main entrance, both off of East Medical Center Drive. Farther to the right is the entrance to the Comprehensive Cancer Center and Geriatrics Center. The helipad on top of the Taubman Center was designed to accommodate two helicopters. Elevators take patients directly from the helipad to the Emergency Department or to the level-one Trauma Burn Center just above it.

much of the United States, Canada, and Mexico. Available twenty-four hours a day, they transport over one thousand patients a year. Affiliations exist with Oakwood Healthcare System (six hospitals, including Oakwood Hospital in Dearborn); Veterans Affairs Medical Center in Ann Arbor; St. Joseph Mercy Hospital at Catherine McAuley Health Center; Chelsea Community Hospital; and hospitals in Jackson, Lansing, Flint, Farmington Hills, and Toledo. There are about twenty-five multidisciplinary centers, research institutes, and patient registries in the health system, including the Breast Care Center,

the Howard Hughes Medical Institute, and the Michigan Kidney Registry.

This brief summary of the growth of the medical center over the past fifty years, however, cannot and should not tell the story of a social institution as vital as the University of Michigan Medical School. If there is a unifying theme to the history of Michigan medicine, it is that this enterprise was fueled by the industry and talents of thousands of men and women.[15] These people, ranging from the Medical School's leaders to the students to the hospital staff, came to work early, stayed late each evening, and devoted their time and energy to the advancement of knowledge, the teaching of medicine, and, above all, the amelioration of disease. Dr. Davenport has demonstrated the roots and origins of our medical institution from its founding to the beginning of World War II. This epilogue, I trust, demonstrates that the proud tradition of excellence has continued to characterize the University of Michigan Medical School.

Abbreviations

Acta Oto-Laryngol.	*Acta Oto-Laryngolica*
Acta Oto-Laryngol. Suppl.	*Acta Oto-Laryngolica, Supplementum*
Acta Radiol.	*Acta Radiologica*
Am. Chem. J.	*American Chemical Journal*
Am. Heart J.	*American Heart Journal*
Am. J. Anat.	*American Journal of Anatomy*
Am. J. Cancer	*American Journal of Cancer*
Am. J. Clin. Pathol.	*American Journal of Clinical Pathology*
Am. J. Dermatol. Genito-Ur. Dis.	*American Journal of Dermatology and Genito-Urinary Diseases*
Am. J. Dis. Child.	*American Journal of Diseases of Children*
Am. J. Insan.	*American Journal of Insanity*
Am. J. Med. Sci.	*American Journal of the Medical Sciences*
Am. J. Ment. Defic.	*American Journal of Mental Deficiency*
Am. J. Obstet.	*American Journal of Obstetrics and Diseases of Women and Children*
Am. J. Obstet. Gynecol.	*American Journal of Obstetrics and Gynecology*
Am. J. Ophthalmol.	*American Journal of Ophthalmology*
Am. J. Orthopsychiatry	*American Journal of Orthopsychiatry*
Am. J. Pharm. Educ.	*American Journal of Pharmaceutical Education*
Am. J. Physiol.	*American Journal of Physiology*
Am. J. Psychiatry	*American Journal of Psychiatry*
Am. J. Psychol.	*American Journal of Psychology*
Am. J. Public Health	*American Journal of Public Health*
Am. J. Roentgenol.	*American Journal of Roentgenology*
Am. J. Roentgenol. Radium Ther.	*American Journal of Roentgenology and Radium Therapy*
Am. J. Surg.	*American Journal of Surgery*
Am. J. Surg. Gynecol.	*American Journal of Surgery and Gynecology*
Am. J. Syph.	*American Journal of Syphilis*
Am. J. Trop. Med.	*American Journal of Tropical Medicine*
Am. Medico-Surg. Bull.	*American Medico-Surgical Bulletin*
Am. Nat.	*American Naturalist*
Am. Rev. Tuberc.	*American Review of Tuberculosis*
Anat. Rec.	*Anatomical Record*
Anesth. Analg.	*Anesthesia and Analgesia*
Ann. Clin. Med.	*Annals of Clinical Medicine*
Ann. Intern. Med.	*Annals of Internal Medicine*
Ann. Med. Hist.	*Annals of Medical History*
Ann. Otol. Rhinol. Laryngol.	*Annals of Otology, Rhinology and Laryngology*
Ann. Surg.	*Annals of Surgery*
Annu. Rev. Biochem.	*Annual Review of Biochemistry*
Annu. Rev. Physiol.	*Annual Review of Physiology*

Arch. Anat. Physiol.	*Archiv für Anatomie und Physiologie*
Arch. Dermatol.	*Archives of Dermatology*
Arch. Dermatol. Syphilol.	*Archives of Dermatology and Syphilology*
Arch. Exp. Pathol. Pharmakol.	*Archiv für experimentelle Pathologie und Pharmacologie*
Arch. Gesamte Physiol.	*Archiv für gesamte Physiologie*
Arch. Int. Pharmacodyn. Ther.	*Archives Internationales de Pharmacodynamie et de Therapie*
Arch. Intern. Med.	*Archives of Internal Medicine*
Arch. Klin. Chir.	*Archiv für klinische Chirurgie*
Arch. Mikrosk. Anat. Entwicklungsmech.	*Archiv für mikroskopische Anatomie und Entwicklungsmechanik*
Arch. Neurol. Psychiatry	*Archives of Neurology and Psychiatry*
Arch. Ophthalmol.	*Archives of Ophthalmology*
Arch. Otolaryngol.	*Archives of Otolaryngology*
Arch. Pathol.	*Archives of Pathology*
Arch. Pediatr.	*Archives of Pediatrics*
Arch. Pediatr. Adolesc. Med.	*Archives of Pediatrics and Adolescent Medicine*
Arch. Phys. Ther.	*Archives of Physical Therapy, X-Ray, Radium*
Arch. Physiol.	*Archiv für Physiologie, physiologische Abteilung des Archives für Anatomie und Physiologie*
Arch. Physiol. Normale Pathol.	*Archives de physiologie normale et pathologique*
Arch. Psychiatr. Nervenkr.	*Archiv für Psychiatrie und Nervenkrankheiten*
Arch. Roentgen Ray	*Archives of the Roentgen Ray*
Arch. Surg.	*Archives of Surgery (Chicago)*
Bacteriol. Rev.	*Bacteriological Reviews*
Biochem. Z.	*Biochemische Zeitschrift*
Bol. Asoc. Med. Puerto Rico	*Boletín de la Asociación Médica de Puerto Rico*
Boston Med. Surg. J.	*Boston Medical and Surgical Journal*
Br. J. Ophthalmol.	*British Journal of Ophthalmology*
Br. Med. J.	*British Medical Journal*
Brain	*Brain*
Bull. Am. Coll. Surg.	*Bulletin of the American College of Surgeons*
Bull. Assoc. Am. Med. Coll.	*Bulletin of the Association of American Medical Colleges*
Bull. Hist. Med.	*Bulletin of the History of Medicine*
Bull. Johns Hopkins Hosp.	*Bulletin of the Johns Hopkins Hospital*
Bull. Med. Libr. Assoc.	*Bulletin of the Medical Library Association*
Bull. N. Y. Acad. Med.	*Bulletin of the New York Academy of Medicine*
Bull. W. H. O.	*Bulletin of the World Health Organization*
C. R. Soc. Biol.	*Comptes Rendus des Séances de la Société de Biologie et de Ses Filiales*
Calif. West. Med.	*California and Western Medicine*
Can. Med. Assoc. J.	*Canadian Medical Association Journal*
Chicago Med. Rec.	*Chicago Medical Recorder*
Colorado Med.	*Colorado Medicine*
Dent. Cosmos	*Dental Cosmos*
Dent. J.	*Dental Journal (Ann Arbor, Mich.)*
Dermatol. Stud.	*Dermatologische Studien*
Dermatol. Wochenschr.	*Dermatologische Wochenschrift*
Detroit Med. J.	*Detroit Medical Journal*
Detroit Rev. Med. Pharm.	*Detroit Review of Medicine and Pharmacy*
Dtsch. Klin.-Ther. Wochenschr.	*Deutsche klinisch-therapeutische Wochenschrift*
Dtsch. Med. Wochenschr.	*Deutsche medizinische Wochenschrift*
Endocrinology	*Endocrinology*
Ergeb. Physiol.	*Ergebnisse der Physiologie*
FASEB J.	*FASEB Journal: Official Publication of the Federation of American Societies of Experimental Biology*

Folia Neuro-Biol.	*Folia Neuro-Biologica*
Harvey Lect.	*Harvey Lectures*
Heart	*Heart*
Int. Clin.	*International Clinics*
Int. J. Lepr.	*International Journal of Leprosy*
Int. J. Surg.	*International Journal of Surgery*
J. Adv. Ther.	*Journal of Advanced Therapeutics*
J. Am. Diet. Assoc.	*Journal of the American Dietetic Association*
J. Am. Med. Assoc.	*JAMA, Journal of the American Medical Association*
J. Am. Pharm. Assoc.	*Journal of the American Pharmaceutical Association*
J. Anat.	*Journal of Anatomy*
J. Anat. Physiol.	*Journal of Anatomy and Physiology*
J. Assoc. Am. Med. Coll.	*Journal of the Association of American Medical Colleges*
J. Bacteriol.	*Journal of Bacteriology*
J. Biol. Chem.	*Journal of Biological Chemistry*
J. Bone Jt. Surg.	*Journal of Bone and Joint Surgery*
J. Cancer Res.	*Journal of Cancer Research*
J. Chem. Educ.	*Journal of Chemical Education*
J. Chir.	*Journal de Chirurgie*
J. Clin. Invest.	*Journal of Clinical Investigation*
J. Comp. Neurol.	*Journal of Comparative Neurology*
J. Exp. Med.	*Journal of Experimental Medicine*
J. Exp. Zool.	*Journal of Experimental Zoology*
J. Gen. Physiol.	*Journal of General Physiology*
J. Hist. Med.	*Journal of the History of Medicine and Allied Sciences*
J. Immunol.	*Journal of Immunology*
J. Indiana Med. Soc.	*Journal of the Indiana Medical Society*
J. Infect. Dis.	*Journal of Infectious Diseases*
J. Iowa State Med. Soc.	*Journal of the Iowa State Medical Society*
J. Lab. Clin. Med.	*Journal of Laboratory and Clinical Medicine*
J. Med. Res.	*Journal of Medical Research*
J. Mich. State Med. Soc.	*Journal of the Michigan State Medical Society*
J. Morphol.	*Journal of Morphology*
J. Nerv. Ment. Dis.	*Journal of Nervous and Mental Disease*
J. Nutr.	*Journal of Nutrition*
J. Oral Surg.	*Journal of Oral Surgery*
J. Pathol. Bacteriol.	*Journal of Pathology and Bacteriology*
J. Pediatr.	*Journal of Pediatrics*
J. Pharmacol. Exp. Ther.	*Journal of Pharmacology and Experimental Therapeutics*
J. Physiol. (London)	*Journal of Physiology (London)*
J. Radiol.	*Journal of Radiology*
J. Tech. Meth. Bull. Int. Assoc. Med. Mus.	*Journal of Technical Methods and Bulletin of the International Association of Medical Museums*
J. Thorac. Surg.	*Journal of Thoracic Surgery*
J. Urol.	*Journal of Urology*
Janus	*Janus; Archives internationales pour l'Histoire de la Médecine et la Geographie Médicale (Amsterdam)*
Johns Hopkins Hosp. Reports	*Johns Hopkins Hospital Reports*
Johns Hopkins Med. J.	*Johns Hopkins Medical Journal*
Lab. Invest.	*Laboratory Investigation*
Lancet	*Lancet*
Laryngoscope	*Laryngoscope*
Med. Age	*Medical Age*
Med. Bl.	*Medizinische Blätter*
Med. Clin. North Am.	*Medical Clinics of North America*

Med. Independ.	Medical Independent
Med. Libr. Hist. J.	Medical Library and Historical Journal
Med. News	Medical News
Med. Surg. Reporter	Medical and Surgical Reporter
Medicine	Medicine (Baltimore)
Mem. Inst. Oswaldo Cruz	Memorias do Instituto Oswaldo Cruz (Rio de Janeiro)
Mich. Alumnus	Michigan Alumnus
Mil. Med.	Military Medicine
Minn. Med.	Minnesota Medicine
Mod. Hosp.	Modern Hospital
Münch. Med. Wochenschr.	Münchener medizinische Wochenschrift
N. Engl. J. Med.	New England Journal of Medicine
N. Y. Med. J.	New York Medical Journal
N. Y. State J. Med.	New York State Journal of Medicine
Ohio State Med. J.	Ohio State Medical Journal
Ophthalmic Rec.	Ophthalmic Record
P. Med. J.	Pennsylvania Medical Journal
Peninsular Independ. Med. J.	Peninsular and Independent Medical Journal
Peninsular J. Med.	Peninsular Journal of Medicine and the Collateral Sciences
Perspect. Biol. Med.	Perspectives in Biology and Medicine
Philos. Trans. R. Soc. London	Philosophical Transactions of the Royal Society of London
Physician Surg.	Physician and Surgeon
Physiol. Rev.	Physiological Reviews
Physiologist	Physiologist
Physiother. Rev.	Physiotherapy Review
Practitioner	Practitioner
Proc. Assoc. Am. Med. Coll.	Proceedings of the Association of American Medical Colleges
Proc. Inst. Med. Chicago	Proceedings of the Institute of Medicine of Chicago
Proc. R. Soc. (London)	Proceedings of the Royal Society of London
Proc. Soc. Exp. Biol. Med.	Proceedings of the Society for Experimental Biology and Medicine
Proc. Victor Vaughan Soc.	Proceedings of the Victor Vaughan Society
Public Health	Public Health
Q. J. Microsc. Sci.	Quarterly Journal of Microscopical Science
R. I. Med. J.	Rhode Island Medical Journal
Radiology	Radiology
Rocky Mount. Med. J.	Rocky Mountain Medical Journal
Science	Science
Sitzungsber. Akad. Wiss. Wien Math.-Naturwiss. Kl. Abt. 2B	Sitzungsberichte der kaiserliche Akademie der Wissenschaften in Wien, mathematisch-naturwissenschaftliche Klasse, Abteilung 2B
Skand. Arch. Physiol.	Skandinavisches Archiv für Physiologie
South. Med. J.	Southern Medical Journal
Stud. Biol. Lab. Johns Hopkins Univ.	Studies from the Biological Laboratory of Johns Hopkins University
Surg. Gynecol. Obstet.	Surgery, Gynecology and Obstetrics
Surg. Neurol.	Surgical Neurology
Surgery	Surgery
Ther. Gaz.	Therapeutic Gazette
Trans. Am. Acad. Ophthalmol. Otolaryngol.	Transactions of the American Academy of Ophthalmology and Otolaryngology
Trans. Am. Assoc. Genito-Ur. Surg.	Transactions of the American Association of Genito-Urinary Surgeons
Trans. Am. Assoc. Stud. Goiter	Transactions of the American Association for the Study of Goiter
Trans. Am. Laryngol. Assoc.	Transactions of the American Laryngological Association
Trans. Am. Laryngol. Rhinol. Otol. Soc.	Transactions of the American Laryngological, Rhinological and Otological Society

Trans. Am. Neurol. Assoc.	*Transactions of the American Neurological Association*
Trans. Am. Otolaryngol. Soc.	*Transactions of the American Otolaryngological Society*
Trans. Am. Otol. Soc.	*Transactions of the American Otological Society*
Trans. Am. Surg. Assoc.	*Transactions of the American Surgical Association*
Trans. Assoc. Am. Physicians	*Transactions of the Association of American Physicians*
Trans. Clin. Soc. Univ. Mich.	*Transactions of the Clinical Society of the University of Michigan*
Trans. Mich. State Med. Soc.	*Transactions of the Michigan State Medical Society*
Trans. Pac. Coast Oto-Ophthalmol. Soc.	*Transactions of the Pacific Coast Oto-Ophthalmological Society*
Univ. Hosp. Bull.	*University Hospital Bulletin*
Univ. Mich. Med. Bull.	*University of Michigan Medical Bulletin*
Univ. Mich. Med. Center J.	*University of Michigan Medical Center Journal*
Urol. Cutaneous Rev.	*Urologic and Cutaneous Review*
Virchows Arch. Pathol. Anat. Physiol.	*Virchows Archiv für pathologische Anatomie und Physiologie und für klinische Medicin*
West. J. Surg. Obstet. Gynecol.	*Western Journal of Surgery, Obstetrics and Gynecology*
Wien. Klin. Wochenschr.	*Wiener klinische Wochenschrift*
Wien. Klin.-Ther. Wochenschr.	*Wiener Klinisch-Therapeutische Wochenschrift*
Wis. Med. J.	*Wisconsin Medical Journal*
Yale J. Biol Med.	*Yale Journal of Biology and Medicine*
Z. Biol.	*Zeitschrift für Biologie*
Z. Hyg. Infektionskr.	*Zeitschrift für Hygiene und Infektionskrankheiten*
Z. Immunitätsforsch. Exp. Ther.	*Zeitschrift für Immunitätsforschung und experimentelle Therapie*
Z. Klin. Med.	*Zeitschrift für klinische Medizin*
Z. Wiss. Mikrosk.	*Zeitschrift für wissenschaftliche Mikroskopie und für mikroskopische Technik*
Zentralbl. Bakteriol. Parasitenk.	*Zentralblatt für Bakteriologie und Parasitenkunde*
Zentralbl. Chir.	*Zentralblatt für Chirurgie*

Notes

Foreword

1. Horace W. Davenport, *The ABC of Acid-Base Chemistry* (Chicago: University of Chicago Press, 1947, 1949, 1950, 1958, 1969, 1974); see also Davenport, *Physiology of the Digestive Tract* (Chicago: Year Book Medical Publishers, 1961, 1966, 1971, 1977, 1982); and *A Digest of Digestion* (Chicago: Year Book Medical Publishers, 1975, 1978).
2. P. Starr, *The Social Transformation of American Medicine* (New York: Basic Books, 1982).
3. See, for example, K. M. Ludmerer, *Learning to Heal: The Development of American Medical Education* (New York: Basic Books, 1985); and Ludmerer, *Time to Heal: Educating Physicians in the Twentieth Century* (New York: Oxford University Press, 1999).

Preface

1. H. W. Davenport, *Fifty Years of Medicine at the University of Michigan, 1891–1941* (Ann Arbor: University of Michigan Medical School, 1986).
2. Letter to Ms. Rebecca McDermott of the University of Michigan Press dated 30 July 1997. Quoted by permission.
3. K. M. Ludmerer, *Learning to Heal: The Development of American Medical Education* (New York: Basic Books, 1985). See also Ludmerer, *Time to Heal: Educating Physicians in the Twentieth Century* (New York: Oxford University Press, 1999).
4. H. W. Davenport, "Physiology, 1850–1923: The View from Michigan," *Physiologist* 25, no. 1, suppl. (1982): 1–96.
5. H. W. Davenport, *Doctor Dock: Teaching and Learning Medicine at the Turn of the Century* (New Brunswick, N.J.: Rutgers University Press, 1987).
6. H. W. Davenport, *University of Michigan Surgeons, 1850–1970: Who They Were and What They Did,* Historical Center for the Health Sciences Monographs, no. 3 (Ann Arbor, 1993).
7. H. W. Davenport, *Victor Vaughan: Statesman and Scientist,* Historical Center for the Health Sciences Monographs, no. 4 (Ann Arbor, 1996).
8. J. D. Howell, ed., *Medical Lives and Scientific Medicine at Michigan, 1891–1969* (Ann Arbor: University of Michigan Press, 1993).

Chapter 1

1. See H. W. Davenport, "Physiology, 1850–1923: The View from Michigan," *Physiologist* 25, no. 1, suppl. (1982): 1–96, for some of the story of Michigan's first forty years.
2. See L. R. Veysey, *The Emergence of the American University* (Chicago: University of Chicago Press, 1965), for an account of this transformation.
3. For a sketch of Sager at Michigan, see Davenport, "Physiology," 4–7.
4. The history of Castleton is in F. C. Waite, *The First Medical College in Vermont* (Montpelier: Vermont Historical Society, 1949). An account of Rensselaer is in P. C. Ricketts, *History of the Rensselaer Polytechnic Institute, 1824–1894* (New York: Wiley, 1895); and in Rensselaer Polytechnic Institute, *The Centennial Celebration of Rensselaer Polytechnic Institute* (Troy, N.Y.: Board of Trustees, 1925).
5. The history of Geneva is in W. H. Smith, *Hobart and William Smith: The History of Two Colleges* (Geneva, N.Y.: Hobart and William Smith Colleges, 1972).
6. See T. N. Bonner, *Becoming a Physician: Medical Education in Britain, France, Germany, and the United States, 1750–1945* (New York: Oxford University Press, 1995), 33–60.
7. K. M. Ludmerer, *Learning to Heal: The Development of American Medical Education* (New York: Basic Books, 1985), is the standard source.
8. John Alexander Campfield Student Notebook, 1860–61, p. 28; George R. Reynolds Student Notebook, 1866–67, [p. 139], Bentley Historical Library, University of Michigan.
9. S. H. Douglas[s], *Guide to a Systematic Course of Qualitative Chemical Analysis, Prepared for the Chem-*

ical Laboratory of the University of Michigan (Ann Arbor: Detroit Free Press, 1864); 2d ed. (Ann Arbor: Schober, 1865); 3d ed. (Ann Arbor: Dr. Chase's Steam Printing House, 1868); and S. H. Douglas and A. B. Prescott, *Qualitative Chemical Analysis: A Guide in the Practical Study of Chemistry and in the Work of Analysis* (Ann Arbor, 1874).

10. P. B. Rose, *Hand-Book of Toxicology* (Ann Arbor: Courier Steam Printing House, 1880).

11. The U.S. edition is G. Harley, *The Urine and Its Derangements; with the Application of Physiological Chemistry to the Diagnosis and Treatment of Constitutional as well as Local Diseases* (Philadelphia: Lindsay and Blakiston, 1872).

12. Douglas[s], *Systematic Course*, 2d ed., 29.

13. See H. W. Davenport, *Victor Vaughan: Statesman and Scientist*, Historical Center for the Health Sciences Monographs, no. 4 (Ann Arbor, 1996), for information on Vaughan's career.

14. V. C. Vaughan, *Lecture Notes on Chemical Physiology and Pathology* (Ann Arbor: Ann Arbor Printing and Publishing, 1878); 2d ed. (Ann Arbor: Ann Arbor Printing and Publishing, 1879); and *Hand-Book of Chemical Physiology and Pathology*, 3d ed. (Ann Arbor: Ann Arbor Printing and Publishing, 1880).

15. H. N. Martin, review of *Lecture Notes on Chemical Physiology and Pathology*, by Victor C. Vaughan, *Am. Chem. J.* 1 (1879): 57–58.

16. Vaughan, *Hand-Book*, 300.

17. F. W. Pavy, *A Treatise on Food and Dietetics, Physiologically, and Therapeutically Considered*, 2d ed. (London: J. and A. Churchill, 1875). Vaughan got his idea from Pavy, "Points Connected with Diabetes," *Lancet* 2 (1878): 1–3.

18. Vaughan, *Hand-Book*, 302.

19. See Davenport, *Victor Vaughan*, 48–57. Vaughan's autobiography, *A Doctor's Memories* (Indianapolis, Ind.: Bobbs-Merrill, 1926), is unreliable.

20. W. Reed, V. C. Vaughan, and E. O. Shakespeare, *Report on the Origin and Spread of Typhoid Fever in U.S. Military Camps during the Spanish War of 1898* (Washington, D.C.: Government Printing Office, 1904).

21. V. C. Vaughan and F. G. Novy, *Ptomaines and Leucomaines, or the Putrefactive and Physiological Alkaloids* (Philadelphia: Lea Brothers, 1888); Vaughan and Novy, *Ptomaïnes, Leucomaïnes, and Bacterial Proteids, or the Chemical Factors in the Causation of Disease*, 2d ed. (Philadelphia: Lea Brothers, 1891); Vaughan and Novy, *Ptomaïns, Leucomaïns, Toxins and Antitoxins: The Chemical Factors in the Causation of Disease*, 3d ed. (Philadelphia: Lea Brothers, 1896); Vaughan and Novy, *Cellular Toxins; or, the Chemical Factors in the Causation of Disease*, 4th ed. (Philadelphia: Lea Brothers, 1902); and Vaughan, *Epidemiology and Public Health: A Text and Reference Book for Physicians, Medical Students, and Health Workers*, 2 vols. (St. Louis: C. V. Mosby, 1922).

22. H. B. Baker, "Poisonous Cheese," in *Twelfth Annual Report of the Secretary of the State Board of Health of the State of Michigan for the Fiscal Year Ending September 30, 1884* (Lansing, 1885), 122–28; V. C. Vaughan, "Poisonous Cheese," in *Thirteenth Annual Report of the Secretary of the State Board of Health of the State of Michigan for the Fiscal Year Ending September 30, 1885* (Lansing, 1886), 221–26; Vaughan, "Report of Progress in Our Knowledge of Tyrotoxicon," in *Fourteenth Annual Report of the Secretary of the State Board of Health of the State of Michigan* (Lansing, 1888), 161–64.

23. Vaughan, "Poisonous Cheese," 225.

24. Ibid., 226.

25. Ibid., 223.

26. Vaughan, "Report of Progress," 162.

27. V. C. Vaughan, "Healthy Homes and Foods for the Working Classes," in American Public Health Association, *Public Health: The Lomb Prize Essays*, 2d ed. (Concord, N.H.: Republican Press Association, 1886), 3–62.

28. J. Eisenberg, *Bakteriologische Diagnostik*, 2d ed. (Hamburg: L. Voss, 1886).

29. W. H. Welch, discussion of "A Bacteriological Study of Drinking-Water" by V. C. Vaughan, *Trans. Assoc. Am. Physicians* 7 (1892): 41–42.

30. V. C. Vaughan, discussion of "A Bacteriological Study of Drinking-Water" by V. C. Vaughan, *Trans. Assoc. Am. Physicians* 7 (1892): 42.

31. D. F. Huelke, "The History of the Department of Anatomy: The University of Michigan. Part I. 1850 to 1894," *Univ. Mich. Med. Bull.* 27 (1961): 1–27. I have relied heavily on Huelke's work in my account of Ford and Michigan's gross anatomy.

32. Huelke, "History," 18.

33. W. P. Lombard, "Henry Sewall and the Department of Physiology," *Physician Surg.* 31 (1909): 114.

34. A. B. Palmer, *A Treatise on the Science and Practice of Medicine, or the Pathology and Therapeutics of Internal Diseases*, 2 vols. (New York: G. P. Putnam's Sons, 1883).

35. Palmer, *Treatise*, 1:229–95 (typhoid fever); 1:308–30 (diphtheria); 1:471–75 (scurvy).

36. There is a fuller account of Allen and his troubles in Davenport, "Physiology," 1–4, 91–92. See also Reuben Peterson Papers, Bentley Historical Library, University of Michigan.

37. Minutes, May 1854, *Regents' Proceedings 1837–64*, 564–67.

38. Winchell, Diary, Alexander Winchell Papers, 1833–91, Bentley Historical Library, University of Michigan.

39. [A. B. Palmer], "Medical Department of the University of Michigan [editorial]," *Peninsular J. Med.* 2 (1854–55): 184, quoting a letter from Regent M. A. Patterson to Palmer.

40. "Two Tickets," *Washtenaw Whig,* 29 March 1854.

41. See Sidney H. Sobel's unpublished Harvard undergraduate thesis of 1957, "John Call Dalton, Jr." I am grateful to Mr. Sobel for giving me a copy. I am also grateful to Chandler McC. Brooks, Dalton's remote successor at Downstate Medical Center, State University of New York, for further information about Dalton and the Long Island Hospital College of Medicine.

42. H. S. Cheever, Report on Work in Therapeutics, Materia Medica, and Physiology, March 1876, Medical School Records, Box 135, Bentley Historical Library, University of Michigan.

43. A. B. Palmer to J. B. Angell, 7 May 1877, James Burrill Angell Papers, 1845–1916, Bentley Historical Library, University of Michigan.

44. H. Sewall, "Experiments on the Preventive Inoculation of Rattlesnake Venom," *J. Physiol. (London)* 8 (1887): 203–10.

45. E. Behring and S. Kitasato, "Ueber das Zustandekommen der Diphtherie-Immunität und der Tetanus-Immunität bei Thieren," *Dtsch. Med. Wochenschr.* 16 (1890): 1113–14.

46. Department of Medicine and Surgery, *Annual Announcement 1877–78,* 2.

47. Department of Medicine and Surgery, *Annual Announcement 1889–90,* 14.

48. Ludmerer, *Learning to Heal.*

49. For Moses Gunn's career, see J. A. Gunn, *Memorial Sketches of Doctor Moses Gunn* (Chicago: W. T. Keener, 1889), and H. W. Davenport, *University of Michigan Surgeons, 1850–1970: Who They Were and What They Did,* Historical Center for the Health Sciences Monographs, no. 3 (Ann Arbor, 1993), 1–12.

50. Daniel Hall Notebook, notes from the lectures of Moses Gunn, January to March 1853, Hall Family Papers, Bentley Historical Library, University of Michigan.

51. Student Lecture Notes, 29 November 1865, and undated notes, Benjamin Thompson Papers, 1865–66, Bentley Historical Library, University of Michigan.

52. M. Gunn, "Removal of the Medical Department [editorial]," *Peninsular Independ. Med. J.* 1 (1858): 109. Earlier editorials by Gunn on this topic are in *Med. Independ.* 3 (1857–58): 414–16, 482–85, 601–3, and 671–72. Detroit population estimates are in editorials by L. G. Robinson in *Med. Independ.* 2 (1856–57): 117; and by Gunn in *Peninsular Independ. Med. J.* 1 (1858–59): 426.

53. These are briefly described in Davenport, *University of Michigan Surgeons,* 12–31.

54. D. Maclean, "A Tabular Statement of the Surgical Work Done in the Department of Medicine and Surgery of the University of Michigan during the School Year of 1881 and 1882," *Physician Surg.* 5 (1883): 385–96; and idem, "A Tabular Statement of the Surgical Work Done in the Department of Medicine and Surgery of the University of Michigan during the School Year of 1882 and 1883," ibid. 5 (1883): 433–44.

55. The argument is in the president's report, October 1888, *Proceedings of the Board of Regents 1886–91,* 261–69.

56. Vaughan, *A Doctor's Memories,* 234.

Chapter 2

1. V. C. Vaughan, *A Doctor's Memories* (Indianapolis, Ind: Bobbs-Merrill, 1926), 214–15.

2. Ibid.

3. H. P. Tappan, *University Education* (New York: G. P. Putnam, 1851), 48.

4. Minutes, July 1890, *Proceedings of the Board of Regents 1886–91,* 425, 429–30. See R. M. Slaughter, "William Cecil Dabney (1849–1894)," in *American Medical Biographies,* ed. H. A. Kelly and W. L. Burrage (Baltimore: Norman, Remington, 1920), 276–77, for a sketch of Dabney and a bibliography showing his mediocrity.

5. There is a bibliography in the obituary "Walter S. Christopher, M.D.," *Chicago Med. Rec.* 27 (1910): 392–95. I paraphrase Christopher's *Summer Complaint and Infant Feeding* (Chicago: Blakely and Rogers, 1892), 37–57.

6. Dock's relations with Osler were described in H. Cushing, *The Life of Sir William Osler,* 2 vols. (London: Oxford University Press, 1940). The book includes the quotation about Pepper (1:235).

7. The three men influenced by Osler when they were young are Wilburt Davison (d. 1972), founding dean of Duke Medical School; Wilder Penfield (d. 1967), neurosurgeon and neurophysiologist; and Emile Holman (d. 1967), professor of surgery at Stanford.

8. These are the accomplishments of Albert Moser, who graduated from Lima (Ohio) High School in 1888. Lima was then a German-American town much like Ann Arbor.

9. Department of Medicine and Surgery, *Annual Announcement 1907–8,* 12.

10. Personal communication from Carl Wiggers, who was Lombard's assistant.

11. The engineers' report is in the Medical School Records, Bentley Historical Library, University of Michigan.

12. A. Flexner, *Medical Education in the United States and Canada: A Report to the Carnegie Foundation for the Advancement of Teaching* (New York: Carnegie Foundation, 1910), 243–44.

Chapter 3

1. There was a general impression that there was a sub rosa quota in Dean Furstenberg's time. I well remember hearing him boast that he had limited enrollment from one of the major eastern sources of Jewish students. Everyone was conscious of Jewishness. When a faculty position was to be filled, letters of recommendation often contained the warning that so-and-so was Jewish, and Medical School correspondence contains occasional assurance that someone with a German name was not Jewish.
2. President's report, October 1887, *Regents' Proceedings 1886–1891*, 159.
3. See H. W. Davenport, "Epinephrin(e)," *Physiologist* 2 (1982): 76–82.
4. D. G. McGuigan, *A Dangerous Experiment: 100 Years of Women at the University of Michigan* (Ann Arbor: Center for the Continuing Education of Women, 1970), 36–37.
5. George Dock Notebooks, 1899–1908, Bentley Historical Library, University of Michigan.
6. A. C. Curtis, "The Woman as a Student of Medicine," *Bull. Assoc. Am. Med. Coll.* 2 (1927): 140–48.
7. The American Medical Association (AMA) did keep records, but the information was supplied to it by the medical schools. Other confounding classifications included "mulatto" and "Oriental"; Asians were occasionally classified as "colored."
8. Department of Medicine and Surgery, *Annual Announcement 1907–1908*, 15, 21.
9. Department of Medicine and Surgery, *Annual Announcement 1909–1910*, 18–19.
10. H. Cabot, "The Premedical Course," *Bull. Assoc. Am. Med. Coll.* 1 (1926): 1–3; and idem, "The Preceptor System at Michigan," ibid. 3 (1928): 37–39. The correspondence with the preceptors is in the Bentley Historical Library, University of Michigan.
11. B. Karpman, "The Student vs. the Faculty: A Psychiatric Appreciation," *Bull. Assoc. Am. Med. Coll.* 2 (1927): 61–67.
12. Medical School, *Annual Announcement 1916–1917*, 67.
13. S. Lewis, *Arrowsmith* (New York: Harcourt Brace, 1925), 17.
14. University of Michigan Medical School, Victor Vaughan Society, *Builders of American Medicine, Being a Collection of Original Papers Read before the Victor C. Vaughan Society of the University of Michigan Medical School* (Ann Arbor: G. Wahr, 1932).

15. Coller's lecture notes on five-by-seven-inch cards are in the Bentley Historical Library. One of his students who inherited his slides confirmed my judgment of the lectures' superficiality.

Chapter 4

1. For a full account of Victor Vaughan's career as a scientist, see H. W. Davenport, *Victor Vaughan: Statesman and Scientist*, Historical Center for the Health Sciences Monographs, no. 4 (Ann Arbor, 1996).
2. V. C. Vaughan, "The Chemistry of Tyrotoxicon: Its Action upon Lower Animals; and Its Relation to the Summer Diarrhœas of Infancy," *J. Am. Med. Assoc.* 9 (1887): 364.
3. V. C. Vaughan and F. G. Novy, *Ptomaines and Leucomaines, or the Putrefactive and Physiological Alkaloids* (Philadelphia: Lea Brothers, 1888), 14.
4. Ibid., 93.
5. Ibid., 92–93.
6. V. C. Vaughan and F. G. Novy, *Cellular Toxins; or, the Chemical Factors in the Causation of Disease*, 4th ed. (Philadelphia: Lea Brothers, 1902).
7. V. C. Vaughan, "How Bacteria Cause Disease," *J. Mich. State Med. Soc.* 13 (1914): 246.
8. V. C. Vaughan, "A Contribution to the Chemistry of the Bacterial Cell and a Study of the Effects of Some of the Split Products on Animals," part 1, *Boston Med. Surg. J.* 155 (1906): 216, 217. A variation of this wording appears in the preface to Vaughan, *Protein Split Products in Relation to Immunity and Disease* (Philadelphia: Lea and Febiger, 1913), iv, v.
9. V. C. Vaughan, *Poisonous Proteins, the Herter Lectures for 1916 Given in the University and Bellevue Medical School, New York* (St. Louis: C. V. Mosby, 1917), 99.
10. Vaughan and Novy, *Cellular Toxins*, 486.
11. Ibid., 487.
12. Vaughan, "How Bacteria Cause Disease," 251.
13. Ibid., 255.
14. Ibid.
15. The nuclein references are V. C. Vaughan and C. T. McClintock, "The Nature of the Germicidal Constituent of Blood-Serum," *Med. News* 63 (1893): 701–7; Vaughan, F. G. Novy, and McClintock, "The Germicidal Properties of Nucleins," *Med. News* 62 (1893): 536–38; Vaughan, "The Nucleins and Nuclein Therapy," *J. Am. Med. Assoc.* 22 (1894): 823–31; Vaughan, "The Treatment of Tuberculosis with Yeast-Nuclein," parts 1 and 2, *Med. News* 65 (1894): 657–59, 675–81; Vaughan, "The Nucleins and Nuclein Therapy," *Trans. Mich. State Med. Soc.* 18 (1894): 22–50; and Vaughan, McClintock, and G. D. Perkins, "The Treatment of Anthrax in Rabbits by the Intravenous Injection of Yeast Nucleinic Acid," *Trans. Assoc. Am. Physicians* 11 (1896): 72–74.

16. Vaughan and McClintock, "Germicidal Constituent of Blood-Serum," 705.

17. Ibid., 706.

18. Vaughan, Novy, and McClintock, "Germicidal Properties of Nucleins," 537.

19. Vaughan, "Nucleins and Nuclein Therapy," 831.

20. H. W. Davenport, *Doctor Dock*, 227.

21. Vaughan, McClintock, and Perkins, "Treatment of Anthrax in Rabbits," 74.

22. Vaughan, "Nucleins and Nuclein Therapy," 831.

23. Vaughan, "Treatment of Tuberculosis," 675.

24. Ibid., 681.

25. Ibid.

26. V. C. Vaughan, *Epidemiology and Public Health: A Text and Reference Book for Physicians, Medical Students and Health Workers*, 2 vols. (St. Louis: C. V. Mosby, 1922).

27. Ibid., 1:4.

28. U.S. Public Health Service, Office of the Surgeon General, *Report on the Origin and Spread of Typhoid Fever in U.S. Military Camps during the Spanish War of 1898*, by W. Reed, V. C. Vaughan, and E. O. Shakespeare (Washington, D.C.: Government Printing Office, 1904), 1:673; Vaughan, "Some Remarks on Typhoid Fever among Our Soldiers during the Late War with Spain," *Trans. Assoc. Am. Physicians* 14 (1899): 67–68; Vaughan, *A Doctor's Memories* (Indianapolis, Ind.: Bobbs-Merrill, 1926), 372.

29. U.S. Commissioner to Investigate Cholera in Europe and India, *Report on Cholera in Europe and India*, by E. O. Shakespeare (Washington, D.C.: Government Printing Office, 1890). This 945-page volume contains "An Inquiry into the Etiology of Asiatic Cholera," by E. Klein and Henneage [*sic*] Gibbes, a reprint of the official report to the British Government (477–515), originally published as E. Klein and H. Gibbes, "An Inquiry by E. Klein, M.D., F.R.S., and Heneage Gibbes, M.D., into the Etiology of Asiatic Cholera," *Cholera: Inquiry by Doctors Klein and Gibbes, and Transactions of a Committee Convened by the Secretary of State for India in Council* ([London], 1885?).

30. Vaughan, *A Doctor's Memories*, 375.

31. G. Dock, "Typho-Malarial Fever, So-Called," *N. Y. Med. J.* 69 (1899): 253–58. Dock said the term *typhomalaria* had been used to describe, in order of importance, a combination of malarial and typhoid fevers, malarial fevers with symptoms of typhoid, and a fever distinct from typhoid, though not necessarily due to malaria (253). In this last sense it was used in northern summer resorts to avoid admission of the presence of typhoid fever (257). See also D. C. Smith, "The Rise and Fall of Typhomalarial Fever," parts 1 and 2, *J. Hist. Med.* 37 (1982): 182–220, 287–321, especially 315–21.

32. U.S. Public Health Service, *Typhoid Fever*, 1:664.

33. Ibid., 674–75.

34. P. F. Clark, *Pioneer Microbiologists of America* (Madison: University of Wisconsin Press, 1961), 237–46, contains a description of Novy by an old friend.

35. F. G. Novy, *Directions for Laboratory Work in Bacteriology* (Ann Arbor: G. Wahr, 1894).

36. F. G. Novy, "Die Kultur anaërober Bakterien," *Zentrabl. Bakteriol. Parasitenk.* 14 (1893): 581–600; and idem, "Die Plattenkultur anaërober Bakterien," ibid. 16 (1894): 566–71.

37. F. G. Novy, "Ein neuer anaërober Bacillus des malignen Oedems," *Z. Hyg. Infektionskr.* 17 (1894): 209–32.

38. W. J. McNeal and F. G. Novy, "On the Cultivation of Trypanosoma lewisi," in *Contributions to Medical Research Dedicated to Victor Clarence Vaughan* (Ann Arbor: G. Wahr, 1903), 549–77.

39. F. G. Novy and W. J. McNeal, "On the Cultivation of Trypanosoma brucei," *J. Infect. Dis.* 1 (1904): 1–30.

40. F. G. Novy, W. J. McNeal, and C. B. Hare, "The Cultivation of the Surra Trypanosome of the Philippines," *Trans. Assoc. Am. Physicians* 19 (1904): 235–46; and idem, "The Cultivation of the Surra Trypanosome of the Philippines," *J. Am. Med. Assoc.* 42 (1904): 1413–17.

41. Novy, "On Trypanosomes," *Harvey Lect.* (1905–6): 33–72.

42. F. G. Novy and R. E. Knapp, "The Cultivation of Spirillum obermeieri," *J. Am. Med. Assoc.* 47 (1906): 2152–54.

43. F. G. Novy, W. A. Perkins, and R. Chambers, "Immunization by Means of Cultures of Trypanosoma lewisi," *Trans. Assoc. Am. Physicians* 27 (1912): 390–406; and idem, "Immunization by Means of Cultures of Trypanosoma lewisi," *J. Infect. Dis.* 11 (1912): 411–26.

44. U.S. Commission on Bubonic Plague in San Francisco, *Report of the Commission Appointed by the Secretary of the Treasury for the Investigation of Plague in San Francisco, under Instructions from the Surgeon-General, Marine-Hospital Service*, by S. Flexner, F. G. Novy, and L. F. Barker (Washington, D.C.: Government Printing Office, 1901).

45. This is a splendid example of the unreliability of testimony of participants. The cigarette story is in J. G. Cumming, "The Plague. A Laboratory Case Report," *Mil. Med.* 128 (1963): 435–39. The student was Charles B. Hare, and James G. Cumming, later director of the Pasteur Institute was his boardinghouse roommate at the time of the infection. Cumming's account, published more than sixty years after the event, says the infection occurred on 1 June 1901.

The student was described as convalescent in Dock's clinic on 26 April 1901. Vaughan said in *A Doctor's Memories* that the student stole the culture. The Lewis-de Kruif-Michigan-Winnemac story is told in M. Schorer, *Sinclair Lewis: An American Life* (New York: McGraw-Hill, 1961).

Chapter 5

1. De Kruif's period at Michigan is briefly described in his autobiography, *The Sweeping Wind, A Memoir* (New York: Harcourt, Brace and World, 1962).

2. P. de Kruif, "Dissociation of Microbic Species. I. Coexistence of Individuals of Different Degrees of Virulence in Cultures of the Bacillus of Rabbit Septicemia," *J. Exp. Med.* 33 (1921): 773–89. There are many more later papers in the same journal, and there are some in the *Journal of General Physiology* written with J. H. Northrop, the Terry Wickett of *Arrowsmith* (New York: Harcourt Brace, 1925), attempting to explain agglutination on a physicochemical basis.

3. W. Braun, "Bacterial Dissociation: A Critical Review of a Phenomenon of Bacterial Variation," *Bacteriol. Rev.* 11 (1947): 75–114.

4. G. Enderlein, *Bakterien-Cyclogenie* (Berlin: W. de Gruyter, 1925), 129: "Die Cyclogenie der Bakterien ist der Kreislauf der morphologischen Entwicklung durch die Summe aller Generationen mit der einfachsten morphologischen Einheit . . . beginnend bis zum höchsten morphologischen Aufbau, welcher der einzelnen Spezies zurkommt, und endet wieder mit der Einheit."

   For Hadley's ideas, see P. Hadley, "Microbic Dissociation: The Instability of Bacterial Species with Special Reference to Active Dissociation and Transmissible Autolysis," *J. Infect. Dis.* 40 (1927): 1–312; Hadley, "The Twort-d'Herelle Phenomenon: A Critical Review and Presentation of a New Conception (Homogamic Theory) of Bacteriophage Action," ibid. 42 (1928): 263–434; and Hadley, E. Delves, and J. Klimek, "The Filterable Forms of Bacteria: I. A Filterable Stage in the Life History of the Shiga Dysentery Bacillus," ibid. 48 (1931): 1–159. The clearest statement of Hadley's views is in Hadley, "Microbic Dissociation," 284–85.

5. Examples: P. Hadley and D. W. Caldwell, "The Bacterial Infection of Fresh Eggs," Bull. 164 (Rhode Island Agricultural Experiment Station, 1916); and Hadley, "Studies on Fowl Cholera. V. The Toxin of Bacillus avisepticus," *J. Bacteriol.* 3 (1918): 277–91.

6. A. Fontes, "Studien ueber Tuberculose," *Mem. Inst. Oswaldo Cruz* 2 (1910): 186–204; F. Arloing and A. Dufourt, "Recherches sur le pouvoir infectant des filtrats de tuberculose aviaire employés en injections sous-cutanées et en ingestion chez le pigéon et la

poule," *C. R. Soc. Biol.* 101 (1929): 455–56; and E. Almquist, "Wuchsformen, Fruktifikation and Variation der Typhusbakterie," *Z. Hyg. Infectionskr.* 83 (1917): 1–18.

7. F. G. Novy and R. E. Knapp, "Studies on *Spirillum obermeierei* and Related Organisms," *J. Infect. Dis.* 3 (1906): 291–393.

8. Hadley, Delves, and Klimek, "Filterable Forms of Bacteria," 1.

9. P. Hadley, "Transmissible Lysis of Bacillus pyocyaneus," *J. Infect. Dis.* 34 (1924): 260–304.

10. J. Barcroft, "Differential Method of Blood-Gas Analysis," *J. Physiol. (London)* 37 (1908): 12–24.

11. O. Warburg, "Versuche an überlebendem Carcinomgewebe. (Methoden.)," *Biochem. Z.* 142 (1923): 317–33.

12. F. G. Novy, H. R. Roehm, and M. H. Soule, "Microbic Respiration. I. The Compensation Manometer and Other Means for the Study of Microbic Respiration," *J. Infect. Dis.* 36 (1925): 109–67.

13. F. G. Novy and M. H. Soule, "Microbic Respiration. II. Respiration of the Tubercle Bacillus," *J. Infect. Dis.* 36 (1925): 168–232. This is Soule's Ph.D. thesis.

14. Ibid., 232.

15. M. Stephenson, *Bacterial Metabolism,* 2d ed. (London: Longmans, Green, 1939), 57.

16. F. G. Novy Jr., "Microbic Respiration. IV. The So-Called Aerobic Growth of Anaerobes: Potato Respiration," *J. Infect. Dis.* 36 (1925): 343–82.

17. W. J. Nungester, "Dissociation of B. anthracis," *J. Infect. Dis.* 44 (1929): 73–125.

18. W. J. Nungester, A. A. Wolf, and L. F. Jourdonais, "Effect of Gastric Mucin on Virulence of Bacteria in Intraperitoneal Injections in the Mouse," *Proc. Soc. Exp. Biol. Med.* 30 (1932): 120–21.

19. W. J. Nungester and L. F. Jourdonais, "Mucin as an Aid in the Experimental Production of Lobar Pneumonia," *J. Infect. Dis.* 59 (1936): 258–65.

20. W. J. Nungester and A. H. Kempf, "The Use of Experimental Pneumonia in Rats for the Evaluation of Therapeutic Procedures," *J. Infect. Dis.* 64 (1939): 288–92.

21. A. H. Kempf and W. J. Nungester, "Action of Antipneumococcus Serum in the Pneumonic Rat and Its Penetration into the Pneumonic Lesion," *J. Infect. Dis.* 65 (1939): 1–11.

22. A. H. Kempf and W. J. Nungester, "Production of Pneumonia in Rats by Intravenous Injection of Pneumococci," *Proc. Soc. Exp. Biol. Med.* 43 (1940): 627–28.

23. W. J. Nungester and R. G. Klepser, "A Possible Mechanism of Lowered Resistance to Pneumonia," *J. Infect. Dis.* 63 (1938): 94–102.

24. M. H. Soule, "Obituary: Dr. Earl Baldwin McKin-

ley," *Ann. Intern. Med.* 12 (1938): 425–28.

25. M. H. Soule and E. B. McKinley, "Cultivation of B. leprae with Experimental Lesions in Monkeys," *Am. J. Trop. Med.* 12 (1932): 1–36; and E. B. McKinley and M. H. Soule, "Studies on Leprosy: Experimental Lesions in Monkeys and Cultivation of Bacillus leprae," *J. Am. Med. Assoc.* 98 (1932): 361–67. These two papers can be told apart only on careful examination.

26. M. H. Soule and E. B. McKinley, "Further Studies on Experimental Leprosy and Cultivation of Mycobacterium leprae," *Am. J. Trop. Med.* 12 (1932): 441–52.

27. M. H. Soule, "Cultivation of Mycobacterium leprae. III," *Proc. Soc. Exp. Biol. Med.* 31 (1934): 1197–99.

28. M. H. Soule, "The Wassermann Reaction and the Kahn Test in Leprosy," *Int. J. Lepr.* 3 (1935): 181–94.

29. J. E. Kempf and M. H. Soule, "Three Strains of Poliomyelitis Virus Isolated from Feces during the 1939 Buffalo and Detroit Epidemics," *J. Infect. Dis.* 68 (1941): 188–92; and idem, "Effect of Chlorination of City Water on Virus of Poliomyelitis," *Proc. Soc. Exp. Biol. Med.* 44 (1940): 431–34.

30. The rest of the story is in the *Regents' Proceedings* for 1951 and the local papers for 5 August 1951.

31. R. L. Kahn, "Department of Clinical Laboratories, University of Michigan Hospital," in *Methods and Problems of Medical Education,* 18th ser. (New York: Rockefeller Foundation, 1930), 75–82.

32. The thesis was published as R. L. Kahn and A. McNeil, "Complement Fixation with Protein Substances," *J. Immunol.* 3 (1918): 277–93.

33. There is a comprehensive discussion of the Wassermann, Kahn, and other tests in H. Eagle, *The Laboratory Diagnosis of Syphilis: The Theory, Technic, and Clinical Interpretation of the Wassermann and Flocculation Tests with Serum and Spinal Fluid* (St. Louis: C. V. Mosby, 1937). Kahn's first description of his test is R. L. Kahn, "A Simple Quantitative Precipitation Reaction for Syphilis: Preliminary Communication," *Arch. Dermatol. Syphilol.* 5 (1922): 570–78. There are any number of subsequent descriptions, including Kahn, *Serum Diagnosis of Syphilis by Precipitation: Governing Principles, Procedure, and Clinical Application of the Kahn Precipitation Test* (Baltimore: Williams and Wilkins, 1925); and Kahn, *The Kahn Test: A Practical Guide* (Baltimore: Williams and Wilkins, 1928). A how-to-do-it guide is Kahn, *Technique of the Standard Kahn Procedure* (Ann Arbor: University of Michigan, 1944). Some history of the Kahn test is in Kahn, *Serology in Syphilis Control: Principles of Sensitivity and Specificity* (Baltimore: Williams and Wilkins, 1942), 53–68. This book also contains a summary of the Wassermann-Kahn comparisons.

34. An early application in 350 cases is H. L. Keim and U. J. Wile, "The Kahn Precipitation Test in the Diagnosis of Syphilis," *J. Am. Med. Assoc.* 79 (1922): 870–74. See also Keim and R. L. Kahn, "Clinical Studies on the Kahn Reaction for Syphilis. I. Diagnostic Value of Test," *Arch. Dermatol. Syphilol.* 10 (1924): 722–33.

35. Eagle, *Syphilis,* 209.

Chapter 6

1. This is one of Vaughan's questions for the National Board of Medical Examiners, of which he was a founding member in 1915.

2. F. G. Novy, *Laboratory Work in Physiological Chemistry,* 2d ed. (Ann Arbor: G. Wahr, 1898). Novy said in his preface: "Every medical student should receive thorough drill in the laboratory, not merely in so-called urine analysis, but in the broader field of physiological chemistry" (3).

3. In the 1920s the University of Michigan was kept busy denying that Koch was associated with the school, as he implied in advertisements for his cancer "cure."

4. See W. C. Rose and M. J. Coon, "Howard Bishop Lewis, November 8, 1887–March 7, 1954," in *Biographical Memoirs,* ed. National Academy of Sciences (Washington, D.C.: National Academy of Sciences, 1974), 44:139–73, for a sympathetic appraisal of Lewis's personality and a description of his hobbies.

5. Donald D. Van Slyke's father, the agricultural chemist Lucius Van Slyke, was a Michigan graduate who earned his Ph.D. in the Chemical Laboratory. Donald D. Van Slyke himself earned his Ph.D. at Michigan working under Moses Gomberg.

6. Medical School Records, Bentley Historical Library, University of Michigan.

7. H. B. Lewis, "The Behavior of Some Hydantoin Derivatives in Metabolism. I. Hydantoin and Ethyl Hydantoate," *J. Biol. Chem.* 13 (1912): 347–56; Lewis, "The Behavior of Some Hydantoin Derivatives in Metabolism. II. 2-Thiohydantoin," ibid. 14 (1912–13): 245–56; and Lewis and B. H. Nicolet, "The Reaction of Some Purine, Pyrimidine, and Hydantoin Derivatives with the Uric Acid and Phenol Reagents of Folin and Denis," ibid. 16 (1913–14): 369–73.

8. H. B. Lewis, "The Behavior of Some Hydantoin Derivatives in Metabolism. III. Parabanic Acid," *J. Biol. Chem.* 23 (1915): 281–86.

9. Altogether Lewis published nine papers on hippuric acid before 1941 from Yale, Pennsylvania, and Michigan. They are listed in the bibliography of Rose and Coon, "Howard Bishop Lewis," 139–73.

10. W. C. Rose, "Recollections of Personalities Involved

in the Early History of American Biochemistry," *J. Chem. Educ.* 46 (1969): 759–63.

11. W. C. Rose, "The Nutritive Significance of the Amino Acids," *Physiol. Rev.* 18 (1938): 109–36.

12. E. Allen and E. A. Doisy, "An Ovarian Hormone: A Preliminary Report on Its Localization, Extraction and Partial Purification, and Action in Test Animals," *J. Am. Med. Assoc.* 81 (1923): 819–21.

13. H. B. Lewis, "Some Contributions of Chemistry to the Art and Science of Medicine," *J. Mich. State Med. Soc.* 24 (1925): 4, 7. There is a description with a picture of students in the laboratory in Lewis, "Department of Physiological Chemistry, University of Michigan Medical School," in *Methods and Problems of Medical Education,* 18th ser. (New York: Rockefeller Foundation, 1930), 55–58.

14. D. A. McGinty, H. B. Lewis, and C. S. Marvel, "Amino Acid Synthesis in the Animal Organism. The Availability of Some Caproic Acid Derivatives for the Synthesis of Lysine," *J. Biol. Chem.* 62 (1924): 75–92.

15. J. P. Chandler and H. B. Lewis, "Comparative Studies of the Metabolism of the Amino Acids. V. The Oxidation of Phenylalanine and Phenylpyruvic Acid in the Organism of the Rabbit," *J. Biol. Chem.* 96 (1932): 619–36.

16. H. B. Lewis, "The Chemistry and Metabolism of the Compounds of Sulfur," *Annu. Rev. Biochem.* 1 (1932): 171–86; idem, "The Chemistry and Metabolism of the Compounds of Sulfur," *Annu. Rev. Biochem.* 2 (1933): 95–108; idem, "The Chemistry and Metabolism of the Compounds of Sulfur," *Annu. Rev. Biochem.* 4 (1935): 149–68; idem, "Sulfur Metabolism," *Physiol. Rev.* 4 (1924): 394–423; and idem, "The Significance of the Sulfur-Containing Amino Acids in Metabolism," *Harvey Lect.* 36 (1941): 159–87.

17. H. B. Lewis, "The Metabolism of Sulfur. I. The Relative Eliminations of Sulfur and Nitrogen in the Dog in Inanition and Subsequent Feeding," *J. Biol. Chem.* 26 (1916): 61–68.

18. T. B. Osborne and L. B. Mendel, "A Comparative Nutritive Value of Certain Proteins in Growth and the Problem of the Protein Minimum," *J. Biol. Chem.* 20 (1915): 351–78.

19. M. Womack, K. S. Kemmerer, and W. C. Rose, "The Relation of Cystine and Methionine to Growth," *J. Biol. Chem.* 121 (1937): 403–10.

20. E. F. Beach and A. White, "Synthesis of Cystine by the Albino Rat," *J. Biol. Chem.* 127 (1939): 87–95.

21. A. E. Garrod, "Inborn Errors of Metabolism," lectures 3 and 4, "Cystinuria," *Lancet* 2 (1908): 142–48, 214–20.

22. H. B. Lewis, "The Occurrence of Cystinuria in Healthy Young Men and Women," *Ann. Intern. Med.* 6 (1932): 183–92.

23. H. B. Lewis and S. A. Lough, "The Metabolism of Sulfur. XIV. A Metabolic Study of a Case of Cystinuria," *J. Biol. Chem.* 81 (1929): 285–97.

24. H. B. Lewis, B. H. Brown, and F. R. White, "The Metabolism of Sulfur. XXIII. The Influence of the Ingestion of Cystine, Cysteine, and Methionine on the Excretion of Cystine in Cystinuria," *J. Biol. Chem.* 114 (1936): 171–84.

25. Lewis and Lough, "Metabolism of Sulfur," 294.

26. Garrod, "Inborn Errors of Metabolism," 147.

Chapter 7

1. Physiology at Michigan through Lombard's time is described in much more detail in H. W. Davenport, "Physiology, 1850–1923: The View from Michigan," *Physiologist* 25, no. 1, suppl. (1982): 1–96.

2. W. H. Howell and F. Donaldson, "Experiments upon the Heart of the Dog with Reference to the Maximum Volume of Blood Sent out by the Left Ventricle in a Single Beat, and the Influence of Variations in Venous Pressure, Atrial Pressure, and Pulse-Rate upon the Work Done by the Heart," *Philos. Trans. R. Soc. London* 175, part 1 (1884): 154, 150.

3. W. H. Howell, "The Life History of the Formed Elements of the Blood, Especially the Red Blood Corpuscles," *J. Morphol.* 4 (1890): 57–116.

4. W. H. Howell, "Observations upon the Occurrence, Structure, and Function of the Giant Cells of the Marrow," *J. Morphol.* 4 (1890): 117–30.

5. W. H. Howell and E. Cooke, "Action of the Inorganic Salts of Serum, Milk, Gastric Juice, etc., upon the Isolated Working Heart, with Remarks upon the Causation of the Heart-Beat," *J. Physiol. (London)* 14 (1893): 198–220. The work of the medical student, Lemuel Churchill, is described in this paper, but Churchill was not given credit as an author.

6. W. H. Howell, with the assistance of S. P. Budgett and E. Leonard, "The Effect of Stimulation and of Changes in Temperature upon the Irritability and Conductivity of Nerve-Fibres," *J. Physiol. (London)* 16 (1894): 317.

7. W. H. Howell, remarks in University of Michigan, *A Memorial of the Seventy-Fifth Anniversary of the Founding of the University of Michigan, Held in Commencement Week, June 23 to June 27, 1912* (Ann Arbor: University of Michigan, 1915), 83.

8. The story of Clark University and its troubles is told in G. S. Hall, *Life and Confessions of a Psychologist* (New York: D. Appleton, 1924); L. R. Veysey, *The Emergence of the American University* (Chicago: University of Chicago Press, 1965); and W. C. Ryan, *Studies in Early Graduate Education, the Johns Hop-*

kins, *Clark University, the University of Chicago* (New York: Carnegie Foundation, 1939), 47–90.

9. H. Schröer, *Carl Ludwig. Begründer der messenden Experimental-physiologie. 1816–1895* (Stuttgart: Wissenschaftliche Verlagsgesellschaft, 1967).

10. W. P. Lombard, "Die räumliche und zeitliche Aufeinanderfolge reflectorisch contrahirter Muskeln," *Arch. Physiol.* (1885): 408–89.

11. W. P. Lombard, "The Variations of the Normal Knee-Jerk and Their Relations to the Activity of the Central Nervous System," *Am. J. Psychol.* 1 (1887): 1–67.

12. W. P. Lombard, "Is the 'Knee-Kick' a Reflex Act?" *Am. J. Med. Sci.* 93 (1887): 88–101; and idem, "On the Nature of the Knee Jerk," *J. Physiol. (London)* 10 (1889): 122–48.

13. Department of Medicine and Surgery, *Annual Announcement 1898–99,* 70.

14. W. P. Lombard, "General Physiology of Muscle and Nerve," in *An American Text-Book of Physiology,* ed. W. H. Howell (Philadelphia: W. B. Saunders, 1896), 32–151.

15. S. Lewis, *Arrowsmith* (New York: Harcourt Brace, 1925), 20.

16. Reuben Peterson to Albert C. Furstenberg, 17 July 1939, Reuben Peterson Papers, Bentley Historical Library, University of Michigan.

17. Personal communication to H. W. D.

18. W. P. Lombard, "A Method of Recording Changes in Body Weight Which Occur within Short Intervals of Time," *J. Am. Med. Assoc.* 47 (1906): 1792.

19. F. G. Benedict and C. G. Benedict, "Perspiratio insensibilis: Ihr Wesen und ihre Ursachen," *Biochem. Z.* 186 (1927): 278.

20. W. P. Lombard, "The Blood Pressure in the Arterioles, Capillaries, and Small Veins of the Human Skin," *Am. J. Physiol.* 29 (1912): 335–62.

21. A. Krogh, *The Anatomy and Physiology of Capillaries* (New Haven: Yale University Press, 1922).

22. T. Lewis, *The Blood Vessels of the Human Skin and Their Responses* (London: Shaw and Sons, 1927).

23. From time immemorial professors retained their chairs out of sheer economic necessity long after they were unable to exercise their functions properly, for if they retired they would be sunk in abject poverty. In 1905 Andrew Carnegie established the Carnegie Foundation for the Advancement of Teaching to provide pensions for long-serving professors such as Lombard. A pension was nearly equal to the last year of the professor's salary. In 1918 the Carnegie Foundation and Carnegie Corporation established the Teachers Insurance and Annuity Association as a successor to the free pension system (W. C. Greenough and F. P. King, *Retirement and Insurance Plans in American Colleges* [New York: Columbia University Press, 1959], 14–21).

24. Albert C. Furstenberg to Reuben Peterson, 13 July 1939, Reuben Peterson Papers, Bentley Historical Library, University of Michigan.

25. J. A. E. Eyster and W. J. Meek, "Instantaneous Radiographs of the Human Heart at Determined Points in the Cardiac Cycle," *Am. J. Roentgenol.* 7 (1920): 471–77.

26. J. Erlanger, "A Physiologist Reminisces," *Annu. Rev. Physiol.* 26 (1964): 1–14.

27. Y. Henderson, "The Volume Curve of the Ventricles of the Mammalian Heart, and the Significance of This Curve in Respect to the Mechanics of the Heart-Beat and the Filling of the Ventricles," *Am. J. Physiol.* 16 (1906): 325–67.

28. R. A. Gesell, "Auricular Systole and Its Relation to Ventricular Output," *Am. J. Physiol.* 29 (1911–12): 32–63. This is the first of four long papers on the same subject. Gesell also used the turtle heart, in which ventricular filling is clearly dependent upon auricular contraction.

29. J. Erlanger et al., "An Experimental Study of Surgical Shock," *J. Am. Med. Assoc.* 69 (1917): 2089–92.

30. R. Gesell, "Studies on the Submaxillary Gland. III. Some Factors Controlling the Volume-Flow of Blood," *Am. J. Physiol.* 47 (1918–19): 438–67.

31. R. Gesell, "Studies on the Submaxillary Gland. IV. A Comparison of the Effects of Hemorrhage and of Tissue-Abuse in Relation to Secondary Shock," *Am. J. Physiol.* 47 (1918–19): 504.

32. E. D. Adrian and D. W. Bronk, "The Discharge of Impulses in Motor Nerve Fibres. Part I. Impulses in Single Fibres of the Phrenic Nerve," *J. Physiol. (London)* 66 (1928): 81–101.

33. Bronk's Ph.D. thesis of 1925 contains the fullest description of his methods, but they are summarized in D. W. Bronk and R. Gesell, "Electrical Conductivity, Electrical Potential, and Hydrogen Ion Concentration Measurements on the Submaxillary Gland of the Dog Recorded with Continuous Photographic Methods," *Am. J. Physiol.* 77 (1926): 570–89.

34. A. S. V. Burgen and N. G. Emmelin, *Physiology of the Salivary Glands* (London: E. Arnold, 1961), 199.

35. J. S. Haldane and J. G. Priestley, "The Regulation of Lung-Ventilation," *J. Physiol. (London)* 32 (1905): 225–66.

36. R. Gesell, "On the Chemical Regulation of Respiration. I. The Regulation of Respiration with Special Reference to the Metabolism of the Respiratory Center and the Coördination of the Dual Function of Hemoglobin," *Am. J. Physiol.* 66 (1923): 5–49.

37. R. Gesell, "Studies on the Submaxillary Gland. II. An Automatic and Bloodless Method of Recording the Volume-Flow of Blood," *Am. J. Physiol.* 47 (1918–19): 428–37. A much improved version is described with photographs in idem, "On the Rela-

tion of Blood Volume to Tissue Nutrition. VI. An Automatic and Bloodless Method of Recording the Volume-Flow of Blood," ibid. 70 (1924): 254–58.

38. R. Gesell and D. W. Bronk, "A Continuous Electrical Method of Recording the Volume-Flow of Blood," *Proc. Soc. Exp. Biol. Med.* 23 (1926): 270–71.

39. R. Gesell, "Studies on the Submaxillary Gland. I. Electrical Deflections in General," *Am. J. Physiol.* 47 (1918–19): 411–27.

40. The department, its equipment, and its program are lovingly described in R. Gesell, "Department of Physiology, University of Michigan," in *Methods and Problems of Medical Education,* 18th ser. (New York: Rockefeller Foundation, 1930), 39–54.

41. R. Gesell and D. A. McGinty, "The Regulation of Respiration. VI. Continuous Electrometric Methods of Recording Changes in Expired Carbon Dioxide and Oxygen," *Am. J. Physiol.* 79 (1926–27): 72–90.

42. R. Gesell, "Regulation der Atmung und des Kreislaufs," *Ergeb. Physiol.* 28 (1929): 340–45.

43. R. Gesell, "A Neurophysiological Interpretation of the Respiratory Act," *Ergeb. Physiol.* 43 (1940): 477–639.

44. D. A. McGinty and R. Gesell, "On the Chemical Regulation of Respiration. II. A Quantitative Study of the Accumulation of Lactic Acid in the Isolated Brain during Anaerobic Conditions and the Rôle of Lactic Acid as a Continuous Regulator of Respiration," *Am. J. Physiol.* 75 (1925–26): 70–83.

45. R. Gesell, "Regulation of Respiration. XIX. Central and Peripheral Action of Sodium Cyanide on Respiratory Movements," *Am. J. Physiol.* 86 (1928): 164–70.

46. J.-F. Heymans and C. Heymans, "Sur les modifications directes et sur la régulation réflexe de l'activité du centre respiratoire de la tête isolée du chien," *Arch. Int. Pharmacodyn. Ther.* 33 (1927): 273–372; and C. Heymans, J. J. Bouckaert, and P. Regniers, *Le sinus carotidien et la zone homologue cardio-aortique* (Paris: G. Doin, 1933).

47. A. B. Hertzman and R. Gesell, "The Regulation of Respiration. XII. The Vagal Reflex Control of the Respiratory Movements of the Isolated Head. Peripheral Mechanical and Peripheral Chemical Factors," *Am. J. Physiol.* 82 (1927): 619–20.

48. R. Gesell, "Respiration and Its Adjustments," *Annu. Rev. Physiol.* 1 (1939): 185–86. See also Gesell, "A Neurophysiological Interpretation"; C. F. Schmidt and J. H. Comroe Jr., "Function of the Carotid and Aortic Bodies," *Physiol. Rev.* 20 (1940): 115–57; and Schmidt, "Respiration," *Annu. Rev. Physiol.* 7 (1945): 231–74.

49. Schmidt and Comroe, "Carotid and Aortic Bodies."

50. C. Heymans and E. Neil, *Reflexogenic Areas of the Cardiovascular System* (London: J. and A. Churchill, 1958).

51. R. Gesell, J. Bricker, and C. Magee, "Structural and Functional Organization of the Central Mechanism Controlling Breathing," *Am. J. Physiol.* 117 (1936): 423–52.

52. T. Lumsden, "Observations on the Respiratory Centres in the Cat," *J. Physiol. (London)* 57 (1922–23): 153–60; and idem, "Observations on the Respiratory Centres," ibid. 57 (1922–23): 354–67.

53. R. F. Pitts, H. W. Magoun, and S. W. Ranson, "Localization of the Medullary Respiratory Centers in the Cat," *Am. J. Physiol.* 126 (1939): 673–88.

54. R. F. Pitts, H. W. Magoun, and S. W. Ranson, "Interrelations of the Respiratory Centers in the Cat," *Am. J. Physiol.* 126 (1939): 689–707.

55. J. M. Brookhart, "The Respiratory Effects of Local Faradic Stimulation of the Medulla Oblongata," *Am. J. Physiol.* 129 (1940): 709–23.

56. Sidney Sobin to H. W. D., 7 February 1977.

57. Gesell's neurological ideas are fully described in Gesell, "A Neurophysiological Interpretation."

58. These comments are from the reports on the curriculum made annually by a committee of senior students. For example, students said that Gesell taught microphysiology whereas they needed macrophysiology. There were details of gas exchange in the lungs but nothing about pressures in the thorax. The faculty attitude that physiology was badly taught is recorded in a survey of faculty opinion made by Dean Furstenberg in 1936.

59. C. S. Sherrington, *Mammalian Physiology: A Course of Practical Exercises* (Oxford: Clarendon Press, 1919), v–vi. Emphasis added.

60. There are pictures of the student laboratory in Gesell, "Department of Physiology."

Chapter 8

1. See J. Parascandola, "John J. Abel and the Early Development of Pharmacology at the Johns Hopkins University," *Bull. Hist. Med.* 56 (1982): 512–27; and idem, *The Development of American Pharmacology: John J. Abel and the Shaping of a Discipline* (Baltimore: Johns Hopkins University Press, 1992) for details of Abel's training and appointment at Ann Arbor. Abel's life and work in Ann Arbor are described in H. H. Swain, E. M. K. Geiling, and A. Heingartner, "John Jacob Abel at Michigan: The Introduction of Pharmacology into the Medical Curriculum," *Univ. Mich. Med. Bull.* 29 (1963): 1–14.

2. J. J. Abel, "Wie verhält sich die negative Schwankung des Nervenstroms bei Reizung der sensiblen und motorischen Spinal-Wurzeln des Frosches?" (Inaug.-Diss. der medicinischen Facultät der Kaiser-Wilhelms-

Universität Strassburg zur Erlangung der Doctor-würde, 1888), in *Collected Reprints of John J. Abel, vol. 1, 1888–1908* (n.p., n.d.), Rare Book Room, Taubman Medical Library, University of Michigan.

3. There are a brief appreciation of Nencki and a long bibliography in J.-F. Heymans, "Marcel von Nencki," *Arch. Int. Pharmacodyn. Ther.* 10 (1902): 1–24. In 1891 Nencki was about to leave Bern for St. Petersburg.

4. J. J. Abel, "Bemerkungen über die thierischen Melanine und das Hämosiderin," *Virchows Arch. Pathol. Anat. Physiol.* 120 (1890): 205.

5. J. J. Abel, "Bestimmung des Molekulargewichtes der Cholalsäure, des Cholesterins und des Hydrobilirubins nach der Raoult'schen Methode," *Sitzungsber. Akad. Wiss. Wien Math.-Naturwiss. Kl. Abt. 2B* 99 (1890): 77–86.

6. J. J. Abel, "On Benzylidenebiuret and Chlorbenzylidenethiobiuret," *Am. Chem. J.* 13 (1891): 114–19.

7. J. J. Abel and E. Drechsel, "Ueber ein neues Vorkommen von Carbaminsäure," *Arch. Physiol.* (1891): 236–43.

8. H. W. Davenport, "Epinephrin(e)," *Physiologist* 25 (1982): 76–82.

9. J. J. Abel and A. Muirhead, "Ueber das Vorkommen der Carbaminsäure im Menschen- und Hundeharn nach reichlichem Genuss von Kalkhydrat," *Arch. Exp. Pathol. Pharmakol.* 31 (1892): 15–29; and the same paper, J. J. Abel, "On the Appearance of Carbamic Acid in the Urine after the Continued Administration of Lime Water, and the Fate of Carbamic Acid in the Body," *Bull. Johns Hopkins Hosp.* 5 (1894): 37–45.

10. A. R. Cushny, "Die wirksamen Bestandtheile des Gelsemium sempervirens," *Arch. Exp. Pathol. Pharmakol.* 31 (1892–93): 49–68; idem, "The Pharmacological Action of Gelsemium sempervirens," *Practitioner* 51 (1893): 38–50; idem, "Ueber die Wirkung des Muscarins auf das Froschherz," *Arch. Exp. Pathol. Pharmakol.* 31 (1892–93): 432–53. Other work done in Strassburg was reported in idem, "On the Action of Piperidine and Some of Its Compounds," *J. Exp. Med.* 1 (1896): 202–10; and idem, "Ueber das Ricinusgift," *Arch. Exp. Pathol. Pharmakol.* 41 (1898): 439–48.

11. Reports of the Hyderabad Chloroform Commissions and Brunton's comments and much discussion are in the 1889, 1890, and 1891 volumes of *Lancet*.

12. A. R. Cushny, "Ueber Chloroform- und Aethernarkose," *Z. Biol.*, n.s., 10 (1891–92): 365–404; and idem, "Some Experiments on Chloroform and Ether," *Lancet* 1 (1891): 593–95.

13. While he was at Michigan Cushny also published on optical isomers: A. R. Cushny, "Atropine and the Hyoscyamines—A Study of the Action of Optical Isomers," *J. Physiol. (London)* 30 (1904): 176–94; and

idem, "The Pharmacologic Action of Drugs; Is It Determined by Chemical Structure or by Physical Characters?" *J. Am. Med. Assoc.* 41 (1903): 1252–55. There are minor papers on alcohol and cocaine.

14. O. Schmiedeberg, "Beiträge zur Kenntniss der pharmakologischen Gruppe des Digitalins," *Arch. Exp. Pathol. Pharmakol.* 16 (1883): 149–87.

15. A. R. Cushny, "On the Action of Substances of the Digitalis Series on the Circulation in Mammals," *J. Exp. Med.* 2 (1897): 233–99.

16. C. S. Roy and J. G. Adami, "Contributions to the Physiology and Pathology of the Mammalian Heart," *Philos. Trans. R. Soc. London,* ser. b, 183 (1893): 199–298.

17. E.-J. Marey, *La circulation du sang à l'état physiologique et dans les maladies* (Paris: G. Masson, 1881), 42.

18. E. Gley, "Recherches sur la loi de l'inexcitabilité périodique du cœur chez les mammifères," *Arch. Physiol. Normale Pathol.,* 5th ser., 1 (1889): 499–507.

19. A. R. Cushny and S. A. Matthews, "On the Effects of Electrical Stimulation of the Mammalian Heart," *J. Physiol. (London)* 21 (1897): 213.

20. J. A. MacWilliam, "On the Rhythm of the Mammalian Heart," *J. Physiol. (London)* 9 (1888): 167–98.

21. O. Langendorff, "Untersuchungen am überlebenden Säugethierherzen," *Arch. Gesamte Physiol.* 61 (1895): 291–332. "Am Säugethierherzen lässt sich dieser wichtige Versuch leicht wiederholen; er ergibt fast genau dasselbe Resultat, wie am Froschherzen" (325).

22. Cushny and Matthews, "Effects of Electrical Stimulation," 219.

23. A. R. Cushny, "On the Interpretation of Pulse-Tracings," *J. Exp. Med.* 4 (1899): 327–47; and idem, "On Intermittent Pulse," *Br. Med. J.* 2 (1900): 892–94.

24. Cushny, "Interpretation of Pulse-Tracings," 340.

25. A. R. Cushny and C. W. Edmunds, "Paroxysmal Irregularity of the Heart and Auricular Fibrillation," *Am. J. Med. Sci.* 133 (1907): 66–77. The same paper was published in *Studies in Pathology,* Aberdeen University Studies, no. 21, ed. W. Bulloch (Aberdeen, 1906). There was a follow-up of Edmunds's patient: G. H. Fox, "The Clinical Significance of Transitory Delirium Cordis," *Am. J. Med. Sci.* 140 (1910): 815–26. The history of Cushny's recognition of auricular fibrillation as a cause of irregular pulse is in M. Block, "The Earliest Correlation of Clinical and Experimental Auricular Fibrillation," *Am. Heart J.* 18 (1939): 684–91, in which the patient's hospital record is reproduced.

26. William Dock, quoted in N. D. Munro, "George Dock, M.D.," *Proc. Victor Vaughan Soc.* 11, part 1

(1939–40). The paper contains other valuable information about Dock.

27. J. Mackenzie, *The Study of the Pulse, Arterial, Venous, and Hepatic, and of the Movements of the Heart* (Edinburgh: Y. J. Pentland, 1902).

28. Ibid., 298; and J. Mackenzie, "The Venous and Liver Pulses and the Arhythmic Contraction of the Cardiac Cavities," parts 1 and 2, *J. Pathol. Bacteriol.* 2 (1894): 84–154, 273–345.

29. Mackenzie, *Study of the Pulse*, 303.

30. J. Mackenzie, "Nodal Bradycardia," *Heart* 1 (1909–10): 23–42.

31. T. Lewis, "Evidences of Auricular Fibrillation, Treated Historically," *Br. Med. J.* 1 (1912): 57–60.

32. *Materia Medica and Therapeutics* was the official name of the department until 1942, but *Pharmacology* was frequently used.

33. A. R. Cushny, *A Textbook of Pharmacology and Therapeutics, or the Action of Drugs in Health and Disease* (Philadelphia: Lea Brothers, 1899).

34. G. B. Wallace and A. R. Cushny, "On Intestinal Absorption and the Saline Cathartics," *Am. J. Physiol.* 1 (1898): 411–34. For many years Wallace was professor of pharmacology at New York University.

35. Wallace and Cushny, "On Intestinal Absorption," 428.

36. A. R. Cushny, *The Secretion of the Urine* (London: Longmans, Green, 1917).

37. A. R. Cushny, "On Saline Diuresis," *J. Physiol. (London)* 28 (1902): 431–47; and idem, "On the Secretion of Acid by the Kidney," ibid. 31 (1904): 188–203.

38. C. Ludwig, "De viribus physicis secretionem urinæ adjuvantibus" (Habilitationsschrift, Marburge Cattorum, 1842); and idem, "Nieren und Harnbereitung," in *Handwörterbuch der Physiologie mit Rücksicht auf physiologische Pathologie*, ed. R. Wagner (Braunschweig: F. Vieweg und Sohn, 1844), 2:628.

39. R. L. Malvin, W. S. Wilde, and L. P. Sullivan, "Localization of Nephron Transport by Stop Flow Analysis," *Am. J. Physiol.* 194 (1958): 135–42.

40. A. R. Cushny, "On Diuresis and the Permeability of the Renal Cells," *J. Physiol. (London)* 27 (1901–2): 439.

41. C. W. Edmunds and A. R. Cushny, *Laboratory Guide in Experimental Pharmacology* (Ann Arbor: G. Wahr, 1905).

42. Cushny, *Textbook*.

43. Ibid., 5.

44. T. L. Brunton, *A Text-Book of Pharmacology, Therapeutics, and Materia Medica* (Philadelphia: Lea Brothers, 1885).

45. Neither, in fact, did Osler.

46. Cushny, *Textbook*, 705.

47. The last edition was C. W. Edmunds and A. R. Cushny, *Laboratory Guide in Experimental Pharma-*

cology (Ann Arbor: G. Wahr, 1939). By that time the book was 262 pages interleaved.

48. C. W. Edmunds, "Pharmacology and the Medical Schools," *J. Am. Med. Assoc.* 95 (1930): 383–85; and idem, "The Teaching of Pharmacology," *J. Assoc. Am. Med. Coll.* 11 (1936): 83–89.

49. T. R. Elliott, "The Action of Adrenalin," *J. Physiol. (London)* 32 (1905): 401–67.

50. C. W. Edmunds and G. B. Roth, "Concerning the Action of Curara and Physostigmine upon Nerve Endings or Muscles," *Am. J. Physiol.* 23 (1908–9): 28.

51. Brunton, *Text-Book*, 130, 297.

52. C. W. Edmunds, "On the Action of Lobeline," *Am. J. Physiol.* 11 (1904): 79–102.

53. C. W. Edmunds, "The Action of the Protein Poison on Dogs: A Study in Anaphylaxis," *Z. Immunitätsforsch. Exp. Ther.* 17 (1913): 105–34; and idem, "Physiological Studies in Anaphylaxis," ibid. 22 (1914): 181–98.

54. Edmunds and Roth, "Action of Curara and Physostigmine," 28–45.

55. H. W. Emerson and G. W. Collins, "Botulism from Canned Ripe Olives," *J. Lab. Clin. Med.* 5 (1919–20): 559–65.

56. G. G. DeBord, R. B. Edmondson, and C. Thom, "Summary of Bureau of Chemistry Investigations of Poisoning Due to Ripe Olives," *J. Am. Med. Assoc.* 74 (1920): 1220–21.

57. C. W. Edmunds and P. H. Long, "Contribution to the Pathologic Physiology of Botulism," *J. Am. Med. Assoc.* 81 (1923): 542–47; Edmunds and G. F. Keiper, "Further Studies on the Action of Botulinus Toxin," ibid. 83 (1924): 495–501.

58. C. W. Edmunds and G. B. Roth, "The Point of Attack of Certain Drugs Acting on the Periphery. I. Action on the Bladder," *J. Pharmacol. Exp. Ther.* 15 (1920): 189–99.

59. Edmunds also published on vasomotor action in the liver, alcohol as a diuretic, tolerance to nicotine, the velocity of blood flow, and leukocytosis following epinephrine administration.

60. C. W. Edmunds and R. G. Smith, "Experimental Adrenal Exhaustion," *Trans. Assoc. Am. Physicians* 46 (1931): 143–49.

61. C. W. Edmunds and R. G. Smith, "Does Digitalis Protect against Diphtheria Toxin?" *J. Pharmacol. Exp. Ther.* 61 (1937): 37–47.

62. C. W. Edmunds, R. G. Smith, and C. A. Moyer, "The Sensitivity of the Diphtheritic Heart to Digitalis," *J. Pharmacol. Exp. Ther.* 61 (1937): 286–92.

63. C. W. Edmunds and F. D. Johnston, "The Relation of the Adrenals to the Circulatory Collapse of Diphtheria," *Am. Heart J.* 4 (1928–29): 16–20; and

C. W. Edmunds, "Circulatory Collapse in Diphtheria," *Am. J. Dis. Child.* 54 (1937): 1066–79.

64. A general description of the program is in C. W. Edmunds, N. B. Eddy, and L. F. Small, "Studies on Morphine Addiction Problem," *J. Am. Med. Assoc.* 103 (1934): 1417–19.

65. R. W. Schwarz, *John Harvey Kellogg, M.D.* (Nashville, Tenn.: Southern Publishing Association, 1970), 37, 245.

66. The coffee papers include K. Horst et al., "The Effect of Caffeine, Coffee and Decaffeinated Coffee upon Blood Pressure, Pulse Rate and Certain Motor Reactions of Normal Young Men," *J. Pharmacol. Exp. Ther.* 52 (1934): 307–21; Horst, R. E. Buxton, and W. D. Robinson, "The Effect of the Habitual Use of Coffee or Decaffeinated Coffee upon Blood Pressure and Certain Motor Reactions of Normal Young Men," ibid. 52 (1934): 322–37; Horst and W. L. Jenkins, "The Effect of Caffeine, Coffee and Decaffeinated Coffee upon Blood Pressure, Pulse Rate and Simple Reaction Time of Men of Various Ages," ibid. 53 (1935): 385–400; and Horst, R. J. Willson [*sic*], and R. G. Smith, "The Effect of Coffee and Decaffeinated Coffee on Oxygen Consumption, Pulse Rate and Blood Pressure," ibid. 58 (1936): 294–304.

67. Deaths—"Charles Wallis Edmunds," *J. Am. Med. Assoc.* 116 (1941): 1176; and "Report of Council on Pharmacy and Chemistry," ibid. 116 (1941): 2400–2401. H. B. Lewis's sympathetic obituary notice in the *American Journal of Pharmaceutical Education* (5 [1941]: 245–48) describes Edmunds's services to the American Society of Pharmacology and Experimental Therapeutics (president, 1921–23, and member of Editorial Board, 1907–37) and his hobbies (painting in the summers on Monhegan Island, Maine, and gardening). C. C. Sturgis's obituary in the *Transactions of the Association of American Physicians* (56 [1941]: 14–15) is routine.

68. C. W. Edmunds, "The Standardization of Cardiac Remedies," *J. Am. Med. Assoc.* 48 (1907): 1744–47; and Edmunds and G. B. Roth, "Physiologic Assay of Nitroglycerine Tablets, Digitalin Tablets and Fluidextract of Ergot," ibid. 51 (1908): 2130–35.

69. Edmunds and Roth, "Physiologic Assay," 2133.

70. Edmunds, "Cardiac Remedies," 1747.

71. C. W. Edmunds, "The Responsibility of the General Practitioner to the Pharmacopoeia," *J. Mich. State Med. Soc.* 21 (1922): 452–55.

72. C. W. Edmunds and W. Hale, *The Physiological Standardization of Digitalis* (Washington, D.C.: Government Printing Office, 1909); and idem, *The Physiological Standardization of Ergot* (Washington, D.C.: Government Printing Office, 1911).

73. Examples: C. W. Edmunds, H. W. Lovell, and S. Braden, "Studies in Bioassays: Tincture of Strophan-

thus," *J. Am. Pharm. Assoc.* 18 (1929): 568–73; Edmunds, Lovell, and Braden, "Studies in Bioassays: Proposed International Standard for Digitalis," ibid. 18 (1929): 778–84; and Edmunds, C. A. Moyer, and J. R. Shaw, "United States Pharmacopœial Standard Digitalis Powder," ibid. 26 (1937): 290–305.

74. Edmunds, "Responsibility of the General Practitioner," 454.

Chapter 9

1. The administrative history and many biographical details are in D. F. Huelke, "The History of the Department of Anatomy, The University of Michigan," parts 1–3, *Univ. Mich. Med. Bull.* 27 (1961): 1–27; 28 (1962): 127–49; 29 (1963): 133–44.

2. W. P. Lombard, "Henry Sewall and the Department of Physiology," *Physician Surg.* 31 (1909): 107–27.

3. I am deeply indebted to Miss Kathleen McMurrich, J. Playfair McMurrich's daughter, for this and other information. In her eighty-seventh year she struggled from her suburban home to the University of Toronto to find the class lists of 1880 and 1881 for me. In contrast, Toronto's professor of anatomy did not answer my letter of inquiry.

4. E. G. Conklin, "The Life and Work of Professor Brooks," *Anat. Rec.* 3 (1909): 1–13.

5. McMurrich's Johns Hopkins thesis was "The Osteology and Myology of *Amiurus catus.* (L.) Gill. 1884," presented in 1885. The animal is the catfish. The *Johns Hopkins University Circular*, no. 321, "Doctors' Dissertations 1878–1919," lists it as having been published in "Canadian inst., Toronto. Proc., n.s., 2:270–310. pl.," but I have not seen it.

6. J. P. McMurrich, "The Ontogeny and Phylogeny of the Hypoglossal Nerve [letter to editor]," *Science* 5 (1885): 374–75. This is the old series of *Science*.

7. See note 8 for chapter 7.

8. McMurrich's papers on invertebrate zoology include "A Contribution to the Embryology of the Prosobranch Gastropods," *Stud. Biol. Lab. Johns Hopkins Univ.* 3 (1884–87): 403–56; "Notes on the Fauna of Beaufort, North Carolina," *Stud. Biol. Lab. Johns Hopkins Univ.* 4 (1887): 55–63; "The Actiniaria of the Bahama Islands, W. I.," *J. Morphol.* 3 (1889): 1–80; "Contributions on the Morphology of the Actinozoa," parts 1–3, *J. Morphol.* 4 (1890–91): 131–50, 303–30; 5 (1891–92): 125–64; "Embryology of Isopod Crustacea," *J. Morphol.* 11 (1895): 63–154; and "The Epithelium of the So-Called Midgut of the Terrestrial Isopods," *J. Morphol.* 14 (1897–98): 83–108.

9. J. P. McMurrich, *A Text-Book of Invertebrate Morphology* (New York: Henry Holt, 1894); 2d ed., 1896.

10. J. P. McMurrich, ed., *Morris's Human Anatomy: A*

Complete Systematic Treatise, 4th ed. (Philadelphia: P. Blakiston's Son, 1907); and J. Sobotta, *Atlas and Text-Book of Human Anatomy,* 3 vols., edited with additions by J. P. McMurrich (Philadelphia: W. B. Saunders, 1909).

11. G. A. Piersol, ed., *Human Anatomy, including Structure and Development and Practical Considerations* (Philadelphia: J. B. Lippincott, 1907).

12. J. P. McMurrich, "Conservatism in Anatomy," *Anat. Rec.* 3 (1909): 15–25.

13. J. P. McMurrich, "The Valves of the Iliac Vein," *Br. Med. J.* 2 (1906): 1699–1700; idem, "Notes on a Pair of Fully-Developed Cervical Ribs," *Anat. Rec.* 1 (1906–8): 76–77; idem, "The Occurrence of Congenital Adhesions in the Common Iliac Veins, and Their Relation to Thrombosis of the Femoral and Iliac Veins," *Am. J. Med. Sci.* 135 (1908): 342–46; and idem, "A Case of Crossed Dystopia of the Kidney, with Fusion," *J. Anat. Physiol.* 32 (1897–98): 652–64. McMurrich got a lot of mileage out of the last, for he published it again as "Some Anomalies of the Kidneys," *Trans. Mich. State Med. Soc.* 22 (1898): 171–76; and "On Fused Kidneys," *Int. J. Surg.* 11 (1898): 335–36.

14. The two papers were published as J. P. McMurrich, "The Present Status of Anatomy," *Am. Nat.* 33 (1899): 185–98; and idem, "Leonardo da Vinci and Vesalius: A Review," *Med. Libr. Hist. J.* 4 (1906): 338–50.

15. J. P. McMurrich, "The Phylogeny of the Forearm Flexors," *Am. J. Anat.* 2 (1902–3): 177.

16. J. P. McMurrich, "The Phylogeny of the Palmar Musculature," *Am. J. Anat.* 2 (1902–3): 463–500; idem, "The Phylogeny of the Crural Flexors," ibid. 4 (1905): 33–76; and idem, "The Phylogeny of the Plantar Musculature," ibid. 6 (1906–7): 407–37.

17. E. Jackschath, "Die Begründung der modernen Anatomie durch Leonardo da Vinci und die Wiederauffindung zweier Schriften derselben," *Med. Bl.* 25 (1902): 770–72. McMurrich also dismissed the contention that the landscape behind the muscle men can be identified, an example of supposed plagiarism brought forward in E. Jackschath, "Zu den anatomischen Abbildungen des Vesal," *Janus* 9 (1904): 238.

18. J. P. McMurrich, *Leonardo da Vinci, the Anatomist* (Baltimore: Williams and Wilkins, 1930).

19. The history of the College of Physicians and Surgeons in Streeter's time can be found in J. Shrady, ed., *The College of Physicians and Surgeons* (New York: Lewis, 1903).

20. This and many details about Streeter are given in G. W. Corner, "George Linius Streeter, 1873–1948," in *Biographical Memoirs* (Washington, D.C.: National Academy of Sciences, 1954), 28:261–87.

21. G. L. Streeter, "The Structure of the Spinal Cord of the Ostrich," *Am. J. Anat.* 3 (1904): 1.

22. G. L. Streeter, "Anatomy of the Floor of the Fourth Ventricle," *Am. J. Anat.* 2 (1902–3): 310.

23. The anatomical collection of Caspar Wistar, the author of the first U.S. textbook of anatomy, went to the University of Pennsylvania on Wistar's death in 1818. The institute was endowed by his great-nephew, General Isaac Wistar, in 1892, and although it was independently chartered the institute was in effect a graduate department of the university.

24. G. L. Streeter, "Technical Experiences: (a) Cataloguing Lantern Slides; (b) Permanent Dry-Mounts of the Laryngeal Cartilages; (c) The Use of Large Tissue Sections for Demonstration Purposes; (d) Degreasing Bones," *Anat. Rec.* 8 (1914): 124–25.

25. Typescript by Rollo McCotter, Bentley Historical Library, University of Michigan.

26. The story is told by Huelke, "Department of Anatomy."

27. G. L. Streeter, "Regarding the Preservation of Anatomical Material," *Anat. Rec.* 5 (1911): 319. The embalming fluid was 6 percent formalin, 4 percent carbolic acid, and 20 percent glycerine. Streeter did not state the pressure used.

28. G. L. Streeter, *Laboratory Guide in Anatomy: An Outline of Dissection Designed for Students of Medicine at the University of Michigan* (Ann Arbor: G. Wahr, 1909). There was also one for dental students, but I have not seen it.

29. G. L. Streeter, "Experimental Evidence concerning the Determination of Posture of the Membranous Labyrinth in Amphibian Embryos," *J. Exp. Zool.* 16 (1914): 149–76. Earlier papers are idem, "Some Experiments on the Developing Ear Vesicle of the Tadpole with Relation to Equilibration," ibid. 3 (1906): 543–58; and idem, "Some Factors in the Development of the Amphibian Ear Vesicle and Further Experiments on Equilibration," ibid. 4 (1907): 431–45.

30. Streeter, "Experimental Evidence," 153–54.

31. G. L. Streeter, "The Development of the Cranial and Spinal Nerves in the Occipital Region of the Human Embryo," *Am. J. Anat.* 4 (1905): 83–116.

32. Streeter said times 100, but this must be wrong ("Cranial and Spinal Nerves," 85).

33. Streeter, "Cranial and Spinal Nerves," 83–84.

34. G. L. Streeter, "On the Development of the Membranous Labyrinth and the Acoustic and Facial Nerves in the Human Embryo," *Am. J. Anat.* 6 (1906–7): 139–65.

35. G. L. Streeter, "The Nuclei of Origin of the Cranial Nerves in the 10 mm. Human Embryo," *Anat. Rec.* 2 (1908): 111–15.

36. G. L. Streeter, "The Peripheral Nervous System in

the Human Embryo at the End of the First Month (10 mm.)," *Am. J. Anat.* 8 (1908): 285–301.

37. F. Keibel and F. P. Mall, eds., *Manual of Human Embryology,* 2 vols. (Philadelphia: J. B. Lippincott, 1910–12).

38. F. P. Mall, "Report upon the Collection of Human Embryos at the Johns Hopkins University," *Anat. Rec.* 5 (1911): 343–57.

39. Ibid., 348.

40. F. P. Mall, "A Plea for an Institute of Human Embryology," *J. Am. Med. Assoc.* 60 (1913): 1599.

41. This is Corner's opinion, and Corner was in a position to know.

42. R. E. McCotter, "The Connection of the Vomeronasal Nerves with the Accessory Olfactory Bulb in the Opossum and Other Mammals," *Anat. Rec.* 6 (1912): 299–318. McCotter's last research paper was on a similar subject, idem, "The Vomero-Nasal Apparatus in Chrysemys punctata and Rana catesbiana," ibid. 13 (1917): 51–67. McCotter made wax reconstructions of the heads of turtles and frogs.

43. R. E. McCotter, "The Nervus Terminalis in the Adult Dog and Cat," *J. Comp. Neurol.* 23 (1913): 145, 147–48. The same volume contains a long paper on the nervus terminalis by a rival at Minnesota.

44. R. E. McCotter, "A Note on the Course and Distribution of the Nervus Terminalis in Man," *Anat. Rec.* 9 (1915): 243–46.

45. G. C. Huber and S. R. Guild, "Observations on the Peripheral Distribution of the Nervus Terminalis in Mammalia," *Anat. Rec.* 7 (1913): 253–72.

46. Ibid., 272.

47. The ignorance is stated in S. W. Ranson, *The Anatomy of the Nervous System: Its Development and Function,* 10th ed., rev. S. L. Clark (Philadelphia: W. B. Saunders, 1959); and in E. C. Crosby, T. Humphrey, and E. W. Lauer, *Correlative Anatomy of the Nervous System* (New York: Macmillan, 1962). However, see L. S. Demski and R. G. Northcutt, "The Terminal Nerve: A New Chemosensory System in Vertebrates?" *Science* 220 (1983): 435–37. "Correlations between terminal nerve projections and neurobehavioral studies suggest that the terminal nerve mediates responses to sex pheromones" (435).

48. This story was still current in the Anatomy Department at Michigan in 1982.

49. McCotter inevitably wrote a laboratory manual: R. E. McCotter, *Dissection Methods in Anatomy* (Ann Arbor: G. Wahr, various dates). The first edition of 78 octavo pages grew to 150 for the fourth edition of 1933.

50. R. E. McCotter and F. B. Fralick, *A Comprehensive Description of the Orbit, Orbital Content, and Associated Structures with Clinical Applications* (n.p.: American Academy of Ophthalmology and Otolaryn-gology, 1938). The thirty-two pages contain seventy-nine figures taken from textbooks and journal articles, but no sources or copyright permissions are given.

51. R. E. McCotter, "On the Occurrence of Pulmonary Arteries Arising from the Thoracic Aorta," *Anat. Rec.* 4 (1910): 291–97.

52. R. E. McCotter, "Regarding the Length and Extent of the Human Medulla Spinalis," *Anat. Rec.* 10 (1916): 559–64.

53. R. E. McCotter: "Three Cases of the Persistence of the Left Superior Vena Cava," *Anat. Rec.* 10 (1916): 371. Also idem, "Demonstration of Three Human Hearts Showing Double Superior Venae Cavae," *J. Mich. State Med. Soc.* 14 (1915): 479–81.

Chapter 10

1. G. C. Huber, "Observations on the Unity of Phthisis and Tuberculosis," *Trans. Mich. State Med. Soc.* 13 (1889): 64–69.

2. A. B. Palmer, *A Treatise on the Science and Practice of Medicine, or the Pathology and Therapeutics of Internal Disease* (New York: G. P. Putnam's Sons, 1883), 2:254.

3. W. H. Howell and G. C. Huber, "Physiology of the Communicating Branch between the Superior and Inferior Laryngeal Nerves," *J. Physiol. (London)* 12 (1891): 5–11.

4. W. H. Howell and G. C. Huber, "A Physiological, Histological, and Clinical Study of the Degeneration and Regeneration in Peripheral Nerve Fibres after Severance of Their Connections with the Nerve Centres," parts 1–3, *J. Physiol. (London)* 13 (1892): 335–56, 357–406; 14 (1893): 1–51.

5. When Huber left for Berlin he was desperately in love with Lulu Parker of Ann Arbor, and he wrote her eight-page love letters every three or four days. They are preserved in the Bentley Historical Library in box 1 of the Gotthelf Carl Huber Papers. I have not struggled through all of them, for the ones I have read contain very little about what Huber actually did at the Physiological Institute. At least he sent Lulu Parker his daily schedule for each of the two terms and something about his relations with Waldeyer and Benda.

6. G. C. Huber, "Observations on the Innervation of the Sublingual and Submaxillary Glands," *J. Exp. Med.* 1 (1896): 281–95.

7. J. Sobotta, *Atlas and Epitome of Human Histology and Microscopic Anatomy,* ed. G. C. Huber, trans. L. M. De Witt (Philadelphia: W. B. Saunders, 1903).

8. G. C. Huber and L. M. De Witt, "A Contribution on the Motor Nerve-Endings and on the Nerve-Endings in the Muscle-Spindles," *J. Comp. Neurol.* 7 (1897):

169–230; and idem, "A Contribution on the Nerve Terminations in Neuro-Tendinous End-Organs," ibid. 10 (1900): 159–208.

9. C. S. Sherrington, "On the Anatomical Constitution of Nerves of Skeletal Muscles; with Remarks on Recurrent Fibres in the Ventral Spinal Nerve-Root," *J. Physiol. (London)* 17 (1894–95): 211–58.

10. G. C. Huber, "Observations on the Degeneration and Regeneration of Motor and Sensory Nerve Endings in Voluntary Muscle," *Am. J. Physiol.* 3 (1899–1900): 339–44.

11. D. Barker, "The Innervation of the Muscle-Spindle," *Q. J. Microsc. Sci.,* 3d ser., 89 (1948): 143–86.

12. G. C. Huber, "The Morphology of the Sympathetic System," *Folia Neuro-Biol.* 7 (1913): 616–39.

13. G. C. Huber, "Lectures on the Sympathetic Nervous System," *J. Comp. Neurol.* 7 (1897): 73–145.

14. J. N. Langley, "The Sympathetic and Other Related Systems of Nerves," in *Text-Book of Physiology,* ed. E. A. [Sharpey]-Schäfer (Edinburgh: Y. J. Pentland, 1898, 1900), 2:616–96.

15. G. C. Huber, "A Contribution on the Minute Anatomy of the Sympathetic Ganglia of the Different Classes of Vertebrates," *J. Morphol.* 16 (1899): 27–90.

16. G. C. Huber, "Observations on the Innervation of the Intracranial Vessels," *J. Comp. Neurol.* 9 (1898): 1–25.

17. Ibid., 22.

18. A. A. Böhm and M. Davidoff, *A Text-Book of Histology,* ed. G. C. Huber, trans. H. H. Cushing, 2 vols. (Philadelphia: W. B. Saunders, 1900). The book was revised and reprinted through 1916.

19. G. C. Huber, "Studies on Neuroglia Tissue," in *Contributions to Medical Research Dedicated to Victor Clarence Vaughan* (Ann Arbor: G. Wahr, 1903), 619. See also idem, "Studies on the Neuroglia," *Am. J. Anat.* 1 (1901–2): 45–61; and idem, "Structure of Neuroglia," *J. Nerv. Ment. Dis.* 30 (1903): 298–300.

20. G. C. Huber, *Directions for Work in the Histological Laboratory for the Use of Medical Classes of the University of Michigan* (Ann Arbor: G. Wahr, 1892).

21. G. C. Huber, "On a Rapid Method of Preparing Large Numbers of Sections," *Z. Wiss. Mikrosk.* 23 (1906): 187–96.

22. Böhm and Davidoff, *Text-Book of Histology.*

23. J. P. McMurrich, *The Development of the Human Body* (Philadelphia: P. Blakiston's Son, 1902).

24. G. C. Huber, "Postgraduate Work for Dental Students," *Dental J.* 8 (1899): 121–24.

25. J. M. Cattell and D. R. Brimhall, eds., *American Men of Science: A Biographical Directory,* 3d ed. (Garrison, N.Y.: Science Press, 1921), 177. Lydia De Witt left Michigan to become a pathologist at Washington University in St. Louis, and she ended her career at the University of Chicago.

26. L. M. De Witt, "Morphology and Physiology of Areas of Langerhans in Some Vertebrates," *J. Exp. Med.* 8 (1906): 193–239. Lydia De Witt did other first-class work on her own at Michigan. An example is L. M. De Witt, "Observations on the Sino-Ventricular Connecting System of the Mammalian Heart," *Anat. Rec.* 3 (1909): 475–97. The paper contains a stereogram of her reconstruction of the ventricular conducting system.

27. In 1920 Frederick Banting read M. Barron, "The Relation of the Islets of Langerhans to Diabetes with Special Reference to Cases of Pancreatic Lithiasis," *Surg. Gynecol. Obstet.* 31 (1920): 437–48, from which he learned that when the pancreatic ducts are ligated the acinar cells degenerate, leaving the islet cells embedded in connective tissue. Barren gave seven references to pancreatic duct ligation, but he did not include De Witt's paper.

28. G. C. Huber and E. W. Adamson, "A Contribution to the Morphology of Sudoriparous and Allied Glands," in *Contributions to Medical Research Dedicated to Victor Clarence Vaughan* (Ann Arbor: G. Wahr, 1903), 365–89.

29. W. J. MacNeal, "Methylene Violet and Methylene Azure," *J. Infect. Dis.* 3 (1906): 412–33.

30. L. A. Hoag, "Histology of the Sensory Root of the Trigeminal Nerve of the Rat (Mus norvegicus)," *Anat. Rec.* 14 (1918): 165–82. There are other papers on the effects of extract of the pituitary gland and the efficacy of injections of absolute alcohol into the thyroid gland as treatment for hyperthyroidism.

31. The standing of a school or department can be judged by where its faculty comes from and where its students go. Of the persons named in this chapter, other than Lydia De Witt, Curtis went to Vanderbilt, Atwell to Buffalo, and Guild to Johns Hopkins. Others in the latter part of Huber's tenure went to Marquette, Ohio University, Temple, Oregon, and Howard.

32. G. M. Curtis, "The Morphology of the Mammalian Seminiferous Tubule," *Am. J. Anat.* 24 (1918): 339–94.

33. W. J. Atwell, "The Development of the Hypophysis Cerebri of the Rabbit (Lepus cuniculus L.)," *Am. J. Anat.* 24 (1918): 271–337; idem, "The Relation of the Chorda Dorsalis to the Entodermal Component of the Hypophysis," *Anat. Rec.* 10 (1915–16): 19–38; and idem, "The Development of the Hypophysis of the Anura," ibid. 15 (1918–19): 73–92.

34. W. J. Atwell, "On the Conversion of a Photograph into a Line Drawing," *Anat. Rec.* 10 (1915–16): 39–41.

35. G. C. Huber and S. R. Guild, "Observations on the Histogenesis of Protoplasmic Processes and of Collaterals, Terminating in End Bulbs, of the Neurones of Peripheral Sensory Ganglia," *Anat. Rec.* 7 (1913): 331–53.

36. S. R. Guild, "War Deafness and Its Prevention—Report of the Labyrinths of the Animals Used in Testing of Preventive Measures," *J. Lab. Clin. Med.* 4 (1918–19): 153–80, is the last of four papers on the subject.

37. G. C. Huber, "On the Relation of the Chorda Dorsalis to the Anlage of the Pharyngeal Bursa or Median Pharyngeal Recess," *Anat. Rec.* 6 (1912): 373–404.

38. The quotation is from a later paper on the same subject: G. C. Huber, "On the Anlage and Morphogenesis of the Chorda Dorsalis in Mammalia, in Particular the Guinea Pig (Cavia cobaya)," *Anat. Rec.* 14 (1918): 262.

39. G. C. Huber, "The Development of the Albino Rat, Mus norvegicus albinus," parts 1 and 2, *J. Morphol.* 26 (1915): 247–358, 359–86. Reprinted as Memoir no. 5 of the Wistar Institute of Anatomy and Biology (1915): 1–142.

40. G. C. Huber, "The Morphology and Structure of the Mammalian Renal Tubule," *Harvey Lect.* (1909–10): 100–149.

41. G. C. Huber, "On the Development and Shape of Uriniferous Tubules of Certain of the Higher Mammals," *Am. J. Anat.* 4, suppl. (1905): 1–98. The original description of the wax plate method is in G. Born, "Die Plattenmodellirmethode," *Arch. Mikrosk. Anat.* 22 (1883): 584–99.

42. G. C. Huber, "On the Morphology of the Renal Tubules of Vertebrates," *Anat. Rec.* 13 (1917): 305–39; and idem, "The Significance of the Structure of the Medullary Loop of the Renal Tubule of Mammalia," *Proc. Soc. Exp. Biol. Med.* 8 (1910–11): 95–96.

43. G. C. Huber, "Renal Tubules," in *Special Cytology,* ed. E. V. Cowdry (New York: P. B. Hoeber, 1928), 1:661–702.

44. Huber, "Morphology and Structure," 148–49.

45. G. C. Huber, "A Study of the Operative Treatment for Loss of Nerve Substance in Peripheral Nerves," *J. Morphol.* 11 (1895): 629–740.

46. G. C. Huber, "Nerve Suturing and Nerve Implantation," *Trans. Mich. State Med. Soc.* 20 (1896): 82; and idem, "Nerve Suturing and Nerve Implantation," part 3, *Int. J. Surg.* 10 (1897): 108.

47. Huber, "Nerve Suturing and Nerve Implantation," *Trans. Mich. State Med. Soc.* 20 (1896): 56; and idem, "Nerve Suturing and Nerve Implantation," part 1, *Int. J. Surg.* 10 (1897): 41.

48. G. C. Huber, "Nerve Suturing and Nerve Implantation," *Trans. Mich. State Med. Soc.* 20 (1896): 56–82.

49. G. C. Huber, "Nerve Suturing and Nerve Implantation," parts 1–3, *Int. J. Surg.* 10 (1897): 41–45, 80–82, 105–8.

50. R. Peterson, "Peripheral Nerve Transplantation," *Am. J. Med. Sci.* 117 (1899): 377–405.

51. Ibid., 378.

52. G. C. Huber, "Experimental Observations on Peripheral Nerve Repair," in *The Medical Department of the United States Army in the World War,* vol. 11, *Surgery* (Washington, D.C.: Government Printing Office, 1927), 1091–283.

53. G. C. Huber, "Transplantation of Peripheral Nerves," article and abstract, *Arch. Neurol. Psychiatry* 2 (1919): 466–80; 3 (1920): 437–38; and "Repair of Peripheral Nerve Injuries," in *Surg. Gynecol. Obstet.* 30 (1920): 464–71.

54. G. C. Huber, "Nerve Degeneration and Regeneration," in *Surgical and Mechanical Treatment of Peripheral Nerves,* by B. Stookey (Philadelphia: W. B. Saunders, 1922), 41–79.

55. B. Stookey, *Surgical and Mechanical Treatment of Peripheral Nerves* (Philadelphia: W. B. Saunders, 1922), 10.

56. G. C. Huber and D. Lewis, "Amputation Neuromas: Their Development and Prevention," *Arch. Surg.* 1 (1920): 113.

57. E. C. Crosby, "The Forebrain of the Alligator mississippiensis," *J. Comp. Neurol.* 27 (1917): 325–402.

58. C. Judson Herrick to G. Carl Huber, La Jolla, California, 17 March 1920, Elizabeth Caroline Crosby Papers, 1918–83, Bentley Historical Library, University of Michigan. For information on Herrick see E. C. Crosby, "Charles Judson Herrick, October 6, 1866–January 29, 1960," *J. Comp. Neurol.* 115 (1960): 3–8. Herrick was "Charles" to his family and friends but "C. Judson" in his publications to avoid confusion with other Herricks.

59. Biographical information is in *J. Comp. Neurol.* 112 (1959): 13–17, 19–29, a special volume honoring Elizabeth Crosby.

60. C. U. Ariëns Kappers, "Principles of Development of the Nervous System (Neurobiotaxis)," in *Cytology and Cellular Pathology of the Nervous System,* ed. W. Penfield (New York: P. B. Hoeber, 1932), 1:43–89. A similar exposition in the joint Ariëns Kappers-Huber-Crosby *Comparative Anatomy of the Nervous System of Vertebrates, Including Man* (New York: Macmillan, 1936), 1:1–134, is clearly by Ariëns Kappers and not by Huber or Crosby. Very much later Crosby, in her *Correlative Anatomy of the Nervous System* (New York: Macmillan, 1962), dismissed neurobiotaxis in a few words.

61. Crosby, "Forebrain of the Alligator," 327, 379, 384.

62. C. J. Herrick, *An Introduction to Neurology* (Philadelphia: W. B. Saunders, 1915).

63. C. J. Herrick and E. C. Crosby, *A Laboratory Outline of Neurology* (Philadelphia: W. B. Saunders, 1918).

64. Ibid., 63.

65. Herrick to Huber, 17 March 1920, Crosby Papers.

66. G. C. Huber and E. C. Crosby, "On Thalamic and Tectal Nuclei and Fiber Paths in the Brain of the American Alligator," *J. Comp. Neurol.* 40 (1926): 99.

67. Ibid., 97–227; G. C. Huber and E. C. Crosby, "The Reptilian Optic Tectum," *J. Comp. Neurol.* 57 (1933): 57–163.

68. G. C. Huber and E. C. Crosby, "The Nuclei and Fiber Paths of the Avian Diencephalon, with Consideration of Telencephalic and Certain Mesencephalic Centers and Connections," *J. Comp. Neurol.* 48 (1929): 1–225.

69. For example, K. S. Lashley found that a rat retained learned habits after he had fried its motor cortex with an electric cautery ("Studies of Cerebral Function in Learning. III. The Motor Areas," *Brain* 44 [1921]: 255–85). Crosby and R. Woodburne observed that Lashley had not studied the course of fibers arising within the structures destroyed. They made similar lesions and followed the degenerating tracts ("Certain Major Trends in the Development of the Efferent Systems of the Brain and the Spinal Cord," *Univ. Hosp. Bull.* 4 [1938]: 125–28).

70. G. C. Huber and E. C. Crosby, "Somatic and Visceral Connections of the Diencephalon," *Arch. Neurol. Psychiatry* 22 (1929): 187–229.

71. E. S. Gurdjian, "Olfactory Connections in the Albino Rat, with Special Reference to the Stria Medullaris and the Anterior Commissure," *J. Comp. Neurol.* 38 (1925): 127–63; idem, "The Diencephalon of the Albino Rat," ibid. 43 (1927): 1–114; and idem, "The Corpus Striatum of the Rat," ibid. 45 (1928): 249–99.

72. D. M. Rioch, "Studies on the Diencephalon of Carnivora. I. The Nuclear Configuration of the Thalamus, Epithalamus, and Hypothalamus of the Dog and Cat," *J. Comp. Neurol.* 49 (1929–30): 1–119; idem, "II. Certain Nuclear Configurations and Fiber Connections of the Subthalamus and Midbrain of the Dog and Cat," ibid. 49 (1929–30): 121–53; and idem, "III. Certain Myelinated-Fiber Connections of the Diencephalon of the Dog (Canis familiaris), Cat (Felis domestica), and Aevisa (Crossarchus obscurus)," ibid. 53 (1931): 319–88. The third paper is from the Ariëns Kappers Institute.

73. E. C. Crosby, "Cornelius Ubbo Ariëns Kappers," *J. Comp. Neurol.* 85 (1946): 309–11.

74. C. U. Ariëns Kappers, *Die vergleichende Anatomie des Nervensystems der Wirbeltiere und des Menschen*, 2 vols. (Haarlem: F. Bohn, 1920–21).

75. C. U. Ariëns Kappers, G. C. Huber, and E. C. Crosby, *The Comparative Anatomy of the Nervous System of Vertebrates, Including Man*, 2 vols. (New York: Macmillan, 1936).

76. C. U. Ariëns Kappers, *Anatomie Comparée du Système Nerveux* (Haarlem: F. Bohn, 1947).

77. A. C. Furstenberg, E. Crosby, and D. Brownell, "Hypertensive Deafness," *Trans. Am. Otolaryngol. Soc.* 27 (1937): 221–39; Furstenberg, Crosby, and B. Farrior, "Neurological Lesions Which Influence the Sense of Smell," *Trans. Am. Laryngol. Rhinol. Otol. Soc.* 48 (1942): 40–55; Furstenberg and Crosby, "Disturbance of the Function of the Salivary Glands," *Ann. Otol. Rhinol. Laryngol.* 54 (1945): 243–64; and Furstenberg and Crosby, "Neuron Arcs of Clinical Significance in Laryngology," *Ann. Otol. Rhinol. Laryngol.* 57 (1948): 298–310.

78. E. C. Crosby and J. W. Henderson, "The Mammalian Midbrain and Isthmus Regions. Part II. Fiber Connections of the Superior Colliculus. B. Pathways Concerned in Automatic Eye Movements," *J. Comp. Neurol.* 88 (1948): 53–91.

79. E. A. Kahn, R. C. Bassett, R. C. Schneider, and E. C. Crosby, *Correlative Neurosurgery* (Springfield, Ill.: C. C Thomas, 1955); 2d ed., 1969; 3d ed., 1982.

80. E. C. Crosby, T. Humphrey, and E. W. Lauer, *Correlative Anatomy of the Nervous System* (New York: Macmillan, 1962).

81. Some of these details are from the Medical School Records, Bentley Historical Library, University of Michigan, and others are from D. F. Huelke, "The History of the Department of Anatomy, The University of Michigan. Part II. 1894 to 1959," *Univ. Mich. Med. Bull.* 28 (1962): 127–49.

82. Loeb's ideas are summarized in J. Loeb, *The Organism as a Whole, from a Physicochemical Viewpoint* (New York: G. P. Putnam's Sons, 1916); and idem, *Forced Movements, Tropisms, and Animal Conduct* (Philadelphia: J. B. Lippincott, 1918).

83. Loeb, quoted in B. M. Patten, "An Analysis of Certain Photic Reactions, with Reference to the Weber-Fechner Law. I. The Reactions of the Blowfly Larva to Opposed Beams of Light," *Am. J. Physiol.* 38 (1915): 318.

84. Loeb, quoted in B. M. Patten, "A Quantitative Determination of the Orienting Reaction of the Blowfly Larva (Calliphora erythrocephala Meigen)," *J. Exp. Zool.* 17 (1914): 215.

85. An additional blowfly paper is B. M. Patten, "The Changes of the Blowfly Larva's Photosensitivity with Age," *J. Exp. Zool.* 20 (1916): 585–98. Patten did similar work with the whip-tail scorpion, and he wrung an additional four papers out of elaboration of Loeb's idea.

86. B. M. Patten, "The Formation of the Cardiac Loop in the Chick," *Am. J. Anat.* 30 (1922): 388.

87. B. M. Patten, "The Closure of the Foramen Ovale,"

Am. J. Anat. 48 (1931): 19–44.

88. B. M. Patten, "The Interatrial Septum of the Chick Heart," *Anat. Rec.* 30 (1925): 56.

89. B. M. Patten, "The Changes in Circulation following Birth," *Am. Heart J.* 6 (1930–31): 192–205; and B. M. Patten, W. A. Sommerfeld, and G. H. Paff, "Functional Limitations of the Foramen Ovale in the Human Foetal Heart," *Anat. Rec.* 44 (1929): 165–78.

90. B. M. Patten, *The Early Embryology of the Chick* (Philadelphia: P. Blakiston's Son, 1920); 2d ed., 1925; 3d ed., 1929; 4th ed., 1951.

91. Patten, *Chick*, 3d ed., vii, viii.

92. B. M. Patten, *Embryology of the Pig* (New York: McGraw-Hill, 1927); 2d ed., 1946; 3d ed., 1948.

93. Some information on Patten and Baldwin is in Huelke, "Department of Anatomy," part 2, 140–41. Some was provided by Theodore Kramer, to whom I am deeply indebted.

94. B. M. Patten, "Microcinematographic and Electrocardiographic Studies of the First Heart Beats and the Beginning of the Circulation in Living Embryos," *Proc. Inst. Med. Chicago* 12 (1939): 369.

95. B. M. Patten and T. C. Kramer, "A Moving-Picture Apparatus for Microscopic Work," *Anat. Rec.* 52 (1932): 169–89.

96. Theodore Kramer very kindly went to the trouble of finding his copies of the two surviving reels on the embryology of the chick and a reel showing Patten and Kramer working together at Western Reserve. He also found two reels of tapes made by Patten to accompany projection of the films. I am grateful for being permitted to see the films and hear the tapes. Shortly before Kramer's death in a nursing home I alerted D. F. Huelke to Kramer's possession of surviving films and tapes and the possibility of their disappearance on Kramer's death, but I do not know whether Huelke was able to rescue them.

97. Patten, in his capacity as a member of the Rockefeller Foundation staff, obtained a copy of a report made by a European professor of anatomy that said that although Ariëns Kappers' institute had a vast collection of brains, it had fallen behind in research. In contrast, the neurological division of the Department of Anatomy at Michigan under Elizabeth Crosby was the best place in the world for research in comparative anatomy. Patten passed a copy of the report to Dean Furstenberg.

98. B. M. Patten, *Human Embryology* (Philadelphia: Blakiston, 1946); and idem, *Foundations of Embryology* (New York: McGraw-Hill, 1958).

Chapter 11

1. H. S. Cheever, "An Anomalous Case of Ovarian Cyst," *Detroit Rev. Med. Pharm.* 2 (1867): 533–35; and idem, "Case of Abscess of the Brain," ibid. 3 (1868): 73–75.

2. Names and dates are given in *The University of Michigan; An Encyclopedic Survey,* ed. W. B. Shaw (Ann Arbor: University of Michigan Press, 1951), 2:886–88.

3. Medical School Records, Bentley Historical Library, University of Michigan. Administrative support was primitive in those days; no one had typists or secretaries. Even the president of the university wrote his own letters in longhand.

4. A. S. Warthin, "Forty Years as a Clinical Pathologist," *J. Lab. Clin. Med.* 16 (1931): 743. Weller, in the *Encyclopedic Survey,* wrote: "[Gibbes's father] intended that his son should prepare for the ministry, but the boy rebelled and at fourteen sailed for the East Indies instead. A period of adventurous living followed, which furnished the material for many tales of the Opium War, of combats with pirates, of shipwreck, and of commanding his own ship at twenty-one" (2:888). Weller must have been recording an oral tradition.

5. The *Who Was Who in America* entry is in volume 1; the obituary is in *J. Am. Med. Assoc.* 59 (1912): 384.

6. E. E. Klein, *Micro-Organisms and Disease: An Introduction into the Study of Specific Micro-Organisms* (London: Macmillan, 1884). The second edition (1885) refers to the "so-called bacilli of cholera."

7. E. Klein and H. Gibbes, "An Inquiry by E. Klein, M.D., F.R.S., and Heneage Gibbes, M.D., into the Etiology of Asiatic Cholera," *Cholera: Inquiry by Doctors Klein and Gibbes, and Transactions of a Committee Convened by the Secretary of State for India in Council* ([London], 1885?). The report is reprinted in U.S. Commissioner to Investigate Cholera in Europe and India, *Report on Cholera in Europe and India,* by E. O. Shakespeare (Washington, D.C.: Government Printing Office, 1890), 477–515, as "An Inquiry into the Etiology of Asiatic Cholera," by E. Klein and Henneage [*sic*] Gibbes. Shakespeare was Vaughan's future colleague on the Typhoid Commission.

8. E. Klein, "The Bacteria in Asiatic Cholera," chapters 1–8, *Practitioner* 37 (1886): 241–58, 334–50, 414–25; and 38 (1887): 4–19, 104–25, 182–201, 267–80, 321–35. The chief *British Medical Journal* article is idem, "The Relation of Bacteria to Asiatic Cholera, *Br. Med. J.* 1 (1885): 289–90. In the same volume, see also "Remarks on the Etiology of Asiatic Cholera," 650–52; and "Some Remarks on the Present State of Our Knowledge of the Comma-Bacilli of Koch," 693–95.

9. Klein, "Bacteria," 344. In the Klein-Gibbes report the last five words are "opposition to the above facts" (37).

10. Ibid., 321.

11. W. Gull, "Transactions of a Committee Convened by the Secretary of State for India in Council," *Cholera: Inquiry and Transactions,* 12 (supplementary note).

12. V. C. Vaughan, *A Doctor's Memories* (Indianapolis: Bobbs-Merrill, 1926), 147. Vaughan continued: "I tried to explain that I was an antagonist to Professor Gibbes' teaching, . . . but I did not succeed in mollifying his anger." Novy wrote in the margin of his copy: "x good story but?"

13. H. Gibbes, *Practical Histology and Pathology* (London: H. K. Lewis, 1880). Second and third editions of 1883 and 1885 were also published in the United States. The book demonstrates that Gibbes was familiar with bacteriological techniques, and in it he quotes Klein's translation of Koch's description of his method of cultivating the tuberculosis bacillus. Gibbes gave directions for demonstrating the bacillus in sputum and tissues.

14. Warthin, "Forty Years," 743.

15. Accounts of conflict are in C. B. Burr, ed., *Medical History of Michigan* (Minneapolis: Bruce Publishing, 1930), 2:722–24. Reports of talks given outside Michigan are H. Gibbes, "Is the Unity of Phthisis an Established Fact?" *Boston Med. Surg. J.* 123 (1890): 608–11; and H. Gibbes, "Pathology of Phthisis Pulmonalis," *J. Am. Med. Assoc.* 16 (1891): 253–58.

16. The Gibbes case is described in detail in V. N. Kobayashi, "From 'Germ Theory' to Bacteriology: A Case of Academic Freedom at the University of Michigan," Bentley Historical Library, University of Michigan. Kobayashi tried to make out that Gibbes's dismissal was a violation of academic freedom and an attempt to impose scientific orthodoxy.

17. G. Dock, "Clinical Pathology in the Eighties and Nineties," *Am. J. Clin. Pathol.* 16 (1946): 671–80.

18. The Warthin Collection is in the Rare Book Room of Michigan's Taubman Medical Library.

19. A. S. Warthin, *The Physician of the Dance of Death* (New York: P. B. Hoeber, 1931), xi.

20. A. S. Warthin, "Some Physiologic Effects of Music in Hypnotized Subjects," *Med. News* 65 (1894): 89.

21. Ibid.

22. Ibid., 90.

23. This is Warthin's mixture of English and German.

24. Warthin, "Some Physiologic Effects," 91.

25. A. S. Warthin, *Old Age: The Major Involution* (New York: P. B. Hoeber, 1929).

26. A comment by A. C. Curtis when he surveyed the curriculum in 1927.

27. Warthin, "Forty Years," 745.

28. A. S. Warthin, *Practical Pathology for Students and Physicians* (Ann Arbor: G. Wahr, 1897). There was a second edition in 1911.

29. E. Ziegler, *General Pathology,* trans. and ed. A. S. Warthin (New York: W. Wood, 1903). This was from the tenth German edition, and there was another from the eleventh edition in 1908.

30. I have seen only the third edition of 1903.

31. *Encyclopedic Survey,* 2:891.

32. Warthin, "Forty Years," 745.

33. M. H. Soule, "Aldred Scott Warthin (1866–1931): An Appreciation," *J. Lab. Clin. Med.* 16 (1931): 1043–46.

34. Warthin, "Forty Years."

35. *Encyclopedic Survey,* 2:891.

36. W. J. Stone, ed., *Contributions to Medical Science Dedicated to Aldred Scott Warthin* (Ann Arbor: G. Wahr, 1927). Warthin dedicated his *Creed of a Biologist: A Biologic Philosophy of Life* (New York: P. B. Hoeber, 1930) "To Those of My Old Students Who Understood."

37. Peyton Rous (1879–1970) won the Nobel Prize in 1969 for his work on cancer viruses, including his discovery of the Rous virus, the first virus shown to cause solid tumors. He also did pioneering work on blood transfusions that led to the establishment of the first blood banks during World War I (P. K. Vogt, "Peyton Rous: Homage and Appraisal," *FASEB J.* 10 [1996]: 1559).

38. Warthin, "Forty Years," 745–46.

39. Ibid., 744.

40. Moses Gomberg, the organic chemist famous for synthesizing the first free radical and a member of the medical faculty until the Chemical Laboratory was converted to the Department of Chemistry in 1910, gave Warthin a pure sample of mustard gas (dichlorethyl sulfide), and Dow Chemical Company gave him an impure sample. Warthin was at first supported by a grant from the regents and then by the Chemical Warfare Service. Warthin and Weller were assisted by George Herrmann, who, as a third- and fourth-year medical student, earned a master's degree in 1918, the same year he received his doctor of medicine. Their six papers describe lesions in animals and humans. The most serious problem was severe secondary infection that could be treated by soaking the lesions in Dakin's solution, 0.5 percent hypochlorous acid. The last paper is A. S. Warthin and C. V. Weller, "The General Pathology of Mustard Gas (Dichlorethylsulphide) Poisoning," *J. Lab. Clin. Med.* 4 (1919): 265–306, and the earlier ones can be found by working back from it.

41. Felix Platter, quoted in J. Ruhräh, *Pediatrics of the Past* (New York: P. B. Hoeber, 1925), 239.

42. E. Boyd, "Growth of the Thymus: Its Relation to Status Thymicolymphaticus and Thymic Symptoms," *Am. J. Dis. Child.* 33 (1927): 867–79.

43. A. S. Warthin, "The Clinical Diagnosis of Enlargement of the Thymus," *Int. Clin.* 1 (1907): 49–66;

Warthin, "The Pathology of Thymic Hyperplasia and the Status Lymphaticus," *Arch. Pediatr.* 26 (1909): 597–617; and in great detail with illustrations, Warthin, "Diseases of the Thymus," in *Modern Medicine,* ed. W. Osler (Philadelphia: Lea Brothers, 1908), 4:779–807. See also D. Marine, "Status Lymphaticus," *Arch. Pathol.* 5 (1928): 661–82. The literature on the subject is enormous, and Warthin was certainly not alone in his belief in the thymicolymphatic constitution.

44. A. Paltauf, "Ueber die Beziehungen der Thymus zum plötzlichen Tod," parts 1 and 2, *Wien. Klin. Wochenschr.* 2 (1889): 877–81; 3 (1890): 172–75.

45. H. B. Dodwell, " 'Status lymphaticus,' the Growth of a Myth," *Br. Med. J.* 1 (1954): 149. The literature of the period contains many articles scoffing at the "thymus vogue" or the "thymus superstition."

46. S. Weiss, "Instantaneous 'Physiologic' Death," *N. Engl. J. Med.* 223 (1940): 797.

47. D. E. Clark, "Association of Irradiation with Cancer of the Thyroid in Children and Adolescents." *J. Am. Med. Assoc.* 159 (1955): 1007–9. However, the first child to receive X-irradiation for a supposedly enlarged thymus lived to old age without developing cancer of the thyroid. (F. N. Silverman, "Thymic Irradiation: A Historical Note," *Am. J. Roentgenol.* 84 [1960]: 562–64.) The Michigan experience is described in H. B. Latourette and F. J. Hodges, "Incidence of Neoplasia after Irradiation of Thymic Region," *Am. J. Roentgenol.* 82 (1959): 667–77.

48. Boyd, "Growth of the Thymus," 879.

49. E. Boyd, "The Weight of the Thymus Gland in Health and Disease," *Am. J. Dis. Child.* 43 (1932): 1214.

50. Weller's lecture to the second-year class on 10 October 1955 is summarized in the Phi Chi notes of that date. I am grateful to Gerald Abrams for lending me a copy of the notes and for introducing me to the status of status lymphaticus at Michigan.

51. A. S. Warthin, "The Constitutional Entity of Exophthalmic Goiter and So-Called Toxic Adenoma," *Ann. Intern. Med.* 2 (1928): 569.

52. A. S. Warthin, "The Nature of Cancer Susceptibility in Human Families," *J. Cancer Res.* 12 (1928): 249–58.

53. A. S. Warthin, "Heredity with Reference to Carcinoma," *Arch. Intern. Med.* 12 (1913): 546–55.

54. A. S. Warthin, "A Further Study of a Cancer Family," *J. Cancer Res.* 9 (1925): 279–86; and idem, "Heredity of Carcinoma in Man," *Ann. Intern. Med.* 4 (1931): 681–96. Warthin published the same data several times in his last years.

55. Warthin, *Creed of a Biologist.*

56. C. V. Weller, "The Blastophthoric Effect of Chronic Lead Poisoning," *J. Med. Res.* 33 (1915): 271–93.

57. C. V. Weller, "Degenerative Changes in the Germinal Epithelium in Acute Alcoholism and Their Possible Relationship to Blastophthoria," *Trans. Assoc. Am. Physicians* 42 (1927): 277–86.

58. Warthin, *Creed of a Biologist,* 53, 57. See also M. S. Pernick, *The Black Stork: Eugenics and the Death of "Defective" Babies in American Medicine and Motion Pictures since 1915* (New York: Oxford University Press, 1996).

59. A. S. Warthin, "The New Pathology of Syphilis," *Harvey Lect.* 13 (1917–18): 67–96.

60. A. S. Warthin and A. C. Starry, "Second Improved Method for the Demonstration of *Spirochaeta pallida* in the Tissues," *J. Am. Med. Assoc.* 76 (1921): 234–37.

61. R. Farrier and A. S. Warthin, "A Study of the Effect of pH upon the Third Improved Warthin-Starry Method for Demonstrating Spirocheta pallida in Single Sections," *Am. J. Syph.* 14 (1930): 394–401, is the last of Warthin's papers on the subject.

62. An example is A. S. Warthin, "The Role of Syphilis in the Etiology of Angina Pectoris, Coronary Arteriosclerosis and Thrombosis and of Sudden Cardiac Death," *Am. Heart J.* 6 (1930): 163–70. Warthin published essentially the same paper several times as named lectures.

63. U. J. Wile, L. Weider, and A. S. Warthin, "Malignant Syphilis, with a New Explanation of the Pathology of the Cutaneous Lesions," *Am. J. Syph.* 14 (1930): 1–34.

64. A. S. Warthin, "The Lesions of Latent Syphilis," *South. Med. J.* 24 (1931): 273–78.

65. Warthin, "Role of Syphilis."

66. Warthin, "Role of Syphilis"; and idem, "Extensive Diffuse Syphilitic Myocarditis Associated with Malignant Syphilis," *Am. J. Syph.* 14 (1930): 35–42.

67. C. V. Weller, "Endometriosis of the Umbilicus," *Am. J. Pathol.* 11 (1935): 281–86.

68. C. V. Weller, "A Distomus; Divergent Duplication of the Lower Portion of the Face," *J. Tech. Meth. Bull. Int. Assoc. Med. Mus.* 16 (1936): 45–50.

69. C. V. Weller, "The Pathology of the Aorta in Haitian Treponematosis," *Am. J. Syph.* 20 (1936): 467–81. The same study also was published as "A Preliminary Report upon 169 Haitian Aortas, with Treponemata Demonstrated in Eighteen Per Cent," *Trans. Assoc. Am. Physicians* 50 (1935): 342–47.

70. C. V. Weller, "The Visceral Pathology in Haitian Treponematosis," *Am. J. Syph.* 21 (1937): 357–69.

71. C. V. Weller and A. Christensen, "The Cerebrospinal Fluid in Lead Poisoning," in *The Human Cerebrospinal Fluid,* ed. C. L. Dana et al. (New York: P. B. Hoeber, 1926); and Weller, "Blastophthoric Effect."

72. A. J. French, "Carl Vernon Weller, a Biographical

Sketch," *Lab. Invest.* 5 (1956): 255. French listed Weller's editorships and participation in national societies.

73. Thomas Weller won the Nobel Prize with his colleagues from Harvard, John F. Enders and Frederick Robbins, for growing polio virus in nonnervous tissue cultures.

74. C. V. Weller and I. Hauser, "A Further Report on the Cancer Family of Warthin," *Am. J. Cancer* 27 (1936): 434–49.

75. C. V. Weller, "The Inheritance of Retinoblastoma and Its Relationship to Practical Eugenics," *Trans. Assoc. Am. Physicians* 55 (1940): 311.

76. J. C. Bugher, "The Probability of the Chance Occurrence of Multiple Malignant Neoplasms," *Am. J. Cancer* 21 (1934): 809–24.

77. C. V. Weller, "On the 'Cause' of Cancer," *Ann. Intern. Med.* 5 (1931): 385–88.

78. C. V. Weller, "The Pathology of Primary Carcinoma of the Lung," *Arch. Pathol.* 7 (1929): 497.

79. C. V. Weller, *Causal Factors in Cancer of the Lung* (Springfield, Ill.: C. C Thomas, 1956), 100.

Chapter 12

1. This and other details in the description of Dock are drawn from a paper by Nathan D. Munro of the class of 1940 read at a Victor Vaughan Society meeting on 12 March 1940 at the home of Dr. Carl Badgley and published as N. D. Munro, "George Dock, M.D.," *Proc. Victor Vaughan Soc.* 11, part 1 (1939–40). This is an example of how a student paper may become a historical document. Frank Wilson, Charles Edmunds, Carl Camp, Frederick Novy, and Mark Marshall, all of whom knew Dock, were present at the meeting.

2. *The University of Michigan: An Encyclopedic Survey*, ed. W. B. Shaw (Ann Arbor: University of Michigan Press, 1958), 4:1654–56; and G. Dock, "The University Hospital: Its Past, Present, and Future," *Mich. Alumnus* 9 (1903): 183–92.

3. The room was called an amphitheater, though it was not double.

4. Dock, "University Hospital," 187.

5. H. W. Davenport, *Doctor Dock: Teaching and Learning Medicine at the Turn of the Century* (New Brunswick, N.J.: Rutgers University Press, 1987), 16; and regents' minutes for June 1910.

6. G. R. Herrmann, *Methods in Medicine, The Manual of the Medical Service of George Dock, M.D., Sc.D.* (St. Louis: C. V. Mosby, 1924).

7. G. Dock, "Spelling as an Index to the Preparation of the Medical Student," *J. Am. Med. Assoc.* 52 (1909): 1176–78.

8. Dr. Koplik (1859–1927) first described in detail "Koplik's spots" and the natural history of measles. H. Markel, "Henry Koplik, MD, The Good Samaritan Dispensary of New York City, and the Description of Koplik's Spots," *Arch. Pediatr. Adolesc. Med.* 150 (1996): 535–39.

9. The distinction between *to lay* and *to lie* has disappeared except among a few of the elite, including myself.

10. G. Dock, *Outlines for Case Taking as Used in the Medical Clinic of the University of Michigan* (Ann Arbor: G. Wahr, 1902). It was based on Strümpell's *Kurzer Leitfaden für die klinische Krankenuntersuchung* (Leipzig: G. C. W. Vogel, 1887).

11. H. W. Davenport, *Doctor Dock*, 20.

12. N. D. Munro, "George Dock," 24.

13. George Dock Notebooks, Bentley Historical Library, University of Michigan.

14. Ibid., 534–35. Spelling of medical terms was often phonetic, but it improved as the year went on. Dock sometimes corrected the typescript in an almost illegible hand.

15. G. Dock, "Clinical Pathology in the Eighties and Nineties," *Am. J. Clin. Pathol.* 16 (1946): 671–80.

16. N. D. Munro, "George Dock," 12.

17. This is obvious from Dock's publications, but it was confirmed by his son.

18. G. Dock, "Endocarditis and Intermittent Fever," *Boston Med. Surg. J.* 133 (1895): 457–61; and idem, "Staphylococcus-aureus Infection with Endocarditis," *N. Y. Med. J.* 65 (1897): 143–47.

19. G. Dock, "Trichomonas as a Parasite of Man," *Am. J. Med. Sci.* 111 (1896): 8. Dock bound a congratulatory note from Osler in his reprint of this paper.

20. G. Dock, "Cancer of the Stomach in Early Life, and the Value of Cells in the Diagnosis of Cancer of the Serous Membrane," *Trans. Assoc. Am. Physicians* 12 (1897): 152–67; and idem, "Chylous Ascites and Chylous Pleurisy, in a Case of Lymphocytoma Involving the Thoracic Duct," *Am. J. Med. Sci.* 134 (1907): 634–43.

21. G. Dock, "Mitosis in Circulating Blood," *Physician Surg.* 26 (1904): 1–10.

22. G. Dock, "Methods, Value and Limitations of the Knowledge of the Gastric Contents," *J. Am. Med. Assoc.* 45 (1905): 1385–87.

23. See J. H. Pratt, *A Year with Osler, 1896–1897* (Baltimore: Johns Hopkins Press, 1949).

24. G. Dock, "Compulsory Vaccination, Antivaccination, and Organized Vaccination," *Am. J. Med. Sci.* 133 (1907): 218–33.

25. G. Dock, "A Case of Infantile Scurvy," *J. Am. Med. Assoc.* 46 (1906): 258–61.

26. G. Dock, "Goitre in Michigan," *Trans. Assoc. Am. Physicians* 10 (1895): 103.

27. T. v. Jürgensen, L. v. Schrötter, and L. Krehl, *Diseases*

of the Heart, ed. G. Dock (Philadelphia: W. B. Saunders, 1908).

28. G. Dock, "Tricuspid Stenosis," *Trans. Assoc. Am. Physicians* 11 (1896): 186–94.

29. G. Dock, "Arteriosclerosis of Nephritic Origin," *J. Am. Med. Assoc.* 43 (1904): 730; and idem, "Sphygmograms from Two Cases of Bradycardia," *Med. News* 87 (1905): 337–39. In the latter paper Dock thanked Cushny for help.

30. G. Dock, "Some Notes on the Coronary Arteries," *Med. Surg. Reporter* 75 (1896): 2.

31. J. B. Herrick, "Clinical Features of Sudden Obstruction of the Coronary Arteries," *J. Am. Med. Assoc.* 59 (1912): 2015–20.

32. For example, see A. Sager, "Report on Obstetrics," *Detroit Rev. Med. Pharm.* 3 (1868): 397–417.

33. A. S. Warthin, "The Medical Library of the University of Michigan," *Bull. Med. Libr. Assoc.* 6 (1917): 46–53.

34. G. Dock, "The Medical Library of the University of Michigan," *Mich. Alumnus* 13 (1907): 240–48. Dock became president of the Association of Medical Librarians. His paper, "Printed Editions of the *Rosa Anglica* of John of Gaddesden," *Janus* 12 (1907): 425–35, records correspondence with librarians all over Europe.

35. Department of Medicine and Surgery, *Annual Announcement 1893–94,* 27.

36. D. M. Cowie et al., "The University of Michigan Summer School," *Physician Surg.* 28 (1906): 454.

37. Ibid.

38. W. Osler, *The Principles and Practice of Medicine,* 6th ed. (New York: D. Appleton, 1906), 731.

39. Cowie et al., "Summer School," 459.

40. Ibid., 462.

41. Ibid.

42. Ibid., 465.

43. Ibid., 458.

44. Ibid., 461.

45. V. C. Vaughan, *A Doctor's Memories* (Indianapolis: Bobbs-Merrill, 1926), 231. His statement that he "never believed in the removal of the Medical School, or even of its clinical teaching, to Detroit" (228) is amply controverted by documents in the medical school files in the Bentley Historical Library. There is even a letter of later date to his son, to be cited later, reporting that he thought Peterson and others were more favorable to the move than they had been and asking his son to stir up those in Detroit whose opinion counted. My assertion in the next section of the chapter that Vaughan had been disingenuous is based upon a letter by Peterson reporting the faculty meeting in which the proposed move had been voted down. There are many newspaper articles on the subject.

46. Dock's opinion is recorded in his clinical notes and was apparently made in response to student grumbling. George Dock Notebooks, Bentley Historical Library, University of Michigan.

47. Reuben Peterson Papers, Bentley Historical Library, University of Michigan.

48. Undated draft of a letter in James Burrill Angell Papers, Bentley Historical Library, University of Michigan.

49. Letter in the Reuben Peterson Papers, Bentley Historical Library, University of Michigan. Dock's letter about the clinical laboratory is in the same file.

50. Dock, "Clinical Pathology." Dock had been offered the job at Jefferson, and he was a candidate for Osler's job at Johns Hopkins in 1905. Peterson said Vaughan was ungracious when Dock left the University of Michigan and that there was lack of appreciation of Dock's work in Ann Arbor. Peterson's frequent critical comments on Vaughan reveal a certain lack of sympathy.

51. This is a paraphrase of a speech given by Cole and quoted in A. McG. Harvey, *Science at the Bedside* (Baltimore: Johns Hopkins University Press, 1981), 66. Cole's career is summarized in W. S. Tillett, "Rufus Cole, 1872–1966," *Trans. Assoc. Am. Physicians* 80 (1967): 9–10.

52. Hewlett always spelled his name in full on the title pages of his books, but his entry in *Who Was Who in America* is headed A(lbion) Walter Hewlett.

53. Biographical details, a bibliography, and a full discussion of Hewlett's career are in A. McG. Harvey, "Albion Walter Hewlett: Pioneer Clinical Physiologist," *Johns Hopkins Med. J.* 144 (1979): 202–14.

54. J. Erlanger and A. W. Hewlett, "A Study of the Metabolism in Dogs with Shortened Small Intestines," *Am. J. Physiol.* 6 (1901): 1–30.

55. See H. Schrörer, *Carl Ludwig* (Stuttgart: Wissenschaftliche Verlagsgesellschaft M.B.H., 1967), for Krehl in Leipzig and his Leipzig papers.

56. A. W. Hewlett, "Ueber die Einwirkung des Peptonblutes auf Hämolyse und Baktercidie," *Arch. Exp. Pathol. Pharmakol.* 49 (1903): 307–23.

57. L. Krehl, *The Principles of Clinical Pathology,* trans. A. W. Hewlett (Philadelphia: J. B. Lippincott, 1905). This is from the third German edition. Krehl published new editions so rapidly that Hewlett gave up after translating the fourth German edition in 1907.

58. J. Erlanger, "A New Instrument for Determining the Minimum and Maximum Blood-Pressures in Man," *Johns Hopkins Hosp. Reports* 12 (1904): 53–110.

59. T. C. Janeway, *The Clinical Study of Blood-Pressure* (New York: D. Appleton, 1904).

60. A. W. Hewlett, "The Clinical Value of the Electrocardiogram," *Physician Surg.* 31 (1909): 322–23.

61. A. Keith and M. Flack, "The Form and Nature of the

Muscular Connections between the Primary Divisions of the Vertebrate Heart," *J. Anat.* 41 (1907): 172–89; and A. W. Hewlett, "Digitalis Heart Block," *J. Am. Med. Assoc.* 48 (1907): 47–50.

62. A. W. Hewlett, "Heart-Block in the Ventricular Walls," *Arch. Intern. Med.* 2 (1908): 139–47.

63. O. Minkowski, "Die Registierung der Hertzbewegungen am linken Vorhof," *Dtsch. Med. Wochenschr.* 32 (1906): 1248–51; and idem, "Zur Deutung von Hertzarrhythmien mittelst des ösophagealen Kardiogramms," *Z. Klin. Med.* 62 (1907): 371–84.

64. C. I. Young and W. Hewlett, "The Normal Pulsations within the Esophagus," *J. Med. Res.* 16 (1907–8): 427–34.

65. J. G. Van Zwaluwenburg and J. H. Agnew, "Some Details of the Auricular Pressure Curves of the Dog," *Heart* 3 (1911–12): 343–52. They determined the resonant frequency of the capsule by its response to the singing voice.

66. Newspaper clipping in George Dock's scrapbook in the Bentley Historical Library, University of Michigan. Dock scorned religion and upset pious students such as Alice Hamilton.

67. A. W. Hewlett, "The Relation of Hospitals to Medical Schools in the United States," *Physician Surg.* 31 (1909): 481–91.

68. Ibid., 484.

69. A. W. Hewlett, Q. O. Gilbert, and A. D. Wickett, "The Toxic Effects of Urea on Normal Individuals," *Arch. Intern. Med.* 18 (1916): 636–51; and idem, "The Toxic Effects of Urea on Normal Individuals," *Trans. Assoc. Am. Physicians* 31 (1916): 311–27.

70. A. W. Hewlett and W. R. P. Clark, "The Symptoms of Descending Thoracic Aneurysm," *Am. J. Med. Sci.* 137 (1909): 792–805.

71. A. W. Hewlett, "A Patient with Extreme Cyanosis," *Physician Surg.* 31 (1909): 509–10.

72. A. W. Hewlett, "Infantilism in Pituitary Diseases," *Arch. Intern. Med.* 93 (1912): 32–43.

73. A. W. Hewlett, "Clinical Effects of 'Natural' and 'Synthetic' Sodium Salicylate," *J. Am. Med. Assoc.* 61 (1913): 315–21.

74. A. W. Hewlett, "A Case of Strychnine Poisoning," *Am. J. Med. Sci.* 146 (1913): 536–41.

75. Hewlett, Gilbert, and Wickett, "Toxic Effects of Urea."

76. A. W. Hewlett, "The Effect of Amyl Nitrite Inhalations upon the Blood Pressures in Man," *J. Med. Res.* 15 (1906): 383–98.

77. J. Barcroft and T. G. Brodie, "The Gaseous Metabolism of the Kidney," *J. Physiol. (London)* 33 (1905): 52–68.

78. T. G. Brodie and A. E. Russell, "On the Determination of the Rate of Blood-Flow through an Organ," *J. Physiol. (London)* 32 (1905): xlvii–xlvix.

79. The history of plethysmography is in H. Barcroft and H. J. C. Swan, *Sympathetic Control of Human Blood Vessels* (London: Edward Arnold, 1953), 139–44.

80. The major papers, not counting duplicate publications, are A. W. Hewlett and J. G. Van Zwaluwenburg, "Method for Estimating the Blood Flow in the Arm," *Arch. Intern. Med.* 3 (1909): 254–56; Hewlett and Van Zwaluwenburg, "The Rate of Blood Flow in the Arm," *Heart* 1 (1909): 87–97; Hewlett and Van Zwaluwenburg, "Comparison between the Blood Flow in the Arm and in the Hand," *Proc. Soc. Exp. Biol. Med.* 8 (1910): 111–13; Hewlett, "The Effect of Room Temperature upon the Blood-Flow in the Arm, with a Few Observations on the Effect of Fever," *Heart* 2 (1910–11): 230–38; Hewlett, Van Zwaluwenburg, and M. Marshall, "The Effect of Some Hydrotherapeutic Procedures upon the Blood Flow in the Arm," *Trans. Assoc. Am. Physicians* 26 (1911): 357–79; Hewlett, Van Zwaluwenburg, and J. H. Agnew, "A New Method for Studying the Brachial Pulse of Man," *Trans. Assoc. Am. Physicians* 27 (1912): 188–92; Hewlett, "The Circulation in the Arm of Man," *Am. J. Med. Sci.* 145 (1913): 656–67; and Hewlett, "Active Hyperemia following Local Exposure to Cold," *Arch. Intern. Med.* 11 (1913): 507–11.

81. G. N. Stewart, "Studies on the Circulation in Man. I. The Measurement of the Bloodflow in the Hands"; "II. The Effect of Reflex Vaso-Motor Excitation on the Blood Flow in the Hand," *Heart* 3 (1911–12): 33–75, 76–84.

82. Papers on this subject include A. W. Hewlett and J. G. Van Zwaluwenburg, "The Pulse Flow in the Brachial Artery," *Arch. Intern. Med.* 12 (1913): 1–23; Hewlett, "The Pulse-Flow in the Brachial Artery," *Arch. Intern. Med.* 14 (1914): 609–19; Hewlett, "The Effect of Pituitary Substance upon the Pulse Form of Febrile Patients," *Proc. Soc. Exp. Biol. Med.* 12 (1914): 61–62; and Hewlett, "The Significance of Pulse Form," *J. Am. Med. Assoc.* 67 (1916): 1134–36.

83. G. E. Burch and N. P. de Pasquale, *A History of Electrocardiography* (Chicago: Year Book Medical Publishers, 1964).

84. F. N. Wilson, "Report of a Case Showing Premature Beats Arising in the Junctional Tissues," *Heart* 6 (1915): 17–26.

85. A. W. Hewlett and F. N. Wilson, "Coarse Auricular Fibrillation in Man," *Arch. Intern. Med.* 15 (1915): 786–92.

86. F. N. Wilson, "Three Cases Showing Changes in the Location of the Cardiac Pacemaker Associated with Respiration," *Arch. Intern. Med.* 16 (1915): 86–97; idem, "A Case in Which the Vagus Influenced the Form of the Ventricular Complex of the Electrocar-

diogram," *Arch. Intern. Med.* 16 (1915): 1008–27; idem, "The Production of Atrioventricular Rhythm in Man after the Administration of Atropin," *Arch. Intern. Med.* 16 (1915): 989–1007; and idem, "Recent Progress in Pediatrics: Résumé on the Circulation," *Am. J. Dis. Child.* 10 (1915): 376–90.

87. A. W. Hewlett, *Functional Pathology of Internal Diseases* (New York: D. Appleton, 1916).

88. Hewlett, *Pathological Physiology of Internal Diseases* (New York: D. Appleton, 1919), iii.

89. Hewlett, *Functional Pathology,* 51, fig. 19.

90. L. Popielski, "β-Imidazolyläthylamin und die Organextrakte. Erster Teil. β-Imidazolyläthylamin als mächtiger Erreger der Magendrüsen," *Arch. Gesamte Physiol.* 178 (1920): 214–36.

91. A. W. Hewlett, "Eight Years in the Department of Internal Medicine," *J. Mich. State Med. Soc.* 15 (1916): 505–8.

92. N. B. Foster, *Diabetes Mellitus* (Philadelphia: J. B. Lippincott, 1915).

93. N. B. Foster, "Demonstration of a Case of Polyserositis," *J. Mich. State Med. Soc.* 16 (1917): 21–22; idem, "Treatment of Chronic Nephritis," ibid. 16 (1917): 217–21; and idem, "Report of Two Cases Where the Symptoms Seemed to be Dependent upon Disease of the Teeth," ibid. 16 (1917): 406–9.

94. N. B. Foster, "Medical Education as Revealed by the War," *J. Am. Med. Assoc.* 72 (1919): 1540–42.

95. *Encyclopedic Survey,* 2:841.

Chapter 13

1. T. Lewis, *Clinical Electrocardiography* (London: Shaw and Sons, 1913) and many subsequent editions. His larger book, *The Mechanism and Graphic Registration of the Heart Beat* (New York: P. B. Hoeber, 1920), must have been in preparation when Frank Wilson was with him.

2. T. Lewis, *The Soldiers' Heart and the Effort Syndrome* (New York: P. B. Hoeber, 1920).

3. S. A. Levine and F. N. Wilson, "Observations on the Vital Capacity of the Lungs in Cases of 'Irritable Heart,'" *Heart* 7 (1916–19): 53–61; and Wilson, Levine, and A. B. Edgar, "The Bicarbonate Concentration of the Blood Plasma in Cases of 'Irritable Heart,'" ibid. 7 (1918–19): 62–64.

4. A. N. Drury, "The Percentage of Carbon Dioxide in the Alveolar Air, and the Tolerance to Accumulating Carbon Dioxide, in Cases of So-Called 'Irritable Heart' of Soldiers," *Heart* 7 (1920): 165–73.

5. F. N. Wilson and R. A. Jamieson, "Musical Diastolic Murmurs in Aortic Insufficiency," *Heart* 7 (1918–19): 71–79.

6. R. A. Jamieson and F. N. Wilson, "The Pistol-Shot Sound in Aortic Disease," *Heart* 7 (1918–19): 66.

7. G. R. Herrmann and F. N. Wilson, "Ventricular Hypertrophy. A Comparison of Electrocardiographic and Post-Mortem Findings," *Heart* 9 (1922): 91–147. Herrmann received his Ph.D. in pathology from Michigan for this work.

8. F. N. Wilson and G. R. Herrmann, "Bundle Branch Block and Arborization Block," *Arch. Intern. Med.* 26 (1920): 153–91; and idem, "An Experimental Study of Incomplete Bundle Branch Block and of the Refractory Period of the Heart of the Dog," *Heart* 8 (1921): 229–96.

9. Wilson and Herrmann, "An Experimental Study," 229.

10. F. N. Wilson, A. G. MacLeod, and P. S. Barker, "The Order of Ventricular Excitation in Human Bundle Branch Block," *Am. Heart J.* 7 (1932): 305–30.

11. F. N. Wilson and P. S. Barker, "The Heart Station of the University of Michigan Hospital," in *Methods and Problems of Medical Education,* 18th ser. (New York: Rockefeller Foundation, 1930), 89–93. The article contains plans, photographs, and a description of the heart station.

12. F. N. Wilson, F. F. Rosenbaum, and F. D. Johnston, "Interpretation of the Ventricular Complex of the Electrocardiogram," in *Selected Papers of Dr. Frank N. Wilson,* ed. F. D. Johnston and E. Lepeschkin (Ann Arbor: Heart Station, University Hospital, 1954), 463. Wilson himself demonstrated that the T wave can be inverted simply by drinking iced water. See Wilson and R. Finch, "The Effect of Drinking Iced-Water upon the Form of the T Deflection of the Electrocardiogram," *Heart* 10 (1923): 275–78.

13. Wilson, Rosenbaum, and Johnston, "Interpretation of Ventricular Complex," 434.

14. F. N. Wilson, A. G. MacLeod, and P. S. Barker, *The Distribution of the Currents of Action and of Injury Displayed by Heart Muscle and Other Excitable Tissues* (Ann Arbor: University of Michigan Press, 1933), 9–10.

15. Ibid., 47.

16. L. A. Woodbury, H. H. Hecht, and A. R. Christopherson, "Membrane Resting and Action Potentials of Single Cardiac Muscle Fibers of the Frog Ventricle," *Am. J. Physiol.* 164 (1951): 307–18. Hans Hecht was Wilson's last pupil at the University of Michigan.

17. W. H. Craib, "Study of Electrical Fields Surrounding Active Heart Muscle," *Heart* 14 (1927): 71–109.

18. W. H. Craib, "A Study of the Electrical Field Surrounding Skeletal Muscle," *J. Physiol. (London)* 66 (1928): 71.

19. A. McGhee Harvey, *Adventures in Medical Research* (Baltimore: Johns Hopkins University Press, 1974), 275. Harvey says that this occurred at a meeting of the American Society for Clinical Investigation. When

queried, he said that the Wilson quotation is inaccessibly buried in the Johns Hopkins archives.

20. Wilson, MacLeod, and Barker, *Distribution of Currents of Action and Injury,* 2 n. 1.

21. F. N. Wilson, "Concerning the Form of the QRS Deflections of the Electrocardiogram in Bundle Branch Block," in *Selected Papers,* 860.

22. F. N. Wilson, "The Origin and Nature of the Progress Made in Our Understanding of the Electrocardiogram during the Last Three Decades," in *Selected Papers,* 20–21.

23. W. Falta, L. H. Newburgh, and E. Nobel, "Ueber Beziehung der Ueberfunktion zur Konstitution," *Z. Klin. Med.* 72 (1911): 97–153.

24. This and other characterizations of Newburgh are in his obituary notice by J. H. Means, *Trans. Assoc. Am. Physicians* 70 (1957): 19.

25. L. H. Newburgh, "The Dietetic Treatment of Constipation," *Boston Med. Surg. J.* 168 (1913): 757–60.

26. L. H. Newburgh, "The Treatment of Cardiac Edema with Alkali and Salt," *Boston Med. Surg. J.* 169 (1913): 40–44.

27. The story of Henderson's relations with Folin is in R. E. Kohler, *From Medicinal Chemistry to Biochemistry; The Making of a Biomedical Discipline* (New York: Cambridge University Press, 1982), 180–82.

28. L. J. Henderson and W. W. Palmer, "On the Intensity of Urinary Acidity in Normal and Pathological Conditions," *J. Biol. Chem.* 13 (1913): 393–405. The clinical paper is Palmer and Henderson, "Clinical Studies on Acid Base Equilibrium and the Nature of Acidosis," *Arch. Intern. Med.* 12 (1913): 153–70.

29. L. J. Henderson, W. W. Palmer, and L. H. Newburgh, "The Swelling of Colloids and Hydrogen Ion Concentration," *J. Pharmacol. Exp. Ther.* 5 (1913–14): 451.

30. L. H. Newburgh, W. W. Palmer, and L. J. Henderson, "A Study of Hydrogen Ion Concentration of the Urine in Heart Disease," *Arch. Intern. Med.* 12 (1913): 146–52.

31. L. H. Newburgh, "The Use of Strychnin and Caffein as Cardiovascular Stimulants in Acute Infectious Diseases," *Arch. Intern. Med.* 15 (1915): 458.

32. L. H. Newburgh and G. R. Minot, "The Blood-Pressure in Pneumonia," *Arch. Intern. Med.* 14 (1914): 48–55.

33. Newburgh, "Use of Strychnin," 469.

34. L. H. Newburgh and W. T. Porter, "The Heart Muscle in Pneumonia," *Boston Med. Surg. J.* 172 (1915): 718–19.

35. One of the last papers is W. T. Porter and L. H. Newburgh, "The Vagus Nerves in Pneumonia," *Am. J. Physiol.* 42 (1916): 175–92.

36. A. Krogh and J. Lindhard, "Measurements of the Blood Flow through the Lungs of Man," *Skand. Arch. Physiol.* 27 (1912): 100–125.

37. J. H. Means and L. H. Newburgh, "Studies of the Blood Flow by the Method of Krogh and Lindhard," *Trans. Assoc. Am. Physicians* 30 (1915): 51–62; and idem, "The Effect of Caffeine upon the Blood Flow in Normal Human Subjects," *J. Pharmacol. Exp. Ther.* 7 (1915): 449–65.

38. L. H. Newburgh and J. H. Means, "The Blood Flow in a Patient with Double Aortic and Double Mitral Disease," *J. Pharmacol. Exp. Ther.* 7 (1915): 441–47.

39. L. H. Newburgh, "Bright's Disease by Feeding High Protein Diets," *Arch. Intern. Med.* 24 (1919): 359.

40. L. H. Newburgh, "The Production of Chronic Nephritis through Feeding High Protein Diets," *J. Mich. State Med. Soc.* 18 (1919): 21.

41. L. H. Newburgh and S. Clarkson, "Renal Injury Produced in Rabbits by Diets Containing Meat," *Arch. Intern. Med.* 32 (1923): 850–69.

42. Newburgh and Clarkson, "Renal Injury," 869.

43. T. L. Squire and L. H. Newburgh, "Renal Irritation in Man from High Protein Diet," *Arch. Intern. Med.* 28 (1921): 15.

44. L. H. Newburgh and S. Clarkson, "The Production of Atherosclerosis in Rabbits by Feeding Diets Rich in Meat," *Arch. Intern. Med.* 31 (1923): 653–76.

45. L. H. Newburgh and P. L. Marsh, "Renal Injury by Amino-Acids," *Arch. Intern. Med.* 36 (1925): 682–711.

46. A. C. Curtis and L. H. Newburgh, "The Toxic Action of Cystine on the Kidney," *Arch. Intern. Med.* 39 (1927): 817–27; and Newburgh and Curtis, "Production of Renal Injury in the White Rat by the Protein of the Diet," ibid. 42 (1928): 801–21.

47. L. H. Newburgh and M. W. Johnston, "High Nitrogen Diets and Renal Injury. The Dependence of the Injury upon the Nature of the Nitrogenous Substance," *J. Clin. Invest.* 10 (1931): 153–60.

48. L. H. Newburgh, M. Falcon-Lesses, and M. W. Johnston, "The Nephropathic Effect in Man of a Diet High in Beef Muscle and Liver," *Am. J. Med. Sci.* 179 (1930): 305–10.

49. Examples: L. H. Newburgh and M. W. Johnston, "The Insensible Loss of Water," *Physiol. Rev.* 22 (1942): 1–18; and Johnston, "The Specific Dynamic Response to Protein of Individuals Suffering from Disease of the Hypophysis," *J. Clin. Invest.* 11 (1932): 437–48.

50. W. O. Atwater and F. G. Benedict, *A Respiration Calorimeter with Appliances for the Direct Determination of Oxygen* (Washington, D.C.: Carnegie Institution of Washington, 1905).

51. L. H. Newburgh and M. W. Johnston, *The Exchange of Energy between Man and the Environment* (Springfield, Ill.: C. C Thomas, 1930), 22.

52. M. W. Johnston and L. H. Newburgh, "The Determination of the Total Heat Eliminated by the Human Being," *J. Clin. Invest.* 8 (1930): 147–60.

53. L. H. Newburgh et al., "A Respiration Chamber for Use with Human Subjects," *J. Nutr.* 13 (1937): 193–201.

54. F. H. Wiley and L. H. Newburgh, "The Relationship between the Environment and the Basal Insensible Loss of Weight," *J. Clin. Invest.* 10 (1931): 689–701; Newburgh, Wiley, and F. H. Lashmet, "A Method for the Determination of Heat Production over Long Periods of Time," *J. Clin. Invest.* 10 (1931): 703–21; Newburgh and M. W. Johnston, "Relation between Dehydration and the Insensible Water Loss," *J. Nutr.* 7 (1934): 107–16; and Newburgh et al., "Further Experiences with the Measurement of Heat Production from Insensible Loss of Weight," *J. Nutr.* 13 (1937): 203–21.

55. F. M. Allen, "The Present Outlook of Diabetic Treatment," *Trans. Assoc. Am. Physicians* 32 (1917): 147.

56. F. M. Allen, "The Role of Fat in Diabetes," *Am. J. Med. Sci.* 153 (1917): 367.

57. Allen, "Role of Fat," 352.

58. L. H. Newburgh and P. L. Marsh, "The Use of a High Fat Diet in the Treatment of Diabetes Mellitus," *Arch. Intern. Med.* 26 (1920): 647–62; and idem, "The Use of a High Fat Diet in the Treatment of Diabetes Mellitus; Second Paper: Blood Sugar," ibid. 27 (1921): 699–705.

59. P. L. Marsh, L. H. Newburgh, and L. E. Holly, "The Nitrogen Requirement for Maintenance in Diabetes Mellitus," *Arch. Intern. Med.* 29 (1922): 97–130.

60. L. H. Newburgh and P. L. Marsh, "Further Observations on the Use of a High Fat Diet in the Treatment of Diabetes Mellitus," *Arch. Intern. Med.* 31 (1923): 455–90.

61. E. P. Joslin, "Ideals in the Treatment of Diabetes and Methods for Their Realization," *N. Engl. J. Med.* 198 (1928): 379–82.

62. E. P. Joslin, *The Treatment of Diabetes Mellitus* (London: Henry Kimpton, 1924), 5–7, 525–32.

63. L. H. Newburgh, "The Dietetic Treatment of Diabetes Mellitus. A Restatement of Fundamental Principles," *Ann. Intern. Med.* 2 (1929): 647.

64. F. N. Allen, "The History of the Treatment of Diabetes by Diet," *J. Am. Diet. Assoc.* 6 (1930): 1–9.

65. R. H. Freyberg, L. H. Newburgh, and W. A. Murrill, "Cholesterol Content of Blood in Diabetic Patients Fed Diets Rich in Fat," *Arch. Intern. Med.* 58 (1930): 589–97.

66. F. H. Wiley and L. H. Newburgh, "The Doubtful Nature of 'Luxuskonsumption,'" *J. Clin. Invest.* 10 (1931): 733–38. See also, K. Voit, *Handbuch der Physiologie des Gesammt-Stoffwechsels und der Fortpflanzung. 1. theil. Physiologie des allgemeinen Stoffwechsels und der Ernährung* (Leipzig: Vogel, 1881); and M. Rubner, *The Laws of Energy Consumption in Nutrition*, trans. A. Markhoff and A. Sandri-White and ed. R. J. T. Joy (Natwick, Mass.: U.S. Army Research Institute of Environmental Medicine; Washington, D.C.: U.S. Army Medical Research and Development Command, 1968).

67. L. H. Newburgh and M. W. Johnston, "The Nature of Obesity," *J. Clin. Invest.* 8 (1930): 197–213; and Newburgh, "The Cause of Obesity," *J. Am. Med. Assoc.* 97 (1931): 1659–61.

68. L. H. Newburgh, "Obesity," *Arch. Intern. Med.* 70 (1942): 1033–96; Newburgh and M. W. Johnston, "Endogenous Obesity—A Misconception," *J. Am. Diet. Assoc.* 5 (1943): 275–85; and Newburgh, "Obesity. I. Energy Metabolism," *Physiol. Rev.* 24 (1944): 18–31.

69. L. H. Newburgh and D. S. Waller, "Studies of Diabetes Mellitus. Evidence That the Disability Is Concerned Solely with the Metabolism of Glucose. The Mode of Action of Insulin," *J. Clin. Invest.* 11 (1932): 995–1002; J. M. Sheldon, M. W. Johnston, and Newburgh, "A Quantitative Study of the Oxidation of Glucose in Normal and Diabetic Men," *J. Clin. Invest.* 16 (1937): 933–36; Johnston, Sheldon, and Newburgh, "The Utilization of Carbohydrate in Human Undernutrition," *J. Nutr.* 17 (1939): 213–22; and J. W. Conn, "Interpretation of the Glucose Tolerance Test. The Necessity of a Standard Preparatory Diet," *Am. J. Med. Sci.* 199 (1940): 555–64.

70. L. H. Newburgh, "Control of Hyperglycemia of Obese 'Diabetics' by Weight Reduction," *Ann. Intern. Med.* 17 (1942): 935–42.

71. L. H. Newburgh et al., "A New Interpretation of Diabetes Mellitus in Obese, Middle-Aged Persons: Recovery through Reduction of Weight," *Trans. Assoc. Am. Physicians* 53 (1938): 245–56.

72. L. H. Newburgh, "Does Insulin Increase Tolerance?" *Boston Med. Surg. J.* 190 (1924): 351–55. One patient was "a young man of unusual intelligence—an instructor in engineering in the University" (352). He was first admitted to the University Hospital on 10 June 1922 and discharged on a diet containing twenty-two hundred calories. In February 1923 he became careless of his diet, and on 3 March 1923 he was admitted in diabetic coma. Newburgh saved his life with some of his first insulin. He was not named in the paper, but he was clearly Franklin Johnston. See the *University of Michigan Medical Center Journal* 31 (1965): 185–86.

73. L. H. Newburgh, "The Dietetic Treatment of Diabetes Mellitus," *Ann. Intern. Med.* 2 (1929): 647.

74. L. H. Newburgh and F. MacKinnon, *The Practice of Dietetics* (New York: Macmillan, 1934); and New-

burgh, M. W. Johnston, and J. D. Newburgh, *Some Fundamental Principles of Metabolism* (Ann Arbor: n.p., 1934).

75. Newburgh and Johnston, *Exchange of Energy*.

76. L. H. Newburgh and A. M. Light, "Teaching Nutrition to Medical Students," *J. Am. Diet. Assoc.* 21 (1945): 9.

77. F. H. Lashmet and L. H. Newburgh, "The Specific Gravity of the Urine as a Test of Kidney Function," *J. Am. Med. Assoc.* 94 (1930): 1883–85; and idem, "An Improved Concentration Test of Renal Function," ibid. 99 (1932): 1396–98.

78. E. M. Isberg and L. H. Newburgh, "An 18-Hour Concentration Test of Kidney Function," *Am. J. Med. Sci.* 211 (1946): 701–4.

79. F. H. Lashmet and L. H. Newburgh, "A Comparative Study of the Excretion of Water and Solids by Normal and Abnormal Kidneys," *J. Clin. Invest.* 11 (1933): 1003–9.

80. L. H. Newburgh, M. W. Johnston, and M. Falcon-Lesses, "Measurement of Total Water Exchange," *J. Clin. Invest.* 8 (1930): 161–87.

Chapter 14

1. A sketch of Warfield's career is in G. C. Robinson, "Louis Marshall Warfield, 1877–1938," *Trans. Assoc. Am. Physicians* 54 (1939): 17–18.

2. L. M. Warfield, "The Cardiovascular Defective," in *Contributions to Medical and Biological Research Dedicated to Sir William Osler* (New York: P. B. Hoeber, 1919), 2:1031–41.

3. L. M. Warfield, *Arteriosclerosis and Hypertension, with Chapters on Blood Pressure* (St. Louis: C. V. Mosby, 1920).

4. L. M. Warfield, "Studies in Auscultatory Blood-Pressure Phenomena. The Experimental Determination of Diastolic Pressure," *Arch. Intern. Med.* 10 (1912): 258–67; G. R. Minot, "Studies in Auscultatory Blood-Pressure Phenomena. The Clinical Determination of Diastolic Pressure," *J. Am. Med. Assoc.* 61 (1913): 1254–55; and Minot, "The Significance of High Pulse Pressure," *J. Am. Med. Assoc.* 68 (1917): 824–26.

5. L. M. Warfield, "Occult Tuberculosis," *Am. Rev. Tuberc.* 11 (1925): 112–21; idem, "The Development of Clinical Tuberculosis from Occult Tuberculosis," ibid. 11 (1925): 122–29; and idem, "Occult Tuberculosis with Gastrointestinal Symptoms," ibid. 11 (1925): 130–38.

6. For example: L. M. Warfield, "How Can We Best Treat Pernicious Anemia?" *N. Y. State Med. J.* 25 (1925): 147–52; and idem, "The Treatment of Chronic Nephritis," *J. Mich. State Med. Soc.* 23 (1924): 377–82.

7. *The University of Michigan: An Encyclopedic Survey,* ed. W. B. Shaw (Ann Arbor: University of Michigan Press, 1951), 2:842.

8. The documents on which this narrative is based are all in the Medical School Records, Bentley Historical Library, University of Michigan. Obituary notices say little about Warfield's death, but there is a copy of a letter by Dean Furstenberg in the records giving details and, characteristically, expressing friendly feelings for Warfield.

9. Cabot had made friends with the chief of surgery at St. Bartholomew's Hospital during World War I, and a number of young men from Bart's who subsequently attained distinction in Great Britain worked under Cabot in Ann Arbor in the 1920s. Mr. Hume was one of them.

10. The beds stayed there until one Christmas vacation about 1960. When they were not filled over the holidays and when the Simpson staff was not looking, the director of the University Hospital snatched them away.

11. J. T. Wearn, "Cyrus Cressey Sturgis, 1891–1966," *Trans. Assoc. Am. Physicians* 80 (1967): 24–26.

12. F. W. Peabody and C. C. Sturgis, "Clinical Studies of the Respiration. VII. The Effect of General Weakness and Fatigue on the Vital Capacity of the Lungs," *Arch. Intern. Med.* 28 (1921): 501–10; and Sturgis et al., "Clinical Studies on the Respiration. VIII. The Relation of Dyspnea to the Maximum Minute-Volume of Pulmonary Ventilation," ibid. 29 (1922): 236–44.

13. P. Roth, "Modifications of Apparatus and Improved Technic Adaptable to the Benedict Type of Respiration Apparatus," parts 1–3, *Boston Med. Surg. J.* 186 (1920): 457–65, 491–501.

14. F. W. Peabody et al., "Epinephrin Hypersensitiveness and Its Relation to Hyperthyroidism," *Am. J. Med. Sci.* 161 (1921): 508–17.

15. C. C. Sturgis and E. M. Tompkins, "A Study of the Correlation of the Basal Metabolism and Pulse Rate in Patients with Hyperthyroidism," *Arch. Intern. Med.* 26 (1920): 467–76; Sturgis, "Observations on One Hundred and Ninety-Two Consecutive Days of the Basal Metabolism, Food Intake, Pulse Rate, and Body Weight in a Patient with Exophthalmic Goiter," *Arch. Intern. Med.* 32 (1923): 50–73; S. A. Levine and Sturgis, "Hyperthyroidism Masked as Heart Disease," *Boston Med. Surg. J.* 190 (1924): 233–37; Sturgis, "Cases of Exophthalmic Goiter Illustrating the Spontaneous Course of the Disease and the Effects of Various Types of Treatment," *Med. Clin. North Am.* 8 (1925): 1465–83; and Sturgis, "Angina Pectoris as a Complication in Myxedema and Exophthalmic Goiter," *Boston Med. Surg. J.* 195 (1926): 351–54.

16. C. C. Sturgis et al., "The Effect of Iodine by Mouth on the Reaction to Intravenous Injections of Thyroxin," *J. Clin. Invest.* 2 (1926): 289–98.

17. C. A. Doan, "Raphael Isaacs, 1891–1965," *Trans. Assoc. Am. Physicians* 80 (1967): 11–12.

18. R. Isaacs, "An Injection Method for Aiding in the Identification of Tapeworm Species," *J. Lab. Clin. Med.* 7 (1922): 691–92. The method was used later by Isaacs, C. C. Sturgis, and M. Smith, "Tapeworm Anemia," *Arch. Intern. Med.* 42 (1928): 313–21.

19. R. Isaacs, "The Alkali Reserve of the Cerebrospinal Fluid in Various States of the Central Nervous System," *Am. J. Med. Sci.* 166 (1923): 237–43.

20. R. Isaacs, "Pathologic Physiology of Polycythemia Vera," *Arch. Intern. Med.* 31 (1923): 289–96.

21. R. Isaacs and B. Gordon, "The Effect of Exercise on the Distribution of Corpuscles in the Blood Stream," *Am. J. Physiol.* 71 (1924): 106–11.

22. R. Isaacs, B. Brock, and G. R. Minot, "The Resistance of Immature Erythrocytes to Heat," *J. Clin. Invest.* 1 (1925): 425–33.

23. R. Isaacs, "Properties of Young Erythrocytes in Relation to Agglutination and Their Behavior in Hemorrhage and Transfusion," *Arch. Intern. Med.* 33 (1924): 197.

24. G. R. Minot and R. Isaacs, "Lymphatic Leukemia: Age Incidence, Duration, and Benefit Derived from Irradiation," *Boston Med. Surg. J.* 191 (1924): 1–9; Minot, T. E. Buckman, and Isaacs, "Chronic Myelogenous Leukemia: Age Incidence, Duration, and Benefit Derived from Irradiation," *J. Am. Med. Assoc.* 82 (1924): 1489–94; and Minot and Isaacs, "Lymphoblastoma (Malignant Lymphoma)," *J. Am. Med. Assoc.* 86 (1926): 1185–89.

25. R. Isaacs, "Blood Changes in the Leucemias and Lymphomata and Their Bearing on Roentgen Therapy," *Am. J. Roentgenol.* 24 (1930): 655.

26. G. R. Minot and W. P. Murphy, "Treatment of Pernicious Anemia by a Special Diet," *J. Am. Med. Assoc.* 87 (1926): 470–76. Raw liver was also effective.

27. E. J. Cohn et al., "The Nature of the Material in Liver Effective in Pernicious Anemia," *J. Biol. Chem.* 77 (1928): 325–58.

28. M. C. Riddle and C. C. Sturgis, "The Effect of Single Massive Doses of Liver Extract on Patients with Pernicious Anemia," *Am. J. Med. Sci.* 180 (1930): 1–11.

29. S. M. Goldhamer, R. Isaacs, and C. C. Sturgis, "The Rôle of the Liver in Hematopoiesis," *Am. J. Med. Sci.* 188 (1935): 193–99.

30. R. Isaacs et al., "The Use of Liver Extract Intravenously in the Treatment of Pernicious Anemia," *J. Am. Med. Assoc.* 100 (1933): 629–33.

31. C. C. Sturgis, "The Present Status of Pernicious Anemia: Experience with 600 Cases over Eight Years," *Ann. Intern. Med.* 10 (1936): 283–89.

32. C. C. Sturgis, "An Analysis of the Causes of Death in 150 Fatal Cases of Pernicious Anemia Observed since 1927," *Trans. Assoc. Am. Physicians* 54 (1939): 46–54.

33. An example with 472 references: C. C. Sturgis et al., "Blood—A Review of the Recent Literature," *Arch. Intern. Med.* 55 (1935): 1001–81. There is also a 302-page book, planned for the use of the general practitioner, by Sturgis and R. Isaacs, *Diseases of the Blood* (New York: National Medical Book, 1937). Sturgis's large *Hematology* (Springfield, Ill.: C. C Thomas, 1948), was written after our period.

34. The first abstract, W. B. Castle and E. A. Locke, "Observations on the Etiological Relationship of Achylia Gastrica to Pernicious Anemia," *J. Clin. Invest.* 6 (1928): 2–3, is remarkable for the amount of information it contains.

35. C. C. Sturgis and R. Isaacs, "Clinical and Experimental Observations on the Treatment of Pernicious Anemia with Desiccated Stomach and with Liver Extract," *Ann. Intern. Med.* 5 (1931): 132. See also idem, "Desiccated Stomach in the Treatment of Pernicious Anemia," *J. Am. Med. Assoc.* 93 (1929): 747–49; and idem, "Treatment of Pernicious Anemia with Desiccated, Defatted Stomach," *Am. J. Med. Sci.* 180 (1930): 597–602.

Chapter 15

1. C. B. G. de Nancrède, "Influences and Conditions Which Should Be Taken into Account Before One Decides to Operate," in *American Practice of Surgery: A Complete System of the Science and Art of Surgery by Representatives of the United States and Canada,* ed. J. D. Bryant and A. H. Buck (New York: William Wood, 1908), 4:107–25.

2. Nancrede's genealogical table in the Bentley Historical Library shows that Charles's great-great-great-grandfather was simply Nicolas Guérard. His son, Jean Guérard de Noyon, was also known as Jean Guérard Chantrème de Guiscard, and he married Marie Josephe Mégret de St. Quentin. Their son was, again, only Jean Joseph Guérard, and he married plain Louise Francoise Gautier. Their son, Paul Joseph Guérard de Nancrède, married Hannah Dixie, and he became plain Joseph Nancrede in the United States. Now, Noyon, Guiscard, and St. Quentin are towns within a few kilometers of each other a bit northeast of Paris. Clearly, *de Noyon, de Guiscard,* and *de St. Quentin* are simply geographical identifications like John Adams *of Quincy* and not territorial designations of aristocratic families. *Nancrede* is not listed in *Gazetteer Number 83, Vol. 2, M–Z, U.S. Board of Geographical Names, France,* but it is a plausible conclusion that when Charles's grandfather called himself

"de Nancrede" he was taking the name of some manor or tiny village in the neighborhood of Noyon, Guiscard, and St. Quentin.

3. C. B. Nancrede, *Essentials of Anatomy and Manual of Practical Dissection*, 3d ed. (Philadelphia: W. B. Saunders, 1890). I have not seen the first edition, and none of the standard bibliographical references lists it. The text is in question-and-answer form.

4. W. W. Keen and J. W. White, eds., *An American Text-Book of Surgery for Practitioners and Students,* 4th ed. (Philadelphia: W. B. Saunders, 1904).

5. C. B. Nancrede, *Questions and Answers on the Essentials of Anatomy Prepared Especially for Students of Medicine* (Philadelphia: W. B. Saunders, 1888).

6. Topics include recurrent epithelioma, tumors of the salivary glands, pathology of the shoulder joint, fractures of the neck of the humerus, tumor of the scapula, fracture of the ankle joint, obstruction of the bowel, foreign bodies in the urethra, fracture of the base of the skull, surgery of the jaw, carcinoma of the breast, nerve suture, surgery of the brain, and appendectomy.

7. F. P. Henry and C. B. Nancrede, "Blood-Cell Counting: A Series of Observations with the Hématimètre of Mm. Hayem and Nachet, and Hæmacytometer of Dr. Gowers," *Boston Med. Surg. J.* 100 (1879): 499.

8. Nancrede's conservatism is amply illustrated and commented upon in M. M. Ravitch, *A Century of Surgery: The History of the American Surgical Association,* 2 vols. (Philadelphia: J. B. Lippincott, 1981). The book also illustrates Nancrede's habit of discussing most papers presented at meetings of the American Surgical Association: "Nancrede's four pages of Discussion on this subject, on which 'I have nothing especially new to offer,' bore witness to the accuracy of his statement" (1:64).

9. The quotation is in H. A. Kelly, ed., *A Cyclopedia of American Medical Biography* (Philadelphia: W. B. Saunders, 1912), 1:366. Nancrede's part in the struggle over listerism and asepsis is described in Ravitch's book, *Century of Surgery.*

10. C. B. Nancrede, *Lectures upon the Principles of Surgery; Delivered at the University of Michigan* (Philadelphia: W. B. Saunders, 1899).

11. W. S. Halsted, "Ligature and Suture Material," *J. Am. Med. Assoc.* 60 (1913): 1119–26. The history of the rubber gloves is in J. F. Mitchell, "The Introduction of Rubber Gloves for Use in Surgical Operations," *Ann. Surg.* 122 (1945): 902–4.

12. C. McBurney, "The Use of Rubber Gloves in Operative Surgery," *Ann. Surg.* 28 (1898): 108–19.

13. A. S. Warthin, R. Peterson, and A. H. Lloyd, "Charles Beylard Guérard de Nancrède, 1847–1921," *Mich. Alumnus* 27 (1921): 567–73.

14. R. H. Fitz, "Perforating Inflammation of the Vermiform Appendix; with Special Reference to Its Early Diagnosis and Treatment," *Trans. Assoc. Am. Physicians* 1 (1886): 107–35.

15. C. B. Nancrede, "The Operative Treatment of Jacksonian and Focal Epilepsy," *Ann. Surg.* 24 (1894): 122–30.

16. C. B. G. de Nancrède, "Should Cholecystitis and Cholelithiasis Be Any Longer Considered Medical Affections, and What Are the Usual Consequences of So Treating Them?" *Ann. Surg.* 47 (1908): 238.

17. Reuben Peterson Papers, Bentley Historical Library, University of Michigan.

18. C. B. Nancrede, "Total Excision of the Lower Jaw for Malignant Disease," *Ann. Surg.* 17 (1893): 295–98.

19. C. B. G. de Nancrède, "The End Results after Total Excision of the Scapula for Sarcoma," *Ann. Surg.* 50 (1909): 22. Warthin had advised against radical treatment.

20. Nancrede, "Total Excision of the Lower Jaw," 295.

21. The 1905 edition of the Cushny-Edmunds laboratory manual has no exercise on chloroform. The 1918 edition has exercises on the use of ether, chloroform, nitrous oxide, and ethyl chloride.

22. R. Peterson, "The Advisability of Making the Practical Administration of Anesthesia a Required Part of the Medical Course," *Surg. Gynecol. Obstet.* 8 (1909): 525–27.

23. F. A. Coller, in *The University of Michigan: An Encyclopedic Survey,* ed. W. B. Shaw (Ann Arbor: University of Michigan Press, 1951), 2:941–44.

24. Nancrede, *Principles of Surgery.*

25. C. B. G. de Nancrède, "Surgical Diseases, Certain Abnormities, and Wounds of the Face," *American Practice of Surgery,* ed. J. D. Bryant and A. H. Buck (New York: William Wood, 1908), 5:417–99. There is a photograph of the results obtained in a patient at the University Hospital after excision and reforming of the lower lip (494).

26. C. J. Lyons, "The History of Oral Surgery and Its Influence on the Profession of Dentistry," *Dent. Cosmos* 76 (1934): 27–40. The other three were Brophy and Gilmore of Chicago and Cryder of Philadelphia. There are some unsatisfactory sketches of Lyons's important career, one being D. H. Bellinger, "The Life and Achievements of Chalmers J. Lyons," *J. Oral Surg.* 2 (1944): 99–105.

27. I. D. Loree and R. W. Kraft, "Results after Prostatectomy," *J. Mich. State Med. Soc.* 15 (1916): 435–36.

28. C. L. Washburne, "Some Phases of the Infantile Paralysis Problem," *J. Mich. State Med. Soc.* 14 (1915): 181.

29. *Encyclopedic Survey,* 2:944.

Chapter 16

1. The word *evaporated* is from A. Lawrence Lowell's introduction to Cabot's *The Doctor's Bill* (New York: Columbia University Press, 1935), xv.

2. H. Cabot, "Medicine—A Profession or a Trade," *Boston Med. Surg. J.* 173 (1915): 687. Much of the preceding paragraph is a paraphrase of this address to a medical society (685–88).

3. H. Cabot, "A Contribution to the Study of Catgut as a Suture and Ligature Material," *Boston Med. Surg. J.* 146 (1902): 327–30; Cabot, "Anterior vs. Posterior Gastro-Enterostomy," *Boston Med. Surg. J.* 151 (1904): 325–26; Cabot and G. S. C. Badger, "The Interrelation of Medicine and Surgery in the Treatment of Gastric Ulcer," *Boston Med. Surg. J.* 151 (1904): 259–64; and Cabot and H. Binney, "Fractures of the Os Calcis and Astragulus," *Ann. Surg.* 45 (1907): 51–68.

4. Frederick A. Coller in *The University of Michigan: An Encyclopedic Survey,* ed. W. B. Shaw (Ann Arbor: University of Michigan Press, 1951), 2:945–50.

5. H. Cabot, "Errors in Diagnosis of Renal and Ureteral Calculus," *Surg. Gynecol. Obstet.* 21 (1915): 403–6.

6. One of many papers on the subject: H. Cabot, "Stone in the Kidney and Ureter. A Critical Review of 157 Cases," *J. Am. Med. Assoc.* 65 (1915): 1233–34.

7. J. R. Herman, "Bladder Stones," chap. 4 in *Urology, A View through the Retrospectroscope* (New York: Harper and Row, 1973), 41–52.

8. H. J. Bigelow, "Lithotrity by a Single Operation," *Am. J. Med. Sci.* 75 (1878): 117–34.

9. H. Cabot, ed., *Modern Urology in Original Contributions by American Authors,* 2 vols. (Philadelphia: Lea and Febiger, 1918). Cabot's own chapters are on stone in the bladder, foreign bodies in the bladder, and stone in the kidney and ureters.

10. H. Cabot, "Varix of Papilla of the Kidney as Cause of Persistent Hematuria," *Am. J. Med. Sci.* 137 (1909): 98–102.

11. H. Cabot, "Diagnosis of Tumors of the Bladder," *N. Y. Med. J.* 25 (1907): 1019–22.

12. H. Cabot, "The Diagnosis and Indications for Operation in Early Hydronephrosis," *J. Am. Med. Assoc.* 60 (1913): 16–20.

13. H. Cabot, "Some Observations upon Diverticulum of the Bladder," *Trans. Am. Assoc. Genito-Ur. Surg.* 7 (1913): 62–72; and the same paper in *Boston Med. Surg. J.* 172 (1915): 300–302.

14. H. Cabot, "Some Observations upon Total Extirpation of the Bladder for Cancer," *Trans. Am. Assoc. Genito-Ur. Surg.* 4 (1909): 125–33.

15. H. Cabot, "Treatment of Stricture of the Bulbar Portion of the Urethra by Resection Partial or Complete," *Boston Med. Surg. J.* 161 (1909): 848–50.

16. H. Cabot and L. T. Brown, "Treatment of Moveable Kidney with or without Infection, by Posture," *Boston Med. Surg. J.* 171 (1914): 369–73.

17. H. Cabot, "Suprapubic Prostatectomy," *Surg. Gynecol. Obstet.* 17 (1913): 213–17; and idem, "Factors Influencing the Mortality of Suprapubic Prostatectomy," ibid. 17 (1913): 689–92.

18. H. H. Young, "A New Procedure (Punch Operation) for Small Prostatic Bars and Contracture of the Prostatic Orifice," *J. Am. Med. Assoc.* 60 (1913): 253–57.

19. H. Cabot, "Subarachnoid (Spinal) Anesthesia," in *Surgery, Its Principles and Practice,* ed. W. W. Keen (Philadelphia: W. B. Saunders, 1912), 8:860–67.

20. L. G. Rowntree and J. T. Geraghty, "An Experimental and Clinical Study of the Fundamental Activity of the Kidneys by the Means of Phenolsulphonephthalein," *J. Pharmacol. Exp. Ther.* 1 (1910): 579–661.

21. H. Cabot and. E. L. Young, "Phenolsulphonephthalin as a Test of Renal Function," *Boston Med. Surg. J.* 165 (1911): 549–61.

22. R. H. Miller and H. Cabot, "The Effect of Anesthesia and Operation on the Kidney Function, as Shown by the Phenolsulphonphthalein Test," *Arch. Intern. Med.* 15 (1915): 369–91.

23. An example reporting 103 cases is E. G. Crabtree, "The End-Results of Seventy Cases of Renal Tuberculosis Treated by Nephrectomy," *Surg. Gynecol. Obstet.* 21 (1915): 669–79.

24. H. Cabot and E. G. Crabtree, "The Etiology and Pathology of Non-Tuberculous Renal Infections," *Surg. Gynecol. Obstet.* 23 (1916): 495–537.

25. H. Cabot, "Undergraduate Teaching of Surgery and Surgical Specialties," *Proc. Assoc. Am. Med. Coll.* 31 (1921): 44–60. This is a committee report, but Cabot published the same ideas elsewhere.

26. *Encyclopedic Survey,* 2:945.

27. H. Cabot, "The Development of Organized Clinical Teaching," *Colorado Med.* 22 (1925): 130–35.

28. H. Cabot, "A Plea for the Further Extension of Clinical Opportunity into Earlier Years of the Medical Course," *Bull. Assoc. Am. Med. Coll.* 2 (1927): 105, 107.

29. H. Cabot, "The Training of the Urologist," *N. Y. Med. J.* 95 (1912): 1077. See also idem, "Surgery and Surgical Specialties," *J. Am. Med. Assoc.* 76 (1921): 870–71.

30. H. Cabot and M. D. Giles, *Surgical Nursing* (Philadelphia: W. B. Saunders, 1931).

31. H. Cabot, "Avoiding Psychological Damage in the Care of Hospital Patients," *Mod. Hosp.* 17 (1921): 164–86.

32. This is clear from a pathetic letter, to be cited later, written by Dunstone to Dean Furstenberg on 27 October 1938.

33. H. Cabot and L. B. Davis, "A Preliminary Report on the Value of Ethylene as a General Anesthetic Based on the Study of 500 Cases," *J. Mich. State Med. Soc.* 23 (1924): 372–76.

34. H. Cabot and H. K. Ransom, "Ethylene as an Anesthetic for General Surgery," *Ann. Surg.* 86 (1927): 255–59.

35. H. Cabot and H. Lamb, "The Choice of Anesthetics with Particular Reference to the Protection of the Patient," *Ohio State Med. J.* 26 (1930): 998.

36. Y. Henderson and H. W. Haggard, "Hyperventilation of the Lungs as a Prophylactic Measure for Pneumonia," *J. Am. Med. Assoc.* 92 (1929): 434–36. This is a review with references.

37. H. Cabot and G. C. Adie, "Etiology of Cancer of the Stomach," *Ann. Surg.* 82 (1925): 86–108. The paper quotes Warthin's views.

38. H. Cabot, "The Department of Surgery," *Mich. Alumnus* 32 (1926): 516.

39. Cabot, "Development of Clinical Teaching," 135.

40. Letters from Cabot in the Medical School files, Bentley Historical Library, University of Michigan.

41. H. Cabot, "Address of the Dean at the Opening of the Medical School—University of Michigan," *J. Mich. State Med. Soc.* 20 (1921): 431–35.

42. H. Cabot, "Compulsory Health Insurance, State Medicine or What?" *Boston Med. Surg. J.* 182 (1920): 595–601. This is a very temperate account of the British and German health insurance schemes that Cabot thought too limited. Many large corporations had provided medical care approaching the ideal by properly paid, well-trained physicians, but Cabot objected on the grounds that the cost was passed on to the community in the heightened cost of production. He repeated his description of a hospital-based health center.

43. Cabot, *The Doctor's Bill*, ix. Although the book was published and perhaps written after Cabot left Ann Arbor, his earlier publications show he had been thinking along these lines for at least twenty years. Lay control of physicians' income was anathema to organized medicine at the time.

44. Minutes, February 1930, *Regents' Proceedings 1929–32*, 169.

45. The *Washtenaw Tribune* published an Extra on the evening of 7 February 1930, and the accounts in the *Ann Arbor News* and the *Detroit Free Press* are in their 8 February issues.

46. C. J. Tupper, who had been Dean Furstenberg's associate dean, gave a circumstantial account of Cabot's dismissal on the occasion of the dedication of the Furstenberg Study Center. I am grateful to him for sending me a copy of his manuscript. The gist of the story is that Cabot, after obtaining the approval of the surgeons, told President Ruthven that the faculty had approved his nominee for the new Department of Anesthesiology. When Cabot asked the faculty for retroactive approval of his communication to President Ruthven the faculty, led by Udo Wile, balked. A deputation of the faculty left the meeting to report to the president that the faculty had taken a vote of no confidence in the dean. It is difficult to reconcile the chronology of this story with documented events.

47. President Ruthven to Abraham Flexner, 24 March 1930, Bentley Historical Library, University of Michigan.

48. Shelby W. Wishart to Reuben Peterson, 11 February 1930, Reuben Peterson Papers, Bentley Historical Library, University of Michigan.

49. Reuben Peterson to Walter H. Sawyer, 4 March 1930, Reuben Peterson Papers, Bentley Historical Library, University of Michigan.

50. H. W. Davenport, *University of Michigan Surgeons, 1850–1970: Who They Were and What They Did*, Historical Center for the Health Sciences Monographs, no. 3 (Ann Arbor, 1993), 79.

51. H. J. S.[edden], "The Late Doctor Cabot," *Lancet* 2 (1945): 354.

52. There is a biographical sketch of Max Peet in F. A. Coller, "Max Minor Peet, 1885–1949," *Trans. Am. Surg. Assoc.* 67 (1949): 569–71. Coller described Peet's eminence as an ornithologist and his desire to shoot one of every species of American birds, and he said Peet had imagination, superb skill, and great daring. Peet was informal and kind, and "[h]e was sure of himself to a point where he had no jealousy of others" (571). Peet's body was cremated, and in an attempt to scatter the ashes over Michigan Eddy Kahn threw them out of his airplane as he was piloting it. They flew back in Kahn's face.

53. E. B. Krumbhaar, J. H. Musser Jr., and M. M. Peet, "The Relation of the Spleen to Blood Destruction and Regeneration and to Hemolytic Jaundice. XIV. Changes in the Blood following Diversion of the Splenic Blood from the Liver. A Control Study of the Effects of Splenectomy," *J. Exp. Med.* 23 (1916): 87–95.

54. O. H. P. Pepper and M. M. Peet, "The Resistance of Reticulated Erythrocytes," *Arch. Intern. Med.* 12 (1913): 81–89.

55. There is a biographical sketch of Frazier in I. S. Ravdin, A. W. Adson, and F. C. Grant, eds., *Surgery in Honor of Charles H. Frazier in Two Parts Comprising Contributions by His Former Students and Associates* (Philadelphia: J. B. Lippincott, 1935). Peet's chapter, "Glossopharyngeal Neuralgia," is on pp. 256–68.

56. C. H. Frazier, "Remarks upon the Surgical Aspects of Tumors of the Cerebellum," in C. K. Mills et al., eds., *Tumors of the Cerebellum* (New York: A. R.

Elliott Publishing Company, 1905), 39–85.

57. J. E. Sweet, M. M. Peet, and B. M. Hendrix, "High Intestinal Stasis," *Ann. Surg.* 63 (1916): 720–28.

58. C. H. Frazier and M. M. Peet, "Experimental Colonic Stasis," *Ann. Surg.* 63 (1916): 729–31.

59. M. M. Peet, "Indications for and Variations in the Technic of Eck Fistula," *Ann. Surg.* 60 (1914): 601–9.

60. C. H. Frazier and M. M. Peet, "Factors of Influence in the Origin and Circulation of the Cerebrospinal Fluid," *Am. J. Physiol.* 35 (1914): 268–82; idem, "The Action of Glandular Extracts on the Secretion of Cerebrospinal Fluid," ibid. 36 (1915): 464–87; and idem, "Influence of Diiodotyrosine and Iodothyrine on the Secretion of Cerebrospinal Fluid," ibid. 38 (1915): 93–97.

61. W. L. Finton and M. M. Peet, "An Experimental Study of the Use of Detached Omental Grafts in Intestinal Surgery," *Surg. Gynecol. Obstet.* 29 (1919): 281–87.

62. The solution of the problem derives from Cannon's demonstration of the law of denervation, and it is described in J. C. White, *The Autonomic Nervous System; Anatomy, Physiology, and Surgical Treatment* (New York: Macmillan, 1935). The second edition is White and R. H. Smithwick, 1941. That Peet made no contribution to the solution of the problem is demonstrated by his comment on Smithwick, "The Problem of Producing Complete and Lasting Sympathetic Denervation of the Upper Extremity by Preganglionic Section," *Ann. Surg.* 12 (1940): 1085–96, in which Peet said that he had visited Smithwick, seen him operate, and adopted his technique.

63. E. A. Kahn, *Journal of a Neurosurgeon* (Springfield, Ill.: C. C Thomas, 1972), 67. The relations with Elizabeth Crosby are dated on p. 83.

64. Peet's papers of this period include M. M. Peet, "Rational Preoperative Treatment with Special Reference to Purgation," *J. Am. Med. Assoc.* 71 (1918): 175–77; idem, "The Problem of Nutrition and a Satisfactory Method of Feeding in High Intestinal Fistulas," *Am. J. Med. Sci.* 158 (1919): 839–44; and idem, "Fracture of the Acetabulum with Intrapelvic Displacement of the Femoral Head," *Ann. Surg.* 70 (1919): 296–304.

65. W. A. Hoyt, "Resection of the Gasserian Ganglion for Trifacial Neuralgia Complicated with Facial Palsy," *J. Mich. State Med. Soc.* 14 (1915): 54–56.

66. C. H. Frazier, "Neuralgias of the Trigeminal Tract and Facial Neuralgias of Other Origin. Impressions Derived from a Survey of 555 Cases," *Am. Otol. Rhinol. Laryngol.* 30 (1921): 855–69.

67. M. M. Peet, "Tic Douloureux and Its Treatment with a Review of the Cases Operated upon at the University Hospital in 1917," *J. Mich. State Med. Soc.* 17 (1917): 91–98. The controversy with Camp is reported at the end of this paper.

68. M. M. Peet, "The Cranial Nerves," chap. 2 in *Practice of Surgery*, vol. 12, ed. D. D. Lewis (Hagerstown, Md.: W. F. Prior, 1954), 1–106. The section on glossopharyngeal nerves is in chapter 2, pp. 84–92.

69. M. M. Peet and E. A. Kahn, "Subdural Hematoma in Infants," *J. Am. Med. Assoc.* 98 (1932): 1851–56.

70. Kahn described his career and his many extramedical activities in his autobiography, *Journal of a Neurosurgeon*. See also J. A. Taren, "Edgar A. Kahn, M.D.," *Surg. Neurol.* 14 (1980): 401–3.

71. M. M. Peet, "The Control of Intractable Pain in the Lumbar Region, Pelvis and Lower Extremities, by Section of the Anterolateral Columns of the Spinal Cord (Chordotomy)," *Arch. Surg.* 13 (1926): 153–204. The paper contains a review of Frazier's cases.

72. M. M. Peet, E. A. Kahn, and S. S. Allen, "Bilateral Cervical Cordotomy for Relief of Chronic Infectious Arthritis," *J. Am. Med. Assoc.* 100 (1933): 488–89; Kahn, "Anterolateral Chordotomy for Intractable Pain," *J. Am. Med. Assoc.* 100 (1933): 1925–28; and Kahn and B. F. Barney, "Anterolateral Chordotomy for Intractable Pain of Tabes Dorsalis," *Arch. Neurol. Psychiatry* 38 (1937): 467–72.

73. E. A. Kahn, "The Treatment of Encapsulated Brain Abscess," *J. Am. Med. Assoc.* 108 (1937): 87–90.

74. E. A. Kahn, "The Treatment of Encapsulated Brain Abscess with Visualization by Colloidal Thorium Dioxide," *Univ. Hosp. Bull.* 4 (1938): 17–19.

75. E. A. Kahn, "Surgical Treatment of Pineal Tumor," *Arch. Neurol. Psychiatry* 38 (1937): 841.

76. Kahn, *Journal of a Neurosurgeon*, 40–60.

77. Ibid., 49.

78. Ibid., 51.

79. Ibid., 55. The parenthetical remark is Kahn's.

80. L. G. Rowntree and A. W. Adson, "Bilateral Lumbar Sympathetic Neurectomy in the Treatment of Malignant Hypertension," *J. Am. Med. Assoc.* 85 (1925): 959.

81. M. M. Peet, "Splanchnic Section for Hypertension: A Preliminary Report," *Univ. Hosp. Bull.* 1 (1935): 17–18.

82. Peet cited A. N. Richards's Beaumont Lecture ("Methods and Results of Direct Investigations of the Function of the Kidney," Beaumont Foundation Lectures, ser. no. 8 [Baltimore: Williams and Wilkins, 1929]), which he may have heard rather than the primary article, Richards and C. F. Schmidt, "A Description of the Glomerular Circulation in the Frog's Kidney and Observations Concerning the Action of Adrenalin and Various Other Substances upon It," *Am. J. Physiol.* 71 (1924): 178–208.

83. H. Goldblatt, J. Lynch, R. F. Hanzal, and W. W.

Summerville, "Studies on Experimental Hypertension. I. The Production of Persistent Elevation of Systolic Blood Pressure by Means of Renal Ischemia," *J. Exp. Med.* 59 (1934): 347–79.

84. Peet, "Splanchnic Section," 18.

85. Smithwick's operation and many of Peet's results are summarized in R. H. Smithwick, *Surgical Measures in Hypertension* (Springfield, Ill.: C. C Thomas, 1951).

86. S. Braden and E. A. Kahn, "The Surgical Treatment of Hypertension: Preliminary Report of Method of Study and Results in 264 Cases," *Yale J. Biol. Med.* 11 (1939): 449–58; M. M. Peet, W. W. Woods, and Braden, "The Surgical Treatment of Hypertension: Results in 350 Consecutive Cases Treated by Bilateral Supradiaphragmatic Splanchnicectomy and Lower Dorsal Sympathetic Ganglionectomy," *J. Am. Med. Assoc.* 115 (1940): 1875–85; Peet and E. M. Isberg, "The Surgical Treatment of Essential Hypertension," *J. Am. Med. Assoc.* 130 (1946): 467–73; and Peet, "Results of Bilateral Supradiaphragmatic Splanchnicectomy for Arterial Hypertension," *N. Engl. J. Med.* 236 (1947): 270–77.

87. F. B. Fralick and M. M. Peet, "Hypertensive Fundus Oculi after Resection of the Splanchnic Sympathetic Nerves. A Preliminary Report," *Arch. Ophthalmol.* 15 (1936): 840–46.

88. R. H. Freyberg and M. M. Peet, "The Effect on the Kidney of Bilateral Splanchnicectomy in Patients with Hypertension," *J. Clin. Invest.* 16 (1937): 49–65.

89. Peet, "Results of Bilateral Supradiaphragmatic Splanchnicectomy," 276.

90. Cameron Haight wrote two biographical sketches: "John Alexander, 1891–1954," *Trans. Am. Surg. Assoc.* 74 (1956): 485–87; and "John Alexander," in *The Surgical Management of Pulmonary Tuberculosis,* ed. J. D. Steele, John Alexander Monograph Series, no. 1 (Springfield, Ill.: C. C Thomas, 1957), x–xiii. The second contains a bibliography.

91. C. Lenormant, "La thoracoplastie extra-pleurale dans le traitement de la tuberculose pulmonaire. Indications et résultats," *J. Chir.* 22 (1923): 240–52.

92. L. Bérard, "Technique de la thoracoplastie extrapleurale dans la tuberculose pulmonaire," *J. Chir.* 22 (1923): 238.

93. C. Georg, "Some Experiments in Lung Surgery," *Trans. Clin. Soc. Univ. Mich.* 7 (1916): 46. Georg used the Meltzer technique of continuous intratracheal insufflation of anesthesia at twenty to twenty-five millimeters of mercury, released about six times a minute. Warthin found the lungs damaged by the anesthesia.

94. J. Alexander, "New Instrument for Subperiosteal Costectomy," *J. Am. Med. Assoc.* 83 (1924): 443.

95. J. Alexander, *The Surgery of Pulmonary Tuberculosis* (Philadelphia: Lea and Febiger, 1925). Chapters were published in four installments in *American Journal of the Medical Sciences* (168 [1924]: 177, 268–83, 412–36, and 574–96).

96. J. Alexander, "Reading and Writing for the Recumbent," *J. Am. Med. Assoc.* 86 (1926): 347.

97. The U.S. practice was not quite so stagnant as Alexander and Cabot implied. In 1924 Alexander published a paper in the *American Review of Tuberculosis* (10 [1924]: 27–34) suggesting that total paralysis of the hemidiaphragm might be useful in treatment of patients with early tuberculosis. His paper was immediately preceded by three papers by U.S. surgeons reporting thoracoplasties.

98. Alexander, *Surgery,* 44.

99. Ibid., 58.

100. Ibid., 19 n. 83.

101. J. Alexander, "The Revolution in the Management of Phthisis," *Surg. Gynecol. Obstet.* 56 (1933): 708–10.

102. J. Alexander, *The Collapse Therapy of Pulmonary Tuberculosis* (Springfield, Ill.: C. C Thomas, 1937).

103. J. Alexander, "Operative Technique of Phrenic Nerve Interruption," *Surg. Gynecol. Obstet.* 49 (1929): 372. See also L. W. Nehil and Alexander, "An Estimate of the Value of Phrenic Nerve Interruption for Phthisis Based on 654 Cases," *J. Thorac. Surg.* 2 (1933): 549–72.

104. J. Alexander, "Temporary Phrenic Nerve Paralysis. Its Advantages over Permanent Paralysis in the Treatment of Phthisis," *J. Am. Med. Assoc.* 102 (1934): 1552.

105. J. Alexander, "Multiple Intercostal Neurectomy for Pulmonary Tuberculosis," *Am. Rev. Tuberc.* 20 (1929): 637–84.

106. J. Alexander, "The Training of a Surgeon Who Expects to Specialize in Thoracic Surgery," *J. Thorac. Surg.* 5 (1936): 579.

107. Technically Alexander's trainees were not residents, but at that time it was the most convenient term for them and others in specialty training.

108. Alexander, "Training of a Surgeon," 581.

109. Alexander's book of 1925, *The Surgery of Pulmonary Tuberculosis,* contains a historical survey. Other examples are J. Alexander, "Some Dramatic Thoracic Operations," *J. Thorac. Surg.* 5 (1935): 1–17; and idem, "Fifty Years of Thoracic Surgery," *Am. J. Surg.* 51 (1941): 217–24.

110. J. Alexander, "Pneumonectomy and Lobectomy [editorial]," *Surg. Gynecol. Obstet.* 60 (1935): 1146; idem, "Total Pulmonary Lobectomy: A Simple and Effective Two Stage Technique," ibid. 56 (1933): 658–73.

111. J. Alexander, "Present Status of Thoracic Surgery," *P. Med. J.* 34 (1930): 302.

112. J. Alexander and W. W. Buckingham, "Treatment of Nontuberculous Suppurative Pneumonitis, Abscess

and Bronchiectasis," *J. Am. Med. Assoc.* 95 (1930): 1483; Alexander, "Abscess of the Lung," *J. Mich. State Med. Soc.* 32 (1933): 637–41; and Alexander, "Abscess of the Lung," *Trans. Am. Laryngol. Assoc.* 58 (1936): 262–72.

113. E. A. Graham, "Cautery Pneumonectomy for Chronic Suppuration of the Lung: A Report of Twenty Cases," *Arch. Surg.* 10 (1925): 397–98.

114. Alexander, "Pneumonectomy," 1147; and idem, "Total Pulmonary Lobectomy," 658.

115. One of Alexander's young men invented a mechanical device for pulling a ligature tight around the hilum: D. Carr, "Automatic Hilar Ligature for Lobectomy," *J. Thorac. Surg.* 4 (1935): 327–28.

116. R. Nissen, "Exstirpation eines ganzen Lungenflügels," *Zentralbl. Chir.* 58 (1931): 3003–6. Nissen published two useful and well-illustrated accounts of the history of thoracic surgery: Nissen, *Erlebtes aus der Thoraxchirurgie* (Stuttgart: Georg Thieme Verlag, 1955); and Nissen and R. H. L. Wilson, *Pages in the History of Chest Surgery* (Springfield, Ill.: C. C Thomas, 1960).

117. C. Haight, "Total Removal of Left Lung for Bronchiectasis," *Surg. Gynecol. Obstet.* 58 (1934): 768–80.

118. E. Windsberg, "Pneumonectomy: Successful Result in a Case of Bronchiectasis," *R. I. Med. J.* 17 (1934): 163–67.

119. E. Windsberg, "Total Removal of the Right Lung for Bronchiectasis," *J. Thorac. Surg.* 4 (1935): 231–35.

120. Haight, "Total Removal," 768.

121. C. Haight, "Congenital Atresia of the Esophagus with Tracheoesophageal Fistula," *Ann. Surg.* 120 (1944): 623–52. Four such patients had been admitted in 1935–38, but Haight did not attempt an operation until 1939.

122. J. Alexander, "Observations on Total Pulmonary Lobectomy and Pneumonectomy," *Ann. Surg.* 101 (1935): 393–406, describes the advantages of a one-stage operation for carcinoma and a two-stage one for abscess. C. Haight, "Complementary Anterior Thoracoplasty for Pulmonary Tuberculosis. A Technic Employing Parasternal Division of the Costal Cartilages," *J. Thorac. Surg.* 5 (1936): 453–70, describes Haight's experience in fifty cases.

123. J. Alexander, "Diagnosis, Operability of Intrathoracic Neoplasms," *Surg. Gynecol. Obstet.* 73 (1941): 554–55. Alexander said the same thing in "Observations on Intrathoracic Neoplasms," *Ann. Surg.* 114 (1941): 734–50; and in idem, "Circumscribed Intrathoracic Neoplasms," *J. Am. Med. Assoc.* 119 (1942): 395–97.

124. Alexander did resect a nonsyphilitic thoracic aneurysm in a young college student: Alexander and F. X. Byron, "Aortectomy for Thoracic Aneurysm," *J. Am. Med. Assoc.* 126 (1944): 1139–45. Those were the days before Teflon sleeves, and Alexander had to rely on the boy's collateral circulation after he divided the aorta just inferior to the left subclavian artery. Alexander also did a single closed mitral valve commissurotomy with Herbert Sloan as his assistant. The patient was operated on again twenty-eight years later. See J. O. Just Viera, "Mitral Valve Commissurotomy by John Alexander: Repeat Surgery 28 Years Later," *Bol. Asoc. Med. Puerto Rico* 73 (1981): 56–58.

125. R. M. Nesbit, Comment, *J. Am. Med. Assoc.* 97 (1931): 1776.

126. T. M. Davis, "Prostate Operation; Prospects of the Patient with Prostatic Disease in Prostatectomy vs. Resection," *J. Am. Med. Assoc.* 97 (1931): 1679.

127. R. M. Nesbit, *Transurethral Prostatectomy* (Springfield, Ill.: C. C Thomas, 1943).

128. H. Cushing, "Electro-Surgery as an Aid to the Removal of Intracranial Tumors; With a Preliminary Note on a New Surgical-Current Generator by W. T. Bovie," *Surg. Gynecol. Obstet.* 47 (1928): 752.

129. R. M. Nesbit, *Your Prostate Gland; Letters from a Surgeon to His Father* (Springfield, Ill.: C. C Thomas, 1950). See also Nesbit, *Prostatabesvær; Brev fra en kirurg til hans far* (Oslo: H. Aschehoug [W. Nygaard], 1960).

130. J. R. Herman, *Urology: A View through the Retrospectroscope* (New York: Harper and Row, 1973), 128.

131. R. M. Nesbit, "A Modification of the Stern-McCarthy Resectoscope Permitting Third Dimensional Perception during Transurethral Prostatectomy," *J. Urol.* 41 (1939): 646–48.

132. Nesbit, *Transurethral Prostatectomy*, 23.

133. R. M. Nesbit, "Transurethral Prostatic Resection: An Evaluation Based upon the Study of Four Hundred Cases," *Urol. Cutaneous Rev.* 38 (1934): 605–10.

134. R. M. Nesbit and K. B. Conger, "Studies of Blood Loss during Transurethral Prostatic Resection," *J. Urol.* 46 (1941): 713–17.

135. E. Davis and R. M. Nesbit, "Comparison of Late Functional Results in Perineal Prostatectomy and Transurethral Resection," *Trans. Am. Assoc. Genito-Ur. Surg.* 33 (1940): 254. Davis, a Nebraska surgeon who did the perineal operations, and Nesbit, who did the transurethral ones, compared results of their last 100 operations. There were essentially no differences.

136. R. M. Nesbit, "The Limitations of Transurethral Prostatectomy," *J. Mich. State Med. Soc.* 38 (1939): 770.

137. Discussion (486) after R. M. Nesbit, "The Treatment of Prostatic Obstruction," *N. Engl. J. Med.* 223 (1940): 481–85.

138. F. E. B. Foley, "The Present Status of Transurethral

Resectionists, Competent or Otherwise," *J. Urol.* 43 (1940): 569.

139. But the word is in medical dictionaries.

140. J. Lapides, ed., *Fundamentals of Urology* (Philadelphia: W. B. Saunders, 1976).

141. R. M. Nesbit, *Fundamentals of Urology* [Ann Arbor: Edwards Brothers, 1942]. The fourth edition is Nesbit, J. Lapides, and W. C. Baum, *Fundamentals of Urology* (Ann Arbor: J. W. Edwards, 1953).

142. F. C. McClellan, *The Neurogenic Bladder* (Springfield, Ill.: C. C Thomas, 1939); R. M. Nesbit and W. G. Gordon, "The Neurogenic Bladder," *P. Med. J.* 43 (1940): 1261–68; Nesbit and Gordon, "The Management of the Urinary Bladder in Traumatic Lesions of the Spinal Cord and Cauda Equina," *Surg. Gynecol. Obstet.* 72 (1941): 328–31; and Nesbit and Gordon, "The Surgical Treatment of the Autonomous Neurogenic Bladder," *J. Am. Med. Assoc.* 117 (1941): 1935–36.

143. D. K. Rose, "Cystometric Bladder Pressure Determinations: Their Clinical Importance," *J. Urol.* 17 (1927): 487–501.

144. L. G. Lewis, "A New Clinical Recording Cystometer," *J. Urol.* 41 (1939): 638–39. Rose (*J. Am. Med. Assoc.* 88 [1927]: 151–56) described a cystometer in which fluid was measured as it was delivered as well as pressure achieved.

145. There is an introduction to the problem in A. L. King and A. G. Lawton, "Elasticity of Body Tissues," in *Medical Physics,* ed. O. Glasser (Chicago: Year Book Publishers, [1950]), 2:303–16.

146. There is a summary in McClellan, *Neurogenic Bladder.*

147. R. M. Nesbit and F. C. McClellan, "Sympathectomy for the Relief of Vesical Spasm and Pain Resulting from Intractable Bladder Infections," *Surg. Gynecol. Obstet.* 68 (1939): 540–46. The innervation of the sphincter is discussed in D. Denny-Brown, "Nervous Disturbances of the Vesical Sphincter," *N. Engl. J. Med.* 215 (1936): 647–50.

148. R. M. Nesbit and W. G. Gordon, "The Uninhibited Neurogenic Bladder. A Clinical Syndrome with Report of Twenty-Five Cases," *Trans. Am. Assoc. Genito-Ur. Surg.* 32 (1939): 213–24.

149. There is a biographical sketch of Coller containing many personal details in G. C. Adie, "Frederick Amasa Coller—Surgeon," *Am. Surg.* 154, suppl. (1961): 18–24. The accompanying bibliography has many errors in volume number and pagination. References in Coller's own papers are not to be trusted implicitly. Another appreciation is P. D. Wilson, "Frederick Amasa Coller. 1887–1964," *Trans. Am. Surg. Assoc.* 83 (1965): 481–87. There is a book about Coller prepared for the Coller-Penberthy Society that is full of ludicrous errors even when it quotes

me. My partially annotated copy is in the Rare Book Room of the Taubman Medical Library.

150. J. F. McClendon, *Iodine and the Incidence of Goiter* (Minneapolis: University of Minnesota Press, 1939).

151. F. A. Coller, "The Inevitable Damage Consequent upon Goiter," *Boston Med. Surg. J.* 193 (1925): 545–50; and Coller and E. B. Potter, "The End-Results of Thyroidectomy," *Ann. Surg.* 94 (1931): 568–81.

152. F. A. Coller and H. B. Barker, "Endemic Goiter, a Precancerous Lesion," *J. Mich. State Med. Soc.* 24 (1925): 413–16; W. M. Simpson, "Clinical and Pathological Study of Fifty-Five Neoplasms of the Thyroid Gland," *Ann. Clin. Med.* 4 (1926): 643–67; and Coller, "Adenoma and Cancer of the Thyroid," *J. Am. Med. Assoc.* 92 (1929): 457–62.

153. F. A. Coller and R. D. Arn, "Thyroidectomy for Goiter without Hyperthyroidism: Post Operative Results in Adenomatous Goiters with Normal and Hypofunction," *West. J. Surg. Obstet. Gynecol.* 39 (1931): 505.

154. Huggins later won the Nobel Prize (in 1966) for his discovery of the endocrine-induced regression of prostate and breast cancer.

155. F. A. Coller and A. M. Boyden, "The Development of the Technique of Thyroidectomy; Presentation of the Method Used in University Hospital," *Surg. Gynecol. Obstet.* 65 (1937): 495–504. The paper is illustrated with nineteen lucid drawings by Jean Young, the Michigan medical illustrator at the time.

156. Coller and Potter, "End-Results of Thyroidectomy."

157. W. G. Maddock, S. Pedersen, and F. A. Coller, "Studies of the Blood Chemistry in Thyroid Crisis," *J. Am. Med. Assoc.* 109 (1937): 2130–35.

158. H. B. Barker, "The Injection of Absolute Alcohol into the Thyroid Gland," *Arch. Surg.* 11 (1925): 160–99.

159. F. A. Coller and H. B. Barker, "Injection of Absolute Alcohol in the Treatment of Hyperthyroidism," *Arch. Surg.* 15 (1927): 918–35.

160. F. A. Coller, "The Use of Iodine in the Treatment of Goiter," *Ann. Clin. Med.* 5 (1926): 92; and Coller and E. B. Potter, "Reaction to Iodine of Goiters from a Goiter Area," *Am. J. Surg.,* n.s., 6 (1929): 609–15.

161. F. A. Coller and C. C. McRae, "Observations on Acute Appendicitis: Factors Influencing Mortality," *J. Mich. State Med. Soc.* 30 (1931): 319–26.

162. F. A. Coller and E. B. Potter, "The Treatment of Peritonitis Associated with Appendicitis," *J. Am. Med. Assoc.* 103 (1934): 1753–58.

163. E. B. Potter and F. A. Coller, "The Treatment of Peritonitis Associated with Appendicitis," *J. Mich. State Med. Soc.* 32 (1933): 573–76. This approach

disappeared for fifty years but has recently returned to use.

164. A. J. Ochsner, "The Cause of Diffuse Peritonitis Complicating Appendicitis and Its Prevention," *Am. J. Surg. Gynecol.* 15 (1902): 84–86.

165. The numerous papers end in B. Steinberg and H. Goldblatt, "Protection of Peritoneum against Infection," *Surg. Gynecol. Obstet.* 57 (1933): 15–20.

166. E. B. Potter and F. A. Coller, "Intraperitoneal Vaccination in Surgery of the Colon," *Ann. Surg.* 101 (1935): 886–90.

167. F. A. Coller and S. Rife, "Immunization of the Peritoneum," *Am. J. Surg.,* n.s., 46 (1939): 61–67.

168. H. C. Jackson and F. A. Coller, "The Use of Sulfanilamide in the Peritoneum: Experimental and Clinical Observations," *J. Am. Med. Assoc.* 118 (1942): 194–99.

169. C. E. Badgley, "The Articular Facets in Relation to Low-Back Pain and Sciatic Radiation," *J. Bone Jt. Surg.* 23 (1941): 481–96.

170. Comment by T. A. Willis (466–67) discussing F. J. Hodges and C. E. Badgley, "Clinical and Roentgenological Study of Low Back Pain with Sciatic Radiation. B. Roentgenological Aspects," *Am. J. Roentgenol.* 37 (1937): 461–66.

171. Introductory remarks to the Carl Badgley Lecture given in Ann Arbor on 22 October 1963 by Sir Herbert Seddon, as quoted in the *University of Michigan Medical Center Journal* 31 (1965): 46.

Chapter 17

1. F. A. Coller and L. Yglesias, "Infections of the Lip and Face," *Surg. Gynecol. Obstet.* 60 (1935): 277–88; and idem, "The Relation of the Spread of Infection to Fascial Planes in the Neck and Thorax," *Surgery* 1 (1937): 323–37. See chapter 23 in this volume for A. C. Furstenberg's part in the work described.

2. F. A. Coller and H. K. Ransom, "The One Stage Procedure of the Treatment of Carcinoma of the Rectum," *Ann. Surg.* 104 (1936): 636–45. A later paper, idem, "Carcinoma of the Rectum. Conclusions Based on 12 Years' Experience with Combined Abdominoperineal Resection," *Surg. Gynecol. Obstet.* 78 (1944): 304–15, describes results of an additional 274 one-stage operations performed between 1936 and 1942.

3. W. E. Miles, "A Method of Performing Abdomino-Perineal Excision for Carcinoma of the Rectum and of the Terminal Portion of the Pelvic Colon," *Lancet* 2 (1908): 1812–13.

4. H. K. Ransom and F. A. Coller, "Intestinal Fistula," *J. Mich. State Med. Soc.* 34 (1935): 281–88.

5. A. M. Boyden, F. A. Coller, and J. C. Bugher, "Riedel's Struma," *West. J. Surg. Obstet. Gynecol.* 43 (1935): 547–63.

6. H. Pinkus, "The Isolation of Pure Strains of Cells from Human Tumors. I. Selection of Specimens and Technic," *Am. J. Cancer* 26 (1936): 521–28; idem, "The Isolation of Pure Strains of Cells from Human Tumors. II. Growth Characteristics of Sarcoma and Two Brain Tumors in Tissue Culture; Conclusions," ibid. 29 (1937): 25–46.

7. H. Pinkus, W. G. Maddock, and F. A. Coller, "Clinical and Experimental Observations on Parathyroid Transplants," *Trans. Am. Assoc. Stud. Goiter* (1937): 65–70.

8. C. F. List and M. M. Peet, "Sweat Secretions in Man. I. Sweating Responses in Normal Persons," *Arch. Neurol. Psychiatry* 39 (1938): 1230.

9. The last paper in the series is C. F. List and M. M. Peet, "Sweat Secretion in Man. V. Disturbances of Sweat Secretion with Lesions of the Pons, Medulla and Cervical Portion of the Cord," *Arch. Neurol. Psychiatry* 42 (1939): 1098–127.

10. For example: V. C. Johnson and C. F. List, "Ventriculographic Localization of Intracranial Tumors. III. Tumors of the Cerebellum and Fourth Ventricle," *Am. J. Roentgenol. Radium Ther.* 43 (1940): 346–55.

11. The financial arrangements and the problems of dealing with both pay and charity patients are described by H. A. Haynes, "The University Hospital, University of Michigan," in *Methods and Problems of Medical Education,* 18th ser. (New York: Rockefeller Foundation, 1930), 59–74.

12. Work done for surgeons is described in R. L. Kahn, "Department of Clinical Laboratories, University of Michigan Hospital," in *Methods and Problems of Medical Education,* 18th ser. (New York: Rockefeller Foundation, 1930), 75–82.

13. G. C. Adie, "Frederick Amasa Coller—Surgeon," *Ann. Surg.* 154, suppl. (1961): 18–24.

14. F. A. Coller and F. L. Troost, "Glucose Tolerance and Hepatic Damage," *Ann. Surg.* 90 (1929): 781–93.

15. F. A. Coller and H. Brinkman, "Studies on the Reaction of the Peritoneum to Trauma and Infection," *Ann. Surg.* 109 (1939): 942–54.

16. F. A. Coller and P. L. Marsh, "Lesions of the Extremities Associated with Diabetes Mellitus," *J. Am. Med. Assoc.* 85 (1925): 168–71.

17. J. J. Morton and W. J. M. Scott, "The Measurement of Sympathetic Vasoconstrictor Activity in the Lower Extremities," *J. Clin. Invest.* 9 (1930): 235–46; Morton and Scott, "Methods for Estimating the Degree of Sympathetic Vasoconstriction in Peripheral Vascular Disease," *N. Engl. J. Med.* 204 (1931): 955–62; and Scott and Morton, "Sympathetic Activity in Cer-

...aseases, Especially Those of the Peripheral Circulation," *Arch. Intern. Med.* 48 (1931): 1065–7.

F. A. Coller and W. G. Maddock, "The Differentiation of Spastic from Organic Peripheral Vascular Occlusion by the Skin-Temperature Response to High Environmental Temperature," *Ann. Surg.* 96 (1932): 719–32. Maddock and Coller, "The Rôle of the Extremities in the Dissipation of Heat," *Am. J. Physiol.* 106 (1933): 589–96, contains some of the control data previously published in the first paper cited and some additional observations correlating basal metabolic rate with skin temperature. Coller and Maddock, "The Function of Peripheral Vasoconstriction," *Ann. Surg.* 100 (1934): 983–92, again contains data published elsewhere and in a note (987) states that Thomas Lewis and George W. Pickering (in "Vasodilation in the Limbs in Response to Warming the Body," *Heart* 16 [1931–32]: 33–51) had done similar experimental warming of their subjects [only after Coller and Maddock had completed the work described in the first reference].

19. L. Buerger, *The Circulatory Disturbances of the Extremities Including Gangrene, Vasomotor and Trophic Disorders* (Philadelphia: W. B. Saunders, 1924).

20. J. W. Bruce, J. R. Miller, and D. R. Hooker, "The Effect of Smoking upon the Blood Pressure and upon the Volume of the Hand," *Am. J. Physiol.* 24 (1909): 104–16.

21. W. G. Maddock and F. A. Coller, "Peripheral Vaso-Constriction by Tobacco Demonstrated by Skin Temperature Changes," *Proc. Soc. Exp. Biol. Med.* 29 (1931): 487–88; and idem, "Peripheral Vasoconstriction by Tobacco and Its Relation to Thrombo-Angiitis Obliterans," *Ann. Surg.* 98 (1933): 70–81. An interesting example of multiple publication of data is C. A. Moyer and Maddock, "Peripheral Vasospasm from Tobacco," *Arch. Surg.* 40 (1940): 277–85, which contains three of the figures and much of the text of the second paper cited here.

22. L. Buerger, "Thrombo-Angiitis Obliterans: A Study of the Vascular Lesions Leading to Presenile Spontaneous Gangrene," *Am. J. Med. Sci.* 136 (1908): 567–80.

23. W. G. Maddock, R. L. Malcolm, and F. A. Coller, "Thrombo-Angiitis Obliterans and Tobacco: The Influence of Sex, Race, and Skin Sensitivity to Tobacco on Cardiovascular Responses to Smoking," *Am. Heart J.* 12 (1936): 46–52.

24. J. C. DaCosta, *Modern Surgery, General and Operative* (Philadelphia: W. B. Saunders, 1919). The book also contains two brief paragraphs on acidosis and alkalosis.

25. The story is told by G. C. Adie, "Frederick Amasa

Coller—Surgeon," 19, and in Coller's lecture notes in the Bentley Historical Library, University of Michigan.

26. Coller gave Newburgh adequate credit by citing many of Newburgh's papers. The major papers on water balance are F. A. Coller and W. G. Maddock, "Dehydration Attendant on Surgical Operations," *J. Am. Med. Assoc.* 99 (1932): 875–80; Coller, "Some Important Factors of Postoperative Treatment," *J. Mich. State Med. Soc.* 32 (1933): 211–14; Coller and Maddock, "Water Balance in Patients with Hyperthyroidism," *West. J. Surg. Obstet. Gynecol.* 41 (1933): 438–52; Coller and Maddock, "Water Requirements of Surgical Patients," *Ann. Surg.* 98 (1933): 952–60; and Coller and Maddock, "Studies in Water Requirements of Surgical Patients," *Anesth. Analg.* 14 (1935): 140–44. Coller, "Studies in Water Balance, Dehydration and the Administration of Parenteral Fluids," *Minn. Med.* 19 (1936): 490–94, is a good example of Coller's many talks to medical societies summarizing his ideas and giving practical advice. All quotations in the section on water balance are from these papers.

27. F. A. Coller and W. G. Maddock, "A Study of Dehydration in Humans," *Ann. Surg.* 102 (1935): 947–60.

28. Coller and Maddock, "Dehydration," 880.

29. Coller and Maddock, "A Study of Dehydration," 947.

30. S. Pedersen, W. G. Maddock, and F. A. Coller, "Serum Sodium in Relation to Liver Damage and Hyperthyroidism," *Proc. Soc. Exp. Biol. Med.* 36 (1937): 491–94. Pedersen also measured serum potassium (Pedersen, Maddock, and S. Winslow, "Serum Potassium in Hyperthyroidism," *J. Lab. Clin. Med.* 23 [1938]: 1123–27), and he found the normal range in seven control subjects to be 20.3–22.2 milligrams percent. That is 4.8 to 5.3 milliequivalents per liter, which is much better than most others could do before the advent of flame photometry.

31. V. S. Dick, W. G. Maddock, and F. A. Coller, "Sodium Chloride Content of Gastro-Intestinal Secretions," *Proc. Soc. Exp. Biol. Med.* 37 (1937): 318–20.

32. R. M. Bartlett et al., "Quantitative Studies on the Replacement of Body Chlorides," *Proc. Soc. Exp. Biol. Med.* 38 (1938): 89–92.

33. R. M. Bartlett, D. L. C. Bingham, and S. Pedersen, "Salt Balance in Surgical Patients," parts 1 and 2, *Surgery* 4 (1938): 441–61, 614–35.

34. Ibid., 441.

35. F. A. Coller, "Acidosis and Alkalosis," in *A Textbook of Surgery by American Authors,* ed. F. Christopher (Philadelphia: W. B. Saunders Company, 1936), 1554–57.

36. Bartlett, Bingham, and Pedersen, "Salt Balance," 616.

37. F. A. Coller et al., "The Replacement of Sodium Chloride in Surgical Patients," *Ann. Surg.* 108 (1938): 769–80.

38. F. A. Coller et al., "The Replacement of Sodium Chloride in Surgical Patients," *Trans. Am. Surg. Assoc.* 56 (1938): 305–16.

Chapter 18

1. A sympathetic view of Dunster is given in R. Peterson, "Edward Swift Dunster, A.M., M.D.: A Biographical Sketch," *Physician Surg.* 27 (1905): 145–56.

2. J. N. Martin, "Tyrotoxicon Poisoning," *Boston Med. Surg. J.* 121 (1889): 512. This is a one-page case report.

3. These data and much else are drawn from Reuben Peterson's article, "Obstetrics and Gynecology," in *The University of Michigan: An Encyclopedic Survey,* ed. W. B. Shaw (Ann Arbor: University of Michigan Press, 1951), 2:858–75. The article is much more than the usual list of names and dates.

4. J. N. Martin, "The Female Perineum," *Trans. Mich. State Med. Soc.* 13 (1889): 33–38.

5. J. N. Martin, "Suffering from Ovarian Trouble, with Illustrative Cases," *Trans. Mich. State Med. Soc.* 15 (1891): 275–88.

6. J. G. Lynds, "The Care of Cases after Labor," *Trans. Mich. State Med. Soc.* 20 (1896): 552–59.

7. J. N. Martin, "Report of Ten Consecutive Laparotomies in Three Months, with Remarks upon the Same," *Trans. Mich. State Med. Soc.* 16 (1892): 305–32.

8. R. Peterson, "A Review of Twenty-Five Consecutive Cases of Abdominal Section," *Trans. Mich. State Med. Soc.* 16 (1892): 364–84.

9. J. N. Martin, "Treatment of Pus in the Pelvis by Abdominal Section; with Hysterectomy," *Trans. Mich. State Med. Soc.* 20 (1896): 616–24.

10. R. Peterson, "Treatment of Pelvic Suppuration by Abdominal Section without Hysterectomy," *Trans. Mich. State Med. Soc.* 20 (1896): 625–31.

11. R. Peterson, "The Treatment of Pus in the Pelvis by Vaginal Incision," *Physician Surg.* 20 (1898): 5–8.

12. R. Peterson, "Suggestions to the Trained Nurse," *Physician Surg.* 31 (1909): 342–47. Peterson described his debt to Boston nurses in this address delivered at the graduation exercises of the Training School for Nurses of the University of Michigan.

13. R. Peterson, "The Need of More Medical Reference-Libraries, and the Way in Which They Can Be Established," *Am. Medico-Surg. Bull.* 8 (1895): 1100–1103.

14. The nature of the polyclinic schools is described in S. J. Peitzman, " 'Thoroughly Practical': America's Polyclinic Medical Schools," *Bull. Hist. Med.* 54 (1980): 166–87.

15. R. Peterson, "Anastomosis of the Ureters with the Intestine," *Am. J. Obstet.* 42 (1900): 95–99. Peterson published at least four papers with the same title.

16. An example: R. Peterson, "Consideration of the Technique of the Radical Abdominal Operation for Uterine Cancer Based upon an Experience with Forty-Four Cases," *Surg. Gynecol. Obstet.* 12 (1911): 152–58, contains ten drawings by E. P. Billings. Many in his style are not signed or are initialed "E.P.B." Billings went into practice in Grand Rapids.

17. J. G. Van Zwaluwenburg and R. Peterson, "Pneumoperitoneum of the Pelvis: Gynecological Studies—A Preliminary Report," *Am. J. Roentgenol.* 8 (1921): 12–19. This paper is in the first person singular, and Peterson's name was obviously tacked on, probably because he referred the patient.

18. R. Peterson, "Suspension of the Retrodisplaced Uterus by the Utero-Ovarian Ligaments. With a Report of Seventeen Cases," *Am. J. Obstet.* 31 (1895): 832–42; and H. A. Kelly, "On Hysterorrhaphy," *Johns Hopkins Hosp. Bull.* 1 (1890): 17–19.

19. R. Peterson, "The Treatment of Retrodisplacements of the Uterus," *Physician Surg.* 24 (1902): 103.

20. R. Peterson, "Two Cases of Cesarean Section following Ventrosuspension of the Uterus," *Physician Surg.* 29 (1907): 529–34.

21. R. Peterson, "A Consideration of Vaginal Cesarean Section in the Treatment of Eclampsia Based upon a Study of Five Hundred and Thirty Published and Unpublished Cases," *Am. J. Obstet.* 64 (1911): 1–56.

22. R. Peterson, "Gall-Stones during the Course of 1,066 Abdominal Sections for Pelvic Disease," *Surg. Gynecol. Obstet.* 20 (1915): 284–91.

23. H. W. Davenport, *Doctor Dock: Teaching and Learning Medicine at the Turn of the Century* (New Brunswick, N.J.: Rutgers University Press, 1987), 183.

24. R. Peterson, "Substitution of the Anal for the Vesical Sphincter in Certain Cases of Inoperable Vesicovaginal Fistulæ," *Surg. Gynecol. Obstet.* 25 (1917): 391–402.

25. R. Peterson, "Tetanus Developing Twelve Days after Shortening of the Round Ligaments—Recovery," *J. Am. Med. Assoc.* 54 (1910): 108.

26. V. C. Vaughan, "The Michigan State Medical Society," *J. Lab. Clin. Med.* 15 (1930): 927.

27. The secretary's resignation in 1908 is gently treated in the *Encyclopedic Survey,* 1:271–72. Accounts in the local papers are more lurid.

28. R. Peterson, *A Manual for a Demonstration Course in Obstetrics* (Ann Arbor, Mich.: Edwards Brothers, 1929). The second and third editions were in 1937 and 1943, the latter with Miller as coauthor.

29. R. Peterson, ed., *The Practice of Obstetrics* (Philadelphia: Lea Brothers, 1907). The ten contributors include G. Carl Huber and Aldred Scott Warthin.

30. H. H. Cummings, "A Review of the Obstetric Work of the University Hospital Maternity for the Year Ending July 1, 1912," *Physician Surg.* 34 (1912): 510–15.

31. D. M. Cowie, "A Graphic Chart Method of Studying and Teaching the Principles of Infant Feeding," *Am. J. Dis. Child.* 4 (1912): 360–77.

32. R. Peterson and N. F. Miller, "Thymus of New-Born and Its Significance to the Obstetrician," *J. Am. Med. Assoc.* 83 (1924): 234–38.

33. R. Peterson, "Under What Circumstances Is Craniotomy on the Living Child Justifiable?" *J. Mich. State Med. Soc.* 14 (1915): 319–24.

34. Ibid., 319.

35. Ibid., 320.

36. R. Peterson, "Points of Contact between Internal Medicine and Obstetrics and Gynecology," *Ann. Clin. Med.* 5 (1926–27): 114.

37. The manuscript is in the Reuben Peterson Papers, Bentley Historical Library, University of Michigan.

38. N. F. Miller, "Gynecological Disturbances of Mechanical Origin," *J. Mich. State Med. Soc.* 25 (1926): 571–74.

39. N. F Miller, "Dysmenorrhœa," *Can. Med. Assoc. J.* 42 (1940): 349–54.

40. N. F. Miller, "Posture Studies in Gynecology," *J. Am. Med. Assoc.* 89 (1927): 1761–65; and idem, "Additional Light on the Dysmenorrhea Problem," ibid. 95 (1930): 1796–1801.

41. N. F. Miller, "Posture and Dysmenorrhea," *Am. J. Obstet. Gynecol.* 27 (1934): 684–91.

42. See W. B. Cannon, *The Mechanical Factors of Digestion* (New York: Longmans, Green, 1911), 48, for the physics of this situation.

43. N. F. Miller, "Retroversion of the Uterus: Factors in Its Production," *J. Iowa State Med. Soc.* 22 (1932): 6–7.

44. Miller, "Dysmenorrhœa," 354.

45. N. F. Miller, "Clinical Aspects of Uterus Didelphys," *Am. J. Obstet. Gynecol.* 4 (1922): 398–408.

46. N. F. Miller, "Atresia Ani Vaginalis, Its Correction: With Report of a Case," *Surg. Gynecol. Obstet.* 43 (1926): 785–89.

47. N. F. Miller, "End-Results from Correction of Cystocele by the Simple Fascia Pleating Method," *Surg. Gynecol. Obstet.* 46 (1928): 403–10.

48. N. F. Miller, "Treatment of Vesicovaginal Fistulas: Past and Present," *Am. J. Obstet. Gynecol.* 30 (1935): 675–95.

49. N. F. Miller, "Some Data on Uterine Cancer," *J. Iowa State Med. Soc.* 23 (1933): 132–35.

50. N. F. Miller and G. H. Sehring, "Uterine Fibroids: The Importance of Diagnostic Curettage in Their Management," *J. Mich. State Med. Soc.* 34 (1935): 4–7.

51. R. G. Dalby, H. W. Jacox, and N. F. Miller, "Fracture of the Femoral Neck following Irradiation," *Am. J. Obstet. Gynecol.* 32 (1936): 50–59.

52. N. F. Miller, "Carcinoma of the Body of the Uterus," *Am. J. Obstet. Gynecol.* 40 (1940): 791–801.

53. N. F. Miller, "The Surgical Treatment of Incontinence in the Female," *J. Am. Med. Assoc.* 98 (1932): 628–32.

54. N. F. Miller and O. E. Todd, "Conization of the Cervix," *Surg. Gynecol. Obstet.* 67 (1938): 265–68.

55. N. F. Miller and C. E. Folsome, "Carcinoma of the Cervix," *Am. J. Obstet. Gynecol.* 36 (1938): 545–58.

56. N. F. Miller, "Pregnancy following Inversion of the Uterus," *Am. J. Obstet. Gynecol.* 13 (1927): 307–22; and idem, "A New Method of Correcting Complete Inversion of the Vagina: With or without Complete Prolapse; Report of Two Cases," *Surg. Gynecol. Obstet.* 44 (1927): 550–55.

57. N. F. Miller and W. Brown, "The Surgical Treatment of Complete Perineal Tears in the Female," *Am. J. Obstet. Gynecol.* 34 (1937): 196–209.

58. Examples: N. F. Miller, "Birth Injuries to Bladder and Bowel," *Calif. West. Med.* 47 (1937): 371–75; idem, "The Uterine Cervix: Its Disorders and Their Treatment," *Calif. West. Med.* 47 (1937): 81–83; and idem, "Vesicovaginal Fistulae: Their Cause and Cure," *N. Y. State Med. J.* 38 (1938): 601–4.

59. N. F. Miller and V. Bryant, *Gynecology and Gynecologic Nursing* (Philadelphia: W. B. Saunders, 1944).

60. N. F. Miller, "A Work Plan for the Section on Gynecology and Obstetrics," *J. Mich. State Med. Soc.* 32 (1933): 1–4.

61. Section on Obstetrics and Gynecology, Committee on Birth Control, "Report," *J. Mich. State Med. Soc.* 33 (1934): 140–45. Another committee made a feeble report on clinical trials, but nothing came of it.

62. A copy of Miller's statement is in the Medical School file in the Bentley Historical Library, University of Michigan.

63. N. F. Miller, "The Obstetric Forceps and Their Use," *J. Mich. State Med. Soc.* 37 (1938): 22–24.

64. Ibid., 22.

65. J. B. DeLee, "The Prophylactic Forceps Operation," *Am. J. Obstet. Gynecol.* 1 (1920): 35.

66. Ibid., 44.

67. N. F. Miller, "The Perpetuation of Error in Obstetrics and Gynecology," *J. Am. Med. Assoc.* 117 (1941): 906–7.

68. J. T. Bradbury, "Study of Endocrine Factors Influencing Mammary Development and Secretion in the Mouse," *Proc. Soc. Exp. Biol. Med.* 30 (1932):

212–13. The paper is the summary of Bradbury's thesis and contains no data whatever.

69. Miller "Perpetuation of Error," 907.

70. U. J. Wile, J. S. Snow, and J. T. Bradbury, "Studies of Sex Hormones in Acne. II. Urinary Excretion of Androgenic and Estrogenic Substances," *Arch. Dermatol. Syphilol.* 39 (1939): 200–210.

71. S. Gardiner and J. T. Bradbury, "Responses of the Human Post-Partum Uterus to Posterior Pituitary Extracts," *Am. J. Obstet. Gynecol.* 39 (1940): 1–10.

72. J. T. Bradbury, "Permanent After-Effects following Masculinization of the Infantile Female Rat," *Endocrinology* 28 (1941): 101–6. The tissues were studied by Lore Marx, an endocrinological pathologist who had fled Germany for Denmark in 1934 and who since 1937 had been at Michigan as a research fellow supported by the Aaron Mendelsohn Fund.

73. W. E. Brown, J. T. Bradbury, and I. Metzger, "Are the Anterior Pituitary-Like Substances Gonadotropic?" *Am. J. Obstet. Gynecol.* 41 (1941): 583. The hormones were still *-tropic* and not *-trophic*. Ida Metzger was a physician at the Ypsilanti State Hospital.

Chapter 19

1. D. M. Cowie to A. W. Hewlett, 12 February 1916, Bentley Historical Library, University of Michigan. Information about Cowie is scattered through many of the library's files.

2. Department of Medicine and Surgery, *Annual Announcement 1905–6* and *1901–2*.

3. The assistants included four women medical graduates, and one was Anne Cooke, whom Cowie married in 1908.

4. For example: Dièreville's *Relation du Voyage du Port Royal de l'Acadie, ou de la Nouvelle France* (Rouen: J. B. Besongne, 1708).

5. Examples: D. M. Cowie, "The Sudan III Stain for the Tubercle Bacillus," *N. Y. Med. J.* 71 (1900): 16–17; idem, "A Preliminary Report on Acid-Resisting Bacilli, with Special Reference to Their Occurrence in the Lower Animals," *J. Exp. Med.* 5 (1900): 205–14; and idem, "Bacilli Which Resemble the Bacillus Tuberculosis," *Physician Surg.* 24 (1902): 8–11.

6. The picture is reproduced in D. M. Cowie, "Two Interesting Cases," *Physician Surg.* 26 (1904): 493.

7. C. von Noorden, "Sitzungsbericht der medicin Gesellschaft zu Giessen," *Arch. Psychiatrie Nervenkrankh.* 18 (1887): 547.

8. C. A. Ewald, *The Diseases of the Stomach*, trans. M. Magnes (New York: D. Appleton, 1894), 414.

9. D. M. Cowie, "Hyperacidity of the Stomach Contents," *Physician Surg.* 23 (1901): 400–411.

10. According to Ewald in *Diseases of the Stomach*: "Titra-
tion is most conveniently performed with a deci-normal solution of caustic soda. . . . As a rule, the acidity of the contents of the stomach obtained one hour after the test-breakfast ranges between 4 to 6 or 6.5 c. c.; results above or below these limits are pathological. It is a matter of convenience to express the acidity in percentage according to the amount of the deci-normal soda solution used; thus, for example, 61 percent acidity would mean that 100 c. c. of filtered stomach-contents were neutralized by 61 c. c. of a deci-normal soda solution" (23).

11. Ewald, *Diseases of the Stomach,* 23, 415.

12. Final results of the work at the asylum were published as D. M. Cowie and F. A. Inch, "Clinical Investigations of the Digestion in the Insane: A Contribution to the Neuroses of the Stomach," *Am. J. Med. Sci.* 130 (1905): 460–92. Florence Allen Inch was the pathologist at the asylum.

13. Cowie, "Hyperacidity of the Stomach Contents," 407–8; and idem, "The Treatment of Hyperacidity of the Stomach Contents, with Special Reference to the Carbohydrate or Meat-Free Diet," *Physician Surg.* 25 (1903): 241–52.

14. Cowie, "Treatment of Hyperacidity," 247.

15. I. P. Pavlov, *Die Arbeit der Verdauungsdrüsen,* trans. A. Walther (Wiesbaden: J. T. Bergmann, 1898); and idem, *The Work of the Digestive Glands,* trans. W. H. Thompson (London: C. Griffin, 1902).

16. D. M. Cowie and J. F. Munson, "An Experimental Study of the Action of Oil on Gastric Acidity and Motility," *Arch. Intern. Med.* 1 (1908): 61–101. Munson had been an instructor at Michigan, and he did a parallel series of experiments in a New York hospital using corn oil rather than olive oil.

17. D. M. Cowie and W. D. Lyon, "An Experimental Study on the Food Reactions in the Infant's Stomach Compared with Those in Vitro," *Arch. Pediatr.* 28 (1911): 100–119.

18. D. M. Cowie, "The Significance of the Pyloric Reflex in True and Pseudopyloric Stenosis in Infants," *Am. J. Dis. Child.* 5 (1913): 225–33.

19. The intestinal gradient is described at length in W. C. Alvarez, *An Introduction to Gastro-Enterology,* 4th ed. (New York: P. B. Hoeber, 1948), 59–136.

20. D. M. Cowie, J. P. Parsons, and F. H. Lashmet, "Studies on the Function of the Intestinal Musculature. I. Longitudinal Muscle of the Rabbit (Gradients)," *Am. J. Physiol.* 88 (1929): 363–68; and Cowie and Lashmet, "Studies on the Function of the Intestinal Musculature. II. Longitudinal Muscle of the Rabbit. Analysis of Curves Produced by Contraction of Excised Segments in Oxygenated Locke's Solution," ibid. 88 (1929): 369–72.

21. D. M. Cowie, "The Gradient Idea in the Vomiting of Infants," *Med. Clin. North Am.* 6 (1923): 1339–47.

22. A. M. Cook and D. M. Cowie, "Rural City Milk Supplies—Their Relation to Infant Feeding—Home Modification versus Laboratory Feeding," *J. Mich. State Med. Soc.* 5 (1906): 415–27.

23. D. M. Cowie, "A Simple, Practical Method for the Feeding of Infants," *J. Mich. State Med. Soc.* 22 (1923): 10–14.

24. The method of measuring acidity but no definition of units is given by Lucius L. Van Slyke, a Michigan Ph.D. who became an eminent agricultural chemist and the father of Donald D. Van Slyke, in his *Modern Methods of Testing Milk and Milk Products* (New York: O. Judd, 1909), 96–112.

25. C. Iverson, "The Relation of Total Acidity to the Bacterial Content of Rural City Milk. A Consideration of the Wyatt Johnston Loop Method of Estimating the Bacterial Content," *Physician Surg.* 33 (1908): 157–64. Christine Iverson did this work in Cowie's private laboratory.

26. L. E. Holt, *The Care and Feeding of Children: A Catechism for the Use of Mothers and Children's Nurses,* 5th ed. (New York: D. Appleton, 1911). This was an assigned textbook at Michigan.

27. J. Brennemann, "Boiled versus Raw Milk: An Experimental Study of Milk Coagulation in the Stomach," *J. Am. Med. Assoc.* 60 (1913): 575–82.

28. D. M. Cowie, "A Graphic Chart Method of Studying and Teaching the Principles of Infant Feeding," *Am. J. Dis. Child.* 4 (1912): 360–77.

29. Ibid., 376.

30. R. Peterson, "The New Contagious Hospital at the University of Michigan and Its Proposed Plan of Operation," *J. Mich. State Med. Soc.* 13 (1914): 323–33. Peterson's paper contains plans and photographs of the hospital, which eventually became an interns' home before being torn down.

31. D. M. Cowie, "The Aseptic Technic Method in the Management of a Contagious Hospital," *J. Mich. State Med. Soc.* 15 (1916): 240–48. There is a copious and informative discussion by Peterson following the article.

32. D. M. Cowie and P. W. Beaven, "Influenza and Influenza Pneumonia. An Analytic Report of the Clinical Findings in 131 Cases of Epidemic Influenza," *J. Mich. State Med. Soc.* 18 (1919): 41–47.

33. D. M. Cowie and P. W. Beaven, "On the Clinical Evidence of Involvement of the Suprarenal Glands in Influenza and Influenzal Pneumonia," *Arch. Intern. Med.* 24 (1919): 78–88.

34. D. M. Cowie, J. P. Parsons, and K. Löwenberg, "Clinico-Pathologic Observations on Infantile Paralysis: Report of 125 Acute Cases with Special Reference to the Therapeutic Use of Convalescent and Adult Blood Transfusions: The Possible Relation of Blood Group to the Severity of the Disease," *Ann. Intern. Med.* 8 (1934): 521–51.

35. D. M. Cowie, "Protection of Monkeys against Intracerebral Inoculation of Virulent Poliomyelitis Virus by Vaccination with Phenolized Poliomyelitis Vaccine," *Proc. Soc. Exp. Biol. Med.* 32 (1934–35): 632–34.

36. D. M. Cowie and P. W. Beaven, "Nonspecific Protein Therapy in Influenzal Pneumonia: A Consideration of the Action of Typhoid Protein," *J. Am. Med. Assoc.* 72 (1919): 1117–21.

37. D. M. Cowie and H. Calhoun, "Nonspecific Therapy in Arthritis and Infections," *Arch. Intern. Med.* 23 (1919): 69–131.

38. D. M. Cowie, "Nonspecific Protein Therapy in Arthritis," *J. Am. Med. Assoc.* 76 (1921): 310–11.

39. D. M. Cowie, "Non-Specific Protein Therapy in Arthritis and Infections. Remarks on the Nature of the Clinical Reaction," *N. Y. State J. Med.* 21 (1921): 395–402.

40. D. M. Cowie, "The Horse Serum (Foreign Protein) Treatment of Pyelitis and Pyuria," *Am. J. Dis. Child.* 24 (1922): 179–85.

41. D. M. Cowie, "Observations on the Bacteriophage," *Ann. Clin. Med.* 5 (1926–27): 57–77.

42. D. M. Cowie and W. C. Hicks, "Observations on the Bacteriophage III. The Treatment of Colon Bacillus Infections of Urinary Tract by Means of Subcutaneous and Intravesicle Injections of Bacteriophage Filtrates. Detailed Case Reports. Methods for Preparation of Filtrates," *J. Lab. Clin. Med.* 17 (1931–32): 681–730.

43. R. M. Olin, "Iodin Deficiency and Prevalence of Simple Goiter in Michigan," *J. Am. Med. Assoc.* 82 (1924): 1328. I am deeply indebted to Howard Markel, my junior colleague for many years in the study of Michigan medicine, for all about iodine in salt that follows. See H. Markel, " 'When It Rains It Pours': Endemic Goiter, Iodized Salt, and David Murray Cowie, MD," *Am. J. Public Health* 77 (1987): 219–29.

44. Marine's career and the background of the Akron experiment are lovingly described in J. Matovinovic, "David Marine (1880–1976): Nestor of Thyroidology," *Perspect. Biol. Med.* 21 (1977–78): 565–89. The Akron experiment is also described in O. P. Kimball, "History of the Prevention of Endemic Goiter," *Bull. W.H.O.* 9 (1953): 241–48.

45. For example: D. Marine and C. H. Lenhart, "Further Observations on the Relation of Iodin to the Structure of the Thyroid Gland in the Sheep, Dog, Hog, and Ox," *Arch. Intern. Med.* 3 (1909): 66–77; Marine and Lenhart, "Colloid Glands (Goitres): Their Etiology and Physiological Significance," *Bull. Johns Hopkins Hosp.* 20 (1909): 131–39; Marine and Lenhart, "On the Occurrence of Goitre (Active Thy-

roid Hyperplasia) in Fish," *Bull. Johns Hopkins Hosp.* 21 (1910): 95–98; Marine and Lenhart, "Observations and Experiments on the So-Called Thyroid Carcinoma of Brook Trout (Salvelinus fontinalis) and Its Relation to Ordinary Goiter," *J. Exp. Med.* 12 (1910): 311–37; and Marine, "The Rapidity of the Involution of Active Thyroid Hyperplasias of Brook Trout following the Use of Fresh Sea Fish as a Food," *J. Exp. Med.* 19 (1914): 376–82.

46. J. F. McClendon, *Iodine and the Incidence of Goiter* (Minneapolis: University of Minnesota Press, 1939).

47. D. Marine, "The Prevention of Goiter," *Public Health* 11 (1923): 23–24.

48. O. P. Kimball, "Endemic Goiter as a Public Health Problem," *Public Health* 12 (1924): 59–64.

49. T. Kocher, "Ueber Jodbasedow," *Arch. Klin. Chir.* 92 (1910): 1166–93. Kocher was dealing with adults, and as Coller observed, a substantial number of Michigan adults with long-established goiters became hyperthyroid when treated with iodine.

50. The beginning of the Akron story is in D. Marine and O. P. Kimball, "The Prevention of Simple Goiter in Man," *J. Lab. Clin. Med.* 3 (1917–18): 40–48. The experiment is summarized in Marine, "Etiology and Prevention of Simple Goiter," *Medicine* 3 (1924): 453–79.

51. Kimball's address to the Michigan State Medical Society is in O. P. Kimball, "The Prevention of Simple Goiter in Man," *J. Mich. State Med. Soc.* 21 (1922): 384–91. His recommendation of iodine in chocolate is in Kimball, "Endemic Goiter," 63. He did not mention iodination of salt in "Endemic Goiter," but he told the medical society that iodine in salt would run to the bottom of the package (Kimball, "Prevention of Simple Goiter," 391).

52. F. B. Miner, "Chairman's Address—Pediatric Section," *J. Mich. State Med. Soc.* 21 (1922): 493.

53. Ibid., 493–95.

54. The minutes of Cowie's committee, copies of his correspondence, and so on, are in the Bentley Historical Library, University of Michigan. The minutes and some correspondence are in "Iodized Salt: Report of the Committee of the Pediatric Section, Michigan State Medical Society," *J. Mich. State Med. Soc.* 23 (1924): 173–82.

55. The attempt to iodinate the water supply of Rochester, New York, is described in L. A. Kohn, "Goiter, Iodine and George W. Goler: The Rochester Experiment," *Bull. Hist. Med.* 49 (1975): 389–99. Kohn said: "A political storm seized on the Akron experiment as an invasion of personal rights, and stopped it," but he gave only a personal communication as reference (391). The truth of the statement could doubtless be tested by consulting the newspa-

pers of the day, but the results were in by the time the experiment was stopped in 1919.

56. Marine, "The Prevention of Goiter," 23.

57. The Swiss experience including the use of iodized salt is described in J. L. Nicod, "Le goitre endémique en Suisse et sa prophylaxie par le sel iodé," *Bull. W.H.O.* 9 (1953): 259–73.

58. J. F. McClendon, "Simple Goiter as a Result of Iodin Deficiency," *J. Am. Med. Assoc.* 80 (1923): 600–601.

59. R. D. McClure, "Thyroid Surgery in Southern Michigan as Affected by the Generalized Use of Iodized Salt," *J. Mich. State Med. Soc.* 33 (1934): 61.

60. D. M. Cowie and J. J. Engelfried, "A Survey of the Iodized Salt Obtained, on the Open Market, from Various Districts of the State of Michigan," *J. Mich. State Med. Soc.* 38 (1939): 1057–64; and idem, "Iodide Content of Iodized Salt: Effect of Storage," ibid. 39 (1940): 784.

61. D. M. Cowie and J. J. Engelfried, "The Iodized Table Salt Carton: Analysis of the Iodide Content of the Pasteboard," *J. Mich. State Med. Soc.* 39 (1940): 785–86.

62. Advisory Committee of the Pediatric Section, Michigan State Medical Society, "A Study of the Effect of the Use of Iodized Salt on the Incidence of Goiter," *J. Mich. State Med. Soc.* 36 (1937): 654.

63. McClure, "Thyroid Surgery," 62.

64. A. F. Abt, ed., *Abt-Garrison History of Pediatrics* (Philadelphia: W. B. Saunders, 1965), 223.

65. Ibid., 149.

66. B. S. Veeder, ed., *Pediatric Profiles* (St. Louis: C. V. Mosby, 1957), 5. The emphasis in the quotation is in the original.

67. Ibid., 136, 261. Thomas B. Cooley was the 1895 graduate of the University of Michigan Medical School and Detroit pediatrician who identified thalassemia.

68. D. M. Cowie, K. M. Jarvis, and M. Cooperstock, "Metabolism Studies in Nephrosis, with Special Reference to the Relationship of Protein Intake to Nitrogen Retention, Edema and Albuminuria," *Am. J. Dis. Child.* 40 (1930): 482.

69. E. H. Starling, "The Properties of Colloids," in *Principles of Human Physiology* (Philadelphia: Lea and Febiger, 1912), 154–61.

70. Medical School Records, Box 6, Bentley Historical Library, University of Michigan.

71. C. F. McKhann Jr., "Coming to Michigan in 1940," in H. Markel and J. Tarolli, eds., *Caring for Children: A Celebration of the Department of Pediatrics and Communicable Diseases,* Historical Center for the Health Sciences Monographs, no. 5 (Ann Arbor, 1998), 93–97.

Chapter 20

1. Greene's name was indifferently spelled, with and without the final *e*.
2. F. Carrow, "Doctor George Edward Frothingham," *Mich. Alumnus* 10 (1904): 443–47.
3. F. Carrow, "Medicine among the Chinese," *Med. Age* 5 (1887): 1–5.
4. Charles L. Patton to Reuben Peterson, 25 June 1939, Reuben Peterson Papers, Bentley Historical Library, University of Michigan.
5. V. C. Vaughan, *A Doctor's Memories* (Indianapolis: Bobbs-Merrill, 1926), 220, 222.
6. F. Carrow, "A Review of a Year's Work in the Treatment of Cataract," *Trans. Mich. State Med. Soc.* 15 (1891): 214–20.
7. F. Carrow, "Adrenalin a Valuable Aid in Surgical Work upon Mucous Surfaces," *Ther. Gaz.* 26 (1902): 300–301.
8. F. Carrow, "Laryngectomy and Partial Excision of the Upper Jaw for the Removal of Pharyngeal Growths," *Trans. Mich. State Med. Soc.* 18 (1894): 301–6.
9. F. Carrow, "Foreign Bodies in, and Injuries to, the Eyeball," *Physician Surg.* 8 (1886): 385–92.
10. F. Carrow, "Some Eye Affections of the Venereal Diseases," *Trans. Mich. State Med. Soc.* 12 (1888): 190–97.
11. F. Carrow and W. H. Sherzer, "The Results of the Examination of the Eyes of 681 Students of the Michigan State Normal School," *Trans. Mich. State Med. Soc.* 18 (1894): 381–82.
12. See note 4 of this section.
13. Richard R. Smith to Reuben Peterson, 2 December 1939, Reuben Peterson Papers, Bentley Historical Library, University of Michigan.
14. Carrow, "Review of a Year's Work," 218.
15. Minutes, June 1904, *Regents' Proceedings 1901–1906,* 368.
16. Ibid., 369.
17. For more details, see J. W. Henderson, *The University of Michigan Department of Ophthalmology: A Proud Heritage* (Ann Arbor: University of Michigan, 1986), 52–54.
18. Minutes, May 1905, *Regents' Proceedings 1901–1906,* 523.
19. Minutes, May 1906, *Regents' Proceedings 1901–1906,* 697.
20. W. R. Parker, "The Teaching of Ophthalmology in This Country," *Arch. Ophthalmol.,* n.s., 9 (1933): 515–22.
21. W. R. Parker, "Tubercular Affections of the Eye," *Ophthalmic Rec.* 15 (1906): 301–9; idem, "A Review of the Study of Conjunctivitis from a Bacteriologic Standpoint," *Physician Surg.* 31 (1909): 49–52; and idem, "The Use of Salvarsan in [Interstitial] Keratitis; Report of Ten Cases," *J. Mich. State Med. Soc.* 11 (1912): 637–40.
22. W. R. Parker, "Report of Case of Dermoid Cyst of the Orbit, Producing Marked Exophthalmos, Relieved by the Krönlein Operation," *J. Mich. State Med. Soc.* 13 (1914): 335–38. Parker used the same procedure: "Neurofibroma of the Orbit: Krönlein Operation," *J. Am. Med. Assoc.* 49 (1907): 17–19.
23. W. R. Parker, "Skin-Grafting," *Physician Surg.* 33 (1911): 247–52; and the same paper, *J. Mich. State Med. Soc.* 12 (1913): 414–17; and idem, "Some Practical Points in Blepharoplasty," *Trans. Am. Acad. Ophthalmol. Otolaryngol.* 36 (1921): 161–76.
24. W. R. Parker, "A Short Review of the Methods of Diagnosis and Treatment of Ocular Muscle Insufficiencies," *Physician Surg.* 19 (1897): 145–49; idem, "In Plain Language What May We Expect from Treatment of Ocular Muscle Errors?" ibid. 24 (1902): 259–62; and idem, "The Management of Crossed Eyes in Children," ibid. 24 (1902): 5–8.
25. W. R. Parker, "Management of Simple Glaucoma. A Clinical Report," *Arch. Ophthalmol.,* n.s., 2 (1929): 174–78; idem, "Sclerocorneal Trephining for Glaucoma," *J. Am. Med. Assoc.* 63 (1914): 215–18; and idem, "The Present Status of the Sclerocorneal Trephine Operation for the Relief of Glaucoma," *Arch. Ophthalmol.* 46 (1917): 1–7.
26. W. R. Parker, "Sclerotrephine Operation for Detached Retina: Clinical Report of Eleven Cases," *J. Am. Med. Assoc.* 65 (1915): 1699–707.
27. W. R. Parker, "The Visual Fields in Hysteria: A Clinical Study of Fifty Cases," *J. Am. Med. Assoc.* 53 (1909): 96.
28. W. R. Parker, "Lessons from Three Hundred Cataract Extractions," *J. Mich. State Med. Soc.* 10 (1911): 112–15; idem, "The Choice of Cataract Operation," ibid. 19 (1920): 550–51; and idem, "Senile Cataract Extraction: A Comparative Study of Results Obtained in One Thousand, Four Hundred and Twenty-One Operations," *J. Am. Med. Assoc.* 77 (1921): 1171–75. The last paper was also published as idem, "Senile Cataract Extraction," *Am. J. Ophthalmol.,* 3d ser., 4 (1921): 650–54.
29. W. R. Parker, "Postcataract Extraction Delirium: Report of Eleven Cases," *J. Am. Med. Assoc.* 61 (1913): 1174–77. The delirium resulted from sensory deprivation from bandaging both eyes for many days.
30. R. H. Elliot, *The Indian Operation of Couching for Cataract* (New York: P. B. Hoeber, 1918).
31. An example: H. Smith, "The Treatment of Immature Cataract," *Lancet* 2 (1908): 452–54. Smith's method is described in an anonymous obituary: "Henry Smith. C.I.E., Lieut.-Col., I.M.S., ret.," *Br. J. Oph-*

thalmol. 32 (1948): 514–15. "Smith made a large section in the corneo-scleral junction; he cut no conjunctival flap; he performed a large iridectomy and delivered the lens by pressure on the lower part of the cornea with the blunt tip of a strabismus hook. The suspensory ligament was ruptured in the first place and the lens either 'tumbled' or pushed straight out" (515). Another obituary, "Henry Smith, I.M.S., 1859–1948," *Arch. Ophthalmol.* 39 (1948): 676–80, describes how in the early days antisepsis was achieved by a stoneware jar filled with dilute mercuric iodide (1:3,000) that hung from the roof and supplied a constant stream to the field of operation. Smith smoked a whacking big cheroot throughout (678–79). Smith is admiringly described in C. B. Meding, "Colonel Henry Smith, C.I.E., I.M.S.," *N. Y. Med. J.* 113 (1921): 582–84.

32. W. R. Parker, "Extraction of Cataract in Its Capsule: Report of Case," *Ophthalmic Rec.* 15 (1906): 162–63.

33. W. R. Parker, "The Relation of Choked Disk to the Tension of the Eyeball," *J. Am. Med. Assoc.* 67 (1916): 1053–58. The experiment is described once more in idem, "The Mechanism of Papilledema," *Arch. Neurol. Psychiatry* 14 (1925): 31–34.

34. W. S. Duke-Elder, *Text-Book of Ophthalmology,* vol. 3, *Diseases of the Inner Eye* (St. Louis: C. V. Mosby, 1941), 2945, 2955.

35. G. E. de Schweinitz, *Diseases of the Eye,* 9th ed. (Philadelphia: W. B. Saunders, 1921), 679, 705.

36. C. A. Clapp, *Cataract: Its Etiology and Treatment* (Philadelphia: Lea and Febiger, 1934).

37. Slocum's background and characteristics are described in W. R. Parker, "George Slocum, 1865–1933," *Am. J. Ophthalmol.,* 3d ser., 16 (1933): 641–42.

38. An example: G. Slocum, "Four Unusual Cases of Strabismus Presented from the Standpoint of Diagnosis," *J. Mich. State Med. Soc.* 13 (1914): 392–97.

39. G. Slocum, "A Report from the Clinic of Ophthalmic Surgery of a Series of Ophthalmoscopic Studies of the Fundus in Cases of Nephritis," *J. Mich. State Med. Soc.* 13 (1914): 534–46; and in a slightly different form with a few more cases: idem, "A Study of Ophthalmoscopic Changes in Nephritis," *J. Am. Med. Assoc.* 67 (1916): 5–12.

40. G. Slocum, "Employment of a Conjunctival Bridge and Suture in Cataract Extraction," *Arch. Ophthalmol.,* n.s., 10 (1933): 329–41.

41. F. B. Fralick, "The Kahn Reaction in the Aqueous Humor: Its Relation to Syphilis of the Eye," *Arch. Ophthalmol.,* n.s., 10 (1933): 745–53.

42. F. B. Fralick, "Luxation of Lens through a Retinal Tear into the Subretinal Space," *Am. J. Ophthalmol.,* 3d ser., 20 (1937): 795–96.

43. F. B. Fralick and R. N. DeJong, "Neuromyelitis Optica," *Am. J. Ophthalmol.,* 3d ser., 20 (1937): 1119–24.

44. F. A. Barbour and F. B. Fralick, "The Posterior Approach for the Removal of Magnetic Intraocular Foreign Bodies," *Am. J. Ophthalmol.,* 3d ser., 24 (1941): 553–56.

45. F. B. Fralick, "The Management of Glaucoma," *J. Mich. State Med. Soc.* 34 (1935): 11–15.

46. F. B. Fralick, "Strabismus," *J. Mich. State Med. Soc.* 37 (1938): 226–29.

47. For example: W. F. Breakey, "The Unsuspected Parasitic Origin of Many Dermatoses," *Physician Surg.* 28 (1906): 385–88. He treated a dozen or more patients with parasitic sycosis caught from cattle, and he identified the parasite by growth on bouillon media.

48. W. F. Breakey, "The Light Cure in Lupus," *Physician Surg.* 23 (1901): 529–32.

49. J. F. Breakey, "Carbon Dioxid as Therapeutic Agent in the Treatment of Skin Diseases," *Physician Surg.* 31 (1909): 3–6.

50. M. Marshall, "A Report of Seven Cases of Syphilis Treated with Salvarsan," *Physician Surg.* 33 (1911): 27–30. There was painful irritation at the site of injection, and one patient required sedation for days.

51. J. F. Breakey, "Demonstration of Two Patients Who Have Received the Salvarsan Treatment," *Physician Surg.* 33 (1911): 98–100.

52. Breakey expressed this opinion several times, notably in W. F. Breakey, "The Elimination and Curability of Syphilis," *Physician Surg.* 23 (1901): 145–51; and idem, "The Management of Suspected Primary Lesions of Syphilis," *Am. J. Dermatol. Genito-Ur. Dis.* 8 (1904): 249–54. An editorial, "The Use of Mercury and the Efflorescence of Syphilis," in the same issue of the *Physician and Surgeon* said mercury should be given early (23 [1901]: 188–89).

53. Breakey, "Elimination and Curability," 151.

54. W. J. Herdman, "The Duty of the Medical Profession to the Public in the Matter of Venereal Diseases and How to Discharge It," *J. Am. Med. Assoc.* 47 (1906): 1246–48.

55. Biographical details are in A. C. Curtis and E. P. Cawley, "Tribute to Dr. Udo Julius Wile," *Arch. Dermatol. Syphilol.* 60 (1949): 139–42; and C. S. Wright and W. N. Sams, "In Memoriam: Udo Julius Wile, MD," *Arch. Dermatol.* 93 (1966): 1–2.

56. There is a Festschrift for P. G. Unna in *Dermatol. Wochenschr.* 71 (1920): 621–38, in which his career is sketched. Unna has a large place in the history of dermatology and Wile a small one. See, for example, H. Goodman, *Notable Contributors to the Knowledge of Dermatology* (New York: Medical Lay Press, 1953).

57. Example: U. J. Wile and H. L. Arnold, "The Senear-Usher Syndrome: Review of the Literature and

Report of Six Cases," *Arch. Dermatol. Syphilol.* 40 (1939): 687–706.

58. U. J. Wile, "The Rigidity of Diagnostic Criteria in Dermatology," *P. Med. J.* 33 (1929–30): 222.

59. U. J. Wile, "Cutaneous Manifestations of Systemic Diseases," *Bull. N. Y. Acad. Med.*, 2d ser., 8 (1932): 289–313.

60. U. J. Wile, "Dermatologic Education: Teaching of Dermatosyphilology (the Educational Background)," *Arch. Dermatol. Syphilol.* 17 (1928): 451–65.

61. U. J. Wile, "Anæmic Infarction of the Adrenal with Thrombosis of the Veins," *N. Y. Med. J.* 85 (1907): 1178–79.

62. U. J. Wile, "Über Granuloma pyogenicum (Pseudo-Botryomykosis)," *Dermatol. Stud.* 20 (1910): 333–47.

63. U. J. Wile, "Familial Study of Three Unusual Cases of Congenital Ichthyosiform Erythroderma," *Arch. Dermatol. Syphilol.* 10 (1924): 487–98.

64. U. J. Wile and F. H. Grauer, "Rosacea-Like Tuberculosis: Review of the Literature with Report of Five Cases," *Arch. Dermatol. Syphilol.* 31 (1935): 174–89.

65. U. J. Wile and F. E. Senear, "Chancre of the Cervix Uteri," *Surg. Gynecol. Obstet.* 21 (1915): 643–46.

66. U. J. Wile and M. G. Butler, "A Critical Survey of Charcot's Arthropathy," *J. Am. Med. Assoc.* 94 (1930): 1053–55.

67. U. J. Wile and E. A. Hand, "Cancer of the Lip: Results of Therapy in Four Hundred and Twenty-Five Cases Followed from One to Ten Years," *J. Am. Med. Assoc.* 108 (1937): 374–81.

68. U. J. Wile, "An Estimate of the Value of the Wassermann Reaction to the General Practitioner," *J. Mich. State Med. Soc.* 13 (1914): 264–66.

69. U. J. Wile, "Comparative Experiments on the Presence of Complement Binding Substances in the Serum and Urine of Syphilitics," *J. Am. Med. Assoc.* 51 (1908): 1142–43.

70. "Franz Blumenthal, zum 75. Geburtstag," *Dermatol. Wochenschr.* 128 (1953): 757–58. The author wrote with geographical insouciance that Blumenthal "um 1934 einem Ruf an die Universität Detroit in Michigan zu folgen, an der er noch jetz tätig ist und die Dermatologische Klinik am Wayne County General Hospital in Ann Arbor leitet" (757).

71. U. J. Wile and C. K. Hasley, "Serologic Cure (?) in the Light of Increasingly Sensitive Wassermann Tests," *J. Am. Med. Assoc.* 72 (1919): 1526–28.

72. H. L. Keim and U. J. Wile, "The Kahn Precipitation Test in the Diagnosis of Syphilis," *J. Am. Med. Assoc.* 79 (1922): 870–74.

73. U. J. Wile, "The Relation of Syphilis to Surgery: A Diagnostic and Prognostic Problem," *J. Mich. State Med. Soc.* 33 (1934): 199–204; and idem, "Syphilis in Relation to Surgical Problems," *Calif. West. Med.* 49 (1938): 7–11.

74. U. J. Wile, "Syphilis of the Liver," *Arch. Dermatol. Syphilol.* 1 (1920): 139–50. The articles continue to volume 4.

75. U. J. Wile and J. S. Snow, "Occult Cardiovascular Syphilis," *Am. J. Med. Sci.* 195 (1938): 240–48.

76. H. Noguchi and J. W. Moore, "A Demonstration of Treponema pallidum in the Brain in Cases of General Paralysis," *J. Exp. Med.* 17 (1913): 232.

77. J. W. Moore, "The Occurrence of the Syphilitic Organism in the Brain in Paresis," *J. Nerv. Ment. Dis.* 40 (1913): 172–79.

78. Noguchi and Moore, "Demonstration," 232.

79. H. Noguchi, "Studien über den Nachweis der Spirochaete pallida im Zentralnervensystem bei der progressiven Paralyse und bei Tabes dorsalis," *Münch. Med. Wochenschr.* 60 (1913): 737–39.

80. H. Noguchi, "The Transmission of Treponema pallidum from the Brains of Paretics to the Rabbit," *J. Am. Med. Assoc.* 61 (1913): 85. Noguchi told the same story at a meeting of the Aertzlicher Verein in Frankfurt am Main: H. Noguchi, "Die Reinzüchtung der Spirochäten," *Münch. Med. Wochenschr.* 60 (1913): 2483.

81. H. J. Nichols and W. H. Hough, "Positive Results following the Inoculation of the Rabbit with Paretic Brain Substance," *J. Am. Med. Assoc.* 61 (1913): 120–21; and H. J. Nichols, "Observations on a Strain of Spirochæta pallida Isolated from the Nervous System," *J. Exp. Med.* 19 (1914): 362–71. The second paper dealt with the problem of a neurotropic strain.

82. E. Forster and E. Tomasczewski, "Nachweis von lebenden Spirochäten im Gehirn von Paralytikern," *Dtsch. Med. Wochenschr.* 34 (1913): 1237.

83. U. J. Wile, "The Demonstration of the Spirochaeta pallida in the Brain Substance of Living Paretics (Forster and Tomasczewski)," *J. Am. Med. Assoc.* 61 (1913): 866.

84. U. J. Wile, "Experimental Syphilis in the Rabbit Produced by the Brain Substance of the Living Paretic," *J. Exp. Med.* 23 (1916): 199–202; and Wile and P. H. de Kruif, "Cultural Experiments with the Spirochaeta pallida Derived from the Paretic Brain," *J. Am. Med. Assoc.* 66 (1916): 646–47. It is noteworthy that the editors of the *Journal of Experimental Medicine* and the *Journal of the American Medical Association* did not raise any question of Wile's ethics when they accepted his papers.

85. [W. B. Cannon], "The Right and Wrong of Making Experiments on Human Beings [editorial]," *J. Am. Med. Assoc.* 67 (1916): 1373.

86. W. W. Keen, "The Inveracities of Antivivisection," *J. Am. Med. Assoc.* 67 (1916): 1390.

87. U. J. Wile, "The Spirochetal Content of the Spinal

Fluid of Tabes, General Paresis, and Cerebrospinal Syphilis," *Am. J. Syph.* 1 (1917): 84–90.

88. U. J. Wile and A. Kirchner, "A New Method for the Demonstration of Spirochaeta pallida in the Spinal Fluid," *Arch. Dermatol. Syphilol.* 8 (1923): 831–36.

89. U. J. Wile and J. A. Elliott, "A Study of Splenic Enlargement in Early Syphilis," *Am. J. Med. Sci.* 150 (1915): 512–18.

90. U. J. Wile and J. A. Elliott, "A Critical Study of One Hundred and Twenty Cases of Late Syphilis, with Particular Reference to Early Treatment," *J. Am. Med. Assoc.* 67 (1916): 1917–18.

91. U. J. Wile and C. H. Marshall, "A Study of the Spinal Fluid in One Thousand Eight Hundred and Sixty-Nine Cases of Syphilis in All Stages," *Arch. Dermatol. Syphilol.* 3 (1921): 272.

92. U. J. Wile and F. E. Senear, "A Study of the Involvement of the Bones and Joints in Early Syphilis," *Am. J. Med. Sci.* 152 (1916): 689–93.

93. U. J. Wile and J. A. Elliott, "Mode of Absorption of Mercury in the Inunction Treatment of Syphilis," *J. Am. Med. Assoc.* 68 (1917): 1024–28.

94. U. J. Wile, "A Preliminary Report on the Employment of Neosalvarsan in Syphilis," *Physician Surg.* 34 (1912): 401–4.

95. U. J. Wile, "The Technic of the Intradural Injections of Neosalvarsan in Syphilis of the Nervous System: Report of Cases," *J. Am. Med. Assoc.* 63 (1914): 137–41. Wile had seen someone else do it in St. Louis.

96. U. J. Wile, "The Principles Underlying the Treatment of Cardiovascular Syphilis," *Ann. Intern. Med.* 15 (1941): 817–20. This is only one of many papers on the subject.

97. U. J. Wile, "The Treatment of the Syphilitic Liver and Heart: A Therapeutic Paradox," *Am. J. Med. Sci.* 164 (1922): 415–28.

98. J. H. Stokes et al., "Standard Treatment Procedure in Early Syphilis," *J. Am. Med. Assoc.* 102 (1934): 1267–72.

99. J. H. Stokes et al., "What Treatment in Early Syphilis Accomplishes. III. Comparison of Bruusgaard's Work and the Three- to Twenty-Year Results of the Coöperative Clinical Group," *Am. J. Med. Sci.* 188 (1934): 678–84.

100. J. H. Jones, *Bad Blood: The Tuskegee Syphilis Experiment* (New York: Free Press, 1981), 1, 204–5.

101. U. J. Wile and L. K. Mundt, "Avoidance of Fatal Complications in Therapeutic Malaria," *Arch. Dermatol. Syphilol.* 44 (1941): 1078–81. Wile's earlier work on malaria therapy can be found by working back from this paper.

102. W. J. Herdman, "The Physician as a Witness in Court," *J. Am. Med. Assoc.* 34 (1900): 650–54.

103. W. J. Herdman, *A Guide to the Dissection of the Human Body* (Ann Arbor: G. Osius, 1883), i.

104. W. J. Herdman, "Tumor at the Base of the Brain," *Trans. Mich. State Med. Soc.* 15 (1891): 195–201.

105. W. J. Herdman, "The Present Campaign against Insanity," *Physician Surg.* 26 (1904): 241–50; and idem, "Reasons Why the Joint Board of the Asylums for the Insane Should Join in the Conduct of the Psychopathic Ward at the University Hospital," ibid. 27 (1905): 97–103.

106. "Deaths—William James Herdman, M.D.," *J. Am. Med. Assoc.* 47 (1906): 2106.

107. W. J. Herdman, "Simple Neuritis," *Trans. Mich. State Med. Soc.* 20 (1896): 416–27.

108. W. J. Herdman, "Primary Lateral Sclerosis," *Trans. Mich. State Med. Soc.* 12 (1888): 174–82.

109. W. J. Herdman, "Exophthalmic Goitre," *Trans. Mich. State Med. Soc.* 14 (1890): 242–53.

110. W. J. Herdman, "Some Forms of Tropho-Neuroses, with an Illustration," *Trans. Mich. State Med. Soc.* 19 (1895): 457–63; 469–71 (discussion).

111. Department of Medicine and Surgery, *Annual Announcement 1900–1901,* 69.

112. Ibid.

113. Department of Medicine and Surgery, *Annual Announcement 1896–97,* 61.

114. Department of Medicine and Surgery, *Annual Announcement 1894–95,* 27.

115. H. M. Hurd, "Practical Suggestions Relative to the Treatment of Insanity," *Physician Surg.* 4 (1882): 390–91.

116. Herdman, "Present Campaign against Insanity," 249.

117. J. H. Talbott, *A Biographical History of Medicine* (New York: Grune and Stratton, 1970), 865.

118. The neurasthenia story is from J. C. Solis, "The Psychotherapeutics of Neurasthenia," *Physician Surg.* 27 (1905): 313.

119. This and much of the next two paragraphs are derived from the textbooks Herdman recommended to his students: T. S. Clouston, *Clinical Lectures on Mental Diseases* (Philadelphia; H. C. Lea's Son, 1884); E. C. Spitzka, *Insanity: Its Classification, Diagnosis and Treatment,* 2d ed. (New York: E. B. Treat, 1887); and H. J. Berkley, *A Treatise on Mental Diseases* (New York: D. Appleton, 1900).

120. S. W. Mitchell, *Fat and Blood: and How to Make Them,* 2d ed. (Philadelphia: J. B. Lippincott, 1878). Solis paraphrased Mitchell.

121. Ibid., 9.

122. Spitzka, *Insanity,* 241–42.

123. Hurd, "Practical Suggestions," 399.

124. The long shelf of books on electrotherapeutics includes the following: A. C. Garratt, *Medical Electricity: Embracing Electro-Physiology and Electricity as a Therapeutic,* 3d ed. (Philadelphia: J. B. Lippincott,

1866); R. Bartholow, *Medical Electricity: A Practical Treatise on the Applications of Electricity to Medicine and Surgery* (Philadelphia: H. C. Lea's Son, 1881); and G. A. Liebig Jr. and G. H. Rohé, *Practical Electricity in Medicine and Surgery* (Philadelphia: F. A. Davis, 1890). Herdman's papers on the subject include "Some Surgical Suggestions," *Trans. Mich. State Med. Soc.* 17 (1893): 163–67; and idem, "Radiant Energy and Ionization: Their Relation to Vital Processes and Their Derangements," *J. Adv. Ther.* 23 (1905): 635–45. There were many symposia on electrotherapeutics, and the gynecologists were particularly enthusiastic.

125. G. Apostoli, *Sur un nouveau traitement de la métrite chronique et en particulier de l'endométrite par la galvano-caustique chimique intra-utérine* (Paris: O. Doin, 1887); and idem, "The Treatment of Salpingo-Ovaritis by Electricity," *J. Am. Med. Assoc.* 13 (1889): 109–19.

126. J. C. Solis, "The Use of Electricity in Inflammatory and Congested Conditions of the Uterus," *Trans. Mich. State Med. Soc.* 18 (1894): 522–28.

127. Solis, "The Psychotherapeutics of Neurasthenia," 316.

128. Liebig and Rohé, *Practical Electricity*, 360.

129. W. J. Herdman and F. W. Nagler, *A Laboratory Manual of Electrotherapeutics* (Ann Arbor: G. Wahr, 1898).

130. An advertisement for Herdman's correspondence course is reproduced in E. R. N. Grigg, *The Trail of the Invisible Light: From X-Strahlen to Radio(bio)logy* (Springfield, Ill.: C. C Thomas, 1965), 644.

Chapter 21

1. *Roentgenology* was the official title of this specialty at Michigan until 1955. The word was seldom spelled *Röntgenology*, but at least once Herdman spelled it *Röentgenology*.

2. R. Brecher and E. Brecher, *The Rays: A History of Radiology in the United States and Canada* (Baltimore: Williams and Wilkins, 1969). The history of X-ray apparatus is in E. R. N. Grigg, *The Trail of the Invisible Light: From X-Strahlen to Radio(bio)logy* (Springfield, Ill.: C. C Thomas, 1965).

3. *The University of Michigan: An Encyclopedic Survey*, ed. W. B. Shaw (Ann Arbor: University of Michigan Press, 1951), 2:931. The skiagrams are reproduced opposite page 268 of the *Michigan Alumnus* 5 (1898–99). They might be the first published in Michigan.

4. C. Georg, "Treatment of Lupus Vulgaris and Inoperable Tumors with the Roentgen Rays," *Physician Surg.* 25 (1903): 61–70.

5. C. B. G. Nancrède, Discussion on surgical affections of the kidney, American Surgical Association meeting, May 1908, *Ann. Surg.* 47 (1908): 1056.

6. V. J. Willey, "Light and Invisible Rays Employed in Medical Practice Considered from a Physical Standpoint," *Physician Surg.* 25 (1903): 337–42; idem, "Principles of Photography for Roentgen Ray Workers," *Physician Surg.* 27 (1905): 538–47; idem, "Modern Skiagraphic Technique," *Physician Surg.* 28 (1906): 193–200; and idem, "Some Experiments with Roentgen Tubes with Respect to the Use of Tubes for Diagnostic Work," *Arch. Roentgen Ray* 12 (1908): 248–60.

7. The history of the controversial Bucky-Potter diaphragm is sketched in Grigg, *Trail of the Invisible Light*, 128–32, and in H. E. Potter, "History of Diaphragming Roentgen Rays by Use of the Bucky Principle," *Am. J. Roentgenol.* 25 (1931): 396–402.

8. The point about Van Zwaluwenburg's knowledge of anatomy is in obituary notices, R. Peterson, D. M. Cowie, and U. J. Wile, "James Gerrit Van Zwaluwenburg, 1874–1922," *Mich. Alumnus* 29 (1922): 757–60; and in R. H. Stevens, "James G. Van Zwaluwenburg—A Memorial," *J. Radiol.* 3 (1922): 73. The latter quotes Cabot's tribute. Another tribute is A. W. Crane, "Dr. James G. Van Zwaluwenburg," *Am. J. Roentgenol.* 9 (1922): 123–25.

9. [F.?] Moritz, "Eine Methode, um beim Röntgenverfahren aus dem Schattenbilde eines Gegenstandes dessen wahre Grösse zu ermitteln (Orthodiographie) und die exacte Bestimmung der Herzgrösse nach diesem Verfahren," *Münch. Med. Wochenschr.* 47 (1900): 992–96. Moritz's initial is not given in his other papers or in reference sources. However, the Groedel article cited in note 10, which follows, cites his papers as by "F. Moritz."

10. F. M. Groedel, "Die Röntgenuntersuchung des Herzens," in *Lehrbuch und Atlas der Röntgendiagnostik*, ed. F. M. Groedel (München: J. F. Lehmann, 1924), 1:349–440.

11. J. G. Van Zwaluwenburg and L. F. Warren, "The Diagnostic Value of the Orthodiagram in Heart Disease," *Arch. Intern. Med.* 7 (1911): 137–52.

12. J. G. Van Zwaluwenburg, "A Plea for the Use of the Fluoroscope in the Examination of the Heart and Great Vessels," *Am. J. Roentgenol.* 7 (1920): 1–6. This is actually a plea for the use of orthodiagramography.

13. J. G. Van Zwaluwenburg, "Correlation of the Roentgenographic and Surgical Findings in Sixty-Two Operated Cases," *J. Mich. State Med. Soc.* 16 (1917): 370–78. Six were removed from consideration on account of imperfect reports.

14. At the first faculty meeting after Van Zwaluwenburg's death the faculty asked the university to continue his salary to his widow for the rest of the school year.

The faculty said he had worked without regard for money.

15. J. G. Van Zwaluwenburg, "The X-Ray Diagnosis of Peptic Ulcer," *J. Mich. State Med. Soc.* 14 (1915): 233.

16. S. W. Donaldson and E. F. Merrill, "The Van Zwaluwenburg Type of Stereoscope," *Am. J. Roentgenol.* 9 (1922): 742–44.

17. J. G. Van Zwaluwenburg, "Greater Certainty in the Localization of Foreign Bodies in the Eye," *Am. J. Roentgenol.* 4 (1917): 512–20.

18. J. G. Van Zwaluwenburg, "The X-Ray Diagnosis of Accessory Sinusitis," *Am. J. Roentgenol.* 9 (1922): 1.

19. J. G. Van Zwaluwenburg and R. Peterson, "Pneumoperitoneum of the Pelvis: Gynecological Studies—A Preliminary Report," *Am. J. Roentgenol.* 8 (1921): 12–19.

20. J. G. Van Zwaluwenburg, "The Capillary Circulation in the Roentgenogram of the Chest," *Am. J. Roentgenol.* 3 (1916): 532–35.

21. J. G. Van Zwaluwenburg and G. P. Grabfield, "The Tonsillar Route of Infection in Pulmonary Tuberculosis," *Am. Rev. Tuberc.* 5 (1921–22): 57.

22. J. G. Van Zwaluwenburg and G. P. Grabfield, "Apical Pleuritis and Its Relationship to Pulmonary Tuberculosis: A Statistical Study of Stereoscopic Roentgenograms of 366 Consecutive Adult Chests," *Am. Rev. Tuberc.* 5 (1921–22): 323–38; and Van Zwaluwenburg, A. D. Wickett, and E. F. Merrill, "Pulmonary Involvement in Nonpulmonary Tuberculosis," ibid. 6 (1922–23): 677–83.

23. J. G. Van Zwaluwenburg and A. D. Wickett, "Apical Pleuritis: A Statistical Study of Stereoscopic Roentgenograms of 267 Presumably Normal Students' Chests," *Am. Rev. Tuberc.* 6 (1922–23): 106–18.

24. The conferences are described in P. M. Hickey and A. S. Warthin, "Roentgenologic-Pathologic Conferences," *J. Radiol.* 4 (1923): 416–23. At the conference used for illustration, six cases involving the Departments of Roentgenology, Dermatology, Internal Medicine, Pediatrics, Surgery, and Pathology were presented in detail.

25. P. M. Hickey, "Plan of Roentgen Department in Hospital," *Am. J. Roentgenol.* 3 (1916): 590.

26. Many appreciations of Hickey include A. W. Crane, "Preston M. Hickey, Pioneer in Roentgenology," *Am. J. Roentgenol.* 27 (1932): 110–12; and L. Edling, "Preston M. Hickey. In Memoriam," *Acta Radiol.* 11 (1930): 658–62.

27. When Van Zwaluwenburg was attempting to make precisely duplicated exposures he stationed a technician to read the ammeter on the transformer and to call out when the load (an elevator?) reduced the current.

28. P. M. Hickey, "Important Considerations in Planning an X-Ray Department," *Radiology* 7 (1926): 104–8; and idem, "The X-Ray Department in the Hospital of the University of Michigan, Ann Arbor, Michigan," in *Methods and Problems of Medical Education,* 12th ser. (New York: Rockefeller Foundation, 1929), 112–25.

29. Hickey's instruments and methods are described in P. M. Hickey et al., "Skin Toleration Doses in Roentgen Units and Their Relation to the Quality of Radiation," *Radiology* 12 (1929): 309–16.

30. A. S. Warthin, "Preston M. Hickey, His Relation to the Medical School, University of Michigan," *Am. J. Roentgenol.* 25 (1931): 158.

31. E. W. Hall, "Hickey, the Teacher," *Am. J. Roentgenol.* 25 (1931): 161.

32. P. M. Hickey, "The First Decade of American Roentgenology [editorial]," parts 1 and 2, *Am. J. Roentgenol.* 20 (1928): 150–57, 249–56.

33. P. M. Hickey, "Treatment of Diphtheria Carriers by Means of the Roentgen Ray," *Am. J. Roentgenol.* 9 (1922): 319–22. Hickey obtained cures in fifteen of nineteen instances.

34. P. M. Hickey, "The Intralaryngeal Application of Radium for Chronic Papillomata," *Am. J. Roentgenol.* 8 (1921): 155–57. A cure in one case.

35. P. M. Hickey, "X-Ray Evidence of Ulcers," *J. Mich. State Med. Soc.* 20 (1921): 8–10.

36. P. M. Hickey, "Stereoscopic X-Ray Work," *Detroit Med. J.* 2 (1920): 513–15; idem, "Scarf Pin in the Right Lung," *Am. J. Roentgenol.* 3 (1916): 536–37; idem, "The Value of the Lateral View of the Hip," *Am. J. Roentgenol.* 3 (1916): 308–9; idem, "Pulmonary Abscess and Its Roentgen Demonstration," *Am. J. Roentgenol.* 3 (1916): 227–28; idem, "Lateral Roentgenography of the Spine," *Am. J. Roentgenol.* 4 (1917): 101–6; idem, "A Simple Method of Immobilization," *Am. J. Roentgenol.* 4 (1917): 131–32; and idem, "Teleoroentgenography as an Aid in Orthopedic Measurements," *Am. J. Roentgenol.* 11 (1924): 232–33.

37. P. M. Hickey, "Peristalsis of the Colon," *Am. J. Roentgenol.* 9 (1922): 260–61.

38. P. M. Hickey, "A Method for Measuring the Lumen of the Esophagus," *Radiology* 13 (1929): 469–71.

39. P. M. Hickey and A. C. Furstenberg, "The Roentgenographic Demonstration of the Trachea and Bronchi," *Am. J. Roentgenol.* 15 (1926): 227–30.

40. G. A. Lindsay, "Studies in the Physics of X-Rays for Students in Medicine," *Radiology* 8 (1927): 387–93.

41. P. M. Hickey, "The Teaching of Roentgenology in the University of Michigan," *Radiology* 6 (1926): 125–26.

42. P. M. Hickey, "The Teaching of X-Ray Anatomy," *Acta Radiol.* 6 (1926): 577.

43. Hall, "Hickey, the Teacher," 164.

44. P. M. Hickey, "Post-Graduate Instruction in Roentgenology," *Radiology* 8 (1927): 379–83; and idem, "Economic Problems of the X-Ray Laboratory," ibid. 15 (1930): 280–83.

45. P. M. Hickey, "Standardization of Roentgen-Ray Reports," *Am. J. Roentgenol.* 9 (1922): 422–25.

46. Ibid., 423.

47. W. F. Manges, Discussion of P. M. Hickey, "Standards in Roentgenology," *J. Am. Med. Assoc.* 89 (1927): 778.

48. An example: M. Fishbein, "The Council on Physical Therapy [editorial]," *J. Am. Med. Assoc.* 86 (1926): 270–74. This and the earlier articles are facetious rather than witty.

49. Activities of the Council on Physical Therapy can be followed in the frequent reports in the *Journal of the American Medical Association*.

50. [A. S. Warthin], "The Teaching of Physical Therapy [editorial]," *Ann. Clin. Med.* 5 (1927): 818.

51. E. A. Pohle and J. M. Barnes, "Clinical and Physical Investigations of the Problem of Dosimetry in Roentgen Therapy," *Radiology* 10 (1928): 300–317.

52. The last of many articles by Pohle on the subject: E. A. Pohle, "Physical and Biological Problems in Heliotherapy. III. The Calibration of the Mercury Vapor Lamp in Reproducible Units for Clinical Purposes," *Am. J. Roentgenol.* 20 (1928): 338–48.

53. E. A. Pohle, "Our Experience with a New Type of Artificial Light," *J. Mich. State Med. Soc.* 24 (1925): 351–52.

54. W. S. Peck, "Education in Physical Therapy," *Physiother. Rev.* 10 (1930): 422–23; and idem, "Educational Problems in Physical Therapy," *Radiology* 16 (1931): 726–29.

55. J. M. Sheldon and W. S. Peck, "Results of Fever Therapy in Severe Incapacitating Intrinsic Asthma," *Univ. Hosp. Bull.* 1 (1935): 18–19. Two papers describing the same patients and procedures in treatment of burns are Peck, "Application of Physical Therapy Measures in the Treatment of Burns," *Arch. Phys. Ther.* 12 (1931): 327–33; and E. B. Potter and Peck, "The Treatment of Extensive Granulating Areas, with Special Reference to the Use of Physical Therapy Measures," *Am. J. Surg.* 14 (1931): 472–76.

56. F. J. Hodges and W. S. Peck, *Introduction to Radiology* (Ann Arbor, Mich.: Edwards Brothers, 1939).

57. P. C. Hodges, "A Comparison of the Teleo-roentgenogram with the Orthodiagram," *Am. J. Roentgenol.* 11 (1924): 466–74; and P. C. Hodges and J. A. E. Eyster, "Estimation of Cardiac Area in Man," ibid. 12 (1924): 252–65.

58. F. J. Hodges and J. A. E. Eyster, "Estimation of Transverse Cardiac Diameter in Man," *Arch. Intern. Med.* 37 (1926): 707–14; and F. J. Hodges, "Roentgenological Examination of the Heart," *Radiology* 7 (1926): 116–18.

59. Hodges and Eyster, "Estimation of Transverse Cardiac Diameter," 714.

60. F. J. Hodges, "The Application of Special X-Ray Methods to Cardiac Diagnosis," *Wis. Med. J.* 25 (1926): 168–70; and idem, "Heart; X-Ray Examination," ibid. 28 (1929): 46.

61. F. J. Hodges, "Determination of Heart Size," *Am. J. Roentgenol.* 42 (1939): 13.

62. *Encyclopedic Survey*, 2:935.

63. "Report of Present X-Ray Situation at the University of Michigan," Fred Hodges to Executive Committee, 16 April 1931 and 4 June 1931, Bentley Historical Library, University of Michigan.

64. F. J. Hodges and J. C. Bugher, "Organized Clinical Investigation of Cancer," *Univ. Hosp. Bull.* 3 (1937): 21–27; and F. J. Hodges, I. Lampe, and L. Barbier, "Fifth Report: Organized Clinical Investigation of Cancer," ibid. 7 (1941): 34–41.

65. F. J. Hodges and I. Lampe, "Filing and Cross-Indexing Roentgen-Ray Records; Demonstration of a Simple and Efficient Method," *Am. J. Roentgenol.* 41 (1939): 1007–18.

66. Ibid., 1018.

67. F. J. Hodges and V. C. Johnson, "Reliability of Brain Tumor Localization by Roentgen Methods," *Am. J. Roentgenol.* 33 (1935): 745.

68. F. J. Hodges, "Diseases of the Colon," *Wis. Med. J.* 34 (1935): 821–25.

69. F. J. Hodges and I. Lampe, "A Comparison of Oral Cholecystographic Findings and Proved Evidences of Gallbladder Disease," *Am. J. Roentgenol.* 37 (1937): 145–53. The same data are in F. J. Hodges, "The Practical Value of Cholecystography in Surgery of the Gall-Bladder," *Am. J. Surg.*, n.s., 40 (1938): 146–51.

70. F. J. Hodges, "Gastro-Intestinal Diagnosis," *Rocky Mount. Med. J.* 39 (1942): 33–35.

71. This is the opinion of H. Richard Crane, who came to Michigan in 1935, ostensibly to work on the cyclotron. He had earned his Ph.D. at the California Institute of Technology in the Kellogg High Voltage Laboratory where cancer patients were treated. I am grateful to him for giving me the initial pages of a talk he gave on his retirement as professor of physics.

72. Correspondence between Hodges and Harrison Randall is in the Physics Department file in the Bentley Historical Library, University of Michigan. Much of it deals with the budget, support for Isadore Lampe, and cost overruns in the travel account.

73. F. J. Hodges, "The Cyclotron as a Medical Instrument," *Radiology* 39 (1942): 440–53.

74. R. E. Zirkle and I. Lampe, "Differences in the Relative Action of Neutrons and Roentgen Rays on Closely Related Tissues," *Am. J. Roentgenol.* 39

(1938): 613. This is Lampe's Ph.D. thesis work. I have not solved the problem of why Zirkle's name was on the paper.

75. I. Lampe and F. J. Hodges, "Differential Tissue Response to Neutron and Roentgen Radiations," *Radiology* 41 (1943): 344–50.

Chapter 22

1. R. N. DeJong, "Carl Dudley Camp, 1880–1955," *Trans. Am. Neurol. Assoc.* 80 (1955): 238–39; and J. W. McConnell, "William Gibson Spiller, 1863–1940," ibid. 66 (1940): 218–22.

2. W. G. Spiller and C. D. Camp, "Multiple Sclerosis, with a Report of Two Additional Cases, with Necropsy," *J. Nerv. Ment. Dis.* 31 (1904): 433–45; C. W. Burr and Camp, "Peripheral Obliterating Arteritis as a Cause of Triplegia following Hemiplegia, and of Paraplegia," *Am. J. Med. Sci.* 129 (1905): 960–66; C. F. Judson and Camp, "Report of a Case of Cerebellar Tumor with Necropsy," *Arch. Pediatr.* 23 (1906): 28–32; and Spiller and Camp, "The Clinical Resemblance of Cerebrospinal Syphilis to Disseminated Sclerosis," *Am. J. Med. Sci.* 133 (1907): 884–92.

3. C. D. Camp, "The Course of Sensory Impulses in the Spinal Cord," *J. Nerv. Ment. Dis.* 36 (1909): 77–96; Camp, "Type and Distribution of Sensory Disturbances Due to Cerebral Lesions," ibid. 37 (1910): 17–26; and W. G. Spiller and Camp, "The Sensory Tract in Relation to the Inner Capsule," ibid. 39 (1912): 92–107.

4. C. D. Camp, "Pathology of Paralysis Agitans," *J. Am. Med. Assoc.* 48 (1907): 1230–39.

5. The *Index Medicus* for 1907 cites the papers as C. D. Camp, "Die Pathologie der Paralysis agitans," *Dtsch. Klin.-Ther. Wochenschr.* 13 (1906): 1181, 1213, 1242, 1272; also *Wien. Klin.-Ther. Wochenschr.* 13 (1906): 1181, 1213, 1243, 1272. I have not seen them.

6. C. D. Camp, *Notes on Dr. Camp's Lectures in Neurology,* arranged by L. Himler (Ann Arbor, Mich.: Edwards Brothers, 1934). Beginning in 1936 examination questions were sent to the dean's office, and bound copies were deposited in the medical library. Questions in neurology were often answerable by quoting Camp's notes.

7. Camp, *Lectures in Neurology,* 89.

8. Camp's early experience with trifacial neuralgia is described in C. D. Camp, "The Causes and Treatment of Trifacial Neuralgia," *Physician Surg.* 31 (1909): 340–41.

9. C. D. Camp, "The Injection of Alcohol into the Gasserian Ganglion in the Treatment of Trifacial Neuralgia," *J. Mich. State Med. Soc.* 13 (1914): 186.

10. C. B. G. de Nancrède, discussion of "The Injection of Alcohol," by C. D. Camp, *J. Mich. State Med. Soc.* 13 (1914): 188.

11. The 1925 hospital had a soundproof room with double doors called the psychoanalysis room, but its couch was used only for a patient to rest on after lumbar puncture. This was told me by Russell DeJong.

12. C. D. Camp, "The Capacity for Medical Study," *Physician Surg.* 35 (1913): 529–34.

13. C. D. Camp, "Remarks on Psychotherapy," *Physician Surg.* 30 (1908): 437.

14. C. D. Camp, "The Distinction between Hysteria, Neurasthenia, Hypochondria and Simulation," *J. Mich. State Med. Soc.* 7 (1908): 531–33.

15. Camp, *Lectures in Neurology,* 239.

16. Ibid., 243–44.

17. Ibid., 236. The same idea is expressed in C. D. Camp, "The Effect of Emotions on Secretions, with Special Reference to the Thyroid Gland," *J. Indiana Med. Soc.* 24 (1931): 204.

18. The quotation is from Camp's part of L. H. Newburgh and C. D. Camp, "The Influence of Anxiety States on the Thyroid Gland," *Ann. Clin. Med.* 4 (1925–26): 1008. Other psychoanalytical experiences are in Camp, "Endocrinal Disturbances of Emotional Origin," *J. Mich. State Med. Soc.* 28 (1929): 92–94.

19. Camp, "Remarks on Psychotherapy," 436.

20. Camp, "The Effect of Emotions," 205.

21. C. D. Camp, "Disturbances of Sleep," *J. Mich. State Med. Soc.* 22 (1923): 133–38; and idem, "The Question of the Existence of a Separate Sleep Center in the Brain," *J. Nerv. Ment. Dis.* 92 (1940): 5–7.

22. R. N. DeJong, "George Huntington and His Relationship to the Earlier Descriptions of Chronic Hereditary Chorea," *Ann. Med. Hist.,* n.s., 9 (1937): 201–10; idem, "The First American Textbook on Psychiatry: A Review and Discussion of Benjamin Rush's 'Medical Inquiries and Observations upon the Diseases of the Mind,'" ibid., 3d ser., 2 (1940): 195–202; and idem, "Migraine: Personal Observations by Physicians Subject to the Disorder," ibid., 3d ser., 4 (1942): 276–83.

23. R. N. DeJong, "Horner's Syndrome; A Report of Ten Cases," *Arch. Neurol. Psychiatry* 34 (1935): 734–43; idem, "Central Nervous System Involvement in Undulant Fever, with the Report of a Case and a Survey of the Literature," *J. Nerv. Ment. Dis.* 83 (1936): 430–42; idem, "Tuberous Sclerosis: Encephalographic Interpretation," *J. Pediatr.* 9 (1936): 203–8; idem, "Central Nervous Complications in Subacute Bacterial Endocarditis," *J. Nerv. Ment. Dis.* 85 (1937): 397–410; and idem, "Delayed Traumatic Intracerebral Hemorrhage," *Arch. Neurol. Psychiatry* 48 (1942): 257–66.

24. R. N. DeJong, "The Guillain-Barré Syndrome,"

Arch. Neurol. Psychiatry 44 (1940): 1044–68; idem, "Vitamin E and alpha-Tocopherol Therapy in Neuromuscular and Muscular Disorders," *Univ. Hosp. Bull.* 7 (1941): 4–5; and idem, "Vitamin E and alpha Tocopherol Therapy of Neuromuscular and Muscular Disorders," *Arch. Neurol. Psychiatry* 46 (1941): 1068–75.

25. Biographical notices of Barrett are C. D. Camp, "Albert Moore Barrett, 1871–1936," *Trans. Am. Neurol. Assoc.* 62 (1936): 183–85; and A. Meyer, "In Memoriam: Albert Moore Barrett, 1871–1936," *Am. J. Psychiatry* 93 (1936): 499–500. The Victor Vaughan Society essay by Donald S. Patterson (*Proc. Victor Vaughan Soc.* 11, part 1 [1939–40]), preserved in the Taubman Medical Library, is particularly useful in containing information about Barrett from those who knew his characteristics.

26. W. J. Herdman, "Reasons Why the Joint Board of the Asylums for the Insane Should Join in the Conduct of the Psychopathic Ward at the University Hospital," *Physician Surg.* 27 (1905): 97–103.

27. A. M. Barrett, "The State Psychopathic Hospital," *Am. J. Insan.* 77 (1920–21): 309–20.

28. [A. Meyer], "Albert M. Barrett, M.D., 1871–1936," *Arch. Neurol. Psychiatry* 36 (1936): 612.

29. Ibid.

30. Twelve papers run from A. M. Barrett, "Disseminated Syphilitic Encephalitis," *Am. J. Med. Sci.* 129 (1905): 390–417, to idem, "Report upon the Clinical Symptoms and Anatomical Findings in Three Cases of Organic Brain Disease Showing Disturbances of an Aphasic and Agnostic Type," *J. Mich. State Med. Soc.* 17 (1918): 330–34.

31. A. M. Barrett, "A Study of Mental Diseases Associated with Cerebral Arterio-Sclerosis," *Am. J. Insan.* 62 (1905–6): 37–62.

32. L. E. Emerson, "Psychoanalysis and Social Service," *Physician Surg.* 33 (1911): 209–19.

33. A. M. Barrett, Discussion of "The Anxiety Neurosis," by L. Miller, *Physician Surg.* 35 (1913): 78. This discussion occurred at a meeting of the Detroit Society of Neurology and Psychiatry on 5 December 1912. Upon reading histories of psychoanalysis in the United States in the early days one would not know that anyone between the eastern shore of the Hudson River and the southwestern shore of Lake Michigan had ever heard of the subject.

34. A. M. Barrett, "Degenerations of Intracellular Neurofibrils with Miliary Gliosis in Psychoses of the Senile Period," *Am. J. Insan.* 67 (1910–11): 503–16.

35. A. M. Barrett, "Psychosis Associated with Tetany," *Am. J. Insan.* 76 (1919–20): 373–92.

36. A. M. Barrett, "The Psychopathic Personality," *Med. Clin. North Am.* 6 (1922–23): 1165–77. A similar attitude is expressed in idem, "Demonstration of Two Patients Showing Abnormalities of Conduct Associated with Psychoneurotic Disorders," *J. Mich. State Med. Soc.* 16 (1917): 273–76.

37. Samples of Barrett's papers on the subject are A. M. Barrett, "Constitution and Disposition in Psychiatric Relations," *Am. J. Psychiatry* 4 (1924–25): 245–60; idem, "Hereditary and Familial Factors in the Development of the Psychoses," *Arch. Neurol. Psychiatry* 13 (1925): 1–25; and idem, "The Significance of Constitutional Factors in Genetic Relations of the Psychoses," *Boston Med. Surg. J.* 195 (1926): 697–703. The last paper was published more fully as idem, "Heredity Relations in Schizophrenia," *Am. J. Psychiatry* 7 (1927–28): 77–104.

38. A. C. Furstenberg to A. G. Ruthven, 18 November 1936. Dean Furstenberg's correspondence and other matters relating to the appointment of Waggoner are in the Bentley Historical Library, University of Michigan. The negotiations were thoroughly confused by misdirection of mail between Ann Arbor and London. The letter offering Waggoner the job was slipped through a mail slot and was buried beneath other mail. Waggoner did not discover it for days.

39. R. W. Waggoner, "Thrombosis of a Superior Cerebral Vein: Clinical and Pathologic Study of a Case," *Arch. Neurol. Psychiatry* 20 (1928): 580–84; and B. J. Alpers and Waggoner, "Extraneural and Neural Anomalies in Friedreich's Ataxia: The Occurrence of Spina Bifida Occulta in Several Members of One Family with Friedreich's Disease," ibid. 21 (1929): 47–60.

40. R. W. Waggoner and W. G. Ferguson, "The Development of the Plantar Reflex in Children," *Arch. Neurol. Psychiatry* 23 (1930): 619.

41. The reference is given in G. P. McCouch, "The Relation of the Pyramidal Tract to Spinal Shock," *Am. J. Physiol.* 71 (1924–25): 137–52, but the device is not illustrated in the paper.

42. W. E. Dandy, "Röntgenography of the Brain after the Injection of Air into the Spinal Canal," *Ann. Surg.* 70 (1919): 397–403.

43. F. C. Grant, "The Value of Ventriculography: A Clinical Experience Based on a Series of Forty Cases," *Arch. Neurol. Psychiatry* 10 (1923): 154–66.

44. R. W. Waggoner, "Encephalography," *Am. J. Med. Sci.* 174 (1927): 459–66.

45. C. D. Camp and R. W. Waggoner, "The Technic of Encephalography," *Arch. Neurol. Psychiatry* 25 (1931): 128. A related paper is Waggoner and L. E. Himler, "Encephalography under Nitrous Oxide Anesthesia," *Am. J. Roentgenol.* 31 (1934): 784–86.

46. R. W. Waggoner and D. M. Clark, "A New Position Used in Encephalography," *Am. J. Roentgenol.* 25 (1931): 533–35.

47. R. N. DeJong and R. W. Waggoner, "The Interpreta-

tion of Encephalograms," *J. Mich. State Med. Soc.* 35 (1936): 652–57.

48. R. W. Waggoner and K. Löwenberg, "Konzentrische Sklerose," *Arch. Psychiatr. Nervenkr.* 101 (1933–34): 184–94; Löwenberg and Waggoner, "Friedreich's Ataxia Associated with Multiple Cerebral Lesions," *J. Nerv. Ment. Dis.* 76 (1932): 467–76; Waggoner and Löwenberg, "Unclassified Organic Psychosis," *Ann. Surg.* 101 (1935): 357–62; Löwenberg and Waggoner, "Familial Organic Psychosis (Alzheimer's Type)," *Arch. Neurol. Psychiatry* 31 (1934): 737–54; Waggoner and Löwenberg, "A Clinicopathologic Study of Astrocytomas," *Arch. Neurol. Psychiatry* 38 (1937): 1208–23; Waggoner, Löwenberg, and K. G. Speicher, "Hereditary Cerebellar Ataxia: Report of a Case and Genetic Study," *Arch. Neurol. Psychiatry* 39 (1938): 570–86; Waggoner and Löwenberg, "Role of Trauma in Amyotrophic Lateral Sclerosis," *Arch. Neurol. Psychiatry* 45 (1941): 296–303 [there is no role]; and Waggoner, Löwenberg-Scharenberg, and M. E. Schilling, "Agenesis of the White Matter with Idiocy," *Am J. Ment. Defic.* 47 (1942–43): 20–24. In that period Waggoner published at least five other neurological papers. Konstantin Löwenberg-Scharenberg eventually became Konstantin Scharenberg. The mutations of his name were explained to me by Raymond Waggoner. The name in Germany was Scharenberg, but as a Jew with that name he could not get his goods out of the country. His wife's name had been Löwenberg, and, as a Gentile, she could emigrate with her belongings; hence her husband's change of name. In the United States he gradually resumed his original name with an intermediate form of the two hyphenated.

49. K. Löwenberg, R. Waggoner, and T. Zbinden, "Destruction of the Cerebral Cortex following Nitrous Oxide-Oxygen Anesthesia," *Ann. Surg.* 104 (1936): 801–10.

50. P. D. Moore, "Observations on Nitrous Oxid-Oxygen in Veterans' Administration Hospitals," *Anesth. Analg.* 13, no. 1 (1934): 35.

51. R. W. Waggoner, "Personality Studies in Children with Particular Reference to Chorea Cases" (thesis, University of Pennsylvania, 1930). I am deeply indebted to Raymond Waggoner for lending me a copy of the thesis. Another version with the psychiatric aspects rather muted is Waggoner, "Sydenham's Chorea," *Am. J. Med. Sci.* 182 (1931): 467–76.

52. R. W. Waggoner and D. A. Boyd Jr., "Juvenile Aberrant Sexual Behavior," *Am. J. Orthopsychiatry* 11 (1941): 275–91.

Chapter 23

1. Appreciations of Canfield include D. M. Cowie, "Roy Bishop Canfield," *Ann. Otol. Rhinol. Laryngol.* 41 (1932): 959–63; and A. C. Furstenberg, in *The University of Michigan: An Encyclopedic Survey,* ed. W. B. Shaw (Ann Arbor: University of Michigan Press, 1951), 2:881–83. Canfield's military record is in R. B. Canfield, "Military Service of Major R. Bishop Canfield, M.C., U.S.A.," *Ann. Otol. Rhinol. Laryngol.* 29 (1920): 104–5. Canfield is said to be the Roscoe Geake of *Arrowsmith* (New York: Harcourt Brace, 1925), perhaps on account of such episodes as the bill rendered Henry Ford, but Lewis omitted his good qualities.

2. R. B. Canfield, "The Application of Conservative and Radical Surgery to Chronic Nasal Accessory Sinus Disease," *Trans. Am. Laryngol. Rhinol. Otol. Soc.* 10 (1904): 287.

3. R. B. Canfield, "Concerning the Radical Treatment of Chronic Diseases of the Antrum with Suggestions for a New Method of Operating by the Submucous Resection of the Lateral Nasal Wall," *Trans. Am. Laryngol. Rhinol. Otol. Soc.* 13 (1907): 384–93, and *Physician Surg.* 31 (1909): 433–39. Another version is Canfield, "The Submucous Resection of the Lateral Nasal Wall in Chronic Empyema of the Antrum, Ethmoid and Sphenoid," *J. Am. Med. Assoc.* 51 (1908): 1136–39.

4. R. B. Canfield, "Concerning the Radical Treatment of Chronic Diseases of the Antrum with Suggestions for a New Method in Operating by the Submucous Resection of the Lateral Nasal Wall," *Laryngoscope* 17 (1907): 614–15. The paper reports the first seven cases.

5. There are at least two denunciations of Furstenberg by patients or patients' relatives in the Medical School files in the Bentley Historical Library, University of Michigan. Copies of Furstenberg's replies, if any, are not there.

6. R. B. Canfield, "Some Remarks on the Course and Management of Acute Mastoiditis," *Physician Surg.* 27 (1905): 245–56.

7. R. B. Canfield, "Some Remarks Concerning the Pathology and Operative Treatment of Chronic Suppurative Otitis Media," *J. Mich. State Med. Soc.* 6 (1907): 161–70.

8. R. B. Canfield, "Diagnosis and Treatment of Suppuration of the Labyrinth," *Trans. Am. Laryngol. Rhinol. Otol. Soc.* 14 (1908): 466–83.

9. R. B. Canfield, "A Case of Otitic Meningitis," *J. Mich. State Med. Soc.* 7 (1908): 53–56.

10. R. B. Canfield, "A Case of Abscess of the Brain in a Child of Four. Operation. Recovery," *Physician Surg.* 33 (1911): 120–22.

11. R. B. Canfield, "Focal Infections in Medical Diseases," *Ann. Clin. Med.* 4 (1926): 1058–67.

12. Cowie, "Roy Bishop Canfield," 960–61.

13. An example: A. C. Furstenberg, "Acute Suppurations

of Throat, Mouth and Cervical Region," *Trans. Pac. Coast Oto-Ophthalmol. Soc.* 21 (1936): 14–25.

14. J. E. McKenty, "Operation of Total Laryngectomy for the Cure of Intrinsic Cancer of the Larynx," *Ann. Otol. Rhinol. Laryngol.* 31 (1922): 1101–17. McKenty habitually gave no references in his papers, but his description of his operation as early as 1916 can be found. He is mistakenly called "George" in a couple of Furstenberg's papers.

15. R. B. Canfield and A. C. Furstenberg, "Clinical Aspects of Laryngeal Cancer," in *Contributions to Medical Science: Dedicated to Aldred Scott Warthin*, ed. W. J. Stone (Ann Arbor: G. Wahr, 1927), 625–37; Furstenberg, "Clinical Aspects of Laryngeal Cancer," *J. Mich. State Med. Soc.* 26 (1927): 94–98; and Furstenberg, "Carcinoma of the Larynx," *J. Mich. State Med. Soc.* 30 (1931): 770–76.

16. A. C. Furstenberg, "The Treatment of Acute Nasal Accessory Sinus Disease," *Ann. Otol. Rhinol. Laryngol.* 47 (1938): 902–9.

17. A. C. Furstenberg, "The Pathology of the Spread of Osteomyelitis of the Skull; Its Relation to Brain Abscess," *Trans. Pac. Coast Oto-Ophthalmol. Soc.* 21 (1936): 111–17.

18. A. C. Furstenberg, "The Pathology of the Spread of Osteomyelitis of the Skull; Its Relation to Brain Abscess," *Trans. Am. Laryngol. Rhinol. Otol. Soc.* 39 (1933): 423–29; idem, "The Pathology of the Spread of Osteomyelitis of the Skull," *Laryngoscope* 44 (1934): 470–76; and idem, "Intracranial Infections and Their Spread from the Ear and Nasal Accessory Sinuses," *Surg. Gynecol. Obstet.* 74 (1942): 585–88.

19. A. C. Furstenberg, "Bone Regeneration in Osteomyelitic Defects of the Cranium," *Trans. Am. Laryngol. Rhinol. Otol. Soc.* 36 (1930): 434–39; and idem, "Osteomyelitis of the Skull. The Osteogenetic Processes in the Repair of Cranial Defects," ibid. 37 (1931): 1–18.

20. A. C. Furstenberg, "The Parotid Gland: Its Common Disorders," *J. Am. Med. Assoc.* 117 (1941): 1594–98.

21. A. C. Furstenberg and L. Yglesias, "Mediastinitis: A Clinical Study with Practical Anatomic Considerations of the Neck and Mediastinum," *Arch. Otolaryngol.* 25 (1937): 540. Much the same paper with fewer illustrations is Furstenberg, "Acute Mediastinal Suppuration," *Trans. Am. Laryngol. Rhinol. Otol. Soc.* 35 (1929): 210–29. Coller's publishing habits are illustrated by F. A. Coller and Yglesias, "The Relation of the Spread of Infection to Fascial Planes in the Neck and Thorax," *Surgery* 1 (1937): 323–37, in which photographs of dissections from the Furstenberg-Yglesias paper are reproduced together with drawings clearly derived from dissections illustrated by photographs in the same paper. Figures "Courtesy of Dr.

A. C. Furstenberg" are also in Coller and Yglesias, "Infections of the Lip and Face," *Surg. Gynecol. Obstet.* 60 (1935): 277–88.

22. Furstenberg, "Acute Mediastinal Suppuration," 210–29.

23. A. C. Furstenberg, "An Anatomical and Clinical Study of Central Lesions Producing Paralysis of the Larynx," *Ann. Otol. Rhinol. Laryngol.* 46 (1937): 39–54. Furstenberg thanked Elizabeth Crosby and Konstantin Scharenberg for help.

24. A. C. Furstenberg, J. H. Maxwell, and G. H. Richardson, "Essential Hypertension from the Standpoint of Otolaryngology," *Trans. Am. Acad. Ophthalmol. Otolaryngol.* 44 (1939): 43–53.

25. A. C. Furstenberg, E. Crosby, and B. Farrior, "Neurological Lesions Which Influence the Sense of Smell," *Trans. Am. Laryngol. Rhinol. Otol. Soc.* 48 (1942): 44.

26. A. C. Furstenberg, F. H. Lashmet, and F. Lathrop, "Ménière's Symptom Complex: Medical Treatment," *Ann. Otol. Rhinol. Laryngol.* 43 (1934): 1038.

27. D. Dederding, "Our Ménière Treatment (Principles and Results)," *Acta Oto-Laryngol.* 16 (1931): 404–15; and idem, "Clinical and Experimental Examinations in Patients Suffering from Mb. Meniéri, Including a Study of the Problem of Boneconduction," vols. 1 and 2, *Acta Oto-Laryngol. Suppl.* 10 (1929): 1–156; 11 (1929): 1–213.

28. Dederding, "Our Ménière Treatment," 404.

29. Furstenberg, Lashmet, and Lathrop, "Ménière's Symptom Complex," 1044. The references to the fundamental Newburgh papers appear to have been omitted as the result of a typographical error. Furstenberg gave Newburgh full credit elsewhere.

30. It remains a standard treatment in the 1990s.

31. A. C. Furstenberg, G. Richardson, and F. D. Lathrop, "Ménière's Disease: Addenda to Medical Therapy," *Arch. Oto-Laryngol.* 34 (1941): 1083–92.

32. R. B. Canfield, "The Present Relation of Otology to the Practice of General Medicine," *Physician Surg.* 27 (1905): 49–54. Canfield said much the same thing in idem, "The Clinical Specialist: His Preparation and Relationship to the General Practitioner," *Mich. Alumnus* 17 (1910): 125–35.

33. *Encyclopedic Survey*, 2:883.

34. A. C. Furstenberg, "Graduate Training in Otolaryngology," *Bull. Am. Coll. Surg.* 24 (1939): 61–64.

35. A. C. Furstenberg, "Critical Comments on the Treatment of Chronic Paranasal Sinusitis," *Trans. Am. Laryngol. Rhinol. Otol. Soc.* 45 (1939): 110.

36. The liberum veto, in Polish history, was "the legal right of each member of the Sejm (legislature) to defeat by his vote alone any measure under consideration." It was first used in 1652 and was abolished in

1791 (*Encyclopaedia Britannica,* 15th ed., *Micropaedia* s.v. "liberum veto").

37. Furstenberg, "Neurological Lesions," 40.

Epilogue

1. University of Michigan, *President's Report for 1943–44,* 97.
2. Ibid., 99.
3. F. J. Hodges, "Origin and Growth of Michigan's Medical Center," *Univ. Mich. Med. Bull.* 16 (1950): 239.
4. Ibid., 242.
5. University of Michigan, *President's Report for 1959–60,* 79.
6. University of Michigan, *President's Report for 1960–61,* 215.
7. University of Michigan, *President's Report for 1962–63,* 81.
8. J. A. Gronvall, President's Report for 1967–68: The Medical School, p. 1, Bentley Historical Library, University of Michigan.
9. R. Fleming, as quoted in Medical Center News, *Univ. Mich. Med. Center J.* 37 (1971): 55.
10. Medical Center News, *Univ. Mich. Med. Center J.* 39 (1973): 94.
11. Ibid.
12. J. W. Dalston, notes on the Replacement Hospital Project development and implementation process [27 May 1986], pp. 31–32, Vice Provost for Medical Affairs Records, Box 47, Bentley Historical Library, University of Michigan.
13. G. D. Zuidema, The University of Michigan Medical Center Archival Report, 1985–1987, Vice Provost for Medical Affairs Records, Box 33, Bentley Historical Library, University of Michigan.
14. G. S. Omenn, "Caring for the Community," Association of American Medical Colleges Robert G. Petersdorf Lecture, 2 November 1998, [online]. Available at http://www.med.umich.edu/1toolbar/omenn.htm. See link at "recent speeches."
15. H. Markel, "'An Example Worthy of Imitation': The University of Michigan Medical School, 1850–2000," Historical Center for the Health Sciences, University of Michigan, 1999.

Index

Page numbers in italics refer to figures.

missal of (1930), xi, 32, 49, 190–91, *192;* education of, 184; on enrollment issues, 29, 30; faculty appointed by, 56, 148–49; hiring of, xi, 181, 182, 183–84; income of, 165; military service by, 183; on pharmacy courses, 86; on preceptorships, 34; research by, 184–85, 188–90; on student loans, 33; as surgery professor, 163, 185–86, 204; as a teacher, 186–88; and teaching of surgical anatomy, 99, 163; on Warfield, 166–67. Works: *Surgical Nursing* (with Giles), 187

cadavers: cost of, 9; disposal of, 9, 99; preparation of, 95, 99; procurement of, 9, 95

caffeine, 88

Cajal, Santiago Ramón y, 105

calcium carbamate, 79

Calmette, Albert, 16

calorimetry, 157–58

Camp, Carl Dudley: education of, 279–80; as neurology professor, 193, 279, 280, 282; research by, 279–80, 281–82; as a teacher, 280–81

cancer: heredity of, 125; intrinsic and extrinsic factors in, 127; radiological treatment of, 276–78; surgical treatment of, 211–13, 230, 292

Canfield, Roy Bishop: death of (1932), 291; education of, 289–90; hiring of, 289; as otolaryngology professor, 137, 252, 290–91; research by, 289–91, 292; as a teacher, 290, 294–95

Cannon, Walter B., 143, 154, 195, 216, 237, 238, 259–60, 272, 273, 274

Capener, Norman, 186

capillary pressure, measurement of, 68

cardiac action potentials, distribution of, 150–51

cardiovascular diseases, 134, 166

cardiovascular research, 139–40, 147–48

Carhart, Henry S., 266

Carnegie Foundation for the Advancement of Teaching, 321n. 23

Carpenter, Thorne, 157

Carrow, Flemming, *251;* education of, 250; as ophthalmology professor, 250; resignation of (1904), 250, 252, 289; as a teacher, 250–51

Carter, W. S., 280

Castle, William, 170

cataract, 253–54

Catherine Street Hospital. *See* University Hospital (Catherine Street)

Catholepistemiad Club, 93

Catholic students, 30

Catron, Lloyd, 127

centennial (1950), 298–99

Central Institute for Brain Research (Amsterdam), 111

cesarean section, 225

Chadbourne, Osbourne F., 23

Chadbourne, Theodore L., 130

charity patients, 189, 227, 232, 235

Cheever, Henry Sylvester, 15, 77, 117

Chemical Laboratory, *2;* autopsies conducted at, 6; construction of (1855–56), 4, 14; development of, 4–7; enlargement of, 15, 27; poisoning analyses at, 7

chemistry: first instruction in, 1, 4–7; in four-year curriculum, 24, *24*

Chemistry-Pharmacy Building, 27

Chicago Neurological and Pathological Societies, 108

children: chorea minor in, 288; feeding of, 239–41; gastric secretion in newborns, 238–39; prevention of congenital deformities in, 207; sudden death of, 123–24. *See also* pediatrics

Chittenden, Russell H., 57

chloroform, 80–81, 188

choked disk, 254

cholera, 118

cholinergic nerves, 102

chorea minor, 288

Christman, Adam, 58

Christopher, Walter S., 22–23, 221, 235

Churchill, Lemuel, 320n. 5

cinemicrophotography, 114

Clark, Jonas Gilman, 63

clinical microscopy: first instruction in, x; in four-year curriculum, 140

Clinical Society, 99, 145, 269

clinical teaching: development of, 18, 19–20, 131–33, 136–38; in tutorials, 34

coffee, 88

Cohn, A. E., 143

Cohn, E. J., 170–71

Cohnheim, Julius, 11

Cole, H. N., 260

Cole, K. C., 151

Cole, Rufus, 138–39, 257

College of Pharmacy: established, 27; management of, 59

Coller, Frederick Amasa, *212;* and blood bank, 232; on Cabot, 184, 186; on Darling, 182; education of, 162, 204; on hiring of Patten, 112; on history of medicine, 37, 212; on McGraw, 19; military service by, 204; research by, 204–6, 214–19, 296; retirement of (1957), 211; as surgery professor, 185, 204–6, 211–14, 219; as a teacher, 211–12; and teaching of anesthesia, 188, 213–14; and teaching of surgical anatomy, 99

Committee on Athletics, 176

Committee on Iodized Salt, 244

comparative neuroanatomy, research in, 109

Comprehensive Cancer and Geriatric Centers, 303

Compton, Arthur H., 274

Comroe, Julius H., 74

Conklin, E. G., 92

Conn, Jerome W., 157

Connors, Edward J., 300

constipation, treatment of, 154, 229

Contagious Hospital, 226, *241,* 241–42

contraception. *See* birth control

Cooley, Mortimer, 226

Cooley, Thomas B., 244, 246

Cooperative Clinical Group, 260–61

Cope, Otis, 70, 105

Corbett, Rupert, 186

coronary occlusion, 134–35

Cowie, Anne Cooke, 353n. 3

housing. *See* student housing
Howard Hughes Medical Institute, 303
Howell, Joel D., xii
Howell, William H.: collaboration with Huber, 101–2; education of, 61–62; as physiology and histology professor, 61, 62. Works: *American Text-Book of Physiology,* 64
Hubbard, William N., Jr., 299–300
Huber, G. Carl, *108;* collaboration with Howell, 101–2; collaboration with Martin, 222; death of (1934), 98, 111; education of, 102–3; as histology professor, 101, *102;* as immunologist, 42; as microscopic anatomy professor, 26, 28, 95, 97, 98, 101, 190; research by, 101–8, 110–11; as a teacher, 104–6. Works: histology laboratory manual, 104; translation of Böhm and Davidoff's *A Text-Book of Histology,* 104; translation of Sobotta's *Atlas and Epitome of Human Histology and Microscopic Anatomy,* 103
Huber, Karl, 119
Huggins, Charles B., 204
human embryology, 96–97, *97*
Hume, Basil, 186
Hunt, Reid, 94
Hunter, John, 134
Huntington, George S., 94
Hurd, Henry Mills, 263
hydantoin, 57
Hyderabad Chloroform Commission, 80
hygiene and public health: department established for, 49; in four-year curriculum, 24; instruction in, 43–44
Hygienic Laboratory: Newburgh's lab in, 155; opening of (1888), 43; as state health laboratory (until 1907), 8, 43
hypertension, surgical treatment of, 194–95
hysterectomy, 223
hysterical blindness, 281–82

idiopathic hydrocephalus, 193
immunology, experiments in, 16, 41–42
Index Medicus, 223
Indian students, 31
infant feeding, proper, 240–41
infections, 185, 236, 292–93
infectious diseases, 39
inflammation, 178
influenza, 242
insanity. *See* psychiatry, instruction in
Institute for Clinical Medical Research, 298
insulin, 161
insurance. *See* health insurance
Integrated Flexible Premedical/Medical School Curriculum (Inteflex program), 301
internal medicine: departmental developments, 171; first instruction in, 11–14; in four-year curriculum, 130–33
International Journal of Surgery, 107
internships, development of, xi, 130, 166, 187, 212
intestinal gradient, 239
intestinal stasis, 191–93
iodine deficiency. *See* goiter
Isaacs, Raphael, 168, 169–71, 277

islets of Langerhans, 105, 159
Iverson, Christine, 354n. 25

Jackschath, E., 94
Jackson, J. Hughlings, 175
Jacobi, Abraham, 235
Janet, Pierre, 281
Jansen, Albert, 289
Japanese students, 31
Jewish students, x–xi, 29–30, 30 (tables)
John E. Weeks Scholarship for Research in Ophthalmology, 255
Johnson, Joseph E., III, 303
Johnston, Franklin, 86, 155, 157, 159, 161
Johnston, Margaret Woodwell, 157
Joint Board of the Asylums for the Insane, 262
Jones, Lafon, 244
Jordan, David Starr, 119
Joslin, Elliott, 159–60, 215
Journal of Experimental Medicine, 82
Journal of Laboratory and Clinical Medicine, 163
Journal of Morphology, 107
Journal of Physiology (London), 16
Journal of the American Medical Association, 259–60, 262, 274, 279
Jung, Carl, 281

Kahn, Albert, 168
Kahn, Edgar A., *112;* education of, 112, 194; as neurosurgery professor, 185, 194, 219; research by, 193, 212. Works: *Correlative Neurosurgery* (with others), 112
Kahn, Reuben, 49, 52–53, 258, 285
Kahn test, 52–53, 255, 258
Keen, William W., 141, 174, 259, 260; *An American Text-Book of Surgery* (with White), 174
Keibel, Franz, *Manual of Human Embryology* (with Mall), 97
Kellogg, John Harvey, 88
Kellogg, W. K., 88, 157
Kellogg Foundation, 247
Kelly, Howard, 225
Kennedy, Foster, 194
Kerlikowske, Albert C., 253, 299
kidneys: embryology of, 106–7; infections of, 185; and nephritis, 156; transplanting of, 300
Kiefer, Hermann, 22, 119
Kimball, O. P., 243–44, 245
Kitasato, Shibasaburo, 16
Klein, Emanuel, 118
Klingman, Theophile, 280
knee jerk reflex, 64, 65, 66, 67
Koch, Robert, 118
Koch, William Frederick, 55
Kocher, Theodor, 244
Koelz, Walter, 254
Kolisko, Alexander, 126
Kollmann, Julius Konstantin Ernst, 104
Kopetsky, Samuel, 294
Koplik, Henry, 131
Kraepelin, Emil, 263, 283, 284

Ringer, Sydney, 66
Rioch, David M., 111
Rittenberg, David, 60
Robert Wood Johnson Scholars Program, 303
Robinson, William D., 37, 88
Rockefeller Foundation, 72, 88, 285
roentgenology: departmental developments, 265, 275–76; in diagnosis, 266; instruction in, x, 265–66, 272–73; research in, 266–68. *See also* X-ray laboratory
Rogoff, J. M., 195
Romberg, Ernst (?), 23
Rose, D. K., 203
Rose, Preston B.: dismissal of (1875), 6; as physiological chemistry professor, 6; as toxicology and urinalysis professor, 4, 6. Works: *Hand-Book of Toxicology*, 6
Rose, William C., 56, 58, 59
Rous, Peyton, 120, 121, 128, 332n. 37
Rowntree, L. G., 185, 194
Roy, C. S., 81
Rubner, Max, 160
Ruthven, Alexander Grant, 49, 115, 191, 295

S. S. Kresge Foundation, 298
Sabin, Florence, 94
Sager, Abram, *3, 5;* hiring of, 2; literature reviews by, 135; as professor of diseases of women and children, 223, 226; qualifications of, 2
St. Joseph Mercy Hospital, 164, 301, 303
saline catharsis, 83–84
salt balance, 217–19. *See also* sodium chloride (salt)
Salt Producers Association, 245
sanitary science. *See* hygiene and public health
Sarton, George, 94
Sauerbruch, Ferdinand, 196, 197
Sawyer, Walter H., 149
Schmidt, Carl F., 74
Schmidt, Harry B., 140
Schmiedeberg, Oswald, 77, 78, 79, 80, 87
Schneider, Richard C., *112,* 213
Schoenheimer, Rudolf, 60
scholarships, 33, 255
School of Dentistry, 20, 104
School of Tropical Medicine (San Juan, Puerto Rico), 51
sciatica, 208
Scott, Merle (W. J. M.), 215
scurvy, 11, 134
Seddon, Sir Herbert, 186, 191, 209
Seevers, Maurice H., 89
senile hypertrophic prostate, 180
serum, 41
Seventeenth International Congress of Medicine (London, 1913), 103
Sewall, Henry: embryos collected by, 97; hiring of, x, 15; as physiology professor, 15–16, 62; plaque commemorating, *16;* resignation of (1889), 16, 21, 61
sex hygiene, instruction in, 44
sexually transmitted diseases. *See* venereal disease, detection and treatment of
Shakespeare, Edward O., 44, 45
Sharp, Elwood A., 171

Shattuck, Frederick Cheever, 185
Sheldon, John, 157, 171
Sherrington, C. S., 64, 103; *Integrative Action of the Nervous System,* 282
Shurly, Ernest L., 271
Simpson, Thomas Henry, 168, 170
Simpson Memorial Institute, *168,* 168–69, 190
skin temperature, 215–16
sleep research, 282
Sloan, Herbert, 347n. 124
Slocum, George, 252, 255
smallpox, 134, 256
Smith, Maj. Henry, 253–54
Smith, Ralph G., 86, 89
Smith, Shirley, 115
Smith-Petersen, Marius, 204, 208
Smithwick, Reginald H., 195, 345n. 62
smoking: linked to cancer, 127; and vasoconstriction, 215–16
Sobotta, J., *Atlas and Epitome of Human Histology and Microscopic Anatomy,* 103, 104
sodium chloride (salt): ingestion of, 161–62, 216–19, 240; iodination of, 244–46
Solis, Jeanne Cady, 262, 264, 280
Sørensen, Soren Peter Lauritz, 84, 154
Soule, Malcolm H.: as bacteriology instructor and research assistant, 49, 50, 51–52; as bacteriology professor, 52; on Warthin, 121
Spanish-American War (1898), 44–45, 173
specialization, xi
Spiller, William G., 194, 279
sports injuries, 207
Starling, Ernest H., 62, 84, 247
Starry, Allen, 126
Steinberg, Bernhard, 205–6
Steiner, David, 106
Stephenson, Marjory, *Bacterial Metabolism,* 51
sterilization (infection), 241, 242
sterilization (reproduction), 228
Sternberg, George Miller, 7
Stewart, George Neil, 142, 195
Stiles, Sir Harold, 206
Stokes, John H., 257, 260
Stowell, Charles, 15
Streeter, George Linius: as anatomy professor, 95–97; collaboration with Patten, 114; education of, 94–95; hiring of, 94; research by, 95–97; staff under, 95; as a teacher, 95. Works: *Laboratory Guide in Anatomy,* 95
Student Health Service, 283
student housing, 35–36
student loans, 33
students: admission requirements for, 1, 23–24; attrition (dropout rate) of, 35; characteristics of, x–xi; class size of, 31; class standing of, 34; discipline of, 32, 35; employment of, 33; exposure to tuberculosis, 36; first class of, 1; grading of, 34–35; interviewing of, 30; out-of-state and foreign, 30–31, 33; on probation, 34; promotion of, 34; punishment of, 32, 35; quotas on, 29–30; relations with faculty, 38. *See also* African Ameri-

Vaughan, Victor Clarence (*continued*)
 prizes awarded to, 7–8; public health work by, 7–8, 43,
 44–45, 163; reforms carried out by, ix, x; research by,
 39–45, 119; retirement of (1921), 6, 49; as a teacher,
 45; and University Hospital construction, 20. Works: on
 cellular toxins, 40; *A Doctor's Memories,* 21; *Epidemiology and Public Health,* 43; *Ptomaines and Leukomaines*
 (with Novy), 7, 39; published lecture notes, 6–7; report
 of Typhoid Commission, 7, 45; textbook on public
 health and epidemiology, 7
venereal disease, detection and treatment of, 43, 52–53,
 227, 255, 256, 258, 298. *See also* gonorrhea; syphilis
Ventriculin, 170–71
Vesalius, 93–94
Veterans Administration Hospital, 299, 301
Veterans Readjustment Center, 298, 299
Victor Vaughan House (dormitory), 36
Victor Vaughan Society, 37
Vienna Pathological Institute, 113
Virchow, Rudolf Ludwig Karl, 23, 119
Visick, Arthur, 186
Voit, Karl von, 6, 160
Vonderlehr, Raymond A., 261

Wade, James Henry, 227
Waggoner, Raymond W.: education of, 285–86; hiring of,
 285; as neurology/psychiatry professor, 280, 285,
 287–88; research by, 282, 286
Wagner, Richard, 120
Waldeyer, Wilhelm, 103
Wallace, George B., 83–84
Waller, Dorothy, 157
Wanstrom, Ruth, 121–22, 127, 128
Wappler, Frederick, 201
Wappler, Reinhold, 201
Warburg, Otto, 49
Ward, Peter, 302
war deafness, prevention of, 105
wards, practical experience in, 24
Warfield, Louis Marshall: death of, 340n. 8; education of,
 166; fundraising by, 157; hiring of, 155, 166–67;
 income of, 165; resignation of (1925), 166, 167, 191
Warnhuis, F. C., 245
Warren, Larry, 303
Warren, Luther F., 140, 268
Warthin, Aldred Scott, *122;* death of (1931), 120, 126;
 education of, 119–20; on Gibbes and pathology course,
 117, 118; on Hickey, 272; hiring of, 119; and history of
 medicine, 37; and medical library, 135; pathology
 museum under, 27, 121; as pathology professor, 26, 28,
 134, 190, 274; research by, 121–26, 188; as a teacher,
 120–21, 129. Works: *Old Age,* 120; pathology laboratory manual, 121; *The Physician of the Dance of Death,*
 119; translation of Ziegler's *General Pathology,* 121
Washburne, Charles, 181–82
Washtenaw Tribune, 192
Wassermann, August von, 43
Wassermann test, 43, 52–53, 227, 256, 258
water balance, 162, 202, 216–17, 294
water loss, insensible, 158–59

Wayne County General Hospital, 301
Weigert, Carl, 23, 119
Weisenburg, T. H., 285
Weiss, Soma, 124
Welch, William Henry, 8, 120, 128, 257
Weller, Carl Vernon, 36, 37, 89, 112, *126;* as pathology pro-
 fessor, 126–27; research by, 124, 125, 127–28, 277; as a
 teacher, 127–28; as Warthin's assistant, 120, 121, 123
Weller, Thomas, 334n. 73
Westland Medical Center, 302
West Ward (vacated Homeopathic Hospital), 129
Whipple, George H., 127
White, Abraham, 59
White, J. William, *An American Text-Book of Surgery* (with
 Keen), 174
Whitman, Charles O., 63
Wiggers, Carl J., 38, 64, 66–67, 68, 85, 121
Wilbur, Ray Lyman, 144
Wilder, Burt Green, 14
Wile, Udo Julius, 214, *257;* education of, 257; hiring of,
 257; opposition to Peterson, 228; research by, 164,
 189, 224, 233, 258–61; as a teacher, 257–58
Willey, Vernon J., 266–68, 280
Willson, J. Robert, 88
Wilms, Max, 197
Wilson, E. B., 92
Wilson, Frank Norman: away from Michigan, 147–48; on
 Cabot, 191; education of, 38, 140; electrocardiographs
 by, 143–44, 149–50; on Foster's resignation, 145; heart
 station of, 148–49, *149;* as internal medicine professor,
 149, 190, 295; research by, 143–44, 148–53, 296
Winchell, Alexander, 14
Windsberg, Eske, 199–200
Wistar, Caspar, 326n. 23
Women's Hospital, 298
women students: segregation of, *26,* 31; at UM, 15; at UM
 Medical School, xi, 15, 16, 31, 95, 302
Woodburne, Russell, 330n. 69
World War I: medical research during, 105, 107–8; medical
 training during, 145
World War II: deferments during, 297; service during,
 297–98
Wünderlich, Karl Reinhold August, 13

X-ray laboratory, 11, 265–66, 269, 271–72. *See also*
 roentgenology

yaws, 127
Yglesias, Luis, 212, 293
Yoakum, Clarence, 247
Young, Hugh, 184
Young, Jean, 348n. 155
Young, Robert, 300
Yutzy, Simon, 95

Zappfe, Fred C., 227
Zeiss, Carl, 148
Ziegler, Ernst, 119; *General Pathology,* 121
zoology, first instruction in, 1
Zuidema, George D., 302